HANDBOOK OF PEDIATRIC SURGICAL PATIENT CARE

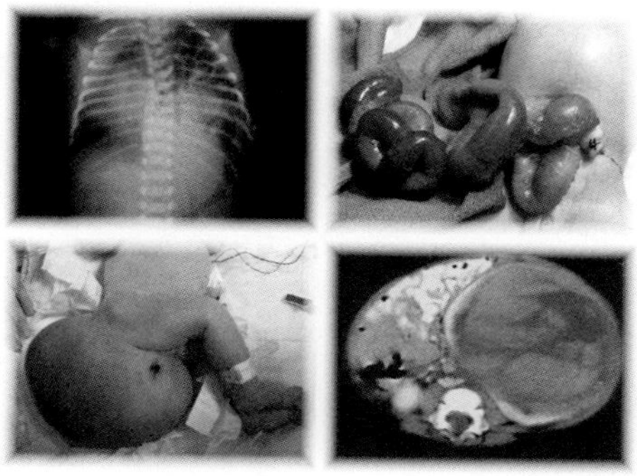

HANDBOOK OF PEDIATRIC SURGICAL PATIENT CARE

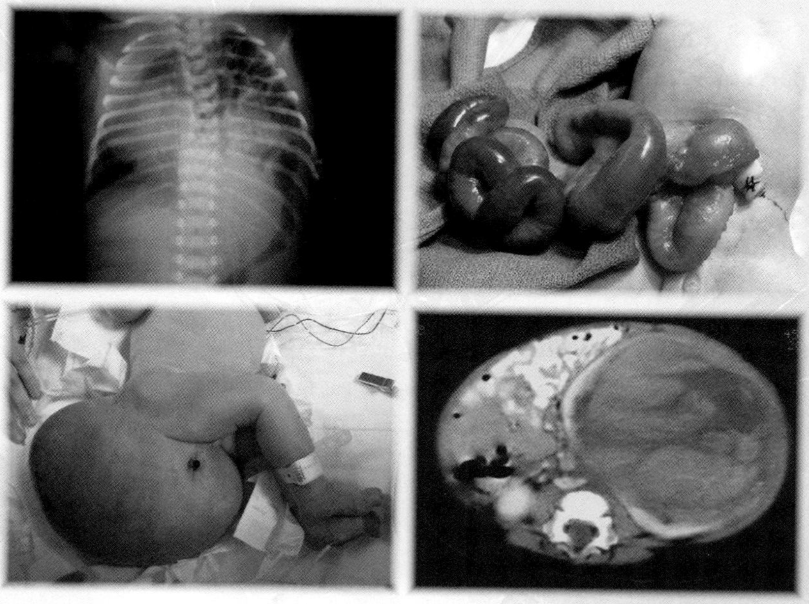

Editors

Alan P. Ladd
Frederick J. Rescorla
Jay L. Grosfeld

Indiana University School of Medicine, USA

World Scientific

NEW JERSEY • LONDON • SINGAPORE • BEIJING • SHANGHAI • HONG KONG • TAIPEI • CHENNAI

Published by

World Scientific Publishing Co. Pte. Ltd.

5 Toh Tuck Link, Singapore 596224

USA office: 27 Warren Street, Suite 401-402, Hackensack, NJ 07601

UK office: 57 Shelton Street, Covent Garden, London WC2H 9HE

British Library Cataloguing-in-Publication Data
A catalogue record for this book is available from the British Library.

HANDBOOK OF PEDIATRIC SURGICAL PATIENT CARE

ISBN 978-981-4287-88-3

Typeset by Stallion Press
Email: enquiries@stallionpress.com

Printed in Singapore by Mainland Press Pte Ltd.

To our wives
Tonya, Mechelle, and Margie
For giving us the opportunity and time to reach for our dreams
And the support to compile this text.

To the children of the world
Whose care we wish to improve with this endeavor.

CONTENTS

CONTRIBUTORS

Laurie L. Ackerman, MD
Assistant Professor of Neurological Surgery
Indiana University/Goodman Campbell Brain & Spine
Riley Hospital for Children/Indiana University Health
Indianapolis, IN

Adam C. Alder, MD
Fellow
Department of Pediatric Surgery
Children's Medical Center
Dallas, TX

Deborah Billmire, MD
Professor of Surgery
Indiana University School of Medicine
Riley Hospital for Children
Indianapolis, IN

Ali Cadili, MD
University of Alberta
Stollery Children's Hospital
Edmonton, Alberta, Canada

Marc Chaet, MD
Orlando, FL

Christine Caltoum, MD
Assistant Professor
Pediatric Orthopedic Surgery
Indiana University
Riley Hospital for Children
Indianapolis, IN

David E. Carney, MD
Associate Professor of Surgery
Mercer University School of Medicine
Memorial Health University Hospital
Savannah, GA

Jenny Cho, MD
Fellow
Division of Vascular Surgery
Department of Surgery
Indiana University School of Medicine

John J. Coleman III, MD
Director of Plastic Surgery
Department of Surgery
Indiana University School of Medicine
Indianapolis, IN

Paul Crisostomo, MD
Fellow
Division of Vascular Surgery
Department of Surgery
Indiana University School of Medicine

Wendy Cruse, MMSc, RD
Pediatric Specialty Dietitian
Transplant and NICU
Riley Children's Hospital at Indiana University Health
Indianapolis, IN

Michael C. Dalsing, MD
E. Dale and Susan E. Habegger Professor of Surgery
Indiana University school of Medicine
Indiana University Health Care System
Indianapolis, IN

Katherine M. DeMasie, MD
Assistant Professor of Clinical Anesthesia
Indiana University School of Medicine
Riley Hospital for Children
Indianapolis, IN

Bryan J. Dicken, MSc FRCSC, FAAP
Assistant Professor of Surgery
University of Alberta
Stollery Children's Hospital
Edmonton, Alberta, Canada

Ann DiMaio, MD
Adjunct Associate Professor of Pediatrics
Saint Louis University College of Medicine
St. Louis, MO

John M. Draus, Jr., MD
Assistant Professor of Surgery
University of Kentucky
Kentucky Children's Hospital
Lexington, Ky

Brian J. Duffy, MD
Assistant Professor of Surgery and Pediatrics
Thomas Jefferson University
Alfred I. DuPont Hospital for Children
Wilmington, DE

James C. Y. Dunn, MD, PhD
Professor of Surgery
University of California, Los Angeles
Mattel Children's Hospital
Los Angeles, CA

Scott A. Engum, MD
Professor of Surgery
Indiana University School of Medicine
Riley Hospital for Children
Indianapolis, IN

Mauricio A. (Tony) Escobar, Jr., MD
Staff Surgeon
Mary Bridge Children's Hospital
Tacoma, WA

Nicholas Fiore, MD
Pediatric Surgery Associates
Las Vegas, NV

Ethan I. Franke, MD
Fellow
Division of Pediatric Urology
Indiana University School of Medicine
Riley Hospital for Children
Indianapolis, Indiana

Julie Fuchs, MD
Associate Professor of Surgery
University of Texas Southwestern Medical Center
Children's Medical Center Dallas
Dallas, TX

Cynthia Gingalewski, MD
Assistant Professor of Surgery and Pediatrics
Children's National Medical Center
Washington, DC

Jay L. Grosfeld, MD
Professor Emeritus,
Lafayette Page Professor of Surgery
Indiana University School of Medicine
Riley Hospital for Children
Indianapolis, Indiana

Miller C. Hamrick, MD
Fellow in Pediatric Colorectal Surgery
Cincinnati Children's Hospital
Cincinnati, OH

Doris M. Hardacker, MD
Clinical Associate Professor
Indiana University School of Medicine
Riley Hospital for Children
Indianapolis, IN

David J. Hobbs, MD
Michigan State University College of Human Medicine
Helen DeVos Children's Hospital
Grand Rapids, MI

Mustafa H. Kabeer, MD
Assistant Professor of Surgery
University of California, Irvine
Attending Surgeon
Children's Hospital of Orange County
Orange, CA

Martin Kaefer, MD
Professor of Urology
Division of Pediatric Urology
Indiana University School of Medicine
Riley Hospital for Children
Indianapolis, IN

Evan R. Kokoska, MD
Clinical Associate Professor of Surgery
Indiana University School of Medicine
Faculty
Peyton Manning Children's Hospital
Indianapolis, IN

Alan P. Ladd, MD
Associate Professor of Surgery
Indiana University School of Medicine
Riley Hospital for Children
Indianapolis, IN

Allen Lee, MD
Resident
University of Texas Southwestern Medical Center
Children's Medical Center Dallas
Dallas, TX

Charles M. Leys, MD, MSCI
Assistant Professor of Surgery
Indiana University School of Medicine
Riley Hospital for Children
Indianapolis, IN

Danny C. Little, MD
Assistant Professor of Surgery
Chief of Pediatric Surgery
Texas A&M Health Science Center
Children's Hospital at Scott & White
Temple, TX

Richard S. Mangus, MD
Assistant Professor of Surgery
Transplant Division, Dept of Surgery
Indiana University School of Medicine
Indiana University Hospital
Indianapolis, IN

Michael S. Mazurek, MD
Associate Professor of Clinical Anesthesia
Indiana University School of Medicine
Riley Hospital for Children
Indianapolis, IN

Rahul Mehan, MD
Resident
Department of Urology
Indiana University School of Medicine
Indianapolis, IN

Kirstan K. Meldrum, MD
Associate Professor of Urology
Division of Pediatric Urology
Indiana University School of Medicine
Riley Hospital for Children
Indianapolis, IN

Kim Molik, MD
Clinical Assistant Professor of Surgery
Kansas University School of Medicine
Wichita, KS

Sarah C. Oltmann, MD
Chief Surgery Resident
University of Texas Southwestern Medical Center
Dallas, TX

Danielle Patterson, MD
Resident
University of California
Los Angeles, CA

Troy Perry, MD
University of Alberta
Department of Surgery
Edmonton, Alberta, Canada

Donald Plumley, MD
Arnold Palmer Hospital for Children
Orlando, FL

Frederick J. Rescorla, MD
Lafayette F. Page Professor of Surgery
Director, Section of Pediatric Surgery
Indiana University School of Medicine
Surgeon-in-Chief
Riley Hospital for Children
Indianapolis, Indiana

Mark Rodefeld, MD
Associate Professor of Surgery
Indiana University School of Medicine
Riley Hospital for Children
Indianapolis, IN

Thomas Rouse, MD
Associate Professor of Clinical Surgery
Indiana University School of Medicine
Riley Hospital for Children
Indianapolis, IN

Rob Russell, MD, MPH
Pediatric Surgery Fellow
Indiana University School of Medicine
Riley Hospital for Children
Indianapolis, IN

L.R. "Tres" Scherer III, MD
Professor of Surgery
Indiana University School of Medicine
Riley Hospital for Children
Indianapolis, IN

David T. Schindel, MD
Associate Professor of Surgery
University of Texas Southwestern Medical School
Children's Medical Center
Dallas, TX

Marc Schlatter, MD
Professor of Surgery
Michigan State University
Helen Devos Children's Hospital
Grand Rapids, MI

Nicole Sharp, MD
Resident
Texas A & M Health Science Center
Scott & White Memorial Hospital
Temple, TX

Michael A. Skinner, MD
Edwin Ide Smith, MD Professor of Pediatric Surgery
University of Texas Southwestern Medical Center
Children's Medical Center
Dallas, TX

Jodi L. Smith, PhD, MD
John E. Kalsbeck Professor and Director of Pediatric Neurosurgery
Associate Professor of Neurological Surgery
Indiana University School of Medicine
Riley Hospital for Children
Indianapolis, IN

Hayden Stagg, MD
Instructor in Surgery
Texas A&M Health Science Center
Scott & White Memorial Hospital
Temple, TX

Gregory A. Stanley, MD
Resident
University of Texas Southwestern Medical Center
Children's Medical Center Dallas
Dallas, TX

James A. Tolley, MD
Assistant Professor of Clinical Anesthesia
Indiana University School of Medicine
Riley Hospital for Children
Indianapolis, IN

Corey Tomlinson, MD
University of Alberta,
Stollery Children's Hospital
Edmonton, Alberta, Canada

Brian A. VanderBrink, MD
Fellow
Division of Pediatric Urology
Indiana University School of Medicine
Riley Hospital for Children
Indianapolis, Indiana

Dennis W. Vane, MD
Professor and Chair of Pediatric Surgery
St. Louis Univeristy
Cardinal Glennon Children's Medical Center
St. Louis, MO

Thomas R. Weber, MD
Professor of Pediatric Surgery
University of Illinois School of Medicine, Chicago
Surgeon-in-Chief
Hope Children's Hospital
Oak Lawn, IL

L. Daniel Wurtz, MD
Associate Professor
Chief, Orthopedic Surgical Oncology
Indiana University School of Medicine
Riley Hospital for Children
Indianapolis, In

Kristen A. Zeller, MD
Assistant Professor of Surgery
Wake Forest University School of Medicine
Brenner Children's Hospital
Winston Salem, NC

Section 1: Physiologic Considerations of Newborn/Child

PEDIATRIC THERMOREGULATION AND METABOLISM

1

David E. Carney and Miller C. Hamrick

NEWBORN AND CHILDHOOD PREDISPOSITION TO HEAT LOSS

The human newborn is a homeotherm desiring to maintain a stable core body temperature over a wide range of environmental changes while minimizing metabolic demand. Hypothermia has been found to increase morbidity and mortality in newborns of all gestational ages and birth weights. The range over which a newborn can maintain body temperature is more limited than that of an adult. The newborn has a high surface area to volume ratio, a distinct lack of subcutaneous fat, poor vasomotor response to cold, and a relative inability to produce heat by shivering.[1] Therefore, equilibrium is maintained by a delicate balance between heat production and heat loss.

TYPES OF HEAT LOSS

Heat loss between the newborn and the environment occurs via four major mechanisms including conduction, convection, radiation, and evaporation (Figure 1).

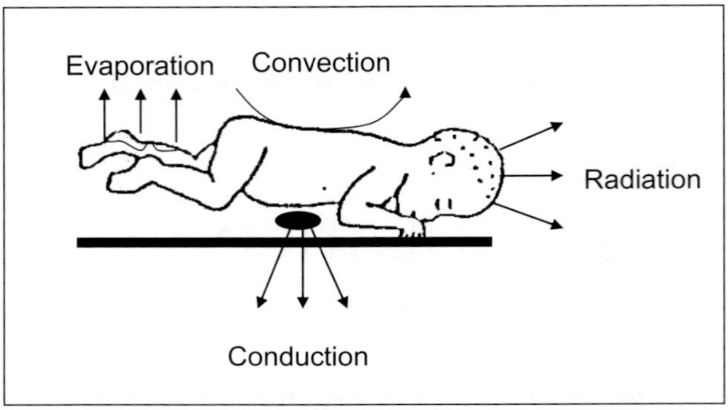

Figure 1. Modes of heat loss in infants and children.

A. Conduction: Involves the transfer of heat from the newborn to a cooler object that is in direct contact with the newborn (e.g. uncovered bed, X-ray plate, scales).
B. Convection: Involves heat loss from the infant due to cool air moving across the skin and dependent on air temperature and the amount of skin exposed; can be prevented by the use of isolette or plastic covering.
C. Radiation: Involves direct transfer of heat from an exposed surface of the newborn to surrounding surfaces and is compounded by moisture on the skin; can be prevented by the use of radiant warmer, hats and bundling.
D. Evaporation: Involves insensible water loss from the skin and respiratory mucosa of the newborn as moisture evaporates; prevented by the use of humidified air and bundling.

MAINTAINING CORE TEMPERATURE

The physiologic mechanisms to produce heat include both voluntary and involuntary actions. In the newborn, the most important of these is non-shivering thermogenesis that utilizes brown fat. Brown fat is located around the muscles and blood vessels of the scapulae, neck, axillae, and mediastinum. It has more mitochondria and a richer blood supply than white fat. Once the hypothalamus receives the message that the infant is cold, norepinephrine stimulates receptors in the brown fat causing oxidation of glycerol and fatty acids producing heat. Alternative mechanisms for maintaining body temperature include peripheral vasoconstriction and central shunting. Proper maintenance of temperature prevents peripheral vasoconstriction and allows for more accurate assessment of resuscitation. All of these mechanisms are important especially in the postoperative period to avoid the development of neonatal cold injury syndrome, which manifests as lassitude, apnea, bradycardia, acidosis, hyperglycemia, hyperkalemia, and oliguria. Prolonged hypothermia increases oxygen consumption, caloric demand, and rapidly decreases glycogen stores. Hypothermia is also associated with an increased rate of wound infections and postoperative sepsis.[2]

The newborn not only has difficulty conserving, but dissipating heat as well. In warm environments, the newborn increases evaporative heat loss by peripheral vasodilatation and sweating, though sweating does not occur in preterm infants. Even so, these mechanisms are often inadequate to prevent a rise in core temperature. Great care must be taken to closely regulate the body temperature of the newborn, with ideal ambient temperature ranging from 35°C (95°F) in preterm and low birth weight infants less than 6 weeks old to 29°C (84°F) for full-term infants heavier than 2–3 kg.

Preventing Heat Loss

Preventing heat loss is of utmost importance, especially in the first 12–24 hrs after birth, as these patients are most at risk for complications related to hypothermia. Multiple factors may predispose certain newborns to difficulties in maintaining normothermia including prematurity and those with CNS problems, sepsis, or prolonged resuscitation at birth. Monitoring of temperature should begin immediately after birth and checked every 4–6 hrs with a goal temperature of 36.7–37.3°C (98–99°F). If the temperature falls out of range, it should be checked every 30 mins until it returns to the target range.[3] It is also important to monitor temperature every 1–2 hrs when a newborn undergoes an environment change for procedural purposes (e.g. imaging, exposure for line placement, surgery). Temperature regulation is most important in preterm and low-birth weight infants as their skin is not yet mature and their ability to initiate nonshivering thermogenesis is very limited.[4] Also, brown adipose tissue begins to be deposited at 28 weeks gestational age; therefore, extremely premature infants have almost no ability to maintain body temperature. At birth, these high-risk infants should be delivered in a room with ambient temperature > 25°C

(77°F) and be covered immediately from the neck down with an occlusive polythene wrapping for transfer to the neonatal ICU.[5] Any infant less than 1.5 kg should be placed in an incubator with humidity levels between 50% and 80%. For those infants >1.5 kg, a radiant warmer should be employed which provides heat by a combination of conduction via a gel mattress and radiation from above.[6] This mechanism is also employed for those infants who require ease of access for procedures such as central line placement or lumbar puncture. Once the infant can maintain normothermia in a 26–28°C room, they can be moved to an open bassinette or crib but should always be covered in blankets and wear a hat. Most infants >4 kg need only bundling and hats to maintain core temperature.

REFERENCES

1. Alden K. (2007) Physiologic and behavioral adaptations of the newborn. In: D Lowdermilk & S Perry (eds.), *Maternity & Women's Health Care,* 9th edition, pp. 639–641. Mosby/Elsevier, St. Louis.
2. Sofer S, Bankovich E. (2000) Severe infantile hypothermia: Short and long-term outcome. *Intensive Care Med* **26**(1):88–92.
3. Cheffer N. (2004) Adaptation to extrauterine life and immediate nursing care. In: S Mattson & J Smith (eds.), *Core Curriculum for Maternal-Newborn Nursing,* 3rd edition, pp. 422–423. Elsevier/Saunders, St. Louis.
4. Sedin G. (2006) Physical environment. Part I: The thermal environment of the newborn infant. In: R Martin, A Fanaroff & M Walsh (eds.), *Fanaroff & Martin's Neonatal-Perinatal Medicine: Diseases of the fetus and infant,* 8th edition. Mosby, Philadelphia.
5. Sherman T, Greenspan J, St. Clair N, *et al.* (2006) Optimizing the neonatal thermal environment. *Neonatal Network* **25**(4):251–260.
6. Williams PR, Oh W. (1974) Effects of radiant warmer on insensible water loss in newborn infants. *Am J Dis Child* **128**:511.

FLUIDS, RESUSCITATION AND ELECTROLYTES 2

David E. Carney and Miller C. Hamrick

INTRODUCTION

The discussion of fluids, resuscitation and electrolyte management in infants and children is broad and a comprehensive understanding is well documented elsewhere.[1–5] Here we briefly review how the newborn physiology varies from older children and adults and the impact of those differences on resuscitation. We then review the generic theme of maintenance fluid replacement and guiding principles to consider during acute resuscitation. Finally, signs of common electrolyte imbalance and treatment are reviewed.

Multiple factors must be assessed in determining the fluid status and fluid requirements of the pediatric population. Total body water in the fetus slowly decreases over time from 80% of total body weight at 32 weeks gestation, to 78% at term, and 60% by 18 months.[6,7] Therefore, the initial duty of the infant kidney is to reduce extracellular fluid volume which begins immediately after birth. This manifests itself as a 4–5% decrease in total body water in the first week of life. Clinically this manifests as a 10% decrease from the initial birth weight. The majority of the total body fluid losses occurring during gestation and early infancy are derived from the extracellular fluid compartment.

The newborn kidney differs from the adult kidney in its ability to manage both fluid shifts and sodium concentration. The glomerular filtration rate of a newborn progresses from 21 mL/min/1.73 m^2 at birth to 60 mL/min/1.73 m^2

by 2 weeks and continues to adult levels (120 mL/min/1.73 m^2) by two years of age. Newborns also have a decreased ability to concentrate urine when compared to adults, likely secondary to an insensitivity of the collecting ducts to antidiuretic hormone. The preterm infant has a high urinary sodium concentration while the term infant has a diminished ability to excrete excess sodium. This makes both term and preterm infants less tolerant of dehydration and greatly affects fluid requirements, especially in the perioperative period.

When initiating resuscitation in the newborn, anticipated fluid losses must be considered including insensible losses from lungs and skin while taking into account the effects of gestational age, body temperature, phototherapy, and the increased metabolic demands of surgical conditions. Accurate measurement of these losses is difficult, yet it is determined that 2–4 mL/kg/hr urine output is required to clear the renal solute load with variability based on individual osmolar load excretion. The demand for urine output falls to 1–2 mL/kg/hr by age one through preadolescence. Children over the age of 12 require adult levels of urine output (0.5–1 mL/kg/hr) to effectively clear renal solute.

Maintenance fluids for a neonate should be initiated with an iso-osmotic solution with dextrose that is hypotonic with respect to saline. A common resuscitative maintenance fluid employed in infants includes 10% dextrose solution with free water or 0.25% normal saline at a rate of 4 mL/kg/hr for those infants less than 10 kg.[8] Older (heavier) infants and children are provided 4 mL/kg/hr for every kilogram up to 10 kg, 2 mL/kg/hr for every kilogram from 10 kg to 20 kg and 1 mL/kg/hr for every kilogram over 20 kg. The goal is to adequately replace both insensible losses as well as urinary losses. It is important to keep in mind that ambient temperature, humidity, and tachypnea can greatly affect insensible losses. In a nonfeeding infant, 10% dextrose solution is critical due to the limited ability of the newborn to utilize fats and protein as substrates for gluconeogenesis. In the early postoperative period, the inherent catabolic state and stress response decreases the dextrose requirement yet these patients still require dextrose-rich hypotonic maintenance fluid. To account for increased fluid requirements and third-space losses by the interstitium and gut, maintenance fluid should be supplemented with isotonic fluid (0.9% normal saline or lactated Ringer's).[9] Additional surgical losses from stomas and drains may be replaced based on an understanding of the electrolyte composition in common bodily fluids (Table 1). There is no clear role for the early use of colloid in the resuscitation of critically ill infants and children.[10]

Table 1. Electrolyte composition in common body fluids and isotonic replacement fluids.

Body/IV fluids	Electrolytes (mEq/L)			
	Na^+	K^+	Cl^-	HCO_3
Gastric	70	5–15	120	0
Pancreas	140	5	75	100
Bile	130	5	100	40
Diarrhea	50	35	40	50
Ileostomy	103	20	120	30
Ringer's lactate	130	4	109	28
0.9% NaCl	154	0	154	0

When considering acute resuscitation of the ill or compromised patient, it is important to appropriately assess the patient's fluid status using standard variables including pulse, blood pressure, urine output, skin turgor, and capillary refill. Knowledge of the circulating blood volume of neonates (80 mL/kg) and infants (75–80 mL/kg) is important to identify the degree of volume depletion. The initial fluid bolus should attempt to replenish the entire circulating volume deficit. In the absence of severe congenital heart disease or renal dysfunction, this aggressive resuscitation is not only well-tolerated but necessary to maintain adequate organ perfusion.

In the setting of a severely dehydrated child, rapid replacement of fluid losses is the foremost priority for the physician. Intravenous rehydration should be initiated at a dosage of 20–40 mL/kg often delivered via a 60-mL syringe as a bolus over 2–3 mins of isotonic fluid. After the initial bolus, if the pulse, blood pressure, and skin tugor do not improve, a second bolus of 20–40 mL/kg should be delivered. The total amount of fluid delivered in the initial 6–12 hrs of resuscitation may exceed 100 mL/kg in a child with severe volume depletion. Serial examinations are important during the initial period of resuscitation with a focused effort to restore pulse rate, blood pressure, and urine output to normal values.

ELECTROLYTE DISTURBANCE AND TREATEMNT

Specific supplementation of electrolytes during the first 24 hours of life is usually not required. Beginning at 24 hours of life, an infant needs

1–2 mEq/kg/day of potassium and 1–3 mEq/kg/day of sodium, assuming urine output is adequate. Consideration should be given to the preterm infant as sodium requirements are increased due to a decreased ability to retain sodium. Also, in the setting of metabolic acidosis, sodium acetate may be the preferred initial resuscitative fluid over sodium chloride as the systemic acidosis in preterm infants is likely secondary to inadequate urinary acidification. The needs for both sodium and potassium increase after the first week of life and appropriate adjustments in supplementation must be made in order to maintain normal levels.

Due to the filtration properties of the newborn kidney, abnormalities in serum sodium are almost universally caused by excessive free water intake (hypervolemic hyponatremia) or inadequate free water intake (hypovolemic hypernatremia). These problems are most common in extremely preterm infants and should be actively corrected when sodium levels fall below 130 mEq/L or rise above 155 mEq/L.[11]

Unlike sodium, potassium is an intracellular ion and serum levels greatly depend on blood pH. For every 0.1 U of pH change, serum potassium levels change 0.3–0.6 mEq/L, with acidosis shifting potassium out of the cell and alkalosis driving potassium into the cell.[12] Hypokalemia becomes concerning when levels fall below 3 mEq/L as it can lead to U waves, flattened T waves, and prolongation of the QT interval. Potassium must be replaced very slowly as bolus replacement can be associated with life-threatening cardiac dysfunction. Hyperkalemia becomes very significant at levels greater than 6 mEq/L in a nonhemolyzed specimen. EKG manifestations include peaked T waves, and widening of the QRS complex. Hyperkalemia may be multifactorial but is worsened by acidosis and renal failure. Rapid action must be taken to normalize the potassium values. Common treatment options include:

(1) Calcium gluconate: 75–100 mg/kg IV (administered slowly over 10 mins) (may use calcium chloride at one-third dose)
(2) Alkalinization: hyperventilation or sodium bicarbonate 0.5–1.0 mEq/kg IV (only if patient has acidemia)
(3) Insulin: 0.1 units regular/kg (administer with 0.5 mg/kg of glucose or 2 mL/kg of 25% glucose concentration)
(4) Nebulized albuterol: 10–20 mg in 4-mL saline over 10–20 mins
(5) Furosemide: 1.0 mg/kg IV
(6) Sodium polystyrene sulfonate (kayexalate): 0.5–1.0 g/kg PO (maximum of 50 g) or 102 g/kg PR (mixed in 70% sorbitol solution)
(7) Dialysis

In general, electrolyte replacement is uncommon outside the neonatal or pediatric intensive care unit with the notable exception of managing children with complex gastrointestinal disorders. Table 2 outlines symptoms of electrolyte depletion and excess. It is generally advised to supplement with oral additives or adjustments to parenteral nutrition when possible before considering intravenous bolus therapy. Table 3 demonstrates options for replacement therapy when acute electrolyte deficiency mandates more aggressive or immediate therapy.

Table 2. Clinical findings associated with electrolyte imbalance.

Electrolyte	Excess	Deficiency
Sodium	Hyperexcitability Hyperreflexia CNS damage	Hypotonia Apnea Seizures
Potassium	Ileus Dysrhythmia Altered renal function	Dysrhythmia (ventricular fibrillation)
Calcium	Vomiting Hypotonia Encephalopathy	Irritability Seizures Stridor Tetany Hypotension
Magnesium	Hypotonia Hyporeflexia Hypotension Apnea Flushing	Persistent hypocalcemia

Table 3. IV Electrolyte replacement guidelines.[13]

Potassium chloride or acetate	0.5–1 mEq/kg/dose (max 20 mEq/dose)
Potassium or sodium phosphate	Low dose: 0.08 mmol/kg Intermediate dose: 0.16–0.24 mmol/kg (use if serum phosphorus level 0.5–1 mg/dl) High dose: 0.36–0.64 mmol/kg (use if serum phosphorus level <0.5) ***Conversion: 3 mmol phos = 4.4 mEq potassium = 4 mEq sodium***

(*continued*)

Table 3. (*Continued*)

Magnesium sulfate	Hypomagnesemia: 25–50 mg/kg/dose (max single dose 2000 mg) Bronchodilation in severe acute asthma: 25 mg/kg/dose (max single dose 2000 mg) over 15–20 mins Treatment of Torsades De Pointes VT: 25–50 mg/kg/dose
Calcium gluconate*	Hypocalcemia: Neonates: 200–800 mg/kg/day divided in 4 doses Infants and children: 200–500 mg/kg/day divided in 4 doses Cardiac arrest: 60–100 mg/kg/dose (max 3 g/dose) Tetany: 100–200 mg/kg/dose, may follow with 500 mg/kg/day in 3–4 divided doses
Calcium chloride*	Hypocalcemia: Manufacturer's recommendations: 2.7–5 mg/kg/dose every 4–6 hrs Alternative dosing: 10–20 mg/kg/dose, repeat every 4–6 hrs prn Cardiac arrest: 20 mg/kg Tetany: 10 mg/kg over 5–10 mins, may repeat after 6 hrs or follow with an infusion with a maximum dose of 200 mg/kg/day

*Do not administer calcium within 48 hrs of intravenous ceftriaxone administration in patients less than 28 days of age. Use extreme caution in all other patients.

REFERENCES

1. Davis ID, Avner ED. (2002) Fluid, electrolytes, and acid-base homeostasis. In: AA Fanaroff & RJ Martin (eds.), *Neonatal-Perinatal Medicine*, 7th edition, pp. 619. Mosby, St. Louis.
2. Ford DM. (1999) Fluid, electrolyte, and acid-base disorders and therapy. In: WW Hay, AR Hayward, MJ Levin & JM Sondheimer (eds.), *Current Pediatric Diagnosis and Treatment*, 14th edition, pp. 1109. Appleton and Lange, Stamford, CT.
3. Hellerstein S. (1993) Fluid and electrolytes: Clinical aspects. *Pediatr Rev* **14**:103.
4. Oh W. (1997) Fluid and electrolyte management. In: AA Fanaroff & RJ Martin (eds.), *Neonatal-Perinatal Medicine: Diseases of the Fetus and Infant*, 6th edition, pp. 622–638. Mosby, St. Louis.

5. Simmons CF Jr. (1997) Fluid and electrolyte management. In: JP Cloherty & AR Stark (eds.), *Manual of Neonatal Care*, 4th edition, pp. 100. Lippincott Raven, New York.
6. Friis-Hansen B. (1961) Body water compartments in children: Changes during growth and related changes in body composition. *Pediatrics* **28**:169.
7. Hartnoll G, Betremieux P, Modi N. (2000) Body water content of extremely preterm infants at birth. *Arch Dis Child Fetal Neonatal Ed* **83**(1):F56–59.
8. Holliday MA, Segar WE. (1957) The maintenance need for water in parenteral fluid therapy. *Pediatrics* **19**:823.
9. Duke T, Molyneux EM. (2003) Intravenous fluids for seriously ill children: Time to reconsider. *Lancet* **362**:1320.
10. So KW, Fok TF, Ng PC, *et al.* (1997) Randomised controlled trial of colloid or crystalloid in hypotensive preterm infants. *Arch Dis Child Fetal Neonatal Ed* **76**(1):43 –46.
11. Finberg L. (1973) Hypernatremic (hypertonic) dehydration in infants. *N Engl J Med* **289**:196.
12. Adrogué HJ, Madias NE. (1981) Changes in plasma potassium concentration during acute acid-base disturbances. *Am J Med* **71**:456.
13. Taketomo CK, Kraus DM, Hodding JH. (2005) *Pediatric Dosage Handbook*, 12th edition. Lexi-Comp Inc., Hudson, OH.

CARDIOVASCULAR PHYSIOLOGY 3

David E. Carney and Miller C. Hamrick

INTRODUCTION

A broad understanding of cardiovascular physiology and pathophysiology is vital to effectively manage the infant or child with surgical pathology. Most entities confounding the pediatric surgeon may be effectively managed with a fundamental knowledge of fetal anatomy and physiology, congenital heart disease, common dysrhythmias, and a basic algorithm for the index evaluation of heart murmurs.

FETAL ANATOMY AND PHYSIOLOGY

The fetal heart is like that of the adult, only it functions as a parallel circuit, made possible through a series of shunts. Alterations in newborn physiology during delivery and in the early postnatal period create the separate systemic and pulmonary systems we find in adults.

As oxygen rich blood diffuses through the placental membrane, it is carried into the fetus via the umbilical vein (Figure 1). This vein enters the abdomen of the fetus and travels directly to the liver. Approximately 50% of the blood that reaches the liver actually passes through the hepatic parenchyma (Figure 1a), while the remaining umbilical blood volume bypasses the liver via the ductus venosus (Figure 1b). The ductus venosus is the first of three shunts in the fetal circulation.[1–3]

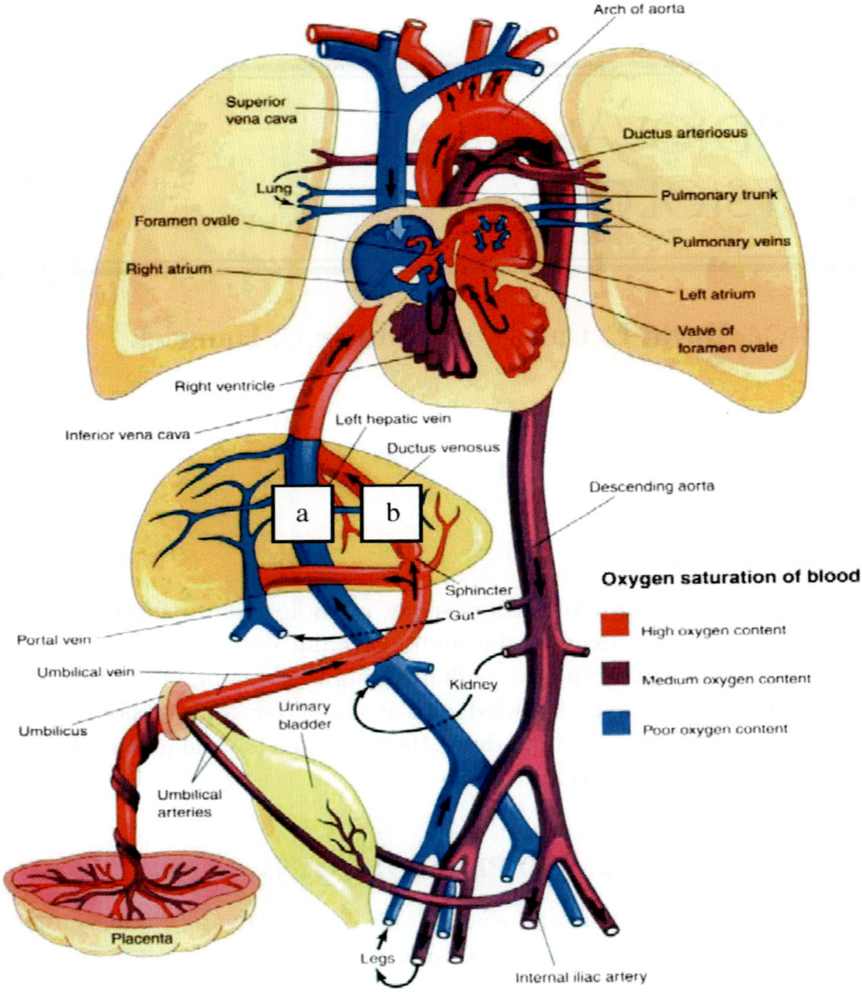

Figure 1. An image of fetal circulation demonstrating umbilical flow (a) traversing the hepatic parenchyma and (b) bypassing the hepatic parenchyma via the ductus venosus. (Reprinted with permission: Moore & Persaud, 1998.)

The second shunt is the foramen ovale. Supported by high pulmonary vascular resistance, the foramen ovale allows passage of blood directly from the right atrium to the left atrium, predominately bypassing the pulmonary circulation. A small valve, the septum primum (valve of foramen ovale), is located on the left side of the atrial septum and prevents the blood from moving in the reverse direction through the foramen ovale. The high oxygen content of placental blood is therefore able to flow directly from the inferior vena cava to the right atrium, on to the left atrium and then into the systemic circulation.

Finally, the third shunt is the ductus arteriosus which connects the pulmonary artery to the descending aorta. The ductus arteriosus allows blood to again bypass the pulmonary circulation, distributing oxygen-rich blood to the visceral circulation before exiting the body via the internal iliac and umbilical arteries.

Within 3–10 days of birth, the ductus venosus typically closes due to loss of blood flow when the umbilical cord is clamped. Also, spontaneous or assisted ventilation of the neonate is associated with a dramatic decrease in pulmonary vascular resistance. This begins the preferential flow from the right atrium to the right ventricle and into the pulmonary arteries. Increased pulmonary venous return increases the volume and subsequent pressure in the left atrium which quickly exceeds the pressure in the right atrium. This pressure difference forces the walls of the atria together, fusing them with the intra-atrial septum. As the changes associated with postnatal circulation begin, endogenous prostaglandin inhibition and an oxygen-induced fall in pulmonary vascular resistance combine to decrease flow through the ductus arteriosus, allowing it to gradually obliterate.[1] In the majority of term and near-term infants, the ductus arteriosus closes within 48 hrs of birth. A ductus that does not close within 72 hrs of birth is considered a persistently patent ductus arteriosus (PDA). The incidence of a patent ductus is inversely proportionate to birth weight. Neonates weighing 1000–1500 g at birth have a 25% incidence of a PDA, while extremely preterm neonates (<1000 g) have a 65% incidence of a patent ductus. In this later group, nearly three-fourths require medical and/or surgical therapy.[4,5]

Failed closure of the ductus is a common issue in the management of the neonate. Although flow through the ductus is often bidirectional, the neonate often becomes compromised by excessive left-to-right shunting that manifests as atrial enlargement, pulmonary over-circulation, pulmonary hemorrhage, and visceral ischemia. Treatment of a PDA is preferably medical, particularly in infants born ≥28 weeks. Medical management includes fluid restriction, diuretic therapy, and often prostaglandin inhibition with indomethacin.[4,6]

For infants <28 weeks gestational age, many institutions administer prophylactic indomethacin within 12 hrs of birth noting that early treatment is associated with increased success of permanent ductal closure.[7] It is important to remember there are frequent contraindications to indomethacin treatment including bleeding, platelets <50,000, low urine output, creatinine >2.0, and suspected necrotizing enterocolitis. This later association of indomethacin with impaired mesenteric blood flow and subsequent necrotizing enterocolitis mandates that infants given indomethacin should be kept NPO for 48 hrs after treatment. Surgery should be considered following failure of indomethacin or in patients with contraindications to its use. In the neonate with a large PDA and evolving necrotizing enterocolitis, semi-urgent surgical ligation may be necessary to prevent advanced intestinal ischemia.[8]

In order to effectively oxygenate the unborn fetus, the shunts of fetal circulation discretely drive oxygen-rich blood to the fetal tissue. To supplement this process, the fetus has adapted qualities to compete with the maternal host for oxygen as blood traverses the placenta. First, the neonate has an elevated hemoglobin level at birth commonly exceeding 18–20 g/dL. Also, the neonate has a very high percentage of fetal hemoglobin (HbF) as compared to adults (75% vs. 1%). The benefit of fetal hemoglobin is an increased affinity for oxygen. Increased affinity is achieved by a fetal hemoglobin subunit gamma maintaining fewer positive charges than the adult hemoglobin beta subunit. Consequently 2,3-bisphosphoglycerate (2,3-BPG) is less electrostatically bound to fetal hemoglobin as compared to adult hemoglobin. Although 2,3-BPG is abundant in fetal red cells, decreased binding with fetal hemoglobin enhances the ability of fetal red blood cells to retain oxygen. In fact, adult hemoglobin alone actually has a higher affinity for oxygen than its fetal equivalent however, enhanced binding to 2,3-BPG reduces affinity. At birth, fetal hemoglobin comprises 50–95% of the child's hemoglobin. These levels have decreased by 6 months as adult hemoglobin synthesis is activated while fetal hemoglobin synthesis is deactivated. Soon after, adult hemoglobin (hemoglobin A in particular) takes over as the predominant form of hemoglobin in normal children. Genetic abnormalities may alter adult hemoglobin synthesis, resulting in a benign condition known as hereditary persistence of fetal hemoglobin.[1,6]

As the infant grows, the cardiac output increases slowly, proportionate to body weight. This increase in cardiac output is accomplished by cardiac growth only, with no initial change in contractility or heart rate. As the infant grows, it gradually gains the ability to venoconstrict in response to catecholamine release, enhancing the ability to augment preload and subsequent cardiac output in times of stress. Consequently, a newborn infant has limited ability to spontaneously augment volume status or contractility in times of stress, making cardiac output dependent on rate. This idea is further supported in the discussion on shock and resuscitation where we emphasize the notion that in healthy infants with hypoperfusion, resolution of tachycardia may be the most reliable indicator of appropriate resuscitation.

When hypotension and other signs of shock are present, resuscitation prioritizes optimizing left ventricular end diastolic volume with fluid boluses, only later supplemented with chronotropic and inotropic agents. In the healthy infant, the utilization of vasopressive agents to increase afterload is reserved only after fluid resuscitation and inotropic/chronotropic agents fail to establish an effective mean arterial pressure.

CONGENITAL HEART DISEASE

The pediatric surgeon must have a basic understanding of congenital heart disease. Specifically, it is helpful to understand which lesions preclude safe, elective surgery. Furthermore, an understanding of the native defect and any surgical reconstruction is paramount to provide effective perinatal and perioperative care. For the purpose of this discussion, we will focus on lesions that require ductal flow and the management of associated pulmonary hypertension. In general, ductal dependent lesions are those that depend on flow via the patent ductus arteriosus in order to maintain systemic, pulmonary, or mixed circulation. Lesions that require right-to-left ductal flow in order to support the systemic circulation include coarctation of the aorta, hypoplastic left heart anomalies, and critical aortic stenosis. These lesions typically present with cyanosis and tachypnea, in the absence of respiratory distress, along with adequate systemic perfusion. Heart failure, decreased global perfusion, acidosis, and cyanosis are late findings secondary to malperfusion as a result of both the primary lesion and failed ductal flow.

Congenital defects that mandate ductal flow to support the pulmonary circulation include critical pulmonary stenosis, transposition of the great vessels, tetrology of fallot, tricuspid/pulmonary atresia, and Ebstein's anomaly. This second group presents with more immediate clinical cyanosis but are often otherwise stable. Irrespective of the etiology, newborn infants with a persistently patent ductus require arterial blood gas sampling, chest radiographic imaging and often an echocardiogram. Once a ductal dependent lesion is presumed, these infants should be immediately administered prostaglandin E2 (10 ng/kg/min), by continuous intravenous drip to maintain patency until diagnostic confirmation with echocardiogram and pediatric cardiology consultation has been obtained. Patients must be monitored closely for side effects of prostaglandin E2 which include apnea and hypotension.[1,4,5,8]

Common Dysrhythmias

Fortunately, most dysrhythmias in the pediatric population are benign, often limited to sinus arrhythmias, wandering atrial pacemaker, isolated premature atrial/ventricular contractions, and first-degree atrioventricular block. These almost never require treatment. Conversely, there are pathologic dysrhythmias in infancy and childhood that require semi-urgent or, rarely, emergent treatment.[5,9,10] Table 1 outlines common dysrhythmias that require treatment. The acute management algorithm for these is best

Table 1. Common cardiac dysrhythmias in children with associated electrophysiologic findings and the recommended management.

Dysrythmia	Incidence	EKG Findings	Treatment
1. Supraventricular tachycardia	Most common Bimodal (0–3 mths/ 8–10 yrs)	Rapid, regular, narrow QRS	Vagal maneuvers, adenosine, cardioversion, amiodarone Chronic Tx: digoxin and B-blockers
2. Third-degree AV block	Common bradycardia assoc. with transposition, maternal SLE	Slow dissociation of P and QRS	Isoproterenol Rarely pacemaker
3. Ventricular tachycardia	Rare, life-threatening	Regular Wide complex AV dissociation	Lidocaine, procainamide, amiodarone Cardioversion Chronic Tx: +/− ablation

guided by a thorough review of the Pediatric Advanced Life Support (PALS) protocol.[11]

Common Murmurs

It is estimated that nearly 60% of all children will have a clinically audible murmur at some point in their life. This finding is often revealed during the newborn examination or in the assessment of patients for elective and urgent surgery. Since over 90% of heart murmurs are normal, it is incumbent upon the pediatric surgeon to recognize common physiologic murmurs and to understand qualities of the examination which may predict a pathologic lesion. Figure 2 demonstrates where common murmurs may be heard. Once a murmur is identified on auscultation, the lesion may be more accurately characterized based on the child's age and the qualities of the murmur (Table 2). Although it remains helpful to be well versed on common "innocent" murmurs, it is of greater importance to be aware of findings elicited during the comprehensive history and physical examination that may suggest a more sinister lesion. Common findings during the

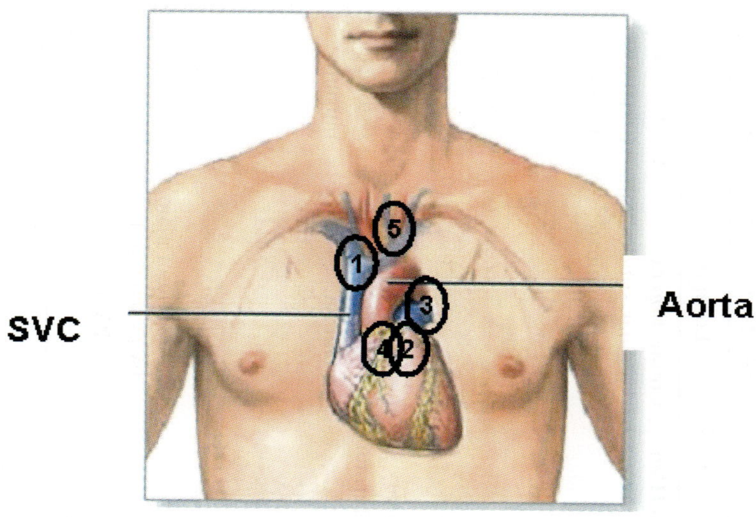

Figure 2. The anatomic location of common "innocent" murmurs in children. (1) Venous hum; (2) Pulmonary flow murmur; (3) Physiologic peripheral pulmonic stenosis; (4) Still's murmur; (5) Supraclavicular systemic bruit.

Table 2. Common characteristics that help differentiate benign pediatric murmurs.

Lesion	Location	Sound	Age	Physical findings	Differential
1. Venous Hum	Connection of jugular, subclavian, and innominate to IVC	Continuous Louder in diastole	Toddler to school age (2–8 yrs)	1. Increased with sitting or standing or if RVOT close to chest wall 2. Decreased in supine position or with compression of neck veins	
2. Pulmonary Flow Murmur	Connection of right ventricle with main PA	Low intensity systolic ejection murmur	School age to young adult	1. Increased with high output states (fever, anemia, sepsis) 2. Decreased with standing or inspiration	ASD, Pulmonic stenosis
3. Physiologic Peripheral Pulmonic Stenosis	Connection of main PA to right and left PA branches	Soft, low pitched systolic ejection murmur	Neonates and infants (birth to 6 mths)	1. Increased in high output states	Pulmonic stenosis, VSD, PDA, pathologic PPS

(Continued)

Table 2. (*Continued*).

Lesion	Location	Sound	Age	Physical findings	Differential
4. Still's murmur	Connection of left ventricle to aorta	Low-pitched early systolic ejection murmur (musical)	Birth to adolescence (often 2–6 yrs)	1. Increased with supine position, anemia, fever 2. Decreased with sitting or standing or with valsalva	VSD, HOCM, Left ventricular outflow obstruction
5. Supraclavicular systemic bruit	Connection of brachiocephalic vessels to aortic arch	Harsh, high-pitched systolic ejection murmur	Children and young adults	1. Decreased with shoulders back. No change with position	Aortic stenosis, supra-aortic stenosis

Table 3. Clinical findings encountered during the cardiac and general physical examination that suggest a pathologic cardiac murmur.

Cardiac examination	General history and physical examination
— Holosytolic murmur	— Chest pain
— Presence of thrill (>III/IV)	— Poor weight gain (growth failure)
— Diastolic murmur	— Cyanosis
— Lncreased intensity with standing	— Tachypnea
— Abnormal S2	— Wheezing
— Early to mid systolic click	— Chronic cough
— Harsh quality	— Syncope
	— Tachycardia
	— Dysmorphic features
	— Additional congenital anomalies
	— Enlarged heart on CXR

focused cardiac examination and the general physical examination that suggest a pathologic murmur are outlined in Table 3. When these findings are revealed on the initial evaluation, a consultative evaluation by pediatric cardiology should precede elective surgery.

Cardiac Metabolism

Unlike the adult heart which uses mainly long-chain fatty acids as fuel, the fetal heart uses lactate derived from the placental circulation. The fetus has a very low supply of fatty acids for fuel and furthermore, high levels of malonyl-CoA inhibit fatty acid uptake into the mitochondria, limiting cellular respiration. After birth, the neonate begins to use glycolysis and glucose oxygenation allowing the newborn heart to effectively utilize fatty acids as a fuel source by the second week of life.[12]

REFERENCES

1. Saltzman DA, Smith SD. (2005) Physiology of the newborn. In: KW Ashcroft, GW Holcomb & JP Murphey (eds.), *Pediatric Surgery*, 4th edition, pp. 3–15. Elsevier, Philadelphia.

2. Yabek SM. (1984) Neonatal cyanosis. *Am J Dis Child* **138**:880.
3. Zuberbuhler JR. Tetralogy of Fallot. In: GC Emmanouilides, TA Riemenschneider, HD Allen & HP Getgesell (eds.), *Heart Disease in Infants, Children, and Adolescents*, 5th edition, pp. 998. Williams and Wilkins, Baltimore.
4. Lees MH. (1970) Cyanosis of the newborn infant. *J Pediatr* **77**:484.
5. Allan LD. (1989) Fetal arrhythmias. In: WA Long (ed.), *Fetal and Neonatal Cardiology*, pp. 180. WB Saunders.
6. Bauer C, Ludwig I, Ludwig M. (1968) Different effects of 2,3-diphospoglycerate and adenosine triphosphate on the oxygen affinity of adult and fetal human hemoglobin. *Life Sci* **7**:1339.
7. Hamrick SEG, Hansmann G. (2010) Patent ductus arteriosus of the preterm infant. *Pediatrics* **125**:1020–1030.
8. Rudolph AM. (2001) Oxygen uptake and delivery. In: AM Rudolph (ed.), *Congenital Diseases of the Heart*, pp. 85. Futura, Armonk.
9. Kleinman CS, Nehgme R, Copel JA. (1999) Fetal cardiac arrhythmias: diagnosis and therapy. In: RK Creasy & R Resnik (eds.), *Maternal-Fetal Medicine*, 4th edition, pp. 301. WB Saunders Co, Philadelphia.
10. McCurdy CM, Reed KL. (1995) Fetal arrhythmias. In: JA Copel JA & KL Reed (eds.), *Doppler Ultrasound in Obstetrics and Gynecology*, pp. 253. Raven Press, New York.
11. Subcommittee on Pediatric Resuscitation (2006) In: M Ralston, *et al.* (eds.), *Pediatric Advanced Life Support Provider Manual*, pp. 98. American Heart Association, Dallas.
12. Rowe MI, O'Neill JA, Grosfeld JL, *et al.* (1995) Endocrine and metabolic response to surgery. In: MI Rowe, JA O'Neill, JL Grosfeld, *et al.* (eds.), *Essentials of Pediatric Surgery*, pp. 25–27. Mosby, St. Louis.

INFECTIOUS CONSIDERATIONS 4

David E. Carney and Miller C. Hamrick

INTRODUCTION

Infection continues to be a major problem in the postsurgical patient. For the pediatric surgeon, infection typically involves neonatal infections or sepsis, perioperative infection, and the management of infection related to indwelling central venous catheters.

The development of a clinically relevant infection requires the breakdown of host defenses and the availability of nutrients for the bacteria to multiply. Without these factors, even virulent bacteria are unable to cause major problems. The postsurgical patient is a prime target for infection as immune defenses are weakened and ability to fight infection is limited.

In the surgical patient, the availability of nutrients for bacterial proliferation is important in the development of infection. Postsurgical fluid collections including hematomas and seromas, as well as necrotic tissue, are perfect media for the growth and propagation of bacteria. It is of utmost importance to limit these factors during and after surgery to minimize the availability of substrate for any bacteria that may be present.

Important consideration should be given to the premature infant for multiple reasons. First, T-cell populations develop and rise throughout gestation and the early postnatal period, reaching adult levels by the age of 9 months. Consequently, premature infants produce lower amounts of TNF-α and IFN-α as compared to term infants. Among the cytokines involved in adaptive immunity, only IL-2 concentrations are comparable in preterm infants while others like IL-5, IL-10, and IL-15, are significantly lower than those in term infants and adults.[1,2] Also, premature infants and neonates are incapable of mounting antigen-specific antibody responses with the same intensity as older children or adults. The limited cytokine production and white cell activity limits the typical proinflammatory response. The result is an immune response in neonates that is both delayed and blunted, only further exacerbated with prematurity.[1]

NEONATAL INFECTIONS

In general, all infants ranging from preterm infants up to 6-week adjusted gestational age require an extensive evaluation for fever or presumed sepsis. Neonatal infections are often best categorized when divided into early- and late-onset sepsis.

Early-onset sepsis is classified as an acute bacterial infection during the first 3 days after birth and occurs in 1–10 per 1000 live births. Although the majority occur in term infants, the likelihood of infection is greater among preterm infants. Culture-proven early-onset sepsis will develop in about 2% of all infants with birth weight less than 1500 g. Risk factors associated with vertical transmission of infectious organisms include:

(1) Premature and/or prolonged rupture of chorioamniotic membranes
(2) Maternal colonization with group B -hemolytic Streptococcus (GBS)
(3) Intrapartum maternal fever
(4) Prematurity
(5) Chorioamnionitis

Since the advent of intrapartum antibiotic prophylaxis to prevent neonatal GBS infection, gram-negative organisms have become the most common pathogens, accounting for nearly two-thirds of all neonatal infections. Among these, Escherichia coli is the most common organism identified, while GBS still remains the organism most often associated with shock and death.[3]

Signs and symptoms of early-onset sepsis are often nonspecific and may include lethargy, hypotonia, irritability, hyperreflexia, seizures, apnea, cyanosis, respiratory distress, acidosis, hypothermia and/or hypo-/hyperglycemia.[4] Early, rapid and thorough evaluation is essential for successful treatment. An asymptomatic term or near-term newborn with even one risk factor for sepsis requires careful physical examination and laboratory assessment that includes blood cultures and a complete blood count with differential. Term infants with symptoms and any risk factor or asymptomatic preterm infants with any risk factor need to be managed with empiric antibiotics. Chest radiographic imaging should be assessed for evidence of pneumonia along with tracheal aspirate for culture if there are signs of respiratory distress. Lumbar puncture is essential in the evaluation of early- and late-onset sepsis of the newborn and in all children less than 6 weeks-adjusted gestational age. While it is optimal to obtain cerebrospinal fluid (CSF) prior to starting antibiotics, do not delay antibiotic therapy if multiple attempts at lumbar puncture are required. Evaluation of CSF should include culture, cell count and differential, protein and glucose. A blood glucose drawn simultaneous may prove helpful in the interpretation of the CSF.[1,5] Although grossly overutilized in older children, serum levels of C-reactive protein (CRP) may prove useful in the evaluation of early-onset sepsis, particularly in preterm infants ≤28 weeks gestational age. If the CRP is <1.0 mg/dL at 12 and 36 hrs following delivery or the onset of symptoms, the likelihood of sepsis is extremely low (0.3%).[6] Treatment should begin as soon as cultures have been obtained. Intravenous ampicillin and gentamicin are the recommended empiric antimicrobial agents with dose and interval based on gestational age (Table 1).

Early-onset sepsis is associated with an increased incidence of respiratory distress syndrome, chronic lung disease, severe intraventricular hemorrhage, and periventricular leukomalacia. Despite diagnostic and therapeutic advances, early-onset sepsis continues to have substantial morbidity and a high mortality with preterm newborns more severely affected. Among extreme preterm infants (birth weight less than 1 kg), mortality approaches 35%.[7,8]

Late-onset sepsis occurs after 3 days of age and incidence among healthy term infants is much less than early-onset sepsis. However, preterm

Table 1. Empiric antibiotic therapy for newborn infants with suspected sepsis.

Age	0–4 wks	<1 wk	≥1 wk
Birth weight	<1200 g	1200–2000 g	>2000 g
Ampicillin	25–50 mg/kg q12hr	25–50 mg/kg q12hr	25–50 mg/kg q6hr
Gentamicin	2.5 mg/kg q18–24hr	2.5 mg/kg q12hr	2.5 mg/kg q8hr

infants and term infants with complex medical or surgical conditions are at greater risk. More than 20% of infants with birth weight less than 1500 g will have at least one episode of late-onset sepsis. Risk factors for late-onset bacterial infection are closely related to horizontal transmission of causative organisms and include tracheal intubation, indwelling urinary and vascular catheters, and lack of enteric feeding. Exposure to broad-spectrum antibiotics increases the risk of late-onset sepsis by altering normal flora, permitting overgrowth and dissemination of fungal species and resistant bacteria.

Two-thirds of cases of late-onset sepsis are caused by gram-positive organisms. Coagulate-negative Staphylococcus is the most common species isolated among preterm infants while gram-negative bacteria (e.g. *E. Coli, Klebsiella pneumoniae, Pseudomonas aeruginosa*) remain abundant. Fungal infections with Candida species occur frequently in extremely low birth weight, preterm infants. Presentation in most cases of late-onset sepsis is gradual, rather than fulminant. The first indications may be subtle signs such as feeding intolerance, need for increased environmental oxygen, persistent tachycardia, or atypical apnea. However, some infants become gravely ill rather quickly (notable with Pseudomonas infections), and the presentation may include signs common to early onset sepsis.

As with early-onset sepsis, it is imperative to perform an early and thorough diagnostic evaluation that should include blood cultures, CBC with differential, and platelet count. Because CNS infection is more likely with late-onset sepsis, lumbar puncture with complete evaluation of CSF is essential. Unlike early-onset disease, urinary infection is common in older infants. Urine should be collected for urinalysis and culture. To prevent contamination of the specimen, a sterile catheter should be used for specimen collection. In the setting of complex obstructive uropathy, a sample may be obtained by suprapubic needle aspiration. Urine by bag collection should never be sent for culture. Again, CRP may be useful to guide therapy. If the CRP is < 1.0 mg/dL at 12 and 36 hrs after the onset of symptoms, the likelihood of proven or probable sepsis is 2.4%.[6] As soon as cultures have been obtained, antibiotic therapy should be instituted without delay. While the spectrum of causative organisms differs from early-onset sepsis, ampicillin and gentamicin remain the antibiotic therapy of choice. Late-onset disease is associated with significant morbidity clinically manifesting as a patent ductus arteriosus, bronchopulmonary dysplasia, and necrotizing enterocolitis. Preterm infants suffer the greatest mortality (20%).

TORCH Infections

Toxoplasmosis, **O**ther (Syphilis), **R**ubella, **C**ytomegalovirus (CMV) and **H**erpes Simplex Virus (HSV) are common neonatal infections that are acquired *in utero* or during birth. Titers for these infections are commonly checked during the first prenatal visit. Toxoplasmosis, syphilis and rubella are typically identified in the prenatal period and are no longer a common source of newborn infections. On the contrary, CMV is the most common congenital viral infection and overt symptoms occur in 5–20% of infants born to mothers with primary infection. A majority of infants infected at birth are asymptomatic but may eventually develop noticeable abnormalities within the first few years of life. Symptoms include jaundice, hepatosplenomegaly, rash, and multiorgan involvement with late complications including hearing loss, visual impairment, and neurological defects. Treatment in asymptomatic patients is not indicated but conservative use of gancyclovir is appropriate for the critically ill newborn.

Herpes simplex virus is transmitted to the infant during birth and risk of transmission reaches 30%. Infected infants develop one of three patterns of symptoms including;

(1) localized lesions of the skin, eyes, and mouth
(2) central nervous system involvement
(3) disseminated multiorgan disease

Diagnosis can be confirmed by culture results taken from lesions on the mouth or eyes, urine, stool, or CSF. Treatment should be initiated with acyclovir and while those with localized disease uniformly survive, mortality rates for patients with disseminated disease approaches 50%.[9]

CENTRAL VENOUS LINE INFECTIONS

Infections related to indwelling central venous lines (CVL) are increasingly more common. Presumed central line infections are best treated with a central and peripheral culture followed by initiation of broad spectrum antimicrobial therapy. A peripheral culture adds to the specificity of the central culture.[10] Although subtleties exist amongst institutions regarding the specific management of CVL infections, there are common guiding principles of treatment.

(1) Presumed infections in temporary venous access catheters should prompt immediate removal of the line. (Temporary venous access catheters include umbilical venous catheters, PICC lines and nontunneled subclavian, jugular or femoral lines.)
(2) Tunneled catheters with documented fungemia should prompt immediate removal of the line.
(3) Tunneled catheters with documented gram-negative bacteria should generally prompt removal of the line. (This is often modified in children with short gut syndrome and complex gastrointestinal disorders who often have limited options for alternative venous access.)
(4) Tunneled catheters with documented gram-positive bacteria may be initially managed with antibiotics in children devoid of congenital heart disease and prosthetic implants (e.g. spinal instrumentation, ventricular-peritoneal shunts). Again, this management is often modified based on the need to maintain central access and the availability of alternative sites.

REFERENCES

1. Bender CM. (2006) Candidacies. In: JS Remington, JO Klein, CB Wilson & CJ Baker (eds.), *Infectious Diseases of the Fetus and Newborn Infant*, 6th edition, pp. 1107. Elsevier Saunders, Philadelphia.
2. Unbar RD, Richardson-de Corral V, O'Malley PJ. (1986) Difficulties in universal application of criteria identifying infants at low risk for serious bacterial infection. *J Pediatr* **109**:483.
3. Baskin MN. (1993) The prevalence of serious bacterial infections by age in febrile infants during the first 3 months of life. *Pediatr Ann* **22**:462.
4. Eschewal EC, Stark AR. (2008) Management and outcomes of very low birth weight. *N Engl J Med* **358**:1700.
5. Belfer RA, Gittelman MA, Muniz AE. (2001) Management of febrile infants and children by pediatric emergency medicine and emergency medicine: comparison with practice guidelines. *Pediatr Emerge Care* **17**:83.
6. Benita WE, Han MY, Madam A. (1998) Serial serum C-reactive protein levels in the diagnosis of neonatal infection. *Pediatrics* **102**:4.
7. Cooper LZ, Alford CA. (2006) Rubella. In: JS Remington, JO Klein, CB Wilson & CJ Baker (eds.), *Infectious Diseases of the Fetus and Newborn Infant*, 6th edition, p. 893. Elsevier Saunders, Philadelphia.
8. Chiu CH, Lin TY, Bullard MJ. (1997) Identification of febrile neonates unlikely to have bacterial infections. *Pediatr Infect Dis J* **16**:59.

9. Schwartz S, Rave D, Taker O, *et al.* (2009) A week-by-week analysis of the low-risk criteria for serious bacterial infection in febrile neonates. *Arch Dis Child* **94**:287.
10. Beets M, Sherman G, Mayfield J, *et al.* (2003) Clinical utility of blood cultures drawn from central vein catheters and peripheral venipuncture in critically ill medical patients. *Chest* **123**(3):854–861.

PEDIATRIC PARENTERAL NUTRITION

5

Wendy Cruse

INTRODUCTION

Parenteral nutrition (PN) is the infusion of a sterile solution of water, protein, fat, carbohydrate, vitamins, trace metals, electrolytes, and minerals administered through the venous system. Parenteral nutrition is utilized when adequate calories and nutrition cannot be provided via the oral/enteral route. This chapter will review the components and most common indications for use of parenteral nutrition in pediatric patients. The nutrition assessment used to determine fluid and nutritional requirements will be discussed. The benefits of delivering enteral nutrition (EN) to supplement PN will also be shared. Guidelines for initiation, advancement and monitoring of PN will be described. Complications associated with the delivery of PN will also be reviewed.

PN is also known as a total nutrient admixture (TNA) and is commonly available as a 3-in-1 formulation in which all components of the macronutrients are included in the mixture. It is also available as a 2-in-1 formulation in which the amino acid and carbohydrate are in the main mixture and the lipid is either administered separately or not included at all. When lipids are infused separately, they may be infused over a shorter period of time. PN may be used to supplement an oral or enteral diet or it may be used to provide total nutrient needs to an individual. PN may be infused via a central or peripheral vein. When infusing IV nutrition into a peripheral vein, special attention needs to be given to the final osmolarity of the mixture with a maximum dextrose concentration of 12.5%.

Table 1. Pediatric indications for PN.

Congenital anomalies
— Volvulus
— Meconium ileus
— Intussusception
— Atresia
— Gastroschisis
— Omphalocele
— Enteric fistula
— Malrotation
— Hirschsprung's disease
Acquired
— NEC
— Inflammatory bowel disease
— Intractable diarrhea
— Radiation enteritis
— Severe trauma or burn injury
— Short-bowel syndrome
— Chronic intestinal pseudo-obstruction

PN is commonly used in preterm infants to meet their high nutritional needs when enteral nutrition is not adequate or tolerated due to their immature gastrointestinal tract and fluid volume is limited. Common congenital anomalies and acquired conditions for use of PN are listed in Table 1.

There are numerous advantages for utilizing enteral nutrition as a supplement when PN is required. EN is less expensive than PN. It prevents gut atrophy by stimulating gut hormones and secretions as well as providing nutrients for enterocytes which may be helpful in supporting normal gastrointestinal mucosa. It is beneficial in decreasing bacterial translocation and may slow the development of cholestatic liver disease. The use of EN as a supplement may reduce the total duration of PN.

Nutritional assessment is used to determine nutritional needs and optimal growth. It consists of a physical assessment, review of laboratory parameters and medical diagnosis, and obtaining a nutritional history and anthropometric measurements. Estimated energy and protein requirements can be established based on the review of this information. Plotting the child's weight, length or height and head circumference on appropriate growth charts and review of

Table 2. Maintenance fluid needs based on Holiday–Segar method.

< 1500 g	130–150 mL/kg/day
1500–2000 g	110–130 mL/kg/day
2–10 kg	100 mL/kg/day
> 10–20 kg	1000 mL for the 1st 10 kg + 50 mL/kg for each kg > 10 kg
> 20 kg	1500 mL for 1st 20 kg + 20 mL/kg for each kg > 20 kg

Table 3. Parenteral calorie goals.

Age	Kcal/kg/day
Preterm neonate	90–120
< 6 months	85–105
6–12 months	80–100
1–7 yrs	75–90
7–12 yrs	50–75
> 12–18 yrs	30–50

Table 4. Parenteral protein requirements.

Age	G/kg
Preterm neonates	3–4
Infants (1–12 mths)	2–3
Children (> 10 kg or 1–10 yrs)	1–2
Adolescents (11–17 yrs)	0.8–1.5

the child's growth will assist in establishing the need for normal growth vs. catch-up growth, thus establishing goals for both weight and growth rate.

Maintenance fluid requirements are typically based on the Holliday–Segar Method as described in Table 2. Fluid volume for the PN mixture is generally determined based on maintenance fluid needs unless patient is fluid restricted or has additional fluid requirements due to enteric or insensible losses.

Initial calorie and protein goals are based on age-based guidelines found in JPEN 2004.[1] These are outlined in Tables 3 and 4. Parenteral calorie and protein goals are approximately 10% lower than enteral goals due to the lack of energy spent on digestion and complete absorption. Calorie and protein goals are adjusted according to the child's growth.

Parenteral carbohydrate source is dextrose. It is 3.4 calories per gram. Total goal is < 60% of calories from dextrose. Glucose infusion rate (GIR) is calculated as mg per kg per minute by the following equation.

$$\text{GIR} = \text{mg/kg/min} = (\text{mL} \times \%\ \text{dextrose}) \times 1000 \div \text{kg} \div \text{minutes}$$

The initial glucose infusion rate is based on the size of the patient. In a newborn infant the initial GIR may be approximately 5–7 mg/kg/min or for an older child it might be 6–9 mg/kg/min and advanced by 2–4 mg/kg/min per day with usual upper limits of 8–18 mg/kg/min. It is important to monitor glucose tolerance and titrate the GIR to better meet calorie needs.

Parenteral fat source is a lipid emulsion. The purpose of providing fat in PN is to meet calorie needs as well as to provide essential fatty acids. It is recommended to provide 0.5–1 g/kg/day or 4% of total calories to prevent essential fatty acid deficiency (EFAD). Lipid infusions at 1 g/kg/day will treat EFAD. A 20% lipid solution provides 2 kcal/mL or 10 kcal/g. Initial dose of lipid is 0.5–1 g/kg/day and can be advanced by 0.5–1 g/kg/day to maximum goal of 2–3 g/kg/day. The final goal will be approximately 30% of the calories or 50% of the nonprotein calories as lipid. The lipid emulsion contains egg so it is important to determine in the diet history if the child has an egg allergy. It is recommended to monitor triglyceride levels daily as lipid is being initiated and advanced. Hypertriglyceridemia is defined as >200 mg/dL. Monitoring weekly once final dose has been achieved is recommended. As previously mentioned, the lipid can be infused separately as a daily infusion over a fewer hours or every other day as indicated. Maximum lipid infusion is 0.125 g/kg/hr to avoid hypertriglyceridemia.

Benefits to adding heparin to the PN are improved activity of the lipoprotein lipase, reduction of phlebitis and maintenance of catheter patency. The concentration of heparin within PN administered via a central venous line is 0.5–1 unit/L.

Carnitine helps mobilize triglyceride into the mitochondria. PN is carnitine-free so if an infant is to receive only PN and not any oral or enteral feedings, then carnitine is added at a dose of 10–50 mg/kg/day. Neonates can quickly develop deficiency in carnitine, so it is important to supplement when indicated.

Parenteral protein is in the form of crystalline amino acids. Both neonatal and standard amino acids are available. Amino acids provide 4 kcal/g and should be provided as 7–20% of the total calories. Typically they are initially given in the amount of 1.5 g/kg/day and advanced by 0.5–1 g/kg/day. The final goal in a term infant will be 2.5–3 g/kg/day and in a preterm infant will be 3.5–4 g/kg/day. In the NICU, the stock solution contains 3 g/kg/day so the initial dose may also be the final goal. The ideal nonprotein calorie to nitrogen ratio (NPC:N) is 150–250:1 for the final PN prescription. If the patient has renal failure, the NPC:N ratio may be administered at greater than 250:1 to provide more calories and less protein. If the patient has suffered trauma or burn injury, the NPC:N ratio may be less than 150:1 to provide more protein for wound healing.

L-cysteine hydrochloride is added to a neonatal prescription as a conditionally essential amino acid. It is added at a dose of 40 mg per gram of amino acid. It is beneficial in many ways, such as improving nitrogen balance and growth. It reduces the pH, thereby improving calcium and phosphorus solubility and allowing for more calcium and phosphorus to be added to the formula. With prolonged metabolic acidosis, the L-cysteine can be removed until resolution of the metabolic imbalance.

The typical ranges of electrolytes and minerals that are added to a PN formula for preterm neonates are found in Table 5 according to JPEN 2004. They are not added initially as infants are born with adequate stores and renal excretion is limited.[1] They are added slowly as tolerated starting on day 2 of life when the neonate is stable and requires close monitoring.

The typical ranges of electrolytes and minerals that are added to a PN formula for infants and children are found in Table 6 according to the JPEN 2004 guidelines.[1] Table 7 lists the typical ranges of electrolytes and minerals for children and adolescents who weigh greater than 50 kg. Monitoring of electrolyte tolerance is critical.

Standard pediatric and adult trace element packages are available. It is important to know what is available in your facility as well as the Home

Table 5. Electrolytes and minerals PN dosage for preterm neonates.

Sodium	2–5 mEq/kg
Potassium	2–4 mEq/kg
Calcium	2–4 mEq/kg
Phosphorus	1–2 mmol/kg
Magnesium	0.3–0.5 mEq/kg

Table 6. Electrolytes and minerals PN dosage for infants and children.

Sodium	2–5 mEq/kg
Potassium	2–4 mEq/kg
Calcium	0.5–4 mEq/kg
Phosphorus	0.5–4 mmol/kg
Magnesium	0.3–0.5 mEq/kg

Table 7. Electrolytes and minerals PN dosage for children and adolescents >50kg.

Sodium	1–2 mEq/kg
Potassium	1–2 mEq/kg
Calcium	10–20 mEq/day
Phosphorus	10–40 mmol/day
Magnesium	10–30 mEq/day

Table 8. Trace element PN dosage for pediatric patients.

Nutrient	Preterm neonates <3 kg (mcg/kg/day)	Term neonates 3–10 kg (mcg/kg/day)	Children 10–40 kg (mcg/kg/day)	Adolescents >40 kg (mcg)
Zinc	400	50–250	50–125	2–5
Copper	20	20	5–20	200–500
Manganese	1	1	1	40–100
Chromium	0.05–0.2	0.2	0.14–0.2	5–15
Selenium	1.5–2	2	1–2	40–60

Care Company if PN is provided at home. Trace element packages typically contain zinc, copper, manganese, chromium, and selenium. Some do not contain selenium and thus it must be added individually. Recent literature suggests reevaluating trace metal delivery including timing of administration and individualized dosage. Trace elements are typically added to PN once it has been administered for about 2 weeks. Trace element dose guidelines according to JPEN 2004 for all pediatric age groups can be found in Table 8.[1] Zinc is added initially. Additional zinc is required if GI losses are excessive. Depending on the patient's disease state and nutritional needs or deficiencies, they can all be added individually. In liver disease or in patients with cholestasis, it is important to monitor copper and manganese serum levels. Copper deficiency can develop if reduced or removed without monitoring serum levels and result in hypochromic anemia, neutropenia or osteoporosis resulting in bone fractures. In renal disease, selenium and chromium are monitored and may be reduced or eliminated accordingly. Standard pediatric dose for patients <20 kg is 0.2 mL/kg/day. Standard dose for patients >20 kg is 1 mL/day of the adult trace element product.

Aluminum is found in PN as a contaminant. It is most commonly found in calcium and phosphate salts, heparin, cysteine, multivitamin and trace element solutions utilized in compounding the PN formula. Preterm infants and those receiving long-term PN support are at risk for aluminum toxicity. The Food and Drug Administration requires aluminum content to be labeled on all products used in the PN preparation in order to determine the total aluminum content. The FDA established a maximum content limit of 25 mcg/L as well as a 5 mcg/kg/day limit. It is critical to monitor the aluminum content of the PN formula.

Parenteral multivitamins are added daily to the PN script. Table 9 provides common MVI dosage for all age groups.

Close monitoring of tolerance to PN is essential. Baseline laboratory parameters are obtained initially. While advancing the PN, daily laboratory values continue to be monitored. Once the final PN script is established, monitoring can be reduced to twice weekly for smaller patients and weekly for older patients. When serum prealbumin is monitored, it is beneficial to also obtain a C-reactive protein to assess for inflammation. Table 10 provides suggested initial and weekly pediatric PN monitoring guidelines.[2] Serum copper and manganese levels need to be obtained in patients receiving PN for greater than 3 months or who have developed cholestasis to assess specific trace metal dosage. If renal insufficiency is present, serum

Table 9. Parenteral multivitamin dose.

	<11 yrs <2.5 kg	<11 yrs >2.5 kg	>11 yrs
Pediatric MVI	2 mL/kg/day	5 mL/day	
Adult MVI			10 mL/day

Table 10. Initial and weekly PN monitoring pediatric guidelines.

Parameter	Initial	Follow-up
BMP	Daily	Included in CMP
CMP	Weekly	Every 1–4 wks
Magnesium	Daily to Weekly	Every 1–4 wks
Phosphorous	Daily to Weekly	Every 1–4 wks
Prealbumin	Weekly	Monthly
Triglycerides	Daily to Weekly	Monthly
PT/INR	Weekly	Monthly
CBC differential/platelets	Weekly	Every 1–4 wks
GGT	Baseline if indicated	Monthly

Table 11. Chronic PN monitor pediatric guidelines.

Parameter	Initial (months)	Follow-up (months)
Iron studies	3	Every 3–6
Zinc	3	Every 3–6
Selenium	3	Every 3–6
Manganese	3	Every 3–6
Copper	3	Every 3–6
Chromium	3	Every 3–6
Vitamins A, D, and E	6	Every 12
Vitamin B-12 and folate	6	Every 12
Carnitine	3	Every 3–12

selenium and chromium need to be monitored. Serum fat-soluble vitamins and zinc should be evaluated in patients receiving chronic PN, malabsorption or liver failure. In a patient whose terminal ileum has been resected, vitamin B12 and RBC folate levels need to be monitored initially at 6 months, then yearly thereafter. Table 11 provides guidelines for patients receiving PN for greater than 3 months.[2]

PN associated complications include metabolic, nutritional, infectious, and mechanical. Metabolic complications include fluid and electrolyte imbalance, hypertriglyceridemia and PN-induced cholestasis. Nutritional complications include nutrient deficiencies or excesses and remain mostly iatrogenic. These deficiencies may include calories, essential fatty acids, electrolytes, minerals, vitamins and trace elements. Monitoring serum levels and physical growth are critical in the management of patients receiving PN. It is important to identify and treat bacterial and fungal infections immediately. Mechanical complications include catheter occlusion, infiltration and embolism. Following careful line care will assist in reducing the occurrences of infection and mechanical complications.

Although PN improves survival of pediatric patients, it also presents many challenges. PN should be reserved for those whose nutritional needs cannot be met enterally or orally. It is important to cycle PN, reduce the number of hours of administration, or discontinue its use once the child is able to meet a percentage of his or her nutritional needs via other routes. When PN is being utilized, it is critical to monitor tolerance and administer trophic enteral feeds as medically able.

REFERENCES

1. Mirtallo J, Canada T, Johnson D, *et al.* (2004) Safe practices for parenteral nutrition. *J Parenter Enteral Nutr* **28**(6):S39–S70.
2. Szeszycki E, Cruse W, Strup M. (2010) Evaluation and monitoring of pediatric patients receiving specialized nutrition support. *The ASPEN Pediatric Nutrition Support Core Curriculum*, pp. 460–476.

ENTERAL NUTRITION 6

Alan P. Ladd

INTRODUCTION

The use of breast milk remains the optimal formula for the caloric management of the newborn or infant. Though its composition fluctuates based on the stage of its production in the postgestational period, the constituents on average consist of approximately 40–45% of calories from carbohydrate, 5% from protein, and approximately 50% from lipid/fat.[1] For most infants, maternal breast milk is the formula of choice in the initiation and maintenance of an enteral diet. However, conditions may arise wherein an infant may have requirements for synthetic formulas when a mother is unable to supply appropriate quantities of milk or when specialized formulas are required, for aspects of intestinal failure, for example. It is for a multitude of reasons that an infant's care may necessitate the use of supplementation or replacement of caloric support with enteral formulas, which is the focus of this chapter.

STANDARD INFANT FORMULAS

Standard formulas are made to mimic the natural composition of human milk to attain appropriate caloric and micronutrient support. On average, the synthetic formulas have a similar composition, with approximately 40–45% of calories from carbohydrate, 8–12% from protein, and 45–50% from fat.[1–6] The actual specific components of each formula differ and thus the utility of any given formula may be defined by the individual patient's enteral tolerance to those given components. The protein component of these formulas often consists of a combination of casein or whey protein, or is present in the form of peptides or pure amino acids, in the more modular formulas. Carbohydrate composition in these formulas is often derived from lactose or corn syrup as forms of glucose, with occasional additives such as sucrose. The fat component of these formulas may also vary among palm, soy, coconut, safflower, or sunflower oils, or may include a combination of them with or without the addition of medium-chain triglycerides (MCT).

For classification purposes as put forth by Joeckel and Phillips, standard formulas are often categorized based upon their protein content, and described by the major categories of cow's milk protein formulas, soy formulas, hydrolyzed protein formulas, and elemental formulas (Table 1).[1–6]

Cow's Milk-based Formula

Milk-based formula is the most common formula provided to infants for either supplementation or as a sole source of caloric support. They often incorporate a higher level of protein than breast milk at 1.45–1.6 g/dL. These types of formulas consist of a combination of casein and whey as their major protein source. The use of partially hydrolyzed protein as the source of protein is also used in special formulations to aid in overall protein digestion for some infants.

Vegetable oil is often the fat source for these formulas, as it is felt to be more easily digested. Contemporary formulas often add long-chain polyunsaturated fats of docosahexaenoic acid (DHA) and arachidonic acid (ARA) to the formulas to better mimic breast milk's composition of these fatty acids and for the belief that they may aid in brain development.

Formulas made of cow's milk protein often include lactose as the source of carbohydrates. Additional varieties of these formulas are also devised without lactose to meet the needs of infants with lactose intolerance, while maintaining the same protein components.

Soy Formulas

The base element for soy formulas is soy protein, and they are constructed lactose-free. Current soy formulas are equally effective to cow's milk-based formulas for term infants, in regards to their growth, bone mineralization,

Table 1. Human milk, infant, preterm infant and pediatric formulas.[2–6]

Formula type	Carbohydrate source	Carbohydrate g/dl	% Carbohydrate energy	Protein source	Protein g/dL	% Protein energy	Fat source	Fat g/dL	% Fat energy	Calcium mg/dl	Osmolality (mOsm/kg water)	Special notations
Human Milk	Lactose	10.8	43	Human Milk	1.05	6	Human Milk	5.7	51	14	290	
Cow's Milk Based												
Enfamil Lipil	Lactose	7.4	43.5	Whey, Nonfat milk	1.4	8.5	Palm olein, soy, coconut, sunflower	3.6	48	53	300	
Similac Advance	Lactose	7.3	43	Nonfat milk and whey	1.4	8	High oleic safflower, soy and coconut oils	3.7	49	52.8	300	
Similac Sensitive (Lactofree) Lipil	Corn maltodextri, sugar	7.2	43	Milk protein	1.4	9	Safflower, soy, coconut oils	3.6	49	57	200	
Enfamil Lactofree Lipil	Corn syrup solids	7.4	44	Milk Protein	1.4	8.5	Palm olein, soy, coconut, sunflower	3.6	48	55	200	
Enfamil AR Lipil	Lactose, rice starch, maltodextrin	7.4	44	Nonfat milk	1.69	10	Palm olein, soy, coconut, sunflower	3.4	46	53	230	Rice Starch additive

(Continued)

Table 1. (*Continued*)

Formula type	Carbohydrate source	Carbohydrate g/dl	% Carbohydrate energy	Protein source	Protein g/dL	% Protein energy	Fat source	Fat g/dL	% Fat energy	Calcium mg/dl	Osmolality (mOsm/kg water)	Special notations
Similac Sensitive RS	Corn syrup, sugar, rice starch	7.2	43	Milk protein	1.4	9	Safflower, soy, coconut oils	3.7	49	57	180	Rice Starch additive
Protein Hydrolysate Based												
Similac Alimentum	Sugar, mod. Tapioca starch	6.9	41	Casein hydrolysate	1.9	11	Safflower oil, 33% MCT, soy oil	3.8	48	71	370	
Enfamil Nutramigen Lipil	Corn syrup solids, corn starch	7	41	Casein hydrolysate, AA	1.9	11	Palm olein, soy, coconut, sunflower	3.6	48	64	300	
Pregestimil Lipil	Corn syrup solids, corn starch	6.9	41	Casein hydrolysate, AA	1.9	11	MCT, Soy, safflower oil	3.8	48	78	330	
Enfamil Gentlease Lipil	Corn syrup solids	7.2	43	Nonfat milk and Whey	1.5	9	Palm olein, soy, coconut, sunflower	3.5	48	55	230	

(*Continued*)

Table 1. (*Continued*)

Formula type	Carbohydrate source	Carbohydrate g/dl	% Carbohydrate energy	Protein source	Protein g/dL	% Protein energy	Fat source	Fat g/dL	% Fat energy	Calcium mg/dl	Osmolality (mOsm/kg water)	Special notations
Gerber Good Start	Whey Protein	7.5	46	Lactose, corn maltodextrin	1.5	8	Palm olein, soy, coconut, sunflower	3.4	46	45		
Soy Protein Based												
Isomil Advance	Corn syrup solids, sugar	7	41	Soy protein isolate	1.7	10	High oleic safflower, soy and coconut oils	3.7	49	71	200	
Enfamil Prosobee Lipil	Corn syrup solids	7.2	42	Soy protein isolate	1.7	10	Palm olein, soy, coconut, sunflower	3.6	48	71	200	
Premature Formula												
Enfamil Premature Lipil (20 cal/oz)	Corn syrup solids and 40% lactose	7.4	44	Nonfat milk and whey	2	12	40% MCT, soy and high ileic vegetable oils	3.4	44	112	240	
Similac Special Care (20 cal/oz)	Corn syrup solids and 50% lactose	7	41	Nonfat milk and whey	2	12	50% MCT, soy, and coconut oils	3.7	47	122	235	

(*Continued*)

Table 1. (*Continued*)

Formula type	Carbohydrate source	Carbohydrate g/dl	% Carbohydrate energy	Protein source	Protein g/dL	% Protein energy	Fat source	Fat g/dL	% Fat energy	Calcium mg/dl	Osmolality (mOsm/ kg water)	Special notations
Premature Discharge Formula												
Enfamil Enfacare Lipil (22 cal/oz)	55% lactose and corn syrup solids	7.7	42	Whey protein and nonfat milk	2.1	11	High oleic vegetable, soy, 20% MCT and coconut oils	3.9	47	89	250	
Similac Neosure (22 cal/oz)	Corn syrup solids and 50% lactose	7.5	40	Nonfat milk and whey	2.1	11	25% MCT, soy oil, coconut oil	4.1	49	78	250	
Amino Acid Based (Infant)												
Elecare	Corn syrup solids	7.2	43	Free L-amino acids	2.1	15	High oleic safflower oil, 33% MCT, soy oil	3.2	42	78	350	unflavored
Neocate Infant	Corn syrup solids	7.8	47	Free L-amino acids	2	12	coconut and soy oil	3	41		342	
Nutramigen AA Lipil	Corn syrup solids	6.9	41	Free L-amino acids	1.9	11	Palm olein, soy, coconut, sunflower	3.5	48	67	320	

(*Continued*)

Table 1. (*Continued*)

Formula type	Carbohydrate source	Carbohydrate g/dl	% Carbohydrate energy	Protein source	Protein g/dL	% Protein energy	Fat source	Fat g/dL	% Fat energy	Calcium mg/dl	Osmolality (mOsm/ kg water)	Special notations
Milk Based (Pediatric)												
Nutren Jr.	Corn maltodextrin, sucrose	11	44	Milk protein and whey	3	12	Soybean, canola, MCT	5	44	100	350	
Protein Hydrolysate Based (Pediatric)												
Vital Jr.	Corn maltodextrin, sugar	13.4	53	Whey hydrolysate, sodium caseinate	3	12	Canola, 50% MCT	4.1	35	106	390	MCT:LCT 50:50
Peptamen Jr.	Corn maltodextrin, cornstarch	13.8	55	Hydrolyzed whey protein	3	12	MCT, soybean, canola	3.8	33	100	260–400	
Amino acid-based (Pediatric)												
Elecare	Corn syrup solids	7.2	43	Free L-amino acids	2.1	15	High oleic safflower oil, 33% MCT, soy oil	3.2	42	78	350	Unflavored or vanilla
Vivonex Pediatric	Corn maltodextrin, mod food starch	13	63	Free amino acids	2.4	12	MCT, soybeal	2.4	25	97	360	AA are 13% glutamine, 22% BCAA

and provision for vitamin and minerals.[1,7] Soy formulas are a safe alternative to milk-based formulas for term infants and preferred in infants with galactosemia. These formulas are effective in infants who have an immunoglobulin E-associated reaction to cow's milk protein; however, they may not be as effective in the treatment of milk protein-induced enteropathy or enterocolitis. Infants with such a reaction to milk protein may also have sensitivity to soy protein in upwards of 30–64%. These infants are often better supported with formulas that utilize hydrolyzed protein or amino acid-based formulas.

The use of soy formulas in preterm, low-weight infants is not recommended. With the demonstration of slower gains in weight and length, and the notation of reduced bone mineralization in preterm infants under 1800 g with soy-based formulas, recommendations are for the use of specialized formulas for premature infants, noted below.[1,2,8]

Despite early concerns of the effect of soy isoflavones, a type of phytoestrogen, on infants who receive soy formulas, numerous studies have looked into its impact in animal and human models. As a result of investigations into the potential effect on growth outcomes, effects on pubertal development, and fertility, there is no conclusive evidence that soy formulas adversely affect development or reproductive health.[1,9]

Hydrolyzed Protein Formulas

Protein hydrolysate formulas consist of a protein source of peptide chains and free amino acids from the result of heat- or enzymatic-processing of casein and/or whey protein. These types of formulas are recommended for the nutritional support of infants who are intolerant to formulas with a protein constitution of either cow's milk or soy proteins. In addition to the favorable construct of protein, these formulas often contain a mixture of long- and medium-chain triglycerides. The metabolism of medium-chain triglycerides does not require the production of micelles in combination with bile salts or the need for pancreatic lipase for their catabolism and absorption. Thus, formulas with MCT are important in infants with conditions such as liver disease, cystic fibrosis, chylothorax, intestinal failure, and lymphangiectasia.[1]

The downside of formulas with protein hydrolysate composition lies in their less palatable nature than standard formulas. Infants with no oral history for the intake of standard formulas will often accept these formulas if introduced as either their first formula or in the first few months of life.

Amino Acid-Based Formulas

Formulas with this composition contain 100% free amino acids as their protein construct. These formulas have been designed only for children with hypersensitivity to more complex protein components. Despite the uniqueness of their protein construct, these formulas are nutritionally complete. The downside to their usefulness for general usage lies in their lack of palatability and in their higher cost.

SPECIALIZED INFANT FORMULAS

In order to provide nutritional support for infants with a varied tolerance to enteral nutrition or to optimize the nutritional absorption of enteral components, a wide range of commercially available formulas have been constructed for home usage. Adjustments in the availability of calcium, phosphorus and some vitamins, along with the increase in protein or carbohydrate composition have been used for the construction of formulas used for premature infants. Additional specialized formulas include variations in the carbohydrate construction for gastrointestinal disorders, protein-altered formulas for inborn errors of metabolism, and protein and electrolyte-altered formulas for renal disease.[1]

Preterm Infant Formulas

Preterm formulas tend to have higher nutritional content including protein, calcium, phosphorus and some vitamins, to meet the specific requirements of the growing preterm infant. These formulas are higher in their composition of MCT at 40–50% of the fat blend than term infant formulas for improved absorption.[3–5] They are also often available in higher caloric concentrations of 24-calorie per ounce concentrations, in addition to the normal 20-calorie per ounce. Their composition of carbohydrate is often a mixture of lactose and glucose polymers, accommodating the lower intestinal lactase activity of premature infants. Additionally, glucose polymers allow the osmolality to remain lower.

Formulas for preterm infants have been constructed for both in-hospital preterm infants and for those postdischarge. The inherent difference in these two formulations lies in the higher composition of certain components in the in-hospital formulation; including 1.5 times the amounts of calcium and phosphorus and 2–2.5 times the amounts of vitamins A and D. These in-hospital formulations are not utilized postdischarge in the larger, former premature infants, as the associated intake quantities by these infants of the higher constructs may potentially lead to toxic intakes of nutrients including vitamin D. The formulation of post–discharge preterm infant formulas can achieve greater growth in terms of weight and length for infants on these formulas for up to 9 months, when compared to preterm infants fed standard formulas.[1,10,11]

Highly Specialized Infant Formulas

Carbohydrate-free infant formulas, which contain either soy or hydrolyzed protein, are available for use by infants with carbohydrate malabsorption. A specific carbohydrate source that is typically glucose or fructose is then added to these formulas to make them complete for consumption. The carbohydrate additive is often begun at a 2–3% weight/volume and increased to the desired caloric concentration.[1]

Nutrient-altered formulas are specifically constructed for the use in highly specialized circumstances. For infants with impaired renal function, a formula may contain lower levels of calcium, phosphorus, iron and potassium than standard formulations, thus adjusting for their reduced needs. Additional formulas may be vitamin D-free for the treatment of infant with hypercalcemia, or formulas with a lower calcium to phosphorus ratio in the treatment of infants with serum calcium disorders.

Prethickened formulas are utilized in the treatment of infants with gastroesophageal reflux. Though available commercially, these formulas may be no more effective than standard formulas with added thickeners of corn starch or rice cereal. They may, however, flow more freely through standard nipples and do not displace nutritional additives .[1,12]

Follow-up infant formulas constructed for utilization by infants 9–24 months of age are specifically made with higher formulations of calcium and phosphorous in amounts 2–3 times that of standard formulas. Increased composition of iron, vitamin E and C and protein are often offered in these formulations.[1] A scientific basis for their utilization has yet to be offered to offset their cost.

PEDIATRIC FORMULAS

In general, pediatric formulas differ from infant formulas by their caloric density and carbohydrate construct. In contrast to the noted calorie-dense infant products, most pediatric formulas are 30 kcal per ounce and roughly 85% water. All pediatric formulas are lactose-free and are appropriate for oral or enteral usage. As described by Joeckel and Phillips, pediatric formulas can be categorized into three groups: polymeric, semi-elemental, and elemental.[1]

These products are devised for usage in children younger than 13 yrs of age. The treatment of older children will often require the usage of adult-type products for more appropriate caloric composition and vitamin and mineral recommended dietary allowances, which often have lower content of calcium, phosphorous and vitamin D.

For children who receive these products enterally as their complete source of nutrition, ongoing monitoring of the feeding regimen is essential in order to optimize nutrient and caloric intake and prevent conditions of osteopenia from inappropriate calcium, phosphorus and vitamin D consumption.

Polymeric Formulas

Polymeric formulas require that the digestive tract is functioning normally. The composition of macronutritients within these polymeric formulas is nearly standardized in providing about 44–53% carbohydrate, 35–45% fat, and 12–15% protein. Each preparation will meet or exceed the recommended dietary allowance for vitamin and mineral content for children.[1]

Fiber-enriched products contain fiber in a range of 5–8 g/L and often have added fructo-oligosaccharides. They are often utilized in children in an attempt to regulate bowel function in addressing diarrhea or constipation. Secondary benefits may include their positive effects on gut-associated lymphoid tissue responses through the production of short-chain fatty acids and in the enhancementof lactic bacteria growth such as lactobacilli.[13]

Semi-Elemental Formulas

These products contain proteins that is similar to infant hydrolyzed-protein products as the protein source is peptides and free amino acids. The intention for the usage of such products is in the treatment of gastrointestinal pathologic conditions that hinder normal bowel function. Macronutrient composition is otherwise similar to that noted in polymeric formulas and a variation in caloric density up to 1.5 kcal/mL is also available.

Elemental Formulas

Elemental formulas have their protein constitution as free amino acids. They are often utilized for children with compromised gastrointestinal tracts, such as in intestinal failure, or in the presence of multiple food-protein allergies. Given the utilization of free amino acids, the osmotic load is often greater in these formulas and approach 600 mOsm/kg water.[1]

PRETERM INFANT NUTRITION CONSIDERATIONS

Enteral nutrition is the preferred method of nutritional support once a baby is stable enough to tolerate feedings. Aspects of feeding infants with prematurity (<38 wks gestation) are confounded by the comorbidities of respiratory insufficiency, higher caloric requirements, and underlying neuromuscular immaturity. Thus, additional vigilance is required in the successful administration of enteral nutrition to the premature infant.[14]

Nutrition should be considered for all infants who maintain clinical stability, including premature infants. As soon as clinically possible, minimal enteral nutrition (MEN) in the form of trophic feedings can be ideally started within the first week of life and continued for 3–5 days or up to 7 days in the extremely low birth weight infant, less than 1000 g. MEN administration tries to achieve low-volume feedings of approximately 10–20 mL/kg/day, administered as either full strength expressed breast milk or as half- or full-strength preterm formula.[14–17]

Once tolerance of basic trophic feedings is shown, enteral feedings are often advanced in administration by 20–35 mL/kg/day up to goals of 150–180 mL/kg/day.[14] This early initiation of enteral feedings is felt to improve intestinal motility and intestinal tolerance, stimulate enterohormone production, and decrease problems associated with parenteral nutrition.

As feedings are advanced, enteral tolerance must be continually assessed. Monitoring of gastric residuals may be the first sign of intolerance to feedings. Concern arises when gastric residuals surpass 20–40% of the previous feeding volume, or if the child has signs of abdominal distension, bloody stool production, or clinical instability. Relative intolerance to feedings may be addressed by a 20% reduction in feeding volumes or increased time intervals between feedings. Utility of glycerin suppositories can be considered for rectal stimulation in order to stimulate gastrointestinal motility.[18]

The use of human milk surpasses the benefits of any other synthetic formula available. However, the quantity of protein and minerals is inadequate for the premature infant. In order to increase the nutrient density of human milk, human milk fortifiers (HMF) are recommended additions to expressed human milk at 1 packet per 25 mL. This may be initiated at a one-half strength formulation of 1 packet to 50 mL of human milk until initial tolerance is proven.[14] HMF is recommended for infants less than 1500 g at birth or less than 34weaks gestation, or in select infants greater than 1500 g at birth with prior use of parenteral nutrition greater than 2 wks, or with limited enteral tolerance to goal feeding volumes.[19] HMF is continued throughout the NICU hospitalization and often continued until infants reach a weight of 3–3.5 kg.[10]

Preterm infants have additional considerations for the supplementation of vitamins and minerals. In preterm infants on enteral nutrition of less than goal volumes or if on unfortified human milk or non-preterm formulas, inadequate intake of micronutrients including iron is likely. Considerations should then be made for the administration of multivitamin supplements that include vitamins A, D, and C and iron.

As most preterm infants have some degree of neuromuscular immaturity, oral feedings are not likely for early enteral nutrition. Nasogastric and orogastric tubes are the most common route for feedings. With eventual growth, the premature infant should eventually be transitioned to oral feedings at the earliest time possible so as to minimize the development of oral aversion during the neonatal period of care. Relative guidelines for the determination of the readiness of oral feedings include achieving 32–34 wks post-gestational age, appropriate signs of oral–motor development through speech therapy or nursing assessment, limited requirements for supplemental oxygen and respiratory rates less than 50 breaths per min without signs of increased work of breathing, and appropriate evidence of rooting and non-nutritive sucking.[14] With these relative considerations, continued trials of oral feedings during a regimen of full enteral feedings will allow for gradual transition to complete oral feeding.

REFERENCES

1. Joeckel RJ, Phillips SK. (2009) Overview of infant and pediatric formula. *Nutr Clin Pract* **24**:356–362.
2. Product Information, Mead Johnson Nutritionals, Mead Johnson and Company, Evansville, IN. http://www.mjn.com.

3. Product Information, Ross Products Division, Abbott Laboratories, Inc., Columbus, OH.
4. Product Information, Nestle Nutrition, Societe des Produits Nestle S.A., Vevey, Switzerland.
5. Product Information, Nutricia North America, Rockville, MD. http://www.shsna.com/pages/neocate_inf_formula.htm.
6. Producti Information, Gerber Division of Nestle Nutrition, Societe des Produits Nestle S.A., Vevey, Switzerland, http://www.gerber.com/allstages/products.aspx.
7. Bhatia J, Greer F. (2008) American academy of pediatrics committee on nutrition. Use of soy protein-based formulas in infant feeding. *Pediatrics* **121**:1062–1068.
8. Callenbach JC, Sheehan MB, Abramson SJ, *et al.* (1981) Etiologic factors in rickets of very low-birth-weight infants. *J Pediatr* **98**:800–805.
9. Strom BL, Schinnar R, Ziegler EE, *et al.* (2001) Exposure to soy-based formula in infancy and endocrinological and reproductive outcomes in young adulthood. *JAMA* **286**:807–814.
10. Picaud JC, Decullier E, Plan O, *et al.* (2008) Growth and bone mineralization in preterm infants fed preterm formula or standard term formula after discharge. *J Pediatr* **153**:616–621.
11. Lucas A, Fewtrell MS, Morley R, *et al.* (2001) Randomized trial of nutrient-enriched formula versus standard formula for postdischarge preterm infants. *Pediatrics* **108**:703–711.
12. Penna FJ, Norton RC, Carvalha AS, *et al.* (2003) Comparison between prethickened and home-thickened formulas in gastroesophageal reflux treatment. *J Pediatr* **79**:49–54.
13. Institute of Medicine. (1997) *Dietary Reference Intakes for Calcium, Phosphorous, Magnesium, Vitamin D and Fluoride.* National Academy Press, Washington DC.
14. Groh-Wargo S, Sapsford A. (2009) Enteral nutrition support of the preterm infant in the neonatal intensive care unit. *Nutr Clin Pract* **24**(3):363–376.
15. Meetze WH, Valentine C, McGuigan JE, *et al.* (1992) gastrointestinal priming prior to full enteral nutrition in very low birth weight infants. *J Pediatr Gastroenterol Nutr* **15**:163–170.
16. Kennedy KA, Tyson JE. (2005) Trophic feedings for parenterally fed infants. *Cochrane Database Syst Rev* **3**:CD000504.
17. Berseth CL, Bisquera JA, Paje VU. (2003) Prolonging small feeding volumes early in life decreases the incidence of necrotizing enterocolitis in very low birth weight infants. *Pediatrics* **11**:529–534.

18. Mihatsch W, von Schoenaich P, Fahnenstich H, *et al.* (2002) The significance of gastric residuals in the early enteral feeding advancement of ELBW infants. *Pediatrics* **109**:457–459.
19. Sapsford AL. (2000) Human milk and enteral nutrition products. In: S Groh-Wargo, M Thompson, JH Cox (eds.), *Nutritional Care for High-Risk Newborns,* 3rd edition, pp. 265–302. Precept Press, Chicago, IL.

PEDIATRIC ANESTHESIA GUIDELINES

7

Doris Hardacker

INTRODUCTION

Advances in pediatric anesthesia have provided for safer anesthesia in all age groups. The incidence of anesthesia-related cardiac arrest is 1.4 in 10,000 anesthetics with a mortality of 26%. Children less than 1 yr of age and those with underlying systemic diseases (ASA PS 3-5, Table 1) have the highest incidence of perioperative cardiac arrest. Causes of cardiac arrest include cardiovascular (41%), respiratory (27%), medication related (18%), and equipment related (5%).[1,2,3] This chapter serves as a guide to assist the surgeon with preoperative patient preparation and provide an understanding of the implications of modern pediatric anesthesia.

NPO GUIDELINES

Pulmonary aspiration of acidic gastric contents can result in a severe chemical pneumonitis requiring mechanical ventilation and intensive postoperative care. Fasting reduces the likelihood of residual gastric contents. The type and amount of oral intake must be considered when determining an appropriate period of preoperative fasting.

Current fasting recommendations for pediatric patient undergoing elective surgical procedures are listed in Table 2. Examples of clear liquids are water, apple juice, carbonated beverages, clear tea, and black coffee.

Table 1. ASA PS classifications from the American Society of Anesthesiologists.

1 Normal healthy patient	No organic, physiologic, or psychiatric disturbance; excludes the very young and very old; healthy with good exercise tolerance
2 Mild systemic disease	No functional limitations; has a well-controlled disease of one body system; controlled hypertension or diabetes without systemic effects, cigarette smoking without chronic obstructive pulmonary disease (COPD); mild obesity, pregnancy
3 Severe systemic disease	Some functional limitation; has a controlled disease of more than one body system or one major system; no immediate danger of death; controlled congestive heart failure (CHF), stable angina, old heart attack, poorly controlled hypertension, morbid obesity, chronic renal failure; bronchospastic disease with intermittent symptoms
4 Severe systemic disease that is a constant threat to life	Has at least one severe disease that is poorly controlled or at end stage; possible risk of death; unstable angina, symptomatic COPD, symptomatic CHF, hepatorenal failure
5 Moribund, not expected to survive without the operation	Not expected to survive >24 hours with or without surgery; imminent risk of death; multiorgan failure, sepsis syndrome with hemodynamic instability, hypothermia, poorly controlled coagulopathy
6 A declared brain-dead patient who organs are being removed for donor purposes	

Table 2. NPO guidelines.

Clear liquids	2 hours
Breast milk	4 hours
Infant formula	6 hours
Non-human milks	6 hours
Light Meal	6 hours
Heavy Meal	8 hours

A light meal consists of dry toast and clear liquids. Routine preoperative administration of medications that block gastric acid secretion in patients who do not have an increased risk for pulmonary aspiration is not routinely recommended.[4]

PREOPERATIVE EVALUATION

Preoperative evaluation of pediatric patients includes a thorough history and physical examination focused on the cardiorespiratory and neurologic systems. Laboratory and radiologic testing may be appropriate in selected patients.

History

The preoperative history should elicit information concerning birth history, gestational age, allergies, current medications, coexisting diseases, previous anesthetics, and family history of anesthetic complications.

Laboratory Testing

Routine preoperative blood testing is of limited value in children undergoing minor surgical procedures and a careful history and physical examination are of greater importance.[5] Most anesthesiologists will accept a hematocrit level in the mid-20s provided there are no other systemic problems. The most common indication to obtain a preoperative hemoglobin and hematocrit is for assessment of allowed blood loss during surgery.[6] Pregnancy screening of menarchal adolescent females is routinely performed in many institutions. The incidence of a positive pregnancy test is 0.5–1.2%.[7]

SPECIAL CONSIDERATIONS

Upper Respiratory Tract Infections

Children with upper respiratory tract infections (URIs) within 4 wks of surgery have a 7–11-times increased risk for perioperative respiratory complications. These complications include oxygen desaturation, laryngospasm, bronchospasm, postintubation croup, airway obstruction, and cough.[8] Patients with reactive airway disease, a history of prematurity, exposure to secondary smoke, nasal congestion, and copious airway secretions are especially likely to have perioperative respiratory complications. Elective surgery in patients with a fever >38.5°C, purulent rhinitis, a productive cough, and rhonchi should be postponed. Most anesthetics, however, can proceed in the presence of clear rhinorrhea and a nonproductive cough.[9]

Reactive Airway Disease

The incidence of reactive airway disease in the pediatric population may be as high as 30%. Prior to elective surgery, the reactive airway disease should be as controlled as possible. Bronchodilators should be administered preoperatively. Hydrocortisone (1 mg/kg IV) should be administered at the time of induction if the child has received corticosteroids in the previous 4–6 months.

Prematurity

Term infants (>37 wks and <44 wks gestation) are at risk for postoperative apnea and should be monitored in the hospital overnight. Preterm infants (<37 wks gestation and <55 wks postconceptual age) should also be monitored overnight.

Congenital Cardiac Disease

The overall incidence of congenital cardiac disease is 0.8%. A cardiology evaluation with a description of the lesion and previous corrective or palliative procedures and interpretation of a recent echocardiogram provide valuable information for planning the anesthetic. A quantitative assessment of left ventricular function is especially helpful. Recommendations for subacute bacterial endocarditis (SBE) prophylaxis have recently changed and only include cardiac conditions associated with the highest risk of adverse outcomes from endocarditis receive prophylaxis (Table 3).[10]

Diabetes Mellitus

Patients with diabetes should ideally be scheduled for surgery as the first case of the day as these patients tolerate fasting and dehydration poorly. Insulin can be administered as an intravenous infusion with glucose or can

Table 3. SBE prophylaxis.

Prosthetic cardiac valve or prosthetic material used for cardiac valve repair
Previous infective endocarditis
Unrepaired cyanotic CHD, including palliative shunts and conduits
Completely repaired congenital heart defect with prosthetic material or device, whether placed by surgery or by catheter intervention, during the first 6 months after the procedure
Repaired CHD with residual defects at the site or adjacent to the site of a prosthetic patch or prosthetic device (which inhibit endothelialization)
Cardiac transplantation recipients who develop cardiac valvulopathy

be administered subcutaneously in the patient's normal manner (one-half the usual morning dose). Blood glucose levels should be measured every 1–2 hrs during the perioperative period. Ideally, blood glucose levels should be maintained at 90–150 mg/dL.[11] This can be challenging if preoperative control is poor.

Neuromuscular Diseases

Children with muscular dystrophy (e.g. Duchenne's, Becker's) often have cardiac and pulmonary dysfunction and may require a preoperative echocardiogram and pulmonary function testing. Halogenated, inhaled anesthetics may trigger rhabdomyolysis that resembles malignant hyperthermia.[12]

Malignant Hyperthermia

Malignant hyperthermia (MH) is a life-threatening genetic disorder triggered by volatile anesthetics and succinylcholine. MH is characterized by extreme hypermetabolism, hyperthermia, muscle rigidity, hypercapnia, tachycardia, acidosis, and rhabdomyolysis. Treatment is directed at control of the hypermetabolism with dantrolene (Table 4).[13]

Cancer

Chemotherapeutic agents, particularly the anthracyclines, are cardiotoxic and can cause restrictive cardiomyopathy 1–6 yrs after treatment.

Table 4. Treatment of malignant hyperthermia.

Discontinuation of all triggering agents
Dantrolene 2.5 mg/kg, repeat up to 30 mg/kg
Bicarbonate 1–2 meq/kg
Insulin 0.1 units insulin/kg and 1 ml/kg 50% glucose
Calcium chloride 10 mg/kg
Lidocaine or other antiarrhythmics as indicated
Cooling to 38 degrees

An echocardiogram and exercise tolerance testing can provide information that will influence the conduct of anesthesia.[14]

Sickle Cell Disease

The goal of perioperative management of the patient with sickle cell disease is avoidance of factors that promote sickling (hypoxemia, hypothermia, dehydration, and acidosis). Preoperative laboratory testing should include a CBC, reticulocyte count, creatinine, urinalysis, and chest radiograph. Although traditional management for major surgery included red blood cell exchange transfusion to reduce the relative amount of hemoglobin S to 30%, more recent guidelines suggest a simple RBC transfusion to achieve a hemoglobin level of 10 g/dL.[15,16] Twenty-two percent of patients with sickle cell disease undergoing elective surgery experience perioperative complications such as acute chest syndrome, pain episodes, hemolytic crisis, aplastic crisis, delayed transfusion reactions, and infection.[17]

PREMEDICATION

The primary purpose of premedication of children prior to surgery is anxiolysis. Toddler aged children are especially apprehensive about parental separation. Although any sedative may provide anxiolysis, the most frequently used drugs are benzodiazepines, opioids, and ketamine (Table 5). The oral route is preferred to intramuscular or rectal routes of administration. If it is anticipated that an intravenous line is required for induction of anesthesia, EMLA cream can be applied to the anticipated insertion site in the pre-anesthetic holding area.

Table 5. Premedication.

Midazolam	0.5–0.75 mg/kg p.o./p.r . 20–30 min prior to induction max 20 mg 0.2–0.3 mg/kg intranasally
Diazepam	0.1 mg/kg p.o. 20–30 min prior to induction
Fentanyl	15–20 mcg/kg
Ketamine	3–6 mg/kg po
EMLA cream	applied topically for I.V. start

Table 6. Stages of anesthesia.

Induction phase	Analgesia, dizziness
Excitement/delirium phase	Amnesia, involuntary muscular activity, potential for vomiting, laryngospasm
Surgical anesthesia	Motionlessness, divided into 4 planes depending on paralysis of respiratory muscles
Overdose/impending death	Weakening of autonomic response

INTRAOPERATIVE MANAGEMENT

The classic four stages of anesthesia that were developed for diethyl ether are not as clearly defined for modern inhaled and intravenous anesthetics (Table 6). During the seconds stage of anesthesia (excitement/delirium) patients may respond to a noxious stimulus with laryngospasm and/or emesis. Patients should not be disturbed (e.g. joints manipulated, abdomen palpated) during the second stage of anesthesia.

Monitoring

American Society of Anesthesiologist standards for monitoring include continuous display of the electrocardiogram, pulse oximetry, and capnography. Core temperature (nasal, esophageal, rectal) is monitored frequently in children. A processed EEG and cerebral oximeter may be used in selected cases.

Induction

Induction of anesthesia for elective surgical procedures is performed by the inhalation or intravenous route. However, an inhalation induction is

Table 7. Induction agents.

Thiopental	4–7 mg/kg
Propofol	2–3 mg/kg
Ketamine	1–3 mg/kg
Etomidate	0.2–0.3 mg/kg

preferred by most children. The most popular inhaled anesthetic for induction is sevoflurane as it is well tolerated with respect to cardiorespiratory function. Isoflurane and desflurane may be used for maintenance of anesthesia, but are not well suited for induction. Parenteral drugs suitable for intravenous induction include thiopental, propofol, ketamine, and etomidate (Table 7). Propofol can cause severe pain upon injection when injected rapidly through small catheters into peripheral veins. Injection pain can be attenuated by the prior administration of lidocaine. If inhaled anesthetics are contraindicated for maintenance of anesthesia, total intravenous anesthesia (TIVA) can be administered. Two types of drugs are required for TIVA: a hypnotic/sedative and an analgesic. Propofol is the most popular sedative used for TIVA. Analgesics for TIVA include remifentanil, fentanyl, and sufentanil. Ketamine has both sedative and analgesic properties.

Muscle Relaxants

Muscle relaxants (neuromuscular blocking agents) can provide excellent relaxation for the surgeon without having to administer large doses of intravenous or inhaled anesthetics. There are two categories of muscle relaxants: depolarizing and non-depolarizing. The only depolarizing muscle relaxant currently in clinical use is succinylcholine. Non-depolarizing muscle relaxants include cis-atracurium, rocuronium, vecuronium, and pancuronium.

Intraoperative Fluid Management

Fluid management can be complicated if patients have underlying fluid and electrolyte deficits and individualization of a fluid management strategy may be required in patients with complex problems. Most pediatric patients, however, can be managed with a standardized approach that provides maintenance and replacement fluids. Lactated Ringers' solution or plasmalyte A are the most suitable intravenous fluids for intraoperative administration. Colloids such as albumin, synthetic starches, or gelatins may be required, but their use is controversial.[18]

RECOVERY ROOM ISSUES

The recovery from an anesthetic is a critical period during which complications can arise. Nausea and vomiting occurs in up to 50% of pediatric patients and its incidence is related to the type of procedure and anesthetic technique. Treatment includes administration of a serotonin 5-HT3 receptor antagonist (ondansetron 0.01 mg/kg) and/or decadron (0.05–0.5 mg/kg). Respiratory events can be secondary to airway obstruction (croup, laryngospasm), hypoxemia (atelectasis, pulmonary edema) and hypercarbia. Additional complications include hypotension, arrhythmias, hypothermia, shivering, residual neuromuscular blockade and pain management.

REFERENCES

1. Morray JP, Geiduschek JM, Ramamoorthy C, Haberkern CM, Hackel A, Caplan RA, Domino KB, Posner K, Cheney FW. (2000) Anesthesia-related cardiac arrest in children: Initial findings of the Pediatric Perioperative Cardiac Arrest (POCA) Registry. *Anesthesiology* **93**(1):6–14.
2. Morray JP, Bhananker SM, (2005) Recent findings from the Pediatric Perioperative Cardiac Arrest (POCA) registry. *ASA Newsletter* **69**(6):10–12.
3. Bhananker SM, Ramamoorthy C, Geiduschek JM, *et al.* (2007) Anesthesia-related cardiac arrest in children: Update from the Pediatric Perioperative Cardiac Arrest Registry. *Anesthesia and Analgesia* **105**: 344–350.
4. Practice Guidelines for Preoperative Fasting and the Use of Pharmacologic Agents to Reduce the Risk of Pulmonary Aspiration: Application to Healthy Patients Undergoing Elective Procedures. (1999) A Report by the American Society of Anesthesiologists Task Force on Preoperative Fasting. *Anesthesiology* **90**: 896–905.
5. Ansermino M, Than M, Swallow D. (1999) Pre-operative blood tests in children undergoing plastic surgery. *J. St Andrew's Ann R Coll Surg England* **81**: 175–178.
6. Patel RI, Hannallah RS. (2000) Laboratory tests in children undergoing ambulatory surgery: A review of clinical practice and scientific studies. *Ambul Surg* **8**: 165–169.

7. Pierre N, Moy LK, Redd S, Emans SJ, Laufer MR. (1988) Evaluation of a pregnancy-testing protocol in adolescents undergoing surgery. *J Pediatr Adolesc Gynecol* **11**(3):139–141.
8. Tait AR, Malviya S, Voepel-Lewis T, *et al.* (2001) Risk factors for perioperative adverse respiratory events in children with upper respiratory tract infections. *Anesthesiology* **95**:299–306.
9. O'Flaherty JE, Yemen TA. (2002) The child with respiratory problems. *Pediatric Anesthesia Handbook.* pp 80–106. McGraw-Hill Companies.
10. Prevention of infective endocarditis. (2007) Guidelines from the American Heart Association. *Circulation* **116**: 1736–1754.
11. Rhodes ET, Ferrari LR, Wolfsdorf JI. (2005) Perioperative management of pediatric surgical patients with diabetes mellitus. *Anesth Analg* **101**: 986–99.
12. Hayes J, Veyckemans F, Bissonnette B. (2008) Duchenne muscular dystrophy: An old anesthesia problem revisited. *Paediatr Anaesth* **18**(2):100–6.
13. Malignant hyperthermia. *Association of the United States.* www.mhaus.org.
14. Kremer L, Caron H. (2004) Anthracycline Cardiotoxicity in Children. *N Engl J Med* 351: 120.
15. Haxby E, Flynn F, Bateman C. (2007) Anaesthesia for patients with sickle cell disease or other haemoglobinopathies. *Anaesthesia & Intensive Care Medicine* **8**:217–219.
16. National Institutes of Health, National Heart, Lung, and Blood Institute, Division of Blood Diseases and Resources. (2002) *The Management of Sickle Cell Disease, 4th edition* Available at: http://www.nhlbi.nih.gov/health/prof/blood/sickle/sc_mngt.pdf
17. Firth PG, Head CA. (2004) Sickle cell disease and anesthesia. *Anesthesiology* **101**: 766–85.
18. Bailey A, McNaull P. Jooste E, Tuchman, JB. (2010) Perioperative crystalloid and colloid fluid management in children: where are we and how did we get here? *Anesthesia and Analgesia* February **110**: 375–390.
19. Gwirtz, K. (1996) Management of Recovery Room Issues. *Anesthesiology Clinics of North America* **14**(2):307–339.

PEDIATRIC AIRWAY MANAGEMENT 8

Katherine M. DeMasie

INTRODUCTION

"Kids are just small adults." This old adage could not be further from the truth when it comes to the pediatric airway. Multiple anatomical and physiological differences exist between the pediatric and adult airways. Knowledge of these differences is critical to the proper management of the pediatric patient. There are many airway maneuvers and adjuncts available to assist the pediatric patient in respiratory distress. An awareness of the equipment needed, an ability to use the equipment appropriately, and an appreciation of one's own limitations are all keys to successful pediatric airway management.

ANATOMY AND PHYSIOLOGY

Anatomical differences between pediatric and adult airways are considerable and are more pronounced the younger the age of the child. A child's airway matures into its adult form by 8 yrs of age. Younger children have a relatively large occiput that leads to more flexion of the neck in the supine position. Their tongues are also proportionally larger. The trachea is more flexible and compressible. Also, adenotonsillar hypertrophy is common in children. All of these differences may promote airway obstruction in the younger child.[1]

Tracheal intubation of the young child is also influenced by pediatric anatomy. The large occiput may make optimal positioning difficult and the large tongue may make direct laryngoscopy more tedious. The larynx is positioned higher (C 3–4 level vs. C 4–5 in adult) and the glottic opening is rotated anteriorly in the pediatric patient. The epiglottis is narrow and acutely angled away from the trachea, making it harder to displace with a laryngoscope blade. The vocal cords are attached at an angle to the trachea in children (vs. perpendicular in adults), which may make it more difficult to pass the tracheal tube. Furthermore, the narrowest diameter of the pediatric airway is at the level of the cricoid ring, compared to the vocal cords of an adult. This means even a tracheal tube that may pass through the child's vocal cords may be too large for the subglottic area (Figure 1).[1,2]

Physiological differences in the pediatric patient make the child more prone to rapid oxygen desaturation when compared to the adult patient. The high metabolic rate of infants dictates a higher minute oxygen consumption of 7 mL/kg/min, vs. 3 mL/kg/min in an adult.[3] Minute ventilation is equal to the product of respiratory rate and tidal volume. Infants have

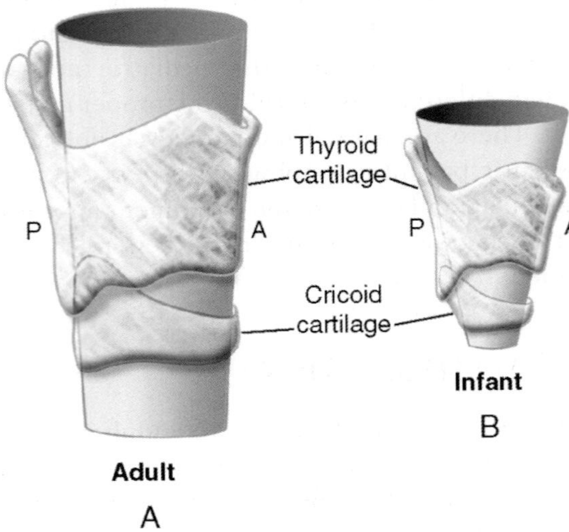

Figure 1. Adult airway vs. pediatric airway. Note the funnel-shaped pediatric airway is narrowest at the level of the cricoids cartilage.[2] (Reprinted from Cote CJ, Lerman J, Todres ID. (2009) The pediatric airway. *A Practice of Anesthesia for Infants and Children*, pp. 237–278. Saunders Elsevier, Philadelphia, with permission from Elsevier.)

a relatively fixed tidal volume and thus can only increase minute ventilation by increasing respiratory rate. Due to an excessively compliant chest wall, the infant has a decreased functional residual capacity, especially in states of decreased muscle tone such as sedation or deep sleep. Thus, the infant has much less oxygen available for gas exchange during the apneic state and arterial oxygen saturation decreases rapidly after ventilation ceases.[1]

In addition to desaturation, anatomical and physiological differences also predispose the pediatric patient to respiratory failure. Type I muscle fibers are more resistant to fatigue. The diaphragm and intercostals muscles of infants have a lower percentage of type I muscle fibers. Glycogen stores in respiratory muscles are also less abundant in infants.[1] Infants have a higher respiratory rate at baseline. It is less efficient for the infant to increase tidal volume, and any increase in minute ventilation is done by increasing the respiratory rate.[3] One must also remember that the pediatric patient has a relatively narrow airway. Poiseuille's law of resistance states that resistance is inversely proportional to the radius ($R \propto 1/r^4$). Thus, small decreases in the radius of a child's airway can lead to large increases in airway resistance.[1] All of these factors predispose the pediatric patient to respiratory failure.

POSITIONING AND AIRWAY-CLEARING MANEUVERS

When respiratory distress has been identified in the pediatric patient, multiple steps should be taken to remedy the situation, ranging from noninvasive measures, such as positioning the patient, to invasive procedures, such as tracheal intubation. Supplemental oxygen should be provided to the child in distress and can be delivered in a variety of ways, including nasal cannula, face mask, or oxygen hut.[1]

Patient positioning is crucial to managing the pediatric airway and may be all that is needed to relieve airway obstruction. The lateral position may be beneficial for the sedated patient or the patient with adenotonsillar hypertrophy and obstructive sleep apnea as it increases the patency of the upper airway by decreasing the gravitational effects on the pharyngeal soft tissues.[4] Recall that younger children have a large occiput. To rectify this natural predisposition to neck flexion and airway obstruction, a shoulder roll should be placed under the patient that allows for neck extension (Figure 2).[1]

If the patient is still experiencing airway obstruction after proper positioning, an airway-clearing maneuver, such as chin lift or jaw thrust, may be beneficial. Chin lift is performed by lifting the inferior border of

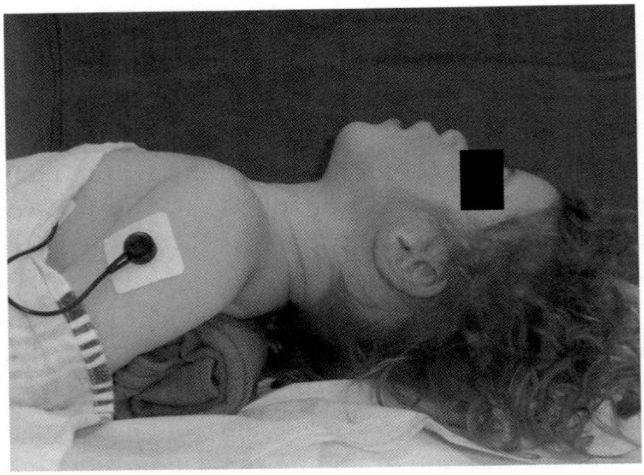

Figure 2. Shoulder roll placement allowing for neck extension.

the mental protuberance. The upper and lower teeth should be in close contact and the jaw should not protrude. This maneuver widens the diameter of the pharyngeal airway. Chin lift may, however, worsen obstruction in the patient with adenotonsillar hypertrophy. Jaw thrust may be preferred for patients with adenotonsillar hypertrophy and is performed by lifting the jaw upward and anterior at the mandibular angles. This action will open the mouth and lift the epiglottis off the posterior pharyngeal wall, thus widening the glottic opening and relieving obstruction.[4] Since jaw thrust can be performed in the head neutral position, it may be preferred if there is suspicion of a cervical spine injury to the patient. However, jaw thrust may completely occlude the airway in patients with cervical masses as the tissues are displaced medially.[5]

PHARYNGEAL AIRWAYS

If ventilation is still difficult following proper positioning and airway-clearing maneuvers, an airway adjunct may be necessary. Placement of a pharyngeal airway (oral or nasal) may be required. The oral airway is best reserved for patients who are sedated/comatose to the point that their gag reflex is lost. Nasal airway should be avoided in patients with a suspected basilar skull fracture, a cerebrospinal fluid leak, or coagulopathy.[1] To determine the appropriate-sized oral airway, place the oral airway on the side of the patient's cheek, with the opening of the oral airway at the patient's lips.

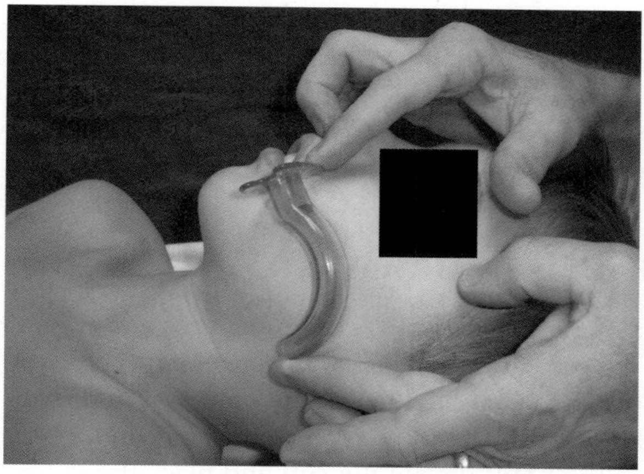

Figure 3. Choosing an appropriate-sized oral airway.

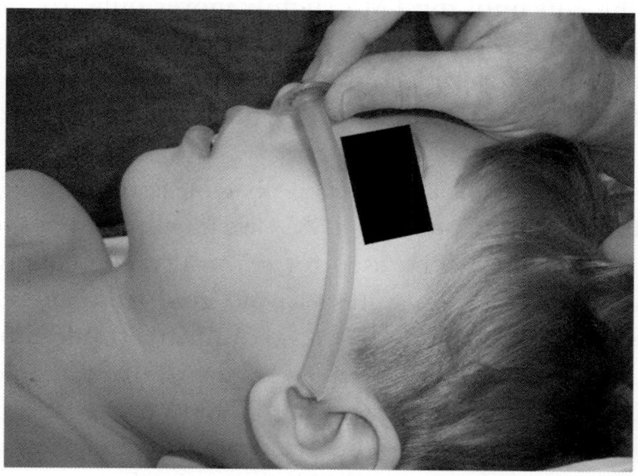

Figure 4. Choosing an appropriate-sized nasal airway.

The tip of a proper-sized airway should lie at the angle of the mandible (Figure 3). For a nasal airway, similarly place the airway starting at the nostril. The tip should extend to the tragus of the ear (Figure 4). An appropriate-sized pharyngeal airway is important. Too small an airway can cause the tongue to push back and worsen obstruction. Too large an airway can force the epiglottis down, thereby obstructing the glottic opening.[3] To insert the oral airway, first place the airway in the mouth "upside down," or such that the distal opening is facing up toward the nose. Once inside the mouth, rotate the airway 180° so that the airway falls back behind the tongue. Prior to insertion of a nasal airway, the trumpet should be well lubricated. Point the bevel away from the septum and slowly insert the nasal airway to avoid trauma to hypertrophied tonsils and adenoids.[1]

LARYNGEAL MASK AIRWAYS

The laryngeal mask airway (LMA) is a supraglottic airway that was invented in 1982 and has revolutionized airway management. The LMA bypasses the tongue and rests just above the glottic opening. It is important to note that the LMA does not provide for a protected airway and aspiration is still a risk.[6] To place the LMA, deflate the cuff and place the index finger at the base of the cuff and the shaft. Glide the LMA along the hard palate around the back of the tongue until the LMA seats at the upper esophageal sphincter.[3] Inflate the cuff until the LMA slightly moves outward and check for adequate ventilation. Disposable LMAs have a weight-based sizing criteria that is printed on the package and on the LMA. There is also a guideline printed on the LMAs for how much air to inflate for a proper seal, although one rarely needs the full amount listed.

Initially regarded as an alternative to bag-mask ventilation, LMAs have become useful in multiple settings. LMAs are ideally used in spontaneously ventilating patients but can be used for controlled ventilation. Care must be taken to ventilate at low pressures to avoid insufflating the stomach. The LMA has become a valuable tool to assist with fiberoptic intubation and diagnostic bronchoscopy. The American Society of Anesthesiologists (ASA) difficult airway algorithm indicates when the LMA may be useful. The LMA is especially recommended in the "cannot ventilate, cannot intubate" scenario prior to cricothyrotomy. LMAs have also been used in the early neonatal resuscitative period where time is essential. An effective airway can quickly be obtained with an LMA while preparing for tracheal intubation.[6]

TRACHEAL INTUBATION

Tracheal intubation may be required and multiple steps must be taken to ensure a smooth and safe transition to securing the airway. Preoxygenation is important to maintain the patient's oxygen saturation during the apneic period of direct laryngoscopy and tracheal tube placement. Proper patient positioning in the sniffing position, which involves elevating the head and extending the head at the atlanto–occipital joint, is key for visualization of the glottic opening. Laryngoscope blades come in two varieties: Straight (Miller or Wis-Hipple) and curved (Macintosh). Straight blades are designed to physically lift the epiglottis to visualize the vocal cords while the curved blades are designed to indirectly lift the epiglottis. The straight blades are generally preferred for children toddler-aged and younger due to their larger, floppier epiglottis (Table 1).[1]

The decision to place a cuffed vs. an uncuffed tracheal tube in the pediatric patient has been a controversial subject for decades.[3] Cuffed tubes in children younger than 8 yrs were feared to increase the risk of damage to the trachea due to ischemia caused by high pressures of the cuff at the cricoid ring. Cuffed tubes have the advantage of more protection from aspiration and allowing more controlled ventilation at higher pressures.[1] Gentle laryngoscopy and the use of better low-pressure cuffed tracheal tubes reduce the likelihood of airway damage. A leak test should be performed after tracheal intubation. If there is a leak around the tracheal tube at 20 cm H_2O, the cuff should be filled with air until the leak just disappears. If there is a leak present between 20 and 30 cm H_2O, no air needs to be placed. If no leak is present at 30 cm H_2O, the tracheal tube should be replaced by a smaller cuffed tube, or an uncuffed tube. It is very important not to overinflate the cuff of a cuffed endotracheal tube. Risk of tracheal ischemia or postextubation stridor is real but can be minimized by following the above guidelines. Capillary pressure in the trachea is approximately 40 cm H_2O, so the goal is to place an endotracheal tube that would not exert a pressure that would compromise this blood flow. In general, the formula for selecting proper tube size, based on internal diameter in millimeters, is (age in years/4) + 4. If using a cuffed tracheal tube, decrease the size by 0.5, i.e. (age in years/4) + 3.5 (Table 2).

Table 1. Guide to selecting laryngoscope blade size.

Age	Blade size
<45 wks postconceptual age	Miller 0
>45 wks postconceptual age–3 yrs	Miller 1, Wis-Hipple 1.5
3–9 yrs	Miller 2, Macintosh 2
>9 yrs	Miller 2, Macintosh 3

Table 2. Guide to selecting tracheal tube size and depth of tube placement.

Age/Weight	Tube Size (ID)	Depth (cm)
<1000 g	2.5 mm uncuffed	7
1000–2000 g	3.0 mm uncuffed	8
2000–3000 g	3.0 mm uncuffed vs. 3.0 mm cuffed	9
Term newborn–4 mths	3.0 mm cuffed	10
4–11 mths	3.5 mm cuffed	11
12 mths–2 yrs	4.0 mm cuffed	12
>2 yrs	Age(yrs)/4 + 3.5 mm cuffed	Age(yrs)/2 + 12

Note: ID = Internal Diameter.

Direct laryngoscopy requires proper technique to help ensure success. With the patient properly positioned, the mouth is opened either by pulling down the chin or using the scissor technique with the thumb and forefinger of the right hand. The laryngoscopist holds the laryngoscope in the left hand. The blade should be inserted into the mouth with the handle slightly angled to the right so that when the handle is brought back to midline, the tongue has been swept to the left by the blade. Once the epiglottis is visualized, it can be lifted directly if using a straight blade, or lifted indirectly by placing a curved blade in the vallecula (the space just above the epiglottis). The laryngoscope should be lifted upward and forward. The wrist should stay neutral throughout the procedure. Attempting to "crank" the wrist back to get a better view may actually worsen the view and damage the patient's teeth. After lifting the epiglottis, the vocal cords should be visualized and the tracheal tube passed between them. The laryngoscope should be carefully removed to avoid damage to the teeth. Always confirm tracheal placement by auscultation of bilateral breath sounds, chest rise, and CO_2 detection. One formula for appropriate depth of a tracheal tube at the lips is (age in years/2) + 12 cm (Table 2).

RAPID SEQUENCE INTUBATION

Pulmonary aspiration of gastric contents is an ever-present risk during tracheal intubation. The risk is further increased in the patient with a full stomach, which will often be the case for the child requiring urgent or

Table 3. Intravenous induction and paralytic agents for rapid sequence intubation (RSI).

Induction Agent*	Dosage (mg/kg)
Propofol	2–3
Thiopental	5
Etomidate	0.4
Ketamine	2
Paralytic Agent	**Dosage (mg/kg)**
Succinylcholine**	2 (4 mg/kg intramuscular)
Rocuronium	1

*Induction agents may not be necessary during RSI if the patient is already deeply sedated/comatose.

**Avoid succinylcholine in patients with a history of myopathy, extensive burns, hyperkalemia, or malignant hyperthermia.

emergent intubation. To decrease the risk of aspiration and increase the chances of successful intubation, rapid sequence intubation (RSI) can be performed. RSI involves the rapid administration of an induction agent and a neuromuscular blocking agent (Table 3). An induction or sedative drug may be omitted if the patient is comatose/unresponsive. Atropine (0.02 mg/kg IV) or glycopyrrolate (0.01 mg/kg IV) may be given as a pretreatment prior to RSI to prevent bradycardia that can be seen in pediatric patients either due to the neuromuscular blocker succinylcholine or to direct laryngoscopy itself. Application of cricoid pressure during induction and intubation may decrease the risk of passive regurgitation and aspiration.[7]

SPECIAL CONSIDERATIONS

Not all intubations are simple procedures. If vocal cords cannot be visualized, blind attempts at tracheal tube passage can cause unnecessary trauma, bleeding, and/or swelling that may decrease chances of success by a more skilled professional in airway management. Insertion of an LMA and waiting for appropriate help to secure the airway may save the patient's life.

There are special cases among pediatric patients that may make intubation extremely difficult. One should have an organized approach in mind when dealing with a difficult airway (Figure 5).[8] Obesity is an increasing

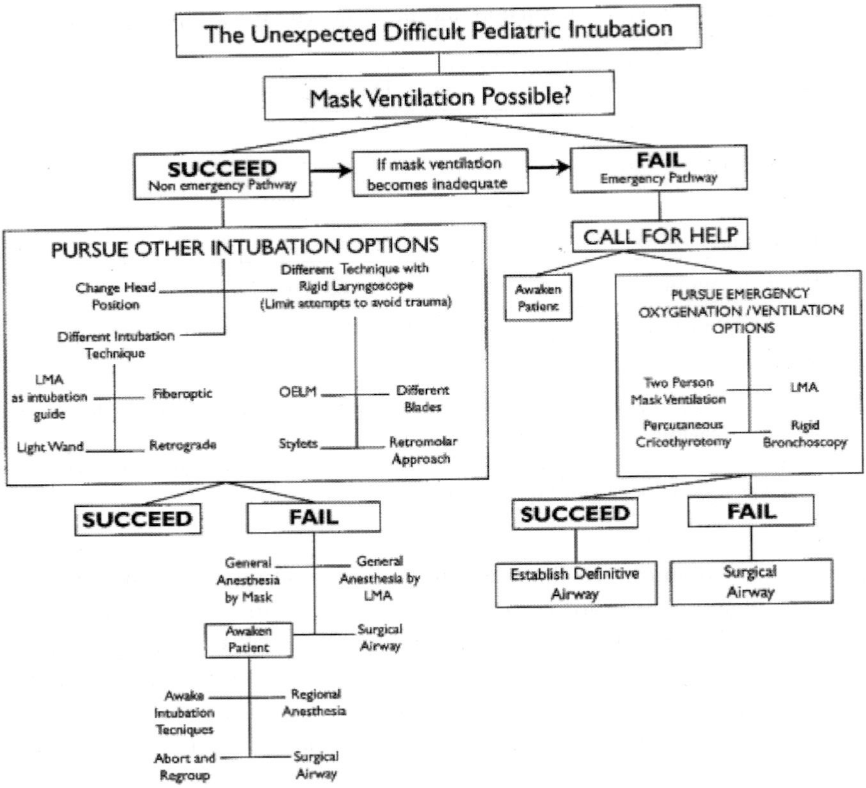

Figure 5. Algorithm for management of the unexpected difficult pediatric airway. LMA = laryngeal mask airway; OELM = optimal external laryngeal manipulation.[8] (Reprinted from Wheeler M. (1998) Management strategies for the difficult pediatric airway. *Anesth Clin North Am* 16:743–761, with permission from Elsevier.)

problem in pediatrics and can make airway management challenging. Many syndromes exist that lead to difficult airway management. Syndromes that include micrognathia, such as Pierre–Robin syndrome or Treacher Collins syndrome, can be very challenging even for experts in airway management. The advent of video laryngoscopes, such as the C-MAC and Glide Scope, have aided in the management of difficult airways. Some patients may require awake fiberoptic intubation to secure their airway. In some situations, patients with difficult airways need to be intubated in the operating room where anesthesiologists and surgeons are both present. Although surgical airways are usually not needed, it is best to be prepared.

CONCLUSION

The pediatric airway is distinct from the adult airway. Proper management of the pediatric patient demands knowledge of the anatomical and physiological differences between these two populations. Successful management of the pediatric airway also requires an understanding of the equipment available as well as the technical skills to use the equipment properly. Above all else, as issues with the airway can be a matter of life and death, one should never hesitate to ask for help.

REFERENCES

1. Santillanes G, Gausche-Hill M. (2008) Pediatric airway management. *Emerg Med Clin N Am* **26**:961–975.
2. Cote CJ, Lerman J, Todres ID. (2009) The pediatric airway. *A Practice of Anesthesia for Infants and Children*, pp. 237–278. Saunders Elsevier, Philadelphia.
3. McNiece WL, Dierdorf SF. (2004) The pediatric airway. *Semin Pediat Surg* **13**:152–165.
4. Von Ungern-Sternberg BS, Erb TO, Reber A, Frei FJ. (2005) Opening the upper airway — Airway maneuvers in pediatric anesthesia. *Pediatr Anesth* **15**:181–189.
5. Von Ungern-Sternberg BS, Erb TO, Frei FJ. (2005) Jaw thrust can deteriorate upper airway patency. *Acta Anaesthesiol Scand* **49**:583–585.
6. Levy RJ, Helfaer MA. (2000) Pediatric airway issues. *Crit Care Clin* **16**:489–504.
7. Sagarin MJ, Chiang V, Sakles JC, *et al.* (2002) Rapid sequence intubation for pediatric emergency airway management. *Pediatr Emerg Care* **18**:417–423.
8. Wheeler M. (1998) Management strategies for the difficult pediatric airway. *Anesth Clin North Am* **16**:743–761.

PEDIATRIC SEDATION 9

Michael Mazurek

INTRODUCTION

A trend in pediatric medical care over the past decade is a significant increase in the number of diagnostic and therapeutic procedures being performed outside the operating room. These areas include cardiac catheterization laboratories; gastroenterology suites; radiology departments such as Magnetic resonance imaging (MRI), Computed tomography (CT), Interventional radiology (IR), Fluoroscopy (Fluoro), Nuclear Medicine (Nuc med); hematology/oncology procedure rooms; emergency departments and the like. The majority of these procedures in children require sedation or anesthesia and many pediatric anesthesia departments across the country may not have the manpower to handle this caseload. Therefore, sedation for a large percentage of these procedures is provided by nonanesthesia medical professionals, and is the driving force affecting development of various types of sedation services. Establishing and maintaining standard in sedation care among different provider types is an important consideration.

LEVELS OF SEDATION

Four levels of sedation have been defined by The Joint Commission on Accreditation of Healthcare Organizations (JCAHO)[1] and American Society of Anesthesiologists Classification (ASA)[2] that include minimal sedation, moderate sedation, deep sedation, and general anesthesia. It is

Table 1. Levels of sedation.

	Minimal sedation	Moderate sedation	Deep sedation	General anesthesia
Patient response	Normal response to verbal stimulation	Purposeful response to verbal or tactile stimulation	Purposeful response following repeated or painful stimulation	Unarousable, even with a painful stimulus
Airway	Unaffected	No intervention required	Intervention may be required	Intervention often required
Spontaneous ventilation	Unaffected	Adequate	May be inadequate	Frequently inadequate
Cardiovascular function	Unaffected	Usually maintained	Usually maintained	May be impaired

important to understand that sedation and analgesia represent a continuum of depth of sedation in relation to the amount of stimulus the patient is receiving and that patients can rapidly pass into a deeper level of sedation than intended. A patient who is moderately sedated during a painful procedure may likely advance into a deeply sedated state once the painful stimulus is removed. Table 1 represents the four levels of sedation as a continuum and demonstrates the deeper level of sedation achieved, the more likely the patient will be less responsive and the airway, ventilation, and cardiovascular function will be adversely affected. When monitoring a sedated patient during a procedure, it is important to recognize when a patient becomes more deeply sedated than intended, so that the care team can act appropriately to prevent cardiorespiratory compromise.

PEDIATRIC SEDATION SERVICES

Whereas most mature adults will tolerate various procedures under minimal or moderate sedation, performing diagnostic and therapeutic procedures usually require deep sedation in pediatric patients. The deeper levels of sedation required for children requires an increased level of care and specialization. As the volume of procedures conducted outside the operating unit has continued to increase, many institutions have developed pediatric sedation services. The continued increase in demand for pediatric sedation services provided by a variety of pediatric sedation practitioners has spawned the development of the Society for Pediatric Sedation (SPS) and the Pediatric Sedation Research Consortium (PSRC). These multispecialty groups are dedicated to improving pediatric sedation care. The SPS provides educational materials through their website, hosts an annual meeting, and sponsors a "listserve" that allows discussion and information exchange between a large group of sedation practitioners. The PSRC is a large quality improvement and research initiative striving to form data-driven recommendations for sedation care and training, and also privileging providers for sedation.

RISKS OF SEDATION

The majority of problems that arise during sedation and analgesia are related to the airway, and include airway obstruction, hypoventilation, apnea, aspiration, and laryngospasm.[3–12] Any of the above noted problems may lead to hypoxia and hypercarbia, and if not recognized promptly, could progress to cardiopulmonary arrest. Primary hemodynamic impairment is less common during sedation and analgesia, occasionally occurring to very ill patients or those with preexisting cardiovascular disease.

Because it is difficult to prospectively study rare events, critical incident analysis has been used to study adverse sedation events.[13] Adverse sedation events reported to the Food and Drug Administration (FDA) over a 30-yr period were reviewed in order to characterize contributing factors that might lead to adverse events. They found that respiratory events were the most frequent initiating factor leading to an adverse outcome. The most common causes of the adverse events were: Combining multiple medications, overdosing the medications, inadequately evaluating the patient before sedation, inadequately monitoring the patient, and inadequately resuscitating the patient during adverse events.

In reviewing medication-related factors, adverse outcome was associated with all routes of drug administration and with all classes of medication, even when given within the recommended dose range.[14] No drug, even those administered at a recommended dose, is safe in all patients. The investigators emphasized that sedation medications should never be given at home prior to coming to the hospital. One of the cases in this series involved a child who received chloral hydrate at home, developed airway obstruction in the car seat, and was dead upon arrival at the hospital. A final recommendation of this study is to avoid premature discharge from the treatment facility, especially when using medications with long half-lives. After a procedure is completed, it is important to place the child in a quiet room with a parent and observe for resedation in the absence of any stimulus.

In two prospective, multicenter studies by the PSRC involving 37 institutions and almost 80,000 sedation/anesthesia encounters, there were no deaths and three instances requiring cardiopulmonary resuscitation.[15,16] Less serious events were more common and included oxygen desaturation, stridor and laryngospasm, unexpected apnea, excessive secretions, and vomiting. It is important to note that the PSRC data listed above showing a very low incidence of serious adverse events comes from a collection of institutions with highly motivated and organized pediatric sedation services.

CONDUCT OF PEDIATRIC SEDATION

The conduct of pediatric sedation can be conveniently divided into presedation, sedation, and postsedation protocols. Presedation protocols include equipment and supply checks, consent, dietary precautions, and a health evaluation.

At every location where sedation and analgesia is provided, it is vital to be prepared for the worst possible scenario, cardiopulmonary arrest. The equipment necessary for resuscitation must be checked and immediately available. An oxygen source and airway equipment of the appropriate size should include patient masks, nasal cannula, oral airways, laryngoscope blades, endotracheal tubes, and a functioning suction source. An age appropriate emergency cart must be immediately available in the sedation location. Monitoring equipment must include a pulse oximeter, noninvasive blood pressure cuff, electrocardiograph (EKG), stethoscope, and a means to monitor continuous ventilation.

JCAHO standards[1] require that consent for sedation and analgesia must be obtained in addition to the consent for the procedure. The potential risks and complications and options other than sedation, such as general anesthesia, should be discussed.

During sedation protective airway reflexes are impaired and vomiting or regurgitation may lead to aspiration of stomach contents. Individual

Table 2. NPO guidelines.

Ingested food	Fasting period (hrs)
Clear liquids	2
Breast milk	4
Infant formula	6
Nonhuman milk	6
Light meal	6
Full meal	8

patient responses vary greatly and it is impossible to guarantee that a particular dose of a certain medication will consistently preserve airway reflexes. Furthermore, there is the possibility that a deeper level of sedation, or even general anesthesia, may be required to complete the procedure. The safest way to avoid aspiration is to adhere to strict NPO guidelines.[17] Table 2 shows the NPO guidelines developed by the ASA. In emergency situations where the procedure needs to be done promptly,[4] the patient's NPO status must be considered on a case-by-case basis.

The sedating physician must perform a presedation health evaluation that includes: A history of problems with sedation or anesthesia, airway problems including obstructive sleep apnea, current medications and drug allergies, a review of systems, obtain vital signs and weight, perform a cardiorespiratory and airway examination and judge the risk classification. While most of the components of the presedation health evaluation seem intuitive, and part of most practitioners' daily practice; the airway examination and the risk classification are more specific to anesthesia practice.

Prior to sedation, one must consider the possibility that the patient might require bag and mask ventilation, or even endotracheal intubation. Therefore, evaluation of the airway is advised to identify anatomical characteristics that might make these difficult. The same characteristics that contribute to difficult bag and mask ventilation and intubation will predispose the patient to airway obstruction with sedation. The importance of an airway examination cannot be overemphasized. Patients with limited ability to open their mouth (mandibular fracture), a large tongue (Down syndrome), limited atlanto–occipital joint extension, and/or micrognathia (Pierre–Robin sequence) will present airway challenges.

Table 3. American society of anesthesiology, physical status.

ASA class	Disease state
Class 1	No organic, physiologic, biochemical, or psychiatric disturbance
Class 2	Mild to moderate systemic disturbance that may or may not be related to the reason for surgery
Class 3	Severe systemic disturbance that may or may not be related to the reason for surgery
Class 4	Severe systemic disturbance that is life-threatening with or without surgery
Class 5	Moribund patient who has little chance of survival but is submitted to surgery as a last resort (resuscitative effort)
Emergency operation (E)	Any patient in whom an emergency operation is required

The final component of the presedation health evaluation is the physical status assessment. The most common physical status assessment system used was developed by the ASA and is represented in Table 3.

While performing the presedation health evaluation, the physician should screen for patients at increased risk. These patients should be referred to physicians with advanced airway training and specialization in sedation or anesthesia. Table 4 shows a list of pediatric patients at increased risk for sedation and analgesia.

Once the physician has completed a thorough presedation health evaluation and developed a sedation plan, the essential requirements for safe sedation should be considered: manpower, monitoring, and documentation.

During every procedure requiring sedation and analgesia, there must be two persons present: one is performing the procedure and another monitoring the patient. During moderate sedation, the monitoring person may assist the proceduralist with short, interruptible tasks. During deep sedation, the monitoring person must have no other duties except monitoring the patient.

Eliciting patient response to commands should be performed frequently during the procedure. A diminished or absent response should alert the caregiver that the patient has become more deeply sedated than anticipated. However, it should be noted that in certain age groups the

Table 4. Risk factors for sedation and analgesia.

Risk factors
Failed sedation
Adverse response to sedation
Obstructive sleep apnea
History of difficult intubation
Anatomical airway abnormality
ASA Class 3 or 4
Delayed gastric emptying or aspiration risk
Severe gastroesophageal reflux
Morbid obesity
Prematurity

process of eliciting a response will interrupt an otherwise adequate level of sedation. Pulse oximetry and monitoring of continuous ventilation is mandatory for all patients. It is important to recognize that the pulse oximeter is not a ventilation monitor. An apneic patient will have a delay of 20–30 secs to register declining oxygen saturations on a pulse oximeter. Monitoring respiratory rate does not monitor ventilation. A completely obstructed patient can still make a respiratory effort and has a normal respiratory rate. Observation, auscultation, and/or palpation by a competent examiner is a reasonable monitor of ventilation. In the patient covered by drapes, ventilation should be monitored by continuous sampling of end tidal carbon dioxide, most commonly via a nasal cannula. The ECG and blood pressure should be monitored for all deeply sedated patients and for moderately sedated patients when indicated.

A flowsheet should be developed that is specific for procedures involving sedation and analgesia and separate it from daily nursing notes. Documentation on the sedation flowsheet should include all medications given including dosages, times, and routes as well as vital signs and level of sedation recorded every 5 mins.

Postsedation protocols apply to patient recovery. Patients should be fully awake, able to perform age-appropriate tasks, breathe deeply and cough. Developmentally delayed patients should be back to presedation status before discharge. If a reversal agent is given, the patient should be observed for at least 1 hr because the sedative agents might outlast the duration of action of the reversal agent. A physician must perform a post-procedure evaluation of the patient prior to discharge and any adverse outcomes should be documented on the sedation flowsheet. Typical adverse outcomes include, but are not necessarily limited to, conversion to general anesthesia, any emergency intervention, respiratory complications and death.

JCAHO standards[1] state that physicians must be qualified and credentialed to administer moderate or deep sedation. JCAHO has given individual institutions the responsibility of determining their own credentialing process.

SPECIFIC DRUGS

When providing sedation and analgesia for procedures, it is better to become knowledgeable and experienced with a few medications than to develop a superficial experience with many medications. Start with small doses and titrate to the desired effect. When combining drugs, decrease the dose of each medication as combinations of drugs will potentiate respiratory depression.[8] Allow sufficient time for drug effect before redosing and tailor medications to need. A mature 8 yr old with a head laceration may only need local anesthetic for analgesia. A child requiring anxiolysis for a head MRI should not need a potentially apnea-producing narcotic for this nonpainful procedure. When used appropriately, local anesthetics will substantially reduce the need for systemic narcotics. Tables 5 and 6 represent a list of commonly used medications for pediatric sedation and analgesia.

Case Example

A 2 yr old girl weighing 15 kg with osteomyelitis needs a temporary central venous line placed for administration of intravenous antibiotics. The venous catheter will be placed in the ward treatment room using sedation and analgesia. The following steps must be completed:

(1) Perform and document a presedation health evaluation with a focus on medical issues that place the child at increased risk for sedation and analgesia.
(2) Obtain a separate consent for the sedation and analgesia.

Table 5. Pediatric sedation medications.

Medication	Route	Dose	Maximum cumulative dose	Onset of action (mins)	Duration	Reversal agents
Chloral hydrate	PO/PR	25–100 mg/kg	100 mg/kg Infants 1 gm/24 hrs Children 2 gm/24 hrs	10–20	4–8 hrs	None
Midazolam (Versed)	PO	0.5 mg/kg	15 mg	20–30	1–2 hrs	Flumazenil (Romazicon)
	IV	0.025–0.075 mg/kg titrating every 5 mins	0.4 mg/kg	1–5	45–60 mins	
	IM	0.1–0.2 mg/kg		5	2–6 hrs	
	IN	0.2–0.3 mg/kg		5	30 mins–1 hr	
Fentanyl	IV	0.5–2 mcg/kg	4 mcg/kg	1–2	30 mins–1 hr	Naloxone (Narcan)
Morphine	PO	0.2–0.5 mg/kg		60	3–5 hrs	Naloxone (Narcan)
	IV	0.05–0.1 mg/kg	0.2 mg/kg	20	3–5 hrs	
	IM	0.05–0.2 mg/kg		30–60	3–5 hrs	
Meperidine (Demerol)	IV	0.5–1 mg/kg	2 mg/kg	2–4	2–3 hrs	Naloxone (Narcan)
	IM	1–2 mg/kg		5	2–4 hrs	
Ketamine	PO	4–6 mg/kg				None
	IV	0.25–0.5 mg/kg	1 mg/kg	1–2	20–60 mins	
	IM	2–3 mg/kg	5 mg/kg	3–4		
Propofol	IV	0.25–0.5 mg/kg 25–100 mcg/kg/min		1–2	5–30 mins	None

Table 6. Pediatric sedation reversal agents.

Medication	Route	Dose (mg/kg)	Maximum cumulative dose	Onset of action (mins)	Duration (hr)
Flumazenil (Romazicon)	IV	0.01	1 mg	1–3	<1
Narcan (Naloxone)	IV	0/0–0.1		2	<1
	IM	0.1		2–5	<1

(3) Check the treatment room for appropriately functioning monitors and equipment.
(4) Make sure a qualified individual is available to monitor the patient during the procedure and until full recovery is achieved.

The health evaluation reveals a previously healthy patient (ASA class 1) who had pedialyte 3 hrs ago and no solid food for 10 hrs. Her airway exam is normal and she has no history of airway problems such as obstructive sleep apnea. She has never had anesthesia or sedation. She is declared an appropriate candidate for sedation and analgesia.

If the patient has an IV, there are several medication options for providing the sedation and analgesia. Drugs with a short duration of action are an attractive choice given that placement of a temporary subclavian vein line in a healthy 2 yr old should be a short procedure. Local anesthetic cream applied to the needle insertion site will help reduce the pain of subcutaneous local anesthesia infiltration if time allows (need 30–45 mins for local anesthetic cream to be effective). Once the patient is in the treatment room, the monitors are applied before initiating sedation including pulse oximeter, blood pressure cuff, ECG, and some means of monitoring continuous ventilation (observing chest rise, stethoscope, end-tidal CO_2 sampling). One sedation option would be to combine local anesthetic cream, subcutaneous local anesthesia infiltration, and IV fentanyl and midazolam. Typical starting doses include 25 mcg/kg midazolam with 0.5 mcg/kg fentanyl. Each component can be redosed as needed every 5 mins until an adequate level of sedation is achieved. Do not exceed 3 mcg/kg of fentanyl or 100 mcg/kg of midazolam. After adequate sedation and analgesia the operator may proceed with subcutaneous local infiltration and the line placement. Another sedation option would include local anesthetic cream, subcutaneous local anesthesia infiltration, and IV atropine and ketamine. Typical starting doses would be 0.01–0.02 mg/kg atropine and 0.25–0.5 mg/kg ketamine. Initially, the ketamine dose may be repeated every 5 mins to achieve a desired level of sedation and then repeated every 15–20 mins to maintain an adequate level of sedation.

REFERENCES

1. Joint Commission on Accreditation of Healthcare Organizations. (2001) Accreditation Manual for Hospitals.
2. American Society of Anesthesiologists. (1999) Approved by the ASA House of Delegates, October 13.
3. Goodson JM, Moore PA. (1983) Life-threatening reactions after pedodontic sedation: An assessment of narcotic, local anesthetic, and antiemetic drug interaction. *J Am Dent Assoc* **107**:239–245.
4. Green SM, Krauss B. (2002) Pulmonary aspiration risk during emergency department procedural sedation — an examination of the role of fasting and sedation depth. *Acad Emerg Med* **9**:35–42.
5. Green SM, Klooster M, Harris T, *et al.* (2001) Ketamine sedation for pediatric gastroenterology procedures. *J Pediatr Gastroenterol Nutri* **32**:26–33.
6. Kennedy RM, Porter FL, Miller JP, *et al.* (1998) Comparison of fentanyl/midazolam with ketamine/midazolam for pediatric orthopedic emergencies. *Pediatrics* **102**:956–963.
7. Marx CM, Stein J, Tyler MK, *et al.* (1997) Ketamine-midazolam versus meperidine-midazolam for painful procedures in pediatric oncology patients. *J Clin Oncol* **15**:94–102.
8. Bailey PL, Pace NL, Ashburn MA, *et al.* (1990) Frequent hypoxemia and apnea after sedation with midazolam and fentanyl. *Anesthesiology* **73**:826–830.
9. Pena BM, Krauss B. (1999) Adverse events of procedural sedation and analgesia in a pediatric emergency department. *Ann Emerg Med* **34**:483–491.
10. Vade A, Sukhani R, Dolenga M, *et al.* (1995) Chloral hydrate sedation of children undergoing CT and MR imaging: Safety as judged by American Academy of Pediatrics guidelines. *AJR* **165**:905–909.
11. Malviya S, Voepel-Lewis T, Tiat R. (1997) Adverse events and risk factors associated with the sedation of children by nonanesthesiologists. *Anesth Analg* **85**:1207–1213.

12. Hoffman GM, Nowakowski R, Troshynski TJ, *et al.* (2002) Risk reduction in pediatric procedural sedation by application of an American Academy of Pediatrics/American Society of Anesthesiologists process model. *Pediatrics* **109**:236–243.
13. Cote CJ, Notterdam DA, Karl HW, *et al.* (2000) Adverse sedation events in pediatrics: A critical incident analysis of contributing factors. *Pediatrics* **105**:805–814.
14. Cote CJ, Karl HW, Notterdam DA, *et al.* (2000) Adverse sedation events in pediatrics: Analysis of medications used for sedation. *Pediatrics* **106**:633–644.
15. Cravero JP, Blike GT, Beach M, *et al.* (2006) Incidence and nature of adverse events during pediatric sedation/anesthesia for procedures outside the operating room: Report from the Pediatric Sedation Research Consortium. *Pediatrics* **118**:1087–1096.
16. Cravero JP, Blike GT, Beach M, *et al.* (2006) The incidence and nature of adverse events during pediatric sedation/anesthesia with propofol for procedures outside the operating room: Report from the Pediatric Sedation Research Consortium. *Anesth Analg* **108**:795–804.
17. American Society of Anesthesiology Task Force. (1999) Practice guidelines for preoperative fasting and the use of pharmacologic agents to reduce the risk of pulmonary aspiration: Application to healthy patients undergoing elective procedures. *Anesthesiology* **99**:896–905.

TREATMENT OF ACUTE POSTSURGICAL PAIN IN THE PEDIATRIC PATIENT 10

James Tolley

The International Association for the Study of Pain defines pain as an "unpleasant sensory and emotional experience associated with actual or potential tissue damage, or described in terms of such damage". While there are many traumatic and pathologic conditions which can cause pain or be perceived as painful, the focus of this chapter will be upon postsurgical pain. The first section will provide a brief overview of nociception providing greater insight into the mechanism of action of the drugs and modalities of treatment discussed later in the chapter. A section on the benefits of the prevention and treatment of postsurgical pain will also be presented as will a brief discussion on patient-controlled analgesia (PCA) and regional analgesia.

Also, there are three tables that are useful for managing postsurgical pain in the pediatric patient. Table 1 contains commonly used oral analgesics, Table 2 lists the opioid agonists and antagonists mentioned in the chapter, and Table 3 lists the maximal amount of various local anesthetics that can be used for infiltration of wounds or peripheral blockade.

NOCICEPTION

Nociception, defined as the perception of a painful stimulus, is a complex process involving many distinct neurotransmitters, receptors, and neurons

Table 1. Commonly used oral analgesics.

Drug	Dose	Frequency (hrs)	Notes
Acetaminophen	10–15 mg/kg up to 1 g	4–6	Max daily dose lesser of 4 g or 100 mg/kg in children; 75 mg/kg in infants; 60 mg/kg in newborns >32 wks gestation
Ibuprofen	10 mg/kg	6	Max daily dose lesser of 2.4 g or 40 mg/kg for children 6 mths–12 yrs
Naproxen	5–10 mg/kg	8–12	Max daily dose 20 mg/kg for children
Ketorolac	0.3–0.5 mg/kg up to 30 mg	6–8	Max daily dose lesser of 120 mg or 2 mg/kg up to 20 doses or 5 days maximum (some would limit ketorolac to 10 mg/dose iv or oral)
Codeine	1 mg/kg	4	Do not exceed maximal acetaminophen dose in combined preparations
Hydrocodone	0.1 mg/kg	4	Do not exceed maximal ibuprofen or acetaminophen dose in combined preparations
Oxycodone	0.1 mg/kg	4	Same as hydrocodone
Tramadol	1–2 mg/kg up to 100 mg	4–6	Max daily dose lesser of 400 mg or 8 mg/kg in children

that can be divided into four distinct steps. Each of these individual processes can serve as the target for various methods and drugs used to interrupt nociception, thus treating or preventing the perception of pain.

Transduction is the process whereby specialized free nerve endings convert a noxious stimulus into an action potential which is *transmitted* to the spinal cord via peripheral nerves. The resulting information is relayed to higher centers of the brainstem and cerebral cortex where it is *perceived* but not without being *modulated* by those same centers.[1]

Table 2. Commonly used intravenous opioid agonists and antagonists.

Drug	Dose	Frequency (hrs)	Notes
Codeine	0.5–1 mg/kg	4–6	Max dose of 60 mg
Tramadol	1–2 mg/kg	4–6	Has been used as an infusion in studies. Limit to maximal oral dose.
Morphine	0.05–0.2 mg/kg	3–4	Used frequently in PCA
Fentanyl	0.5–2 mcg/kg	1–2	Used frequently in PCA
Hydromorphone	10–20 mcg/kg	3–6	Used frequently in PCA
Naloxone	0.01 mg/kg up to 0.1 mg/kg up to 2 mg for resp depression	Titrate to effect	Lower dose post operatively to retain analgesia

Table 3. Maximal amount of various local anesthetics for infiltration or peripheral blockade.

Local anesthetic	Maximal dose in mg/kg
2-Chloroprocaine	8–10
Mepivacaine	5–6
Lidocaine	5–7
Bupivacaine	2–3
Levobupivacaine	2.5–4
Ropivacaine	2.5–4

In the tissues are nociceptors which respond to mechanical, thermal, and chemical stimuli. Surgery will result in mechanical injury to cells with the resultant inflammatory mediators leading to chemical stimuli in the immediate and surrounding areas. As a result of this chemical stimulus, peripheral sensitization will result such that the response threshold to other stimuli is decreased, the magnitude is increased, and the receptive field size is enlarged leading to primary hyperalgesia.[2]

Information regarding the injurious stimulus is transmitted along thinly myelinated A-delta fibers and unmyelinated C fibers to the cell bodies located in the dorsal horn of the spinal cord. These cell bodies synapse with nociceptive specific cells.[3] They will also synapse with wide dynamic range (WDR) cells which receive input from both noxious and non-noxious stimuli. These WDR neurons can also exhibit "wind-up" with an increase in the graded response to stimuli, both noxious and non-noxious, along with spontaneous firing.[4] This process is known as central sensitization and leads to secondary hyperalgesia.[2]

Modulation of the spinal cord activity from the brainstem centers can be both inhibitory and excitatory.[3] Two of the more well studied excitatory factors include glutamate acting through the N-methyl D-aspartate (NMDA) receptor and the peptide, substance P. Inhibitory factors include the endogenous endorphins that bind to opioid receptors, norepinephrine, and serotonin.[5]

PHYSIOLOGIC RESPONSE TO PAIN AND THE BENEFITS OF POSTSURGICAL ANALGESIA

Increasingly, pain is being understood as a component of the body's interoceptive homeostatic afferents,[6] and the physiologic response is a part of the body's attempt to maintain homeostasis and promote healing. However, given the severe injury that can occur with certain surgical procedures, the surgical stress response can lead to many undesirable effects.

The surgical stress response is a cascade of inflammatory, metabolic, and hormonal changes that result primarily from the systemic activation of the sympathetic nervous system. The resultant increase of pro-inflammatory mediators, cytokines, and catecholamines can result in immunosuppression, protein catabolism, a hypercoagulable state, and gastrointestinal dysfunction.[7,8]

General anesthetics alone are not effective in suppressing the surgical stress response. The addition of opioids or other systemic medications such as clonidine is necessary in order to have a moderate reduction in the response[7] while regional analgesia has the most profound effects in reducing the body's sympathetic response to surgical stimuli.[8]

In fact, epidural anesthesia and analgesia reduce perioperative cardiac morbidity, postsurgical pulmonary complications such as infection and embolism, improve gastrointestinal function, as well as reduce length of ICU and hospital stays.[8] The profound effect on the stress response, however, is associated with the use of local anesthetics.[9] Addition of opioid to the local anesthetic mixture confers no additional suppression of the surgical stress response as demonstrated in the systemic level of stress hormones.[10]

These observations should not be surprising in light of the fact that local anesthetics will interrupt afferent pain transmission while opioids will only have an impact on modulation of painful stimuli after the fact. Furthermore, continued suppression of the stress response is dependent upon ongoing transmission blockade in the presence of continued afferent impulses which may occur for several days following significant surgical trauma.[1]

THE LADDER APPROACH TO RATIONAL POSTOPERATIVE PAIN MANAGEMENT

Given the above basic physiologic information, one can take the World Health Organization's guidelines for analgesic use in cancer pain[11] and adapt the same "ladder" approach to treating surgical pain. Minimal surgical trauma would be expected to result in little homeostatic change in the patient and thus minimal amounts of pain and physiologic consequence. A large amount of surgical trauma would be expected to result in significant afferent impulses resulting in a dramatic surgical stress response and a multi-modal approach to postoperative pain management would seem most logical. The remainder of this chapter will examine the drugs and methods used to treat increasingly severe postsurgical pain.

Acetaminophen and other Nonsteroidal Anti-inflammatory Drugs

Acetaminophen is the most widely used nonsteroidal anti-inflammatory drug (NSAID) for mild pain. It is an inhibitor of the cyclooxygenase (COX) enzyme in the central nervous system but not peripherally. Thus, it lacks many of the adverse effects of COX inhibition such as bleeding, gastric ulceration, and renal failure. Acetaminophen is currently available in oral, rectal or intravenous preparations. Careful attention should be paid to dosing as acetaminophen overdose can result in hepatic failure. A decreased daily dosing regimen is necessary for infants, neonates, and premature neonates.[12,13]

Ibuprofen is another commonly used NSAID for mild to moderate pain in pediatric surgical patients. It is also a COX inhibitor that acts in the periphery at the site of inflammation and pain. In contrast with acetaminophen, ibuprofen should be used with caution in patients at risk for gastrointestinal or surgical bleeding, renal failure, or asthma.[14] Naproxen is another NSAID with a similar mechanism of action and side effect profile to ibuprofen. One major difference is that the half-life of naproxen is longer allowing for dosing every 8 to 12 hrs. Also, its safety in infants and newborns has not been adequately studied.[13]

Ketorolac is another NSAID that is available for intravenous use in the treatment of pain in pediatric patients. It can be used to treat moderate amounts of pain and is as effective as morphine in various pediatric surgical procedures.[13,15] Because of the increased risk of acute renal failure, ketorolac should not be used for greater than 5 days.[16]

As the surgical insult increases, the amount of postoperative pain would be expected to increase necessitating the addition of other drugs or modalities to the analgesic regimen such as weak opioids or regional analgesic techniques appropriate for outpatient procedures.

Opioids

Codeine is an opioid receptor agonist that is commonly combined with acetaminophen for use in the outpatient setting to treat mild or moderate postsurgical pain. The majority of codeine's analgesic effects are dependent upon on O-demethylation in the liver to morphine. Up to 10% of the Caucasian population lacks the enzyme responsible for this conversion and therefore, derive no analgesic benefit from codeine. Codeine is associated with significant gastrointestinal side effects such as nausea and vomiting and may be poorly tolerated.[12,13,14]

Hydrocodone and oxycodone are semi-synthetic opioids that are used for moderate to severe pain either alone or in combination with acetaminophen, aspirin, or ibuprofen. They are 10 times as potent as codeine but have a similar bioavailability with an onset time of 20–30 mins and a clinical duration of approximately 4 hrs. One must keep in mind when prescribing combined preparations not to exceed the maximal singular or daily dose of acetaminophen, aspirin, or NSAID.[12,14]

Tramadol is a synthetic derivative of codeine which acts as a mu receptor agonist but also inhibits reuptake of both norepinephrine and serotonin in the central nervous system. Tramadol is metabolized in the liver, and its active metabolite is six times as potent and has an affinity for the mu receptor that is 200 times greater.[12,14] Tramadol has a similar side effect profile as other opioids with nausea and vomiting being the most common adverse events.[17] In contrast to other opioids, it has negligible respiratory effects[17] but has been associated with seizures.[12]

Morphine is the prototypical opioid and is used extensively in postoperative pain management in pediatric patients. It can be used orally, intramuscularly, intravenously, intraarticularly, epidurally, and intrathecally. Its most common side effects include nausea, vomiting, and sedation when used intravenously. Pruritis, urinary retention and respiratory depression can also be a concern especially when administered neuraxially.[18] Morphine is not superior to other methods of pain control except when given in the intrathecal space.[18] Care should be used when giving morphine to premature neonates as the free fraction of drug in plasma is increased, elimination half-life is prolonged, and clearance is decreased compared to older children.[13]

Fentanyl is a synthetic opioid that is more potent than morphine by a factor of 100. It is highly lipophilic with a short duration of action secondary to redistribution. However, it is possible to saturate peripheral redistribution sites giving fentanyl a half-life of over 3 hrs in infants and children. Fentanyl can also be given through multiple routes including orally, transmucosally, nasally, intravenously, transdermally, intravenously, epidurally, and intrathecally.[12,13]

Hydromorphone is a semi-synthetic derivative of morphine that is approximately five times as potent.[13] It can be administered orally, intramuscularly, intravenously or epidurally and has fewer side effects such as nausea and pruritis than morphine.[19]

Naloxone is an opioid receptor antagonist that is used to counter-act the sedative and respiratory depressant effects of opioids. Titration of the naloxone dose is suggested in the postoperative period so as not to antagonize the beneficial effects of opioid analgesia.[20] Because the half-life of naloxone is shorter than the opioids it is meant to antagonize, the patient should be observed for a return of opiate side effects.[13] Naloxone should be made readily available for any patient who has received opiates regardless of the means of administration.

PATIENT, PARENT, OR NURSE CONTROLLED ANALGESIA

Intravenous PCA is safe and effective in pediatric patients as young as 5 yrs old[21] and has become a routine component of postoperative care at many pediatric hospitals. Parent-controlled or nurse-controlled analgesia is also effective for younger patients or patients who are developmentally delayed although it is highly recommended that adequate education of both nurses and parents, strict adherence to established protocols, and adequate patient monitoring be instituted to ensure patient safety and minimize adverse reactions.[22]

Patient-controlled epidural analgesia (PCEA) is a newer modality that allows a patient to administer additional bolus doses of analgesic through an epidural catheter in addition to any background infusion that may be running. PCEA has been studied on a limited basis in pediatric patients but has been shown to be safe and effective with a high degree of patient satisfaction.[23]

REGIONAL ANALGESIA

The use of regional analgesia in pediatric patients has increased due to recognition of improved outcomes[8,24] and has shifted from primarily neuraxial techniques to include a wide range of peripheral nerve blocks using single injection techniques for mild pain as well as catheter placement and subsequent continuous infusion for more extensive and painful surgical procedures.[24,25] Furthermore, the use of ultrasound guidance for needle placement offers the promise of increased safety and improved efficiency over other techniques such as using anatomic landmarks or nerve stimulation.[24,25]

Local anesthetics interfere with the neural transmission and action potentials that would normally result from the application of noxious stimuli to the tissues. Preventing information regarding noxious stimuli from arriving at the level of the spinal cord minimizes the amount of "wind-up" that can occur[3] which is likely clinically manifest by the decreased stress response from surgical stimulation.[8] It is important, however, to maintain blockade of transmission for the duration of the most severe painful stimuli in order to maintain this benefit.[1]

The mechanism of action of local anesthetics is through inactivation of activated sodium channels along the nerve axon.[26] Excitable nervous tissue in the central nervous system and cardiac conduction system can also be affected by local anesthetics explaining the signs and symptoms associated with local anesthetic toxicity.[26] It is important that both anesthesiologists and surgeons are cognizant of the maximal doses of the various local anesthetics that should be used for neural blockade to minimize the risk of toxicity (Table 3).

In an effort to prolong the effective duration of pain relief following peripheral and neuraxial local anesthetic blockade, several adjuvants have been studied. Some of those studied include epinephrine, opioids, clonidine, ketamine, midazolam, neostigmine, and corticosteroids. This is still an area of active investigation and controversy but it appears that epinephrine and clonidine are effective adjuncts in the epidural space.[27,28] Epinephrine also prolongs the clinical effects of local anesthetics in peripheral nerve blocks but the effect is less well established with clonidine.[29]

SUMMARY

Historically, pain in pediatric patients has been underappreciated and undertreated. The recognition that pain can have adverse physiologic and psychological consequences has led to increased research and interest in the postsurgical treatment of pediatric pain.

Adequate treatment of postsurgical pain requires preparation that begins in the preoperative period. Treatment that is appropriate for the expected insult, individualized to the needs of the patient, and multimodal in its approach is essential. Furthermore, communication between the patient, family, surgeon, and anesthesiologist is required in order to achieve the best possible outcome.

Patients with physiologic or anatomic conditions that would preclude certain pain treatments should be managed with alternative approaches that still consider the extent of the expected pain and anticipated physiologic derangements. Patients with a history of chronic pain should be treated for the acute pain that occurs as a result of surgery above and beyond their baseline pain disorder.

Pain after surgery is one of the greatest fears that patients, adult and children alike, face. By recognizing these fears and addressing them in a compassionate manner and demonstrating a thoughtful approach in managing these concerns, the pediatric surgeon can decrease some of the anxiety associated with surgery and facilitate the healing process before surgery even begins.

REFERENCES

1. Kelly DJ, Ahmad M, Brull SJ. (2001) Preemptive analgesia I: Physiological pathways and pharmacological modalities. *Can J Anesth* **48**:1000–1010.
2. Brennan TJ, Zahn PK, Pogatzki-Zahn EM. (2005) Mechanisms of incisional pain. *Anesthesiol Clin N Am* **23**:1–20.
3. D'Mello R, Dickenson AH. (2008) Spinal cord mechanisms of pain. *Brit J Anaesth* **101**:8–16.

4. Chu KL, Faltynek CR, Jarvis MF, *et al.* (2004) Increased WDR spontaneous activity and receptive field size in rats following a neuropathic or inflammatory injury: Implications for mechanical sensitivity. *Neurosci Lett* **372**:123–126.
5. Meyr AJ, Steinberg JS. (2008) The physiology of the acute pain pathway. *Clin Pediatr Med Surg* **25**:305–326.
6. Craig AD. (2003) Pain mechanisms: Labeled lines versus convergence in central processing. *Annu Rev Neurosci* **26**:1–30.
7. Miner JR. (2008) The surgical stress response, preemptive analgesia, and procedural sedation in the emergency department. *Acad Emerg Med* **15**:955–958.
8. Moraca RJ, Sheldon DG, Thirlby RC. (2003) The role of epidural anesthesia and analgesia in surgical practice. *Ann Surg* **238**:663–673.
9. Teyin E, Derbent A, Balcioglu T, *et al.* (2006) The efficacy of caudal morphine or bupivacaine combined with general anesthesia on postoperative pain and neuroendocrine stress response in children. *Pediatr Anesth* **16**:290–296.
10. Erol A, Tuncer S, Tavlan A, *et al.* (2007) Addition of sufentanil to bupivacaine in caudal block effect on stress responses in children. *Pediatr Int* **49**:928–932.
11. Ventafridda V, Saita L, Ripamonti C, *et al.* (1985) WHO guidelines for the use of analgesics in cancer pain. *Int J Tissue React* **7**:93–96.
12. Brislin RP, Rose JB. (2005) Pediatric acute pain management. *Anesthesiol Clin N Am* **23**:789–814.
13. Kraemer FW, Rose JB. (2009) Pharmacologic management of acute pediatric pain. *Anesthesiol Clin* **27**:241–268.
14. Tobias JD. (2000) Weak analgesics and nonsteroidal anti-inflammatory agents in the management of children with acute pain. *Pediatric Clin N Am* **47**:527–543.
15. Kokki H. (2003) Nonsteroidal anti-inflammatory drugs for postoperative pain: A focus on children. *Pediatr Drugs* **5**:103–123.
16. Rocca GD, Chiarandini P, Pietropaoli P. (2005) Analgesia in PACU: Nonsteroidal anti-inflammatory drugs. *Current Drug Targets* **6**:781–787.
17. Finkel JC, Rose JB, Schmitz ML, *et al.* (2002) An evaluation of the efficacy and tolerability of oral tramadol hydrochloride tablets for the treatment of postsurgical pain in children. *Anesth Analg* **94**:1469–1473.
18. Duedahl TH, Hansen EH. (2007) A qualitative systematic review of morphine treatment in children with postoperative pain. *Pediatr Anesth* **17**:756–774.
19. Quigley C, Wiffen P. (2003) A systematic review of hydromorphone in acute and chronic pain. *J Pain and Symptom Manag* **25**:169–178.
20. Hasan RA, Benko AS, Nolan BM, *et al.* (2003) Cardiorespiratory effects of naloxone in children. *Ann Pharmacother* **37**:1587–1592.

21. Shin D, Kim S, Kim CS, *et al.* (2001) Postoperative pain management using intravenous patient-controlled analgesia for pediatric patients. *J Craniofac Surg* **12**:129–133.

22. Czarnecki ML, Ferrise AS, Jastrowski-Mano KE, *et al.* (2008) Parent/Nurse-controlled analgesia for children with developmental delay. *Clin J Pain* **24**:817–824.

23. Saudan S, Habre W, Ceroni D, *et al.* (2008) Safety and efficacy of patient controlled epidural analgesia following pediatric spinal surgery. *Pediatr Anesth* **18**:132–139.

24. Ivani G, Mossetti V. (2008) Regional anesthesia for postoperative pain control in children: Focus on continuous central and perineural infusions. *Pediatr Drugs* **10**:107–114.

25. Rochette A, Dadure C, Raux O, *et al.* (2009) Changing trends in paediatric regional anaesthetic practice in recent years. *Curr Opin Anaesthesio* **22**:374–377.

26. Tetzlaff JE. (2000) The pharmacology of local anesthetics. *Anesthesiol Clin N Am* **18**:217–233.

27. Dalens B. (2006) Some current controversies in paediatric regional anaesthesia. *Curr Opin Anaesthesiol* **19**:301–308.

28. Ansermino M, Basu R, Vandebeek C, *et al.* (2003) Nonopioid additives to local anaesthetics for caudal blockade in children: A systematic review. *Paediatr Anaesth* **13**:561–573.

29. McCartney CJL, Duggan E, Apatu E. (2007) Should we add clonidine to local anesthetic for peripheral nerve blockade? A qualitative systematic review of the literature. Reg Anesth and Pain Medicine **32**:330–338.

THE EX-UTERO TREATMENT (EXIT) PROCEDURE

11

Cynthia Gingalewski, Sarah Oltmann and David Schindel

INTRODUCTION

Advances in the prenatal identification and diagnosis of congenital malformations of the neck, in particular tumors, and lymphatic malformations have allowed maternal fetal medicine specialists and pediatric surgeons to identify those fetuses that pose an immediate threat of hypoxia and death. The Ex-Utero Intrapartum Treatment (EXIT) procedure was described in the 1990s as a treatment option for high risk infants who could potentially develop devastating, life threatening complications at birth secondary to their prenatally diagnosed congenital anomalies. Initially deemed the operating on placental support (OOPS) procedure by Skarsgard, it quickly became apparent that in addition to retaining the umbilical cord intact, the procedure also required maintenance of the placental blood flow.[1] The EXIT procedure combines a cesarean section delivery and an operation on the newborn to correct a problem which would otherwise compromise the infant's survival. It is a highly coordinated effort requiring two full operative teams working in the same space and demands a high level of expertise and planning before undertaking.

The EXIT procedure was described in detail during the clinical trails of tracheal clip occlusion for congenital diaphragmatic hernia.[2,3] Maintenance of utero–placental blood flow was critical until the tracheal clips could be removed and an airway secured by endotracheal intubation. Prevention of uterine contractions and maintenance of uterine volume are key principles in the maintenance of placental blood flow. Therefore, controlled uterine hypotonia is the key to EXIT procedure.

At present, the experience of several fetal centers with the EXIT procedure have allowed indications for its use to be expanded to include giant fetal neck masses, congenital high airway obstruction syndrome (CHAOS), congenital pulmonary airway malformations (CPAM) and mediastinal masses, as well as rarer indications such as EXIT to extracorporeal membrane oxygenation. In summary, an EXIT procedure should be considered whenever it is anticipated that establishing an airway in a newborn may be difficult.

PRINCIPLES OF THE EXIT PROCEDURE

The EXIT procedure, as mentioned previously, involves more than leaving the umbilical cord intact, nor is it merely a cesarean section. Instead, the EXIT procedure involves the maintenance of uterine hypotonia and the orchestrated care of the fetus and mother involving maternal and pediatric anesthesiologists, a maternal–fetal medicine specialist, the appropriate pediatric surgical services (general surgery, ENT, cardiac), a neonatologist, and two surgical teams of nurses and technicians. The goals of the procedure are to use deep general anesthesia on the mother to allow for uterine hypotonia and preserved utero–placental circulation while maintaining the normal maternal blood pressure, preventing placental abruption by maintaining uterine volume, and to achieve fetal anesthesia without cardiac depression. The team must ensure that there are no other lethal fetal anomalies. Each case requires careful planning during team meetings of all individuals involved.

The Decision Making Process

The EXIT procedure was designed to remove tracheal clips placed for infants with severe congenital diaphragmatic hernia. Since then its indications have been broadened to include other diagnosis for which there is potential for fetal airway compromise (Table 1). Prenatal diagnosis of potential airway obstructions can be made by prenatal ultrasound and fetal MRI. When a fetus is identified as a potential candidate for an EXIT procedure,

Table 1. Indications for consideration of EXIT procedure.

Airway compromise	Cardiac compromise
Neck masses	Severe aortic stenosis
Cervical teratoma	Hypoplastic left heart syndrome
Lymphatic malformations	
Hemangioma	
Congenital goiter	
Tumor (PNET, neuroblastoma)	
Lung masses	
Congenital pulmonary airway malformations (CCAM, sequestration, lobar emphysema)	
Foregut anomalies	
Intrinsic airway obstruction	
Tracheal stenosis/web	
Laryngeal stenosis/web	

a multidisciplinary group comprising pediatric surgeons, maternal fetal medicine specialists or obstetricians, anesthesiologist, neonatologists, and pediatric/fetal radiologists should be convened to decide what options are in the best interest of the fetus and mother. Decisions will need to be taken regarding the best way to handle the fetal airway while on placental support: intubation or tracheotomy.

Delays in obtaining an airway secondary to neck masses and inability to ventilate the newborn is a significant cause of death secondary to unnecessary hypoxia, acidosis and anoxic brain injury. Giant neck masses distort the anatomy and may make routine intubation difficult. Airway obstruction can occur by means of external compression and distortion or internal obstruction of the trachea or larynx.

Fetal neck masses have increased in their diagnosis due to better and more frequent prenatal imaging techniques. The vast majority of these are lymphatic malformations. Other, much rarer causes include cervical teratomas, neuroblastoma, primitive neurectodermal tumors, disorders of the fetal thyroid gland (goiter, cyst, tumors), and hemangiomas.

Once the airway is successfully established, the neck mass can be dealt with. This may be immediate or at a later procedure depending upon the complexity and urgency of the subsequent surgery.

Extrinsic Compression of the Airway: Lymphatic Malformations

Cervical lymphangiomas have different prognosis and survival rates depending upon gestational age at diagnosis and location. Those lymphangiomas diagnosed earlier are typically located within the posterior triangle of the neck and are associated with chromosomal abnormalities and other structural anomalies in 60% of the cases. They are associated with a high mortality secondary to nonimmune hydrops formation, but are less likely to compromise the airway.

Lymphatic malformations diagnosed in the third trimester are usually located anteriorly in the neck, they are much less likely to be associated with other anomalies, but have an increased risk of airway distortion. The prognosis is much better and these infants may require an EXIT procedure to secure the airway for postnatal intervention by sclerotherapy or resection.

Fetal MRI is the best diagnostic modality for neck masses. It provides better detail about the size and position of the mass and its anatomic relationship to the airway than standard prenatal ultrasonography (Figure 1). Fetal MRI gives improved visualization of the mass to the entire airway, and may be better at predicting those fetuses which require an EXIT for airway procedure.

Compression of the fetal esophagus causes polyhydramnios in fetuses with large neck masses. Close monitoring of these infants after 23 weaks gestation is critical for development of preterm labor, hydrops, or cardiac compromise. With progression of hydrops, the fetus may require open fetal surgery if less than 30 weaks, in order to salvage in the baby. After 30 weaks gestation, EXIT strategies are employed.

The timing of the EXIT procedure is often dictated by the degree of polyhydramnios and the ensuing preterm labor. The mean gestational age of fetuses requiring EXIT procedures is 34 weaks. The surgeons must be prepared for every possible airway contingency.

Intrinsic Obstruction of the Airway

CHAOS is a rare prenatally diagnosed constellation of complete or near complete airway obstruction which prevents the egress of lung fluid from the tracheobronchial tree and the development of hydrops. Many of these fetuses die *in utero*, or are stillborn. There are multiple etiologies; however, the clinical presentation is similar with bilaterally enlarged echogenic lungs, flat diaphragms, fetal ascites, and hydrops (Table 2).

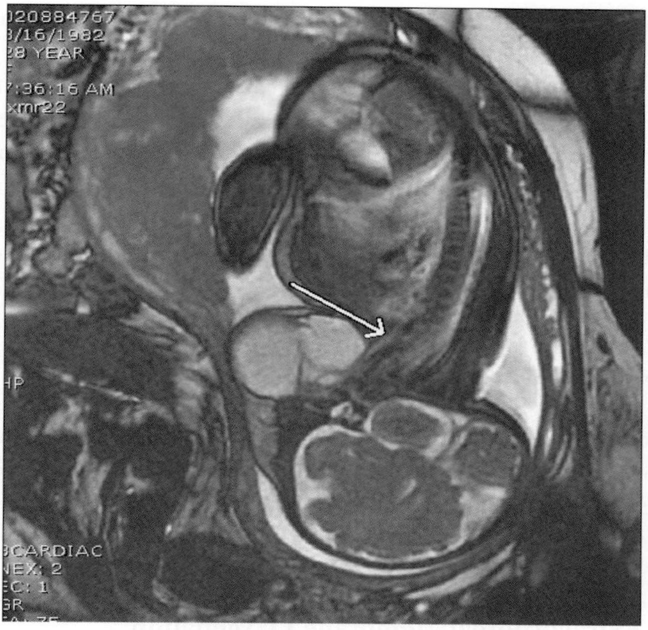

Figure 1. Prenatal imaging of fetus by MRI.

Note: Fiesta series ultrafast MRI demonstrates a large cervical lymphangioma. MRI is also able to identify the trachea to help ascertain if there is luminal compromise (arrow).

Table 2. Causes of congenital high airway obstruction syndrome.

Tracheal atresia
Tracheal web
Laryngeal stenosis
Laryngeal cyst
Laryngeal web

It is important to screen for other malformations when CHAOS is diagnosed. These include genitourinary malformations, cardiac anomalies, esophageal atresia, absent radii, anophthalmia, and Fraser syndrome (hidden eyes (cryptophthalmos) because the skin of their eyelids is partially or fully sealed shut, syndactyly, and abnormalities of the genitalia). Neurologic abnormalities associated with the vertebrae, anus, trachea, esophagus and renal (kidneys) (VATER) syndrome are missing.

The EXIT procedure for CHAOS can be employed if the airway obstruction is high enough to be bypassed by a tracheotomy. If the intrinsic obstruction is low in the trachea then EXIT to extra corporeal membrane oxygenation (ECMO) can be considered to stabilize infant for definitive procedure while on ECMO bypass. This may be considered to be heroic by many. Infants with CHAOS require prolonged ventilation and definitive reconstruction of the airway.

SPECIFIC, UNIQUE CONSIDERATIONS

In addition to the EXIT procedure for securing a newborn airway, the EXIT procedure can be used as an adjunct to other life saving procedures, such as EXIT to ECMO or EXIT to lung/mass resection, and EXIT to catheterization lab.

EXIT to Extracorporeal Membrane Oxygenation

EXIT to ECMO is reserved for those fetuses with severe cardiac or pulmonary malformations in which separation from the placental blood flow would lead to immediate instability of the fetus. In these cases, EXIT to ECMO allows for the infant to obtain a secure airway and undergo arterial and venous ECMO cannulation while on placental support. In a select number of fetal centers, this strategy is employed for infants with congenital diaphragmatic hernias and a head:lung ratio < 1.0 with liver herniation into the chest or those with congenital diaphragmatic hernias and congenital heart disease. These babies maintain the highest mortality risk.

EXIT to ECMO is also valuable for those infants diagnosed with severe aortic stenosis or hypoplastic left heart syndrome that is accompanied by a restrictive atrial septum. This allows the neonate to be stabilized and transported to the catheterization laboratory to allow for emergent atrial septostomy. A team of Pediatric cardiologists and cardiac surgeons needs to be intimately involved in the care of these infants.

EXIT to ECMO avoids any periods of neonatal hypoxia or acidosis, allows for stabilization of the neonate and potential for therapeutic intervention.

EXIT to Resection

The EXIT to resection strategy allows for lung or mass resection while on placental support to aid in the ability to ventilate and oxygenate these infants postnatally. This strategy can be used for those congenital lung lesions that are large and causing significant mediastinal shift *in utero* and with mediastinal masses that compresses the trachea. Although the majority of thoracic masses remain asymptomatic at birth, those with a volume to head circumference ratio of > 1.6 are at significant risk for development of fetal hydrops as well as pulmonary compromise at birth.

PREPARATION FOR SURGERY

The EXIT procedure takes into account the two patients involved in the procedure, where anesthetic considerations are critical for both. In general fetal, gas exchange can be supported on placental circulation for approximately 60 mins (although there have been cases described of longer times, up to 2.5 hrs).[4,5]

Fetal Anesthesia

Fetal well-being throughout the EXIT procedure is dependent upon maintenance of the utero–placental gas exchange.[6] This relies upon both the umbilical arteries and the uterine arteries. Inhalation anesthetics decrease uterine tone but also decrease maternal blood pressure and thus placental blood flow. Maintenance of maternal blood pressure is critical to fetal oxygenation during the EXIT procedure, and this is accomplished by using vasoconstrictor agents such as ephedrine. Ephedrine selectively acts on maternal peripheral vascular resistance, while preserving placental circulation.

Umbilical blood flow is dependent upon fetal cardiac output, which is directly dependent upon fetal heart rate. Inhalation anesthetics can cause fetal myocardial depression and vasodilatation which may lead to fetal instability.

Fetal anesthesia is provided by the transplacental passage of the volatile anesthetic gas. Supplementation with intramuscular injection of atropine, fentanyl, and vecuronium to the fetus can also be given.

Maternal Anesthesia

The EXIT procedure requires two anesthesiologists, one for the mother and one for the fetus. Unlike standard obstetrical anesthesia, the EXIT procedure requires general anesthesia rather than regional anesthesia. The pregnancy itself places the mother at several risks including aspiration due to increased gastric acid production, decreased lower esophageal pressures and compression of the gravid uterus upon the stomach. In addition, hypotension easily occurs due to uterine compression of the IVC, expanded blood volume with a lower hematocrit and increased peripheral vasculature capacity.

Maternal anesthesia is induced via a rapid sequence of techniques followed by endotracheal intubation and maintenance of inhalation anesthesia.[7] The doses of volatile anesthetic agents during an EXIT procedure are much higher than for routine surgical procedures (2.5 MAC). Paralytic agents are essential. There have been reports of performing EXIT procedures under a combined spinal epidural anesthesia, although in general this is not preferred.[8]

There are two phases of anesthesia during an EXIT procedure, the first is induction and maintenance using either isoflurane or desflurane. This has to be deepened just prior to the maternal incision and again just before the hysterotomy to achieve uterine relaxation. Tocolytic agents can be used to help maintain uterine relaxation during the procedure and this includes terbutaline, indomethacin, or nitroglycerine. Uterine volume maintenance by amnioinfusion of Lactated Ringers solution and preventing the fetus from complete delivery are also critical in preventing uterine contractions.

The second critical timing in anesthesia comes at the anticipation of the end of the EXIT and the cord clamping. The coordination between surgery and anesthesia is critical at this point to prevent uterine atony and maternal hemorrhage. When it is anticipated that the surgeons will clamp the cord, the inhalation anesthetic is significantly decreased to allow uterine tone to return to normal and oxytocin is given via a IV infusion. Other measures to prevent uterine atony include uterine massage, and injection of methergine into the myometrium.

Intraoperative Considerations

Monitoring

Both maternal and fetal monitoring is required during an EXIT procedure. Maternal monitoring should include an arterial line for blood pressure monitoring, continuous EKG, pulse oximetry and end-tidal CO_2 monitoring as well. Fetal monitoring is critical during an EXIT and should include continuous pulse oximetry with a probe wrapped around the fetal hand.[9] Normal fetal saturation should remain 60–70%. Continuous fetal echocardiography is used to monitor cardiac function. Intravenous access is obtained and arterial and venous blood gases can be monitored via umbilical vessel puncture if necessary.

Procedure

The incision of choice is a low transverse abdominal incision; however this may need to be altered to a midline depending upon placental lie and indication for the EXIT. Before the hysterotomy the uterine tone is examined and inhalation anesthetics are adjusted accordingly. The placental edge should be mapped out using intraoperative ultrasound to avoid injury and hemorrhage. The positioning of the hysterotomy is determined by the placental lie. The hysterotomy is done using specially designed uterine staples to decrease bleeding. If polyhydramnios is present, it should be reduced by amnioreduction before the EXIT procedure. Polyhydramnios can flatten the placenta and can make mapping of the placenta difficult. In addition, placental separation and cord prolapse may occur when there is a sudden release in a large amount of amniotic fluid.

After the fetus is exposed, maintenance of uterine volume by amnioinfusion is critical to the remainder of the procedure to prevent contractions. This is accomplished by the continuous infusion of warmed Lactated Ringers solution.[10] Fetal exposure should be minimized and only the head, neck, and shoulders should be delivered to secure the airway (Figure 2).

After securing the airway, its position should be confirmed by flexible bronchoscopy. Surfactant can then be administered, if necessary, and the fetus is hand ventilated. Umbilical artery and venous catheters can then be placed as the cord is clamped. This is the critical moment during the procedure to prevent maternal complications. The newborn is then taken either to a second operating room for additional procedures or transferred to the neonatal intensive care unit for resuscitation and further management. Umbilical cord blood gases have been evaluated and have been shown to be normal, providing evidence that the utero–placental gas exchange is preserved during the EXIT procedure.[11]

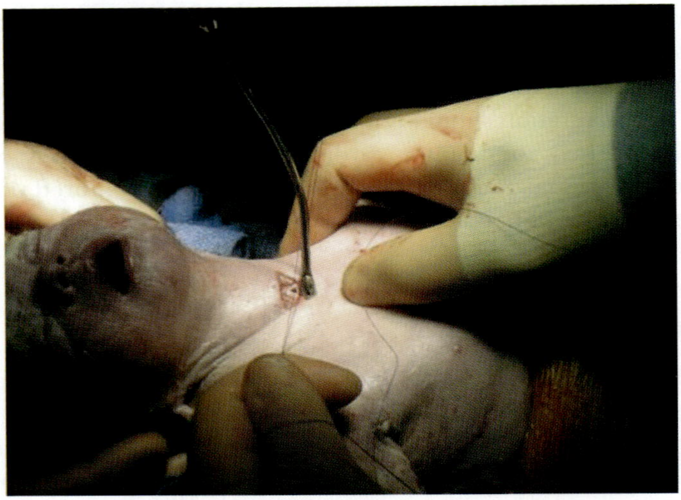

Figure 2. EXIT to airway procedure.

Note: The fetal head, shoulders and upper chest are delivered as the fetus remains connected to placental support and the airway is secured by tracheostomy.

Potential Pitfalls

The EXIT procedure adds a secondary operative risk to the mother as well as the fetus. There is an increased risk of maternal hemorrhage secondary to uterine hypotonia. Uterine hypotonia as previously mentioned is necessary for the procedure to maintain placental flow and oxygenation of the fetus, and is induced by using high concentrations of inhalation anesthetics. Reassuring prompt return of uterine tone minimizes maternal bleeding and in general, the blood loss for an EXIT procedure is equivalent to that of a caesarian section. Uterine atony is a major risk, and requires hysterectomy.

In addition, the risk of wound infections is higher after an EXIT procedure when compared to its caesarian-section counterpart.

The EXIT procedure is tailored to optimize fetal outcomes; however, there is the potential for fetal complications as well. Failure to preserve the utero–placental gas exchange can occur under a variety of conditions but are most likely secondary to placental abruption, loss of myometrial relaxation or kinking of the cord.

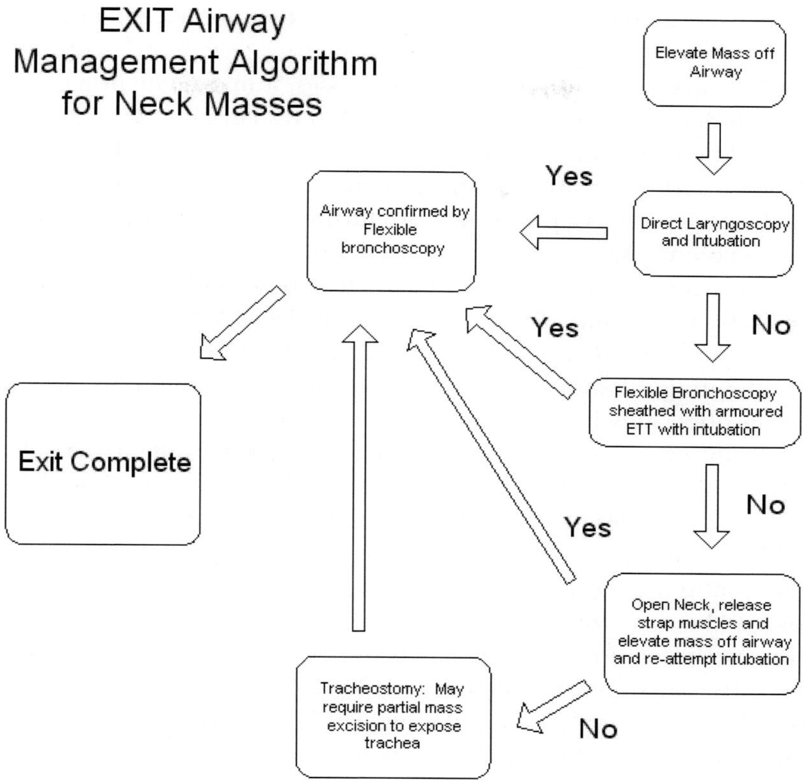

Figure 3. Algorithm for airway assessment during EXIT procedure.

The most important point in securing a fetal airway is to be prepared for anything and everything! Never assume that the fetus will be able to undergo direct laryngoscopy and endotracheal tube placement. Therefore, the following should always be planned for, "in case": Rigid bronchoscopy (2.5 and 3.0 scopes), flexible bronchoscopy, and a neck dissection with tracheotomy and/or mass resection. In some cases where laryngoscopy is not successful in allowing an endotracheal tube to pass, then a fiberoptic-guided intubation should be the next option. If both of these conservative approaches to the airway fail then a tracheotomy is the next step to secure an airway. Proper positioning of the tracheotomy is essential. If tracheotomy is necessary, care should be taken not to place the tracheotomy tube below the third tracheal ring. Remember that giant neck masses can pull the carina to the level of the thoracic inlet with neck hyperextension.

When managing obstructive neck masses, a management algorithm originally described by the Cincinnati Children's Hospital Medical Center and modified from our experience is efficiently followed.[12] Direct laryngoscopy is performed and an attempt to intubate is made. If unsuccessful, flexible endoscopy is performed to further assess laryngeal and tracheal anatomy. An appropriately sized armored endotracheal tube is sheathed over the endoscope to facilitate tube placement under direct visualization once the airway has been visualized. An armored endotracheal tube is used to avoid endotracheal tube collapse by tumor compression. Elevating the mass away from or off the trachea or larynx by gentle traction often aids in visualizing the airway, allowing successful intubation. If an adequate airway remains elusive, an assessment is made to whether the mass can be lifted away from the trachea following division of the strap muscles of the neck or whether a formal tracheostomy, with or without partial mass resection performed in order to visualize the trachea, is most appropriate. Additionally, an airway obstructed by a cystic mass may be visualized by simply aspirating the cystic component of the lesion. Such decisions are facilitated by preoperative knowledge of the fetus' airway anatomy obtained by fetal MRI. Once an appropriate airway is obtained at any stage along the algorithm and confirmed by flexible bronchoscopy, the EXIT procedure is terminated and the baby is transported to the neonatal intensive care unit (NICU) for further care and assessment.

SUMMARY

The EXIT procedure is an adjunct in the care of the fetus prenatally diagnosed with congenital anomalies of the neck and chest. It requires a well orchestrated group of maternal fetal medicine specialists, anesthesiologists, and pediatric surgeons. It has allowed for infant survival in what was previously considered fatal fetal conditions. The indications for the EXIT procedure are increasing as the safety to the mother and infant continue to improve. The EXIT procedure requires significant preoperative planning from all members of the multidisciplinary team, and every possibility must be taken into consideration prior to the elective scheduling of the procedure.

REFERENCES

1. Skarsgrad ED, Chitkara U, Krane EJ, *et al.* (1996) The OOPS procedure (operation on placental support): *In utero* airway management of the fetus with prenatally diagnosed tracheal obstruction. *J Pediatr Surg* **31**(6):826–828.
2. Mychaliska GB, Bealer JK, Graf JL, *et al.* (1997) Operating on placental support: The ex utero Intrapartum treatment procedure. *J Pediatr Surg* **32**(2):227–331.
3. Harrison MR, Adzick NS, Flake AW. (1996) Correction of congenital diagphragmatic hernia *in utero* VIII: Response of the hypoplastic lung to tracheal occlusion. *J Pediatr Surg* **31**:1119–1348.
4. Rahbar R, Wilkins-Haugh L, Levine D, *et al.* (2005) A new era in the diagnosis and management of fetal airway obstruction because of advances in prenatal imaging. *Arch Otol-Head and Neck Surg* **131**:393–398.
5. Hirose S, Sydorak RM, Tsao L, *et al.* (2003) Spectrum of intrapartum management strategies for giant fetal cervical teratoma. *J Pediatr Surg* **38**:446–450.
6. Gaiser RR, Kurth CD. (1999) Anesthetic considerations for fetal surgery. *Semin Perinatol* **23**:507–514.
7. Restrepo CE, Gomez ME, Puerta JJ, *et al.* (2006) Anaesthesia for the EXIT procedure: The value of fast track anaesthesia. *Internat J Clin Anesth* **15**:S43.
8. George RB, Melnick AH, Rose EC, *et al.* (2007) Case series: Combined spinal epidural anesthesia for caesarean delivery and ex utero intrapartum treatment procedure. *Canadian J Anaesth* **54**:218–222.
9. Marwan A, Crombleholme TM. (2006) The EXIT procedure: Principles, pitfalls and progress. *Semin Ped Surg* **15**:107–115.
10. Schwartz DA, Moriarty KP, Tashjian DB. (2001) Anesthetic management of the exit (*in utero* extrapartum treatment) procedure. *J Clin Anesth* **13**:387–391.
11. Bouchard S, Johnson MP, Flake AW, *et al.* (2002) The EXIT procedure: Experience and outcome in 31 cases. *J Pediatr Surg* **37**:418–426.
12. Marwan A, Crombleholme TM. (2006) The EXIT procedure: Principles, pitfalls, and progress. *Semin Pediatr Surg* **15**:107–115.

Section 2:
Trauma

EVALUATION AND RESUSCITATION OF THE INJURED CHILD

12

Thomas M. Rouse

INTRODUCTION

Every year thousands of children and adolescents die from injury, and permanent disability is suffered by many thousands more. Most of the disability is neurologic or orthopedic and may permanently change a life. Despite attempts at injury prevention, more children die from trauma than from all other causes. Once the child is injured, the aspect of trauma management that offers the greatest chance of limiting poor outcomes is rapid and effective resuscitation.

Resuscitation of the injured child includes the identification of all critical injuries, and the necessary interventions to reverse and stabilize the physiologic changes that occur as a result of the trauma. It begins with the recognition of a serious injury at the scene, stabilization in the field by Emergency Medical Services (EMS), ongoing evaluation in the emergency department, and definitive stabilization in the operating room and intensive care unit. This involves the ongoing reassessment for physiologic stability. Resuscitation is not complete until all life-threatening injuries have been definitively treated and the child displays physiologic stability without continued intervention.

Despite the frequency in which injured children are cared for in emergency departments, most injuries do not threaten the child's life. Only a fraction of children who present to emergency departments for evaluation and management of injury require admission, and approximately 10–15% have serious injuries. Nationally, fewer than 2% of injured children admitted to a hospital expire, mostly from overwhelming brain injury. The leading cause of fatal, unintentional injury among children is motor vehicle occupant injury (28%), followed by drowning (16%) and airway obstruction injury (14%). Falls are the leading cause (36%) of nonfatal injuries seen in hospital emergency rooms.

Intentional injury and death may result from homicide, child abuse, or suicide. Suspicion of any of these requires referral to Child Protective Services for investigation. The resuscitation of abused children is frequently difficult because there is often a delay in the child's presentation for medical care, with depletion of the child's physiologic reserve.

Most children die from their injuries within hours or days of the trauma. The late deaths from ongoing systemic inflammatory response syndrome (SIRS), as is seen in adults, is rare in children.

Resuscitation and Impact on Outcome

Resuscitation of an injured child includes the steps needed to reverse the alterations that occur as a result of injury, and then maintain the child's physiologic homeostasis. Resuscitation is not complete until all life-threatening injuries have been definitively treated, and the child shows ongoing physiologic stability.

Resuscitation of the injured child should follow the American College of Surgeons ATLS (Advanced Trauma Life Support) protocols of prioritizing the identification and treatment of life-threatening injuries. These priorities of treatment are derived from knowledge of injuries that may cause death within minutes to hours of injury. These injuries involve the CNS, chest, abdomen, and vascular systems. They require prompt and effective treatment during the "golden hour" after injury. The mechanism of injury is blunt in over 90% of injured children. The vast majority of seriously hurt children have multisystem injuries. Within the emergency department, the ATLS protocols can be implemented by a team trained in the rapid assessment and treatment of these injuries. The team leader is most often a pediatric surgeon or a surgeon credentialed in pediatric trauma care.

THE PRIMARY SURVEY

The ATLS protocol starts with a primary and secondary survey. The primary survey follows the "ABCDE" steps that lead to the diagnosis and initial treatment of life-threatening injuries. The priorities are the same for all injured patients, but there are important aspects of pediatric care that will be emphasized.

Airway and Cervical Spine Control

A patent and stable airway is the most important priority of pediatric trauma care. The inability to establish and maintain a child's airway, leading to hypoxia and inadequate ventilation, is the most common cause of cardiorespiratory arrest and death. Hypoxia is suspected when oxygen saturation is less than 93%. The assessment starts with evaluating for a patent airway. If a child is alert, breathing normally, and without stridor or distress, no airway intervention is needed. If the airway is not normal, inspection of the oral cavity is required with removal of debris, loose teeth and soft tissue fragments; and aspiration of blood and secretions with mechanical suction. Airway patency can be improved in a spontaneously breathing child by the use of jaw thrust or chin lift maneuvers.

An injured child who is in a coma, combative, in shock or has evidence of direct airway trauma requires endotracheal intubation. Nasal pharyngeal or oral pharyngeal airways may improve bag-valve mask ventilation, but this is a temporizing measure only, until definitive control is established. In most cases, oral tracheal intubation with in-line cervical stabilization is performed to establish airway control. Nasal tracheal intubation is rarely performed in injured children, even when a cervical spine injury is suspected.

Pediatric airway anatomy is unique and knowledge of this leads to efficient and safe endotracheal intubation. The child's larynx is anatomically more proximal and more anterior than in the adult, an upward angulation of the laryngoscope is needed to place the endotracheal tube properly. Removing the anterior half of the rigid cervical collar allows access to the neck for gentle cricoid pressure. The pediatric epiglottis is shorter, more flexible, and tilted posteriorly over the glottis. Because of this, direct control of the epiglottis with the straight blade is usually necessary for visualizing the vocal cords. The vocal cords themselves are fragile and easily damaged.

The narrowest point of the pediatric airway is the subglottic trachea at the cricoid ring, as opposed to the glottis in the adult patient. Therefore, passage of the endotracheal tube through the vocal cords does not guarantee safe advancement into the trachea. The correct-sized endotracheal tube selection must be placed. The internal diameter can range from 3.0 to 3.5 mm in newborns to 4.5 mm at 1 to 2 yrs of age. After 2 yrs, the internal diameter can be estimated by the following formula: **internal diameter = (age divided by 4) + 4**. Approximating the diameter of the patient's little finger is also useful. Because of the narrow subglottic trachea, an uncuffed endotracheal tube is indicated in children 8 yrs of age or younger.

The technique of intubation depends on the urgency of establishing an airway. In a hypotensive, hypoxic, or comatose child, oral tracheal intubation is performed after a short period of bag-valve mask ventilation with 100% oxygen. The most experienced physician in airway management should perform this intubation. In-line stabilization of the cervical spine is performed by another member of the trauma team.

In a more controlled situation, a rapid sequence induction is used to establish a stable airway. Following preoxygenation using bag-valve mask ventilation, children should receive atropine (0.01 to 0.02 mg/kg) to ensure that the heart rate remains stable during intubation, as the cardiac output is dependent on heart rate. Also, children should be premedicated with intravenous sedatives and muscle relaxants. Appropriate sedatives include short-acting barbiturates such as thiopental sodium (5.0 mg/kg) if the volume status is normal or a benzodiazepine such as midazolam (0.1 mg/kg) if hypovolemia is suspected. Fentanyl (1 mcg/kg) may also be used.

Muscle relaxation is achieved with short-acting nondepolarizing agents (vecuronium bromide 0.1 mg/kg) or short-acting depolarizing agents (succinylcholine chloride 1.0 mg/kg). The presence of burns and devitalized tissue precludes the use of succinylcholine because of the risk of hyperkalemia. Continuous monitoring of an intubated child with pulse oximetry is essential.

It is rare that endotracheal intubation is not possible; it may occur with severe maxillofacial trauma with hemorrhage or a laryngeal injury. In these circumstances a surgical airway is indicated. A surgical cricothyroidotomy is the preferred approach in children older than 10 yrs. The cricothyroid membrane is easily exposed through a transverse skin incision to accommodate placement of a small, uncuffed endotracheal tube. Morbidity is lower than with an emergency tracheostomy because of the superficial location of the cricothyroid membrane. The cricothyroidotomy should be converted to a formal tracheostomy when the child is stabilized, to avoid subglottic stenosis.

In smaller children, the cricoid cartilage is a delicate structure and provides the majority of support to the trachea. Injury to this membrane during emergency cricothyroidotomy can lead to significant morbidity and lifelong laryngotracheomalacia. To avoid this complication, children younger than 10 yrs should undergo needle cricothyroidotomy with jet insufflation of the trachea. A 16- to 18-gauge intravenous catheter is used to access the tracheal lumen through the cricothyroid membrane and is connected to a 100% oxygen source at a high flow rate of 10 to 12 L/min. Needle jet ventilation is limited in children by hypocarbia that occurs in about 30 mins; therefore, this method is effective for only a short time. Following stabilization of the child, endotracheal intubation or formal tracheostomy is necessary.

Breathing

Compromised breathing and ventilation in an injured child are usually the result of either head injury (decreased ventilatory drive) or thoracic injury (impaired lung expansion). Following chest injury, air, fluid, or viscera can compromise the pleural space. Compression of the pulmonary parenchyma can result in impaired gas exchange that is sufficient to produce respiratory distress. Mechanical ventilatory failure is life threatening and requires immediate treatment during the primary survey. Recognition of ventilatory compromise is usually not difficult. The sound of air movement at the mouth and nares are assessed as are the rate, depth, and effort of respiration. Asymmetrical excursion of the chest wall with inspiration suggests a ventilatory abnormality. Percussion shows hypo- or hyper-resonance, depending on the presence of fluid or air, respectively, in the pleural space, and breath sounds are decreased. With tension pneumothorax or hemothorax mediastinal shift is detected by tracheal deviation, displacement of the cardiac impulse, and distended neck veins from impaired venous return.

All injured children require supplemental oxygen by nasal cannula, mask, or endotracheal tube. Endotracheal intubation and assisted ventilation are sufficient to treat hypoventilation due to head injury, pain from rib fractures, flail chest and pulmonary contusion. Simple pneumothorax may be well tolerated with supplemental oxygen until tube thoracostomy can be performed after the primary survey. In cases of hemopneumothorax causing compromised ventilation or hypotension, tube thoracostomy is required, combined with endotracheal intubation and intravenous access for rapid fluid infusion.

If tension pneumothorax is present, the hemodynamic derangements can be minimized by needle thoracostomy in the second intracostal space at the mid-clavicular line, followed by thoracostomy tube placement in the anterior axillary line of the fifth intercostal space. A chest tube of adequate caliber to evacuate blood and air should be inserted into the pleural space. The narrow intercostal space of a small child usually limits the size of the tube, the largest caliber tube that can be placed should be used. The tube is placed in the mid-axillary line at the nipple level (fourth or fifth intercostal space), to avoid intraabdominal placement through an elevated diaphragm. The tube is directed posterior and towards the apex of the chest, to evacuate both blood and air, and is connected to a closed suction drainage system set at −15 cm of water. Initial drainage of greater than 20 mL/kg requires emergent chest exploration. Persistent hemorrhage from a thoracostomy tube is uncommon in children; however, drainage of 1 to 2 mL/kg/hr for 2 hrs is a sign of significant ongoing bleeding from a vascular or mediastinal injury that may require a thoracotomy to identify and control.

In traumatic rupture of the diaphragm, loss of muscular integrity also has a direct effect on lung expansion. The child's mediastinum is extremely mobile; as pressure increases in the pleural space, the mediastinum is displaced to the opposite side, causing compression of the contralateral lung. The distortion of mediastinal vascular structures, along with elevated intrathoracic pressures, can result in a critical reduction in venous return and refractory hypotension. Urgent laparotomy is indicated for a diagnosed traumatic rupture of the diaphragm, as intraabdominal injuries are commonly identified.

Loss of chest wall integrity from flail chest impairs ventilation and oxygenation. Consequently, paradoxical chest wall movement occurs during inspiration, preventing lung expansion. Intubation and assisted positive pressure ventilation is the best treatment. Because of the flexible nature of the child's chest, the substantial force required to fracture multiple ribs is transmitted to the underlying lung parenchyma, resulting in a pulmonary contusion. Parenchymal hemorrhage and edema impair ventilation perfusion mismatch, decrease pulmonary compliance, and result in an increase in the work of breathing, each leading to ventilatory failure.

Circulation and Vascular Access

The third priority in the primary survey is the rapid assessment of circulation and the establishment of venous access. Seriously injured children often have normal vital signs, even with a significant decrease in circulating blood volume; their cardiovascular reserve delays the early hemodynamic signs of hypovolemia until late in the resuscitation phase. A high index of suspicion based on the mechanism of injury and continuous careful evaluation of physiologic parameters and clinical signs are necessary to minimize morbidity.

Normal mental status is a reliable sign of adequate profusion. As the child is resuscitated, clinical signs of an adequate resuscitation should be monitored. Improvement in the physical signs correlates with hemodynamic stability and effective resuscitation. These include slowing down of the heart to less than 100 beats/min, increased systolic pressure to >90 mm Hg, improved capillary refill to <2 secs, clearing of the sensorium, increased warmth of the extremities, increased pulse pressure(<20 mm Hg), and adequate urinary output.

After establishment of an adequate airway, obtaining secure venous access in a hypovolemic child is often a challenge. Two functioning intravenous catheters are needed when there is significant injury. Optimally, venous access should be achieved above and below the diaphragm, given the potential for extravasation of resuscitation fluid from an intraabdominal venous injury. However, in small children any peripheral venous access is useful.

Two to three attempts should be made to place a large bore peripheral line in the upper extremities. If percutaneous placement is unsuccessful, insertion of an interosseous line is useful in a child younger than 6 yrs. An interosseous line is a simple, reliable, and safe route for the administration of fluids, blood products, and medications. This technique is applicable to children who are 6 yrs of age and younger because the marrow is well perfused in early childhood. The preferred site for interosseous insertion is through the flat anterior medial surface of the tibia about to 3 cm below the tibial plateau. The needle is angled 60° from horizontal and pointed toward the foot. The cortex is penetrated and the marrow cavity is detected by aspirating blood and particulate material. Alternative sites include the midline distal femur, 3 cm above the condyles directed proximally in small children and the distal tibia above medial malleolus. Specifically designed interosseous needles should be available in the pediatric resuscitation room to facilitate this maneuver. The complication rate is low, but includes osteomyelitis, cellulitis, fracture, growth plate injury, fat embolism, and compartment syndrome.

In children older than 6 yrs, a venous cut down can be performed at the ankle. The greater saphenous vein is easily exposed through short transverse incisions 0.5 to 1 cm proximal and anterior to the medial malleolus. The exposed vein is suspended by the ligature and the largest appropriate intravenous catheter is introduced into the vessel lumen under direct vision. Central venous catheterization can result in significant complications, such as laceration of the subclavian or femoral artery or vein, making it a less useful technique that should be used with caution. The femoral route is often preferred because of ease of access. If subclavian access is necessary, the child should be placed in the Trendelenburg position with the head maintained in a neutral position without the placement of a posterior shoulder roll. In experienced hands, central venous catheters provide secure venous access and can be placed with acceptable morbidity. Physicians with limited experience with this procedure in infants and small children should not attempt placement.

As soon as vascular access is established, fluid resuscitation with a bolus of fluid is begun. Generally, isotonic crystalloid solution, such as Lactated Ringers is administered in 20 mL/kg increments. If evidence of hypovolemia persists after resuscitation of 40 mL/kg has been given, transfusion of ABO-matched packed red blood cells is initiated in a bolus of 10 mL/kg. All fluids (crystalloid, colloid, and blood) should be warmed during infusion. This is best accomplished using inline, fluid warming devices.

It is important to continually reassess the child's response to resuscitation, to characterize the extent of the injuries, and to avoid the complications of excessive fluid resuscitation. As perfusion is restored, the rate of fluid infusion is gradually reduced. If hemodynamic instability persists with crystalloid and blood resuscitation, hemorrhage is likely from intraabdominal or pelvic source. In children, scalp and facial lacerations can bleed in large volumes and contribute to hypotension. If these sites are bleeding, secure rapidly with staples or temporary sutures.

When hypotension persists in the emergency department, the operating room should be placed on alert for a possible laparotomy or thoracotomy. A focused abdominal sonography in blunt abdominal trauma (FAST) of the abdomen and pericardium should be performed. If there is fluid in the pericardium, fluid resuscitation should continue and a pericardiocentesis is performed. If blood is aspirated, an urgent thoracotomy in the operating room is indicated to repair the injury, usually a cardiac rupture. If moderate to large amounts of fluid are seen in the abdomen with ongoing hypotension, a laparotomy is indicated.

Other causes of hypotension include cardiac dysfunction due to myocardial contusion, tension hemothorax or pneumothorax that has developed after initial examination, severe brain and spinal cord injuries; and profound hypothermia.

Disability

A rapid neurologic assessment is part of the primary survey to evaluate gross cerebral function. The alert, voice, pain, unresponsive (AVPU) pneumonic details the level of alertness, voice response, and pain response. Pupillary response is also documented. The findings may indicate life-threatening central nervous system (CNS) injury. Pupillary dilation and loss of light reflex may indicate transtentorial herniation, but occurs with direct eye injury. Decorticate or decerebrate posturing is seen in loss of brain function, either cerebral or global, and is associated with elevated intracranial pressure (ICP). Children with these findings need urgent endotracheal intubation, controlled moderate hyperventilation (pCO_2 30–35 mm Hg), fluid resuscitation to establish normal hemodynamics, and intravenous mannitol (0.25 g/kg). Urgent evaluation by a neurosurgeon is required.

Exposure

A complete physical examination is required, and exposure of the child's body is necessary for this. In the alert child, this is best performed in stages and the child does not need all clothing removed at the same time. Hypothermia is an important factor in the effective resuscitation of the pediatric patient, especially small children. Warming the resuscitation room and intravenous fluids are helpful. Overhead radiant warmers can be used for infants, but forced air warmers are used in older children.

Resuscitation Phase

Essential to resuscitation is ongoing evaluation of the child's response to treatment. Deterioration at any point requires a thorough reevaluation with the primary survey. Once the ABCDE's are complete and life-threatening injuries are stable, a gastric tube and urinary catheter is placed, followed by the drawing of blood for analysis and placement of a cardiac monitor. In children, acute gastric dilatation can cause both respiratory compromise and vagal-mediated bradycardia and gastric decompression to evacuate the stomach and reduce the risk of vomiting with aspiration, especially those with a decreased level of consciousness. Assessment for midface fractures and for the presence of cerebrospinal fluid rhinorrhea is necessary before the placement of a nasogastric tube for decompression. If the assessment is abnormal, an orogastric tube is placed. A urinary catheter is also placed after a thorough perineal assessment, including a rectal examination. In instances of a high riding prostate, meatal bleeding, perineal or scrotal ecchymosis, or unstable anterior pelvic fracture, a retrograde urethrogram is indicated before insertion of a catheter.

An electrocardiogram is used to monitor cardiac rhythm. Abnormalities are occasionally seen and include sinus bradycardia due to advanced shock; electromechanical dissociation from hypovolemia, tension pneumothorax, or pericardial tamponade; and ventricular fibrillation due to hypothermia or acidosis. Ventricular dysrhythmia, low voltages, and signs of ischemia occur with myocardial contusion. Diffuse low voltage may be the first indication of a hemopericardium. After vascular access is obtained, blood and urine are sent for laboratory analyses, including complete blood count, urinalysis, and arterial blood gas analysis. Blood alcohol level and toxicology screen are routinely obtained in children over 12 yrs of age in many pediatric trauma centers. Blood should be sent for type and cross match.

SECONDARY SURVEY

After the primary survey and life-threatening injuries have been stabilized, a detailed search for specific injuries is performed. If, at any time during this activity, the child deteriorates, the primary survey is repeated to stabilize the patient. The secondary survey is a head to toe examination. Life-threatening injuries that evolve over a few hours from injury must be identified. These most often involve the CNS, chest, abdomen, and skeleton.

CNS Injuries

The goal of resuscitation of the child with a brain injury is to prevent secondary brain injury. The initial brain injury occurs with the traumatic event, the secondary injury is most often due to hypoxia, hypotension, or cerebral edema. Early intubation with controlled ventilation improves oxygenation, fluid resuscitation improves blood pressure and perfusion to the brain, and moderate hyperventilation (pCO_2 30–35 mm Hg) can lessen cerebral edema. The Glasgow Coma Score (GCS) measures the severity of the brain injury. Ongoing resuscitation attempts to maximize cerebral perfusion pressure (CPP) by normalizing mean arterial pressure (MAP), and lowering ICP. Seizures are treated with intravenous Dilantin (10 mg/kg). Prompt neurosurgical consultation is critical.

Spinal cord injuries are uncommon in children, especially less than 8 yrs. They can occur without radiologic abnormality (SCIWORA). The signs of spinal cord injury include paralysis and lack of sensation below the level of injury, hypotension, loss of rectal tone, and priapism. Blunt spinal cord injuries are treated with methylprednisolone within the initial 8 hrs after injury. The initial dose is 30 mg/kg over 30 mins, followed in 45 mins with an infusion of 5.4 mg/kg/h for 23 hrs.

Clinical signs or symptoms that suggest an intracranial injury include a skull fracture, loss of consciousness, altered mental status, focal neurologic findings, age less than 3 months, and lack of a history consistent with physical findings. An urgent computed tomography (CT) of the head should be performed for those indications.

Chest Injuries

Most (85%) thoracic injuries in children can be identified and treated at the bedside. These include airway obstruction, tension pneumothorax, hemothorax, and cardiac tamponade. Fifteen to twenty percent of seriously injured children have a chest injury, so these are a marker for more severely injured children. The blunt force that causes most pediatric chest injuries is initially absorbed by the chest wall. Since the ribs are more flexible in children than adults, rib fractures occur less often. The force is then absorbed by the lungs and pulmonary contusions are common in children. Traumatic asphyxia from chest compression is seen with some frequency in children, and this is associated with thoracic and abdominal injuries. The child's mobile mediastinum leads to a higher incidence of tension pneumothorax in children.

Important aspects of chest injuries in children:

(1) Hemothorax — place a thoracostomy tube that is the appropriate size in the child's fifth intercostals in the mid-axillary line. If a large hemothorax is present, establish secure IV access before placing the tube. Thoracotomy is indicated for initial volume greater than 20 mL/kg, or for ongoing bleeding greater than 2 mL/kg for 2 hrs.
(2) Massive subcutaneous emphysema, hemoptysis, and dyspnea are signs of an airway injury. A large pneumothorax that does not resolve with thoracostomy tube placement may indicate an airway injury as well. Cardiopulmonary collapse with intubation and mechanical ventilation may occur with these injuries and this may be temporized by positioning the endotracheal tube distally in the trachea or in the mainstem bronchus opposite to the pneumothorax. Bronchoscopy and repair is urgently performed.
(3) Blunt aortic tear is uncommon in children and when seen, it is most often in adolescents. Rapid deceleration is the mechanism of injury. Chest X-ray findings are not diagnostic but the following require further evaluation: Widened mediastinum, loss of the aortic knob contour, depressed left mainstem bronchus, deviation of the trachea or esophagus to the right, left apical cap, and left hemothorax. A spiral CT with IV contrast is the most available screening exam.
(4) Cardiac contusion occurs with blunt trauma to the chest. These are not common but usually present with arrhythmias. When suspected, the child needs continuous EKG monitoring and an echocardiogram is obtained.
(5) A child less than 3 yrs with two or more rib fractures should be evaluated for nonaccidental injuries.
(6) Blunt cardiac rupture, when not fatal at the scene, presents as refractory hypotension despite ongoing resuscitation, muffled heart tones, and jugular venous distension. A FAST examination is performed. If hemopericardium is present, blood is aspirated via a subxiphoid approach and urgent thoracotomy is performed.

ABDOMINAL INJURIES

The evaluation for abdominal injuries includes physical examination to evaluate for abrasions, contusions, distension, and tenderness. Gastric decompression should be performed early. Most injuries are from blunt mechanisms and multisystem injuries are again common. The following are important in the diagnosis of abdominal injuries:

(1) Placement of Nasogastric (NG)/Orogastric (OG) tube and placement of foley if no sign of urethral injury.
(2) CT scan for suspicion of abdominal injury.
(3) FAST for rapid evaluation, especially if child remains hypotensive with resuscitation.
The need for transfusion in the emergency department (ED) indicates significant blood loss of at least 25% of the blood volume. If not obvious by exam, it is most likely a solid organ injury — liver, spleen, or kidney — or a pelvic fracture. It is less likely to be due to long bone fractures.
(4) Repeat physical examination is an essential component of care of the injured child.
(5) Certain mechanisms of injury cause patterns of abdominal injury that must be recognized forearly diagnosis.

The compression injury that seatbelts — especially poorly fitting belts — is associated with hollow viscous injury and lumbar spine injuries. The bowel trauma may be perforation with early signs and symptoms, mesenteric tears with only a small amount of bleeding that result in delayed perforation due to ischemia, or bowel obstruction from a stricture usually 2–4 wks after injury.

The lumbar vertebral injury is often a compression fracture or a fracture dislocation with neurologic deficit. The neurologic deficit may be present on arrival to the ED, but may only occur with movement in the hospital if "spine precautions" are not initiated until the spine is evaluated.

Handlebar injury due to direct compression by the end of the bar into the abdominal wall is associated with hollow viscous and pancreatic injuries. A high index of suspicion is required for early diagnosis.

EXTREMITY INJURIES

At least 40% of injured children have orthopedic injuries. During the secondary survey, it is essential that those bone or joint injuries that are life- or limb-threatening are identified and treatment initiated.

Important aspects of skeletal injuries include:

(1) 40% of children hospitalized with traumatic injury will have a fracture or other orthopedic injury.
(2) Signs of child abuse include rib fractures, long bone injuries, and multiple fractures of differing ages. There is often a vague or varying history of injury from the same or multiple caregivers.
(3) Open fractures are common and require incision and drainage and stabilization within 8 hrs of injury. This includes any fracture with a skin laceration that is near the injury. Antibiotics are started — usually a cephalosporin and aminoglycoside. Penicillin is added with a highly-contaminated wound, as in a farm-related injury. Tetanus status should be confirmed, and if in doubt, a booster should be given.
(4) Fractures of the mid- or distal humerus and femur are associated with vascular injuries, as are dislocations of the knee. The vascular status of the injured extremity must be evaluated and documented. Fractures should be splinted and stabilized in the position of injury. If there is a pulse deficit the fracture should be splinted in anatomic position. If a pulse deficit remains, urgent vascular repair is indicated with fracture stabilization.
(5) Compartment syndrome may result from crush injury or from prolonged or ongoing ischemia of an injured extremity. Pain with movement is often extreme. Other signs of ischemia are the five "P"s of pallor, pulselessness, paresthesias, and paralysis. A high level of suspicion for the development of ischemia is the key to early detection. Compartment pressures that are measured at the bedside above 30 mm Hg require an urgent four compartment fasciotomy.

SUMMARY

Unintentional injury is the leading cause of death and permanent disability in children. Blunt trauma occurs in 90% of children hospitalized for their injuries. Some are so severely injured that they die at the scene or in emergency departments. Ten to fifteen percent of injured children are hospitalized with life-threatening injuries and the prompt and careful evaluation and treatment of these injuries will minimize morbidity and reduce mortality.

REFERENCES

1. Cooper A. (2010) Early assessment and management of trauma. In: GW Holcomb III, JP Murphy (eds.), *Ashcraft's Pediatric Surgery,* 5th edition, pp. 167–181. Saunders, Philadelphia.
2. Lukish JL, Eichelberger MR. (2006) Accident victims and their emergency management. In: JL Grosfeld, JA O'Neill Jr, EW Fonkalsrud, AG Coran (eds.), *Pediatric Surgery,* 6th edition, pp. 265–274. Mosby, Philadelphia.

THORACIC INJURIES IN CHILDREN 13

L. R. "Tres" Scherer

Traumatic injuries remain a primary mode of morbidity and mortality in children. There are a number of important clinical differences that must be recognized between adult and pediatric trauma patients, and these differences make the evaluation and management of the injured child a challenge for the general clinician and pediatric trauma specialists.

Chest trauma comprises less than 5% of pediatric injuries, but it is the second leading cause of death in pediatric trauma. The clinician must have the knowledge of the pathophysiological changes of the chest, lungs, and heart as they affect the airway, breathing, and hemodynamics of the injured child. This chapter will delineate these life-threatening injuries into the respiratory, chest wall, and mediastinal trauma.

EPIDEMIOLOGICAL FACTORS AND PATTERNS OF INJURIES

Despite growing national attention, traumatic injury remains the single most common source of morbidity and mortality in children age 1 to 14 yrs. Although thoracic injury accounts for only 5–12% of the admissions to trauma centers, it may be associated with greater lethality.[1–3] In isolation, thoracic trauma in children carries a 5% mortality. However, this increases to 25% when head or abdominal injuries are superimposed. The combined presence of head, chest, and abdominal injuries may be fatal in nearly 40%.[2,4]

Despite geographical differences in modes of injuries, most chest injuries in children result from blunt trauma. Infants and toddlers are most often the victim of blunt trauma due to motor-vehicle-related injuries, falls or intentional (abusive) injury, whereas school-aged children are frequently injured because of transport-related mechanisms, such as bicycles, scooters, automobiles, or off-road vehicles.[5] Teenagers are more likely to be injured in high-energy motor and off-road vehicle collisions, sports injuries, personal violence, and suicide. Their risk is amplified by the coincident use of illegal drugs and alcohol. The evolution of "extreme" sports may carry greater risk of profound injury. These activities of the mountains, deserts, and water are characterized by increased physical risk due to the potential for high-energy impacts, limited safety precautions, and medical attention requiring long transport. Such a difference can be noted on the winter slopes; 6.1% of injured snowboarders sustained chest trauma, whereas only 2.7% of skiers had similar injuries.[6]

Children undergo constant growth and change and consequently have anatomic, physiologic, psychological, and epidemiologic differences through childhood. They have age-related limitations on their ability to comprehend their injuries, cooperate with care, and to communicate. Thus, any consideration of their care must pay attention to age-specific variations, the potential for recovery via growth, and the implications for a lifetime of recovery and productivity.[3,5]

PATHOPHYSIOLOGY OF CHEST INJURIES

Chest wall, mediastinal, and intrathoracic injuries may present in children as isolated or combined injuries. Children have a unique response to thoracic trauma, perhaps because of differences in anatomy, physiology, and mechanisms of injury. It is important to keep in mind that children physiologically compensate hemodynamically despite significant blood loss, although they are more at risk to hypoxemia. Cardiac output is largely determined by heart rate and preload because contractility is largely fixed. Hence, circulatory compromise is heralded by tachycardia and hypoxia long before hypotension. This concept is of paramount importance when gauging the cardiopulmonary status of the pediatric trauma patient. Rare pediatric injuries, such as cardiac trauma and great vessel injury, may remain undiagnosed because of the paucity of presenting symptoms.[2] Holmes in 2002 revealed six predictors of thoracic injury in children sustaining blunt trauma to the torso to include: (1) Low-systolic blood pressure, (2) Tachypnea, (3) Abnormal thoracic examination findings, (4) Abnormal chest auscultation findings, (5) Femur fracture, and a (6) Glasgow coma scale score of less than 15.[7] Children with any of these predictors of thoracic injury should undergo chest radiography. Conversely, children without any of the predictors have a very low likelihood of thoracic injury. Infants and children have more compliant or elastic chest walls and a mobile mediastinum. Due to greater elasticity of the chest wall in children, traumatic force to the chest wall permits transmission of intrathoracic energy without resulting in rib fractures. Consequently, pulmonary contusions are more common and rib fractures occur less frequently.[3]

Importantly, although thoracic trauma in children is an infrequent but potentially lethal injury, coexistent injuries are frequent. Injury to the central nervous system is the most common injury that increases the morbidity and mortality of chest trauma. Thoracic injuries are therefore a reliable marker for injury severity in children. Significant injuries to vital thoracic structures are associated with mortality rates in excess of 20%.[2]

LIFE-THREATENING CHEST INJURIES

Pulmonary Contusion

Pulmonary contusions are the most commonly encountered thoracic injury in children.[8] Direct lung injury usually manifests as nonanatomic areas of consolidation not associated with rib fractures, chest wall bruising, or other external manifestations of trauma. It most commonly occurs after a motor-vehicle injury and is associated with rapid deceleration of the thorax.

Pulmonary contusions are produced by a combination of shearing and bursting effects on the lung parenchyma that result in alveolar disruption, alveolar hemorrhage, and interstitial edema.[2] Progressive inflammation and edema of the lung parenchyma occurs within the first 24 to 48 hrs after injury and can result in ventilation/perfusion mismatch, intrapulmonary shunting, increased lung water, decreased lung compliance, atelectasis, and pulmonary consolidation. Clinically significant pulmonary contusions present with hypoxemia, hypercarbia, and tachypnea, but their presentation may range from simple abnormalities seen on a chest X-ray to severe respiratory distress. The clinical course of pulmonary contusion varies with the extent of injury. Initial chest X-rays are diagnostic in 85–97% of children, but a normal X-ray does not exclude this injury. Radiographic changes may not become apparent for 4 to 6 hrs after injury and include consolidation or edema of the lung parenchyma. Helical chest computerized tomography (CT) can demonstrate pulmonary contusions not evident on chest X-rays.[9] Past studies have correlated with the findings on chest CT with the need of ventilator support, finding injury to more than 28% of the lung is predictive of the need for ventilatory support.[8] A more recent study in children reveals the severity of lung contusion determined by chest radiograph, not CT, correlates with impairment of oxygenation, CO2 exchange and duration of ventilator support.[10] The treatment for pulmonary contusions is usually supportive, consisting of adequate analgesia, supplemental oxygen, chest physical therapy, and good pulmonary toilet. Judicious fluid resuscitation and strict attention to fluid management may limit alveolar edema. With appropriate treatment, most pulmonary contusions resolve in 7 to 10 days. Overall 20% to 37% of children with pulmonary contusions require mechanical ventilation.[9] Conventional ventilator support is adequate in most cases though occasionally high frequency oscillatory ventilation, inhaled nitric oxide, or extracorporeal life support are necessary.[2]

Secondary complications of pulmonary contusion remain disturbingly common. Half of those who develop respiratory insufficiency will do so in the first few hours after injury. Approximately 20% of affected children develop pneumonia, and this may progress to respiratory failure. True adult respiratory distress syndrome occurs in 5–20% of cases.[2] Death directly attributable to pulmonary contusion and its complications is fortunately rare in children.

Pneumothorax and Hemothorax

Lung contusions and penetrating injuries may be accompanied by pneumothorax and/or hemothorax as a consequence of air or blood leaking from the injured parenchyma into the pleural space. In almost half the cases, these lesions are associated injuries. Other intrathoracic injuries causing pneumothorax or hemothorax include tracheobronchial injuries, intercostal, or mammary vessel injury, heart puncture and/or major vessel injury. Prompt diagnosis is therefore necessary. Minor pneumothorax produces relatively mild clinical symptoms that are mixed with those of lung parenchymal damage: tachypnea, distress, decreased saturation. These injuries may have no clinical symptoms and noted only by CT scan.

However, if the involved hemithorax is distended, hyperresonant to percussion and without breath sounds or crackles on auscultation prompt drainage by thoracostomy is required. When there is tension pneumothorax, distension is massive, there is major distress, the mediastinal structures are displaced to the contralateral side, and venous return may be compromised.[3]

Tension pneumothorax is a life-threatening condition, and needle or tube thoracostomy should be carried out expeditiously. Rapid drainage of the pressurized air usually provides immediate relief of symptoms and improvement of the associated signs. As noted by the physical findings, if suspected, treatment of tension pneumothorax should be instituted before obtaining a chest radiograph. Other conditions may mimic tension pneumothorax, including pulmonary embolism, hemothorax, right mainstem intubation, and cardiac tamponade.

Hemothorax occurs in 13% to 29% of children with blunt chest injuries and is associated with 57% mortality. The most common sources for significant intrapleural blood are lacerated intercostal vessels or pulmonary parenchymal lacerations, but hemothorax may also be indicative of a great vessel injury. In the pediatric patient, each hemithorax has the capacity to hold 40% of a child's blood volume, and 14% of pediatric blunt chest injuries result in clinically relevant hemothorax with hemodynamic changes.[2] When diagnosed, blood should be promptly evacuated from the pleural space with tube thoracostomy. Whereas plain film radiography does not allow for estimation of the volume of blood loss in a hemothorax and a CT of the chest provides no further clinical information, a thoracostomy provides a means for accurate measurement of the volume of blood and monitoring of the rate of blood loss. Furthermore, tube thoracostomy enables the clinician to make appropriate decisions regarding resuscitation and the need for operative repair. Retained hemothorax may lead to the development of an empyema or fibrothorax. Retained intrathoracic blood should be evacuated early by thoracotomy or thoracoscopy.[9]

Traumatic Asphyxia

Traumatic asphyxia is characterized by cyanosis, subconjunctival hemorrhages, facial edema and petechial hemorrhages on the chest, face, and neck. Intrathoracic pressure increases suddenly and forces venous blood in the chest into the great veins of the head and arms, producing petechial hemorrhages. The most common mechanism of injury is motor-vehicle-related, followed by falls and compression due to a heavy object.[9]

Rarely, children may present with neurological deficits and coma due to cerebral edema and hypoxia and hypoventilation due to sustained compression to the chest wall. However, almost all cases of traumatic asphyxia are self-limited and reversible and are rarely life-threatening.[4]

INJURIES TO THE THORACIC CAGE

Rib Fractures

Rib fractures rarely occur in the pediatric patient, likely due in part to increased elasticity of the pediatric rib cage, occurring in only 1–2% of trauma victims, and flail chest occurring in only 1–2% of children with rib fractures. However, their presence may be associated with other severe injuries. Rib fractures, when they do occur in children, result from significant forces, including automobile collisions, pedestrian crashes and intentional injury.[9] Seventy percent of children with two or more rib fractures had multisystem injuries, compared to 12% of children with one rib fracture. Rib fractures that occur in children less than 12 mths of age should alert the clinician to the possibility of birth trauma, child abuse, or bone fragility.[11] Rib fractures associated with abusive trauma are believed to result from anterior–posterior compression of the chest, typically during shaking. Posterior rib fractures are thought to be specific for child abuse. However, it is important to point out that rib fractures secondary to birth trauma are often posteriorly located near the costovertebral junction. Rib fractures in children under 3 yrs of age are highly suggestive of intentional injury and are nearly 100% predictive when causes of unintentional injury and medical conditions have been excluded.[11] Multiple rib fractures are a marker of severe injury in children and have been associated with high mortality rates (40–50%) and rises to over 70% when they occur with traumatic brain injury. In fact, the risk of death increases with the number of fractured ribs. In addition, the likelihood of hepatic or splenic injury was found to be greater for patients with multiple rib fractures.

The diagnosis of rib fractures is often made through the use of plain radiographs of the chest. However, to complete the diagnostic evaluation of injuries associated with broken ribs may require computerized tomography without or with angiography.[2] The management of rib fractures is primarily supportive. The goal is to prevent atelectasis and pneumonia, which is usually best achieved with analgesia and deep-breathing measures such as incentive spirometry. It may also be necessary to drain intrathoracic collections of air or fluid if pulmonary expansion is compromised.

MEDIASTINAL INJURIES

Pericardial Tamponade

Pericardial tamponade is a life-threatening condition and must be recognized and treated immediately. Blood accumulating within the pericardial sac leads to decreased cardiac output. Importantly, the findings of muffled heart tones, distended neck veins, and hypotension may be difficult to recognize in the emergent setting. Pericardial tamponade may be accompanied by syncope, altered mental status or severe agitation.[12,13] The evaluation for suspected cardiac tamponade begins with the suspicion of hypovolemia, shock and poor cardiac output not responsive to volume replacement. The definitive test is cardiac ultrasound.[12] Early use of echocardiography may improve survival. Pericardiocentesis is a resuscitative intervention for pericardial tamponade prior to pericardial window and mediastinal exploration.

Cardiac Contusion

The most common cardiac injury to occur in children is cardiac contusion. Cardiac contusion often occurs from direct blows or trauma associated with motor-vehicle collision. Cardiac contusion may present as chest pain, arrhythmia, or unexplained hypotension. Although cardiac-specific enzymes such as cardiac troponin I may be diagnostic[13,14] elevated levels of the "cardiac enzyme" creatinine kinase are considered not predictive of cardiac contusion, and neither are predictive of severity or management. Twelve-lead electrocardiography may show ST ischemic changes, premature beats, sinus tachycardia, or atrial arrhythmias. Echocardiography is instrumental in the presence of arrhythmia or hypotension. It is helpful in determining cardiac performance and evaluating for structural injury.[14,15]

The management of cardiac contusion is mainly supportive. It is rare for hemodynamically stable patients who present with a normal sinus rhythm at admission to develop subsequent cardiac arrhythmia or cardiac failure. Thus, stable patients who do not require monitoring for other injuries should only be monitored in an inpatient setting if there are abnormalities on electrocardiogram. In that case, children should be placed on a continuous cardiac monitor with frequent measurement of blood pressure. Significant hemodynamic changes should prompt the use of echocardiography to determine the extent of cardiac injury. Inotropic agents may be necessary to reestablish normal perfusion, but these agents can increase myocardial oxygen consumption and irritability.[2,14,15]

Great Vessels

Great vessel injuries in young children are substantially rarer than in adolescents and adults. The mean age of children sustaining blunt aortic injury is 12 yrs, and less than 10% of cases occur in children less than 10 yrs. Sixty to eighty percent of children with aortic injury have sustained additional non-thoracic injuries.[15] Almost all injuries are associated with motor-vehicle impact as a passenger, driver or pedestrian, and a severe deceleration force. Other causes include falls and severe off-road crashes. The diagnosis remains elusive due to the rarity of this injury. The mechanism of injury and an abnormal chest radiograph demonstrating a wide mediastinum, loss of the aortic knob or strip, deviation of the esophagus or first rib fracture are signs of an injury. Helical CT of the chest with intravenous contrast is sensitive and provides an accurate negative prediction when normal.[16] Transesophageal echocardiography may be helpful, and arch aortography remains the gold standard in defining the injury, most commonly at the level of the ligamentum arteriosum of the descending aorta. Operative intervention is the mainstay of therapy in the stable patient with techniques including clamp and sew vs. left sided bypass to maintain distal perfusion. In children the surgeon may consider primary anastomosis over synthetic graft if the child has significant growth potential. Newer management techniques include beta-blockade to minimize shear stress of the arterial wall and stabilize the risk of rupture while treating other life-threatening injuries.[16,17]

Tracheobronchial Disruption

Injuries to the trachea or bronchi normally result from blunt trauma. These injuries are unusual in children but can be rapidly fatal (up to one third within an hour of injury) requiring high index of suspicion and urgent evaluation. The rarity of the injury is probably a result of the flexibility and mobility of the pediatric mediastinum. Most injuries occur close to the carina, involving either the distal trachea or proximal bronchi.[3]

Bronchial injuries will usually present with massive pneumothorax, subcutaneous emphysema, hemoptysis, and hypotension. Rupture involving more distal structures may present as a tension pneumothorax. Most children will present with history of high acceleration or deceleration injury. The diagnosis of a bronchial injury is usually made via plain chest radiograph, chest CT scan, and/or bronchoscopy.[18] The presence of a continuing massive air leak after tube thoracostomy, pneumomediastinum, and cervical subcutaneous air signals the presence of this injury.[2] Whereas distal bronchial tears will often seal spontaneously, more proximal injuries usually require direct surgical repair by thoracotomy. If respiratory compromise requires intubation, flexible bronchoscopy can be diagnostic and therapeutic to avoid further bronchial injury and selective intubation of the uninvolved bronchus.[18,19] Tracheobronchial disruption has been associated with a mortality rate of 30%, with severe associated injuries occurring in 50% of cases.

Esophageal Rupture

Esophageal perforations from blunt trauma are extremely rare. The most common cause of an esophageal rupture, however, is a penetrating injury. Esophageal perforation due to blunt trauma is usually caused by the sudden passage of gastric contents into the esophagus. This results in a linear tear in the distal esophagus. Esophageal ruptures may result in mediastinitis and contamination of the pleural space.[9]

The presence of both mediastinal and subcutaneous air is suggestive of the diagnosis. In addition, children may complain of chest or epigastric pain.[2] Confirmation of an esophageal rupture can be made by the use of a water-soluble contrast study and esophagoscopy.

The treatment of esophageal rupture is thoracotomy, drainage of the mediastinum, and primary repair of the esophagus. With severe contamination of the mediastinum, exclusion of the esophagus may be required. Broad-spectrum intravenous antibiotics should be instituted once the diagnosis is suspected.[20]

Diaphragm

Blunt diaphragmatic rupture has a prevalence of 1–2% in pediatric thoracic trauma and involves the left hemidiaphragm in two thirds of cases.[9] Clinical findings include: respiratory distress, chest pain, absent breath sounds on the affected side, and bowel sounds in the chest in half of the patients. Radiographic signs of diaphragmatic injury after blunt injury include a high-riding diaphragm, abnormal contour of the diaphragm, and questionable overlap of abdominal visceral shadows. Although results may be normal in the presence of injury, CT and ultrasound are also used to diagnose diaphragmatic injury.[21] Turning of a nasogastric tube into the hemithorax, associated intestinal obstruction, or frank visceral herniation are diagnostic. This injury may not be recognized for weeks or years later; 40% to 50% of blunt injury to the diaphragm is not diagnosed in the acute setting of trauma.[22] Therefore, suspicion of diaphragmatic rupture warrants surgical exploration to avoid associated late complications such as herniation or strangulation of hollow viscera and lung compression. Laceration of the diaphragm should be considered in the presence of penetrating trauma inferior to the nipple line. After ascertaining whether other life-threatening injuries to the heart, lung, liver, spleen, or gastrointestinal tract exist, consideration should be given to operative exploration and approach including thoracotomy, thoracoscopy, laparotomy, or laparoscopy.[2]

REFERENCES

1. Peterson RJ, *et al.* (1994) Pediatric and adult thoracic trauma: Age-related impact on presentation and outcome. *Ann Thorac Surg* **58**(1):14–18.
2. Bliss D, Silen M. (2002) Pediatric thoracic trauma. *Crit Care Med* **30**(11 Suppl): S409–S415.
3. Tovar JA. (2008) The lung and pediatric trauma. *Semin Pediat Surg* **17**(1):53–59.
4. Black TL, *et al.* (1996) Significance of chest trauma in children. *Southern Med J* **89**(5):494–496.
5. Samarasekera SP, *et al.* (2009) Epidemiology of major paediatric chest trauma. *J Paediatr Child H* **45**(11):676–680.
6. Machida T, *et al.* (1999) Snowboarding injuries of the chest: Comparison with skiing injuries. *J Trauma* **46**(6):1062–1065.
7. Holmes JF, *et al.* (2002) A clinical decision rule for identifying children with thoracic injuries after blunt torso trauma. *Ann Emerg Med* **39**(5):492–499.
8. Pitetti RD, Walker S. (2005) Life-threatening chest injuries in children. *Clin Pediatr Emerg Med* **6**:16–22.
9. Sartorelli KH, Vane DW. (2004) The diagnosis and management of children with blunt injury of the chest. *Semin Pediat Surg* **13**(2):98–105.

10. Wylie JMD, *et al.* (2009) Lung contusion in children-Early computed tomography versus radiography. *Pediatr Crit Care Me* **10**(6):643–647.
11. Barsness KA, *et al.* (2003) The positive predictive value of rib fractures as an indicator of nonaccidental trauma in children. *J Trauma* **54**(6):1107–1110.
12. Roland J, *et al.* (2009) Right atrial rupture from blunt thoracic trauma in a 4-year-old child. *Pediat Emerg Care* **25**(3):188–189.
13. Bromberg BI, *et al.* (1996) Recognition and management of nonpenetrating cardiac trauma in children. *J Pediatr* **128**(4):536–541.
14. Dowd MD, Krug S. (1996) Pediatric blunt cardiac injury: Epidemiology, clinical features, and diagnosis. *J Trauma* **40**(1):61–67.
15. Tiao GM, *et al.* (2000) Cardiac and great vessel injuries in children after blunt trauma: An institutional review. *J Pediatr Surg* **35**(11):1656–1660.
16. Allison ND, *et al.* (2009) Outcomes of truncal vascular injuries in children. *J Pediatr Surg* **44**(10):1958–1964.
17. Cox CS, *et al.* (1998) Operative treatment of truncal vascular injuries in children and adolescents. *J Pediatr Surg* **33**(3):462–467.
18. Cosper GH, Dassinger MS. (2009) Tracheobronchial injury diagnosed by computed tomography scan: a case report. *J Pediatr Surg* **44**(3):648–650.
19. Dango S, *et al.* (2008) Successful repair of a subtotal rupture of distal tracheobronchial tree with complete abridgment of the right bronchus in a 4-year-old child. *Ann Thorac Surg* **86**(3):1020–1022.
20. Engum SA, *et al.* (1996) Improved survival in children with esophageal perforation. *Arch Surg* **131**(6):604–611.
21. Sharma AK, *et al.* (2002) Rupture of the right hemidiaphragm due to blunt trauma in children: a diagnostic dilemma. *Pediatr Surg Int* **18**(2):173–174.
22. Mihos P, *et al.* (2003) Traumatic rupture of the diaphragm: Experience with 65 patients. *Injury* **34**(3):169–172.

ABDOMINAL TRAUMA 14

Dennis Vane

Abdominal trauma is relatively rare in children although it makes up a significant portion of admissions to hospitals. The management of children with abdominal trauma is surgical without regard to the mechanism of injury. In general abdominal injuries are separated into penetrating vs. blunt as etiologies since the management protocols are very different for these two entities. For this reason they will be treated independently in this review.

PENETRATING ABDOMINAL INJURIES

Penetrating abdominal injury (as well as penetrating injury of any sort) is relatively rare in children representing only about 10% of admissions to most pediatric centers. They do however represent a disproportionate severity of injury accounting for about 20% of deaths in this age group.[1] Firearm injuries are the most common type of penetrating injury sustained by children and occur predominantly in adolescents and older teenagers.[2] Impalement injuries are uncommon, but carry a significant mortality due to their mechanism.[3]

Evaluation of the child with penetrating abdominal trauma follows the guidelines established by the Committee on Trauma of the American College of Surgeons in their Advanced Trauma Life Support Course. The child is evaluated for hemodynamic stability and delay for diagnostic evaluation is only considered when no physiologic derangement is encountered. Focused abdominal sonographic evaluation of the abdomen or Focused

Abdominal Sonography for Trauma (FAST) provides a rapid noninvasive method to determine the presence of fluid in the abdominal cavity but cannot ascertain what kind of fluid is present (blood vs. succus).[4] Plain films of the abdomen may allow the clinician to determine the trajectory of the penetrating object, but depending on what type of object caused the penetration this may not be useful. Bullets carry with them an impact of force field and may cause significant damage to surrounding tissue from this field rather than by direct penetration. In general all abdominal penetrating wounds are explored because of the frequency of associated hollow viscus and vascular injury.[1,5]

Preparation of the child for abdominal exploration after penetrating injury is identical to preparation of any patient for exploration for any reason. Adequate vascular access is mandated (usually two large bore intravenous (IV) lines), appropriate availability of blood products and IV fluids, and adequate hemodynamic monitoring tools. Laparoscopy appears to be of limited value to ascertain and treat penetrating injuries other than to identify violation of the peritoneal cavity.[6] However, recent publications have advocated for this approach. These studies selected less severely injured children for laparoscopic evaluation and found the most benefit from this procedure was determining the need for open laparotomy.[7]

In general broad spectrum antibiotics are recommended prior to proceeding with laparotomy for penetrating injury because of the high association with hollow viscus injury. Exploration is carried out systematically to assure complete evaluation of the abdominal cavity including the diaphragms and entire bowel (including duodenum). Vascular injuries are usually repaired primarily, however in some cases of extreme hemodynamic instability ligation of the vena cava with later repair has been successfully carried out. Injuries to the intestine are commonly repaired primarily particularly in the small intestine and right colon. In cases where vascular compromise of the intestine is identified, multiple injuries are found, or the patient demonstrates hemodynamic instability a decompressive enterostomy should be considered. In cases where the child is extremely unstable hemodynamically, may have an uncorrected coagulopathy, or may be extremely cold, the surgeon should minimize operative time. This may entail simply stapling off enterotomies and planning a return to the operating room when the child is better resuscitated for definitive intervention.

Penetrating injury to the duodenum and head of the pancreas are often problematic. Primary pancreatico–duodenectomy carries a high mortality and temporizing procedures such as duodenal exclusion should be considered in these emergency operations. As a rule, minimal operations in unstable or physiologically deranged children should be undertaken. Primary repairs of significant injuries must be reserved for stable patients who have the optimal ability to heal their injuries.

In summary, although there have been some reports of successful nonoperative management of penetrating injuries in children this is not a widely accepted practice.[4,8] Any attempt to treat a child without an exploration assuring that the peritoneal cavity has not been violated or that a hollow viscus has not been perforated cannot be supported. Operative approach should assure the safety of the child. Interventions should be limited to control of bleeding and enteric contamination in an unstable patient. Formal repair can be undertaken if no significant metabolic derangement is present, or at a later time after the child has been returned to a safe physiologic state.

BLUNT ABDOMINAL INJURY

Where abdominal exploration is the rule in penetrating injury in children nonoperative management predominates with blunt injury. It is critical however for any surgeon caring for injured children to remember that every child with an abdominal injury is a surgical candidate and may require exploration and surgical management of their injury at any time.

When a surgeon encounters a child sustaining blunt injury to the abdomen a surgical algorithm for care opens. The first decision to be made is whether or not the child should be taken immediately to the operating room. This decision is based entirely on the hemodynamic status of the patient, and whether or not a surgical condition exists within the abdominal cavity. In a hemodynamically unstable child the surgeon must decide if there is bleeding within the abdominal cavity. Historically this was done by performing a diagnostic peritoneal lavage or aspiration of the peritoneal cavity. More recently this has been replaced with the FAST examination of the abdomen. The use of ultrasound to ascertain whether or not fluid (blood) is present in significant volume within the abdominal cavity is simple, painless, and quick. The procedure is quickly learned and performed by an experienced physician in less than 3 minutes. The specificity and sensitivity are excellent, when used properly. FAST is not designed to diagnose the specific injury to an intraabdominal organ. Its sole purpose it to ascertain whether or not there is a significant amount of fluid within the abdominal cavity. This coupled with a hemodynamically unstable child mandates immediate transfer to the operating room and an abdominal exploration. FAST may discern the difference between intraabdominal fluid and the accumulation of blood in the retroperitoneum secondary to a pelvic fracture. In the later case opening the abdominal cavity can potentially release the tamponade effect of the peritoneal cavity and increase mortality and morbidity in these patients.

If an immediate surgical intervention is not mandated due to the initial hemodynamic status of the child and they have been stabilized, other diagnostic parameters may be considered. Computerized Tomography (CT) of the abdomen is really the gold standard for evaluation of blunt trauma. The test is extremely accurate, and can in most centers be done expeditiously. However, a child who has not been stabilized should never be taken to the radiology department for a diagnostic CT scan. Scans are generally done with IV contrast. If done properly in the arterial phase the test can identify vascular injuries as well as vascular compromise in the intestine and other solid organs. A delayed series is an excellent evaluation of the renal system and its function as well. Historically, there has been some question regarding the accuracy of identifying intestinal injury and injury to the pancreas and duodenum. It appears though that with the advent of more sensitive scanning equipment, these issues have been resolved. The only remaining question appears to be in the evaluation of the duodenum in an acute blunt injury. The use of a small amount of oral contrast may be beneficial if this injury is suspected and this does not require the large volumes of oral contrast and long wait times previously recommended for evaluation of the intestine.

As with penetrating trauma to the abdomen the determination of what operation to perform in a child with blunt injury to the abdomen and perforation or damage to the hollow viscus is determined by the physiologic and hemodynamic state of the child. Children in shock, or who are hemodynamically unstable should have damage control only with minimal operations to prevent continued soiling of the abdominal cavity. Primary repair of intestinal injuries take longer and are not likely to remain intact in a child who is hemodynamically unstable and potentially in shock. Subsequently continued contamination of the abdominal cavity may occur. Safety mandates that primary repair only be undertaken in patients who are not impacted by extending the length of surgery for primary repairs and who are physiologically and hemodynamically stable enough to clot their blood and perfuse their organs. Closing an unstable patient after bleeding and contamination of the abdomen are controlled, then taking that patient to the Pediatric Intensive Care Unit (PICU) for improvement of their overall state, and then returning to the operating room at a later time is often the safest course of action.

SOLID ORGAN INJURY

Blunt injury to the abdomen most often involves the solid organs. In children it is often advisable to treat these injuries with nonoperative management. This approach has been shown to be safe, effective, and carry less morbidity than operative management in select cases. In all instances the surgeon must remember that in order to manage a child with a blunt solid organ injury without operation that child must be (and remain) hemodynamically and physiologically stable. If at any time the child becomes unstable, intervention must be considered.

THE SPLEEN

The spleen is the most frequently injured solid organ in children who sustain blunt abdominal trauma.[9] The anatomic location of the spleen under the ribs give it a somewhat protected location from blunt abdominal trauma, however, the pliability of the child's thoracic cavity throughout early teenage allow for this organ to be frequently injured. The spleen is essentially a collection of soft tissue and blood vessels covered by a thin membrane. It functions as a filter to remove abnormal, damaged, or retired red blood cells and encapsulated bacteria and store white blood cells. It does produce immunoglobulins but this function is redundant to other organs in the body. Loss of the spleen has been implicated in the development of "postsplenectomy sepsis", a severe form of sepsis with an extremely high mortality. Mechanism of injury is similar in all solid organs of the abdomen in children with motor vehicles (either as a passenger or pedestrian) being the most common etiology followed by falls and sporting events.[9] Physical examination is often problematic to ascertain whether or not a splenic injury has occurred. Pain and tenderness in the left upper quadrant are often present in children with an isolated splenic injury; however, multiple injuries to the abdomen can cloud this presentation. A direct bruise in the left upper quadrant is suspicious but again not specific. The presence or absence of a significant amount of blood in the peritoneal cavity may cause localized peritoneal signs to be inconstant as well.

Blunt injury to the spleen has been graded by the American Association for the Surgery of Trauma into five categories which define severity and allow the clinician to more readily standardize outcomes and potential therapies.[10] (Table 1) The grades are determined by CT scan and theoretically might be used to determine treatment. In children over 90% of grade I–IV splenic injures are successfully treated without intervention.[11] Grade V injuries are more likely to undergo operation or other intervention. Convention states that the grade of injury is advanced one grade (up to grade III) when multiple injuries are sustained.

Observation of splenic injuries, although common place, suffers from a lack of consensus on details of management. All authors agree that hemodynamic stability is a precursor of nonoperative management. In this author's opinion hemodynamic stability is defined by several parameters. First, the child's blood pressure is maintained in the normal range for their age. Second, although some tachycardia is to be expected, particularly in children whose hematocrits are purposefully allowed to decrease below normal ranges, this stabilizes after initial resuscitation. And finally, the child's hemoglobin and hematocrit stabilize after initial resuscitation.

When these criteria are met the child is admitted to the hospital for observation. Laboratory evaluation of a child with a splenic injury is limited to determination of the hemoglobin and hematocrit. These are done serially after admission to ascertain the potential for continued bleeding from the spleen. The schedule of evaluation is somewhat controversial and will be discussed later. All grades of splenic injury have been reported to

Table 1. Spleen injury.[10]

Grade	Injury
I	Subcapsular hematoma < 10% of surface or capsular tear < 1 cm in depth
II	Subcapsular hematoma 10—50% of surface or < 5 cm in diameter Capsular tear 1—3 cm in depth not involving a trabecular vessel
III	Subcapsular hematoma > 50% surface area or expanding hematoma; ruptured subcapsular or parenchymal hematoma, or intraparenchymal hematoma > 5 cm or expanding; > 3 cm depth laceration potentially involvintg a trabecular vessel
IV	Laceration involving a segmental or hilar vessel with devascularization of > 25% of the spleen
V	Shattered spleen Hilar devascularization of the spleen

have necessitated operative intervention. This is particularly true in children suffering multiple injuries.

On occasion initial CT scanning of the abdomen will reveal a splenic blush or "pseudoaneurysm" associated with the spleen. Historically, in the adult literature this has indicated the need for exploration, repair, or splenectomy. This has not been found to be the case in children. In children, the single indication for intervention remains the hemodynamic status of the child. CT and other diagnostic findings indicating pseudoaneurysm and splenic blush are not by themselves indications for intervention, but rather simply indications that intervention may be warranted or to increase the level of concern for the clinician that at the point of the examination some active bleeding was present.[12,13]

Should the child develop hemodynamic instability then intervention is warranted. Historically this required surgical intervention for either splenectomy or splenorraphy. Today, since intervention is usually reserved for spleens that are significantly damaged, splenorraphy is less common than splenectomy. The question becomes how much spleen is necessary for effective immunologic functioning and which vessels need to remain intact. It appears from very early experimental work that preservation of the splenic artery is critical for effective prevention of postsplenectomy sepsis.[14] Subsequently, trauma surgeons dealing with pediatric patients have not routinely used splenic artery embolization for traumatized spleens. This therapeutic modality is effective however in selected cases where an operation may cause unwanted morbidity.[15] The treating surgeon must take into consideration that embolization of the splenic artery may render the child immunologically compromised and mandates appropriate immunizations. In short, most splenic injuries in children can be safely treated with observation. Should the child develop continued bleeding or other hemodynamic instability, then an intervention should be undertaken. If the child is considered adequately stable or has a contraindication for laparotomy, arteriography, and splenic artery embolization may be considered. If laparotomy is undertaken the surgeon may elect to attempt a splenorraphy, or splenectomy. There is information that indicates tying off of the splenic artery leaves the child essentially asplenic and that should be considered by the surgeon, particularly if the child has other injuries that may impact their physiologic state at a later time. Splenectomy should never be delayed or avoided if an injured spleen does not stop bleeding spontaneously. Splenic artery embolization or ligating the splenic artery should be accompanied with appropriate postsplenectomy immunizations and the child treated as if they were asplenic.

Discharge after an acute injury to the spleen without a period of observation to ascertain any change in the child's physiological condition is unwise. At the present time there is controversy as to the optimal management of blunt injury to the spleen regarding hospitalization and return to activities.

THE LIVER

The liver is the largest solid abdominal organ in children. Its large size coupled with its thin capsule make it particularly susceptible to blunt traumatic injury.[16] The liver is second only to the spleen, as the most common solid abdominal organ injured in children, occurring in 2% to 3% of children with blunt abdominal trauma.[17,18] Most solid organ injuries in children are the result of blunt trauma, with only 1% to 10% of injuries resulting from penetrating trauma.[19] Injury to the right lobe of the liver is most frequent, however lacerations along the attachment of the falciform ligament are also common.[16,17] Fortunately, despite making up nearly one-third of all traumatic abdominal organ injuries, most children who sustain liver injuries and arrive at the hospital alive have excellent outcomes, with only 2.5% to 10 % requiring operative intervention.[18,20–23] The current standard of care for hemodynamically stable children with isolated liver injury is nonoperative management with success rates reported in excess of 90% by several centers.[18,20,22,24,25]

As with the spleen most liver injuries in children occur as the result of motor vehicle crashes where they are passengers or pedestrians.[17,20,23,26] Gross *et al.* report in a single institutional 13-yr review of pediatric liver injuries, 39% and 34% of children with liver injury were pedestrians struck by a motor vehicle and occupants of a motor vehicle, respectively.[17] Falls, bicycle accidents, and nonaccidental blunt trauma are also significant causes of liver injury in children.[17,27]

Physical Examination

The elastic nature of the pediatric body (particularly the thoracic cavity) can often mask internal injuries from blunt mechanisms, therefore despite a normal physical examination; significant intraabdominal injuries in children can be present.[17,28] The most common physical exam signs of significant liver injury in children include; right upper quadrant abdominal tenderness, hypoactive bowel sounds, external abdominal trauma (e.g. "seat-belt sign"), abdominal distention and shoulder pain.[17,18,29] These findings should raise suspicion of significant liver injury and prompt further evaluation with diagnostic imaging and/or repeated serial examinations. As with the spleen the amount of intraabdominal blood can cloud the examination.

Although not directly related to the severity of liver injury, an accurate Glasgow Coma Score (GCS) should also be noted on physical exam, as decreased GCS is associated with a significant mortality increase in children with liver injury.[16,30]

Laboratory Evaluation

Several studies have looked at the utility of liver function tests (LFT) in the evaluation of pediatric trauma patients with suspected liver injury. Despite the lack of a clear consensus on the sensitivity and specificity of LFTs, many authors agree that elevated LFTs in the setting of blunt abdominal trauma in a child should trigger further evaluation with CT to assess for specific liver injury.[16,28,31,32] However, it is also noteworthy that although the degree of LFT elevation may correlate with injury severity, increased LFTs have not been shown to be an accurate predictor for the need for surgical intervention.[17] In addition to LFTs, frequent serial hematocrits are also useful in the evaluation of liver injury as they may determine the existence of persistent bleeding from the liver.[29]

Radiology

With advancements in technology and increasing accessibility, CT has become the imaging modality of choice for the grading (Table 1) and identification of blunt liver injury in hemodynamically stable children.[17,21,28] CT imaging has the advantage of not only detecting liver injury but also injuries to other intraperitoneal organs. It is generally accepted that the use of IV contrast will improve the accuracy of imaging but it is not required and institutional experience with contrast protocols will likely guide the decision to use contrast.[21] On the other hand, enteral contrast is not recommended as it increases the delay to diagnosis and significantly increases the risk of aspiration.[21] Despite its radiologic accuracy at identifying liver injury, CT scanning has been repeatedly shown not to reliably predict patient mortality or hospital course and radiologic findings seldom affect the decision to operate.[17,26,30,33,34] This can be partially attributed to the inability of CT scans to reliable characterize the more severe juxtahepatic injuries or expanding hematomas, and emphasizes the overriding principle that clinical status and patient physiology drive successful management of blunt abdominal injury.[26]

In addition to CT, other initial imaging modalities, specifically plain X-ray and ultrasound may offer some preCT information that could suggest liver injury. Classically, X-ray findings in the presence of liver injury have been nonspecific, but may include right-sided rib fractures, right pleural effusion, elevated right hemidiaphragm, ileus, and irregularity of the liver contour.[29] B-mode ultrasound or FAST exam may also be useful for screening children for intraabdominal bleeding from blunt abdominal trauma because of their high specificity in experienced hands.[19,21]

Associated Injuries

The frequency of associated injuries with liver injury is significant, with over half of all patients sustaining multisystem injury.[16,17] Several centers have reported nervous system injury (i.e. traumatic brain injury) as the most common associated injury, while thoracic and musculoskeletal injuries are also frequent.[16,17,22,26,35] Nervous system injury is also believed to be most significant predictor of mortality in the pediatric population. Decreased GCS has been shown to correlate better with patient mortality than the severity grade of liver injury.[1,12,15] Fortunately, concomitant hollow viscus injuries are rare and reported to occur only 2.5% to 3.2% of the time.[16,36]

Management

Management of hepatic injuries in children has significantly evolved over the past several decades. Since the sentinel report of Upadhyaya and Simpson describing the successful selective nonoperative management of splenic injuries in children in 1968, the indications for operative management of solid abdominal organ injuries in children have become exceedingly stringent.[37] The management of blunt hepatic injuries is no exception to this rule.

Nonoperative Management

Several centers have reported successful nonoperative management rates of pediatric liver injury from 72% to 97%.[2,3,5,7,9,10] Historically, concerns over lengthened hospital stays, transfusion requirements, and delayed complications of nonoperative management of liver injuries have deterred surgeons from committing to nonoperative management schemes. However, a growing body of literature has now challenged these early claims. Today, most hemodynamically stable children who present with liver injuries can expect shorter hospital and intensive care unit lengths of stays, less transfusions and less complications than their operative counter-parts.[2,3,29,38,39] In fact, transfusion rates for children with isolated liver injuries has fallen below 10%. This is partially because most centers are now no longer transfusing children based on low hematocrit "triggers" but rather evidence of continued blood loss.[39,40] In addition, recent prospectively validated evidence based guidelines by the American Pediatric Surgical Association (APSA) Trauma Committee have set-forth an expectation of decreased hospital and intensive care unit lengths of stay for hemodynamically stable children with spleen or liver injuries (Table 2). The guidelines propose that children with blunt liver injury only require a number of days of bed rest to equal the grade of injury plus 1 day. Exceptions to this guideline include hemodynamically unstable patients or patients with ongoing bleeding or evidence of grade V injuries.[40] However,

Table 2. Liver injury.[10]

Grade	Injury
I	Subcapsular hematoma <10% of surface or capsular tear <1cm in depth
II	Subcapsular hematoma 10–50% of surface or <10 cm in diameter Capsular tear 1–3 cm in depth <10 cm length
III	Subcapsular hematoma>50% surface area or expanding hematoma; ruptured subcapsular or parenchymal hematoma, or intraparenchymal hematoma>10 cm or expanding; >3 cm depth laceration
IV	Parenchymal disruption 25–75% of a hepatic lobe or 1–3 Couinaud's segments
V	Parenchymal disruption>75% of a hepatic lobe or>3 Couinaud's segments within a lobeRetrohepatic vena cava or central major hepatic vein injury
VI	Hepatic avulsion

despite the utility of these recent guidelines it is important to recognize that patients with hepatic injuries, the severity of injury (i.e. ISS) and the number of associated injuries are often more predictive of outcome than the injury grade.[1,26] The use of nonoperative interventions such as angiographic embolization has also led to increased nonoperative success rates. Small case series now describe the successful use of angiographic embolization in children with evidence of ongoing hemorrhage and a blush seen on CT.[15,41,42,43]

Operative Management

Commonly accepted criteria for operative management of children with suspected or known liver injury include; persistent hemodynamic instability despite 20 to 30 cc/kg of initial fluid resuscitation, worsening peritonitis with evidence of persistent intraabdominal hemorrhage, or transfusion requirements greater than one-third to one-half of estimated blood volume (25 to 40 cc/kg).[2, 4, 23,29,44] Requiring greater than 25 cc/kg in the first 2 hrs has also been shown to be 88% and 95% predictive of the need for surgical intervention and major hepatic vascular injury, respectively.[2] It is now recognized that children who require operative intervention declare themselves early in their hospital course, usually within 12–24 hrs, with a peak of nonoperative management failure at 4 hrs.[1,5,29,33] Unfortunately, when operative intervention is undertaken associated mortality significantly increases. Although, institutional experience varies, most authors have reported at least 40% mortality for children who require surgery for major hepatic vascular or severe parenchymal injury.[2,27,29] In light of the significant morbidity associated with operative repair of liver injuries, several operative strategies have been proposed to deal with these very complex injuries.

Surgical Options

The most common aim of operative exploration for hepatic injuries is hemorrhage control.[3] Most often this can be achieved with a combination of debridement of devitalized tissues and manual compression, topical hemostatic agents (thrombin, microfibrillar collagen), or suturing.[28,36] Large mattress sutures through Glisson's capsule are used to control simple lacerations of the liver surface, while direct suture vessel ligation is more commonly used to control hemorrhage from deep parenchymal lacerations.[45] When these approaches fail to control bleeding, early and aggressive abdominal packing ("damage control") should be utilized to stop life-threatening hemorrhage with the plan to return to the operating room for inspection and removal of packs in 24–48 hrs later.[4] If "damage control" is undertaken, large sump drains and a compressive suction dressing are typically applied to temporarily provide decompression and closure of the abdominal wall, but it is importation to remember that despite the placement of drains, children are still at risk for developing an abdominal compartment syndrome. Several key signs of a developing compartment syndrome include; increased abdominal distention, increased intraabdominal pressures in the range of 25–35 mm Hg, respiratory insufficiency secondary to restricted diaphragmatic movement, hemodynamic instability due to inferior vena caval compression, and impaired renal function from renal vein compression.[36] When abdominal compartment syndrome is recognized decompression of the abdomen is required to minimize further multi-system failure.

Other less commonly utilized methods for hemorrhage control include the use of a liver mesh wrap and formal hepatic resection.[23] In the setting of trauma, formal hepatic resection has been associated with a 70% mortality and is now considered a last resort maneuver to deal with extensive hemorrhage and devitalized tissue.[28]

Complications

Complications of nonoperative management of hepatic injuries are rare. Initial studies reported liver-related complications rates in the range of 20% to 50%, however this has significantly improved over the past several decades and most recent studies describe complication rates in the range of <1% to 12%.[2,22,33] It is generally accepted that children with higher grade liver injuries (grade III or higher) or injuries that involve greater than 50% of the liver are at a greater risk for complications.[22] Common symptoms of complications include; new onset fever, persistent right abdominal or shoulder pain, worsening food intolerance or ileus, abdominal distention, and persistently elevated LFTs (GGT and alkaline phosphatase).[22,33]

The most commonly encountered liver-related complication is biloma formation. Bilomas are encapsulated pockets of bile that may form after liver injury secondary to bile duct disruptions. These pockets are at risk for infection and abscess formation, peritonitis from rupture, and fistulization. Giss *et al.* reported that bilomas comprised 71% of their total liver-related complications.[22] Bilomas are commonly diagnosed by CT or if persistent biliary leak is suspected cholescintography (HIDA scans). Fortunately, most bilomas and bile leaks can be successfully managed with ultrasound- or CT-guided percutaneous drainage procedures and endoscopic retrograde cholangiopancreatography (ERCP)-guided biliary stent placement and do not require surgery.[22,29]

The most worrisome liver-related complication is delayed hemorrhage. The exact etiology of delayed-hemorrhage is still unclear, but may involve unrecognized pseudoaneurysm rupture. Children who present with delayed-hemorrhage may present anywhere from 3 days to 6 wks postinjury and several studies now report 1% to 3% of incidence of delayed-hemorrhage after initial nonoperative management of hepatic injuries.[33] In the past two decades only two deaths have been reported as a result of delayed-hemorrhage and both of these deaths occurred after attempted operative management of delayed hemorrhage.[33] Confirmation of the diagnosis of delayed-hemorrhage is commonly achieved with contrast enhanced CT or angiography. Fortunately, most hemodynamically stable patients with delayed-hemorrhage can be successfully managed nonoperatively with angioembolization and do not require surgery.[29,33] Other reported liver-related complications after nonoperative management of hepatic injuries have included duodenal obstruction from liver hypertrophy and right pleural effusions.[33]

Posthospitalization Care

The appropriate activity restrictions and imaging following successful management of hepatic injuries is still under debate. However, many authors do not recommend routine follow-up imaging of asymptomatic children.[27,33,39,40] In addition, liver appearance on imaging does not seem to reflect the organ's integrity and therefore is not a reliably tool on which to recommend activity restrictions after injury.[27,39,40] Generally, low grade hepatic injuries will heal in less than 4 wks, while injuries of greater severity (≥grade III) may require at least 6 wks to completely heal.[27,33] Therefore, children are now typically counseled to return to school upon hospital discharge to minimize the number of school days missed, but to refrain from full contact activity for at least 5 wks for grade III injuries or higher (Table 2).[32,33,39,40]

THE PANCREAS

Injury to the pancreas while uncommon in children is certainly not rare. The function of the pancreas and its unique architecture allow it to formulate enzymes and other by products which have the ability to be extremely destructive to the body when exposed to environments and conditions that cause their activation. Pancreatic enzymes with the potential to essentially "digest" the body are created in a contained alkali milieu which when disturbed exposed to the normal pH of the body (7.4) become activated and can cause destruction.

Fortunately, injury to the pancreas is relatively uncommon representing the fourth most commonly injured solid organ of the body after the spleen, liver, and kidneys.[46] The incidence of injury to the pancreas is reported to occur in between 3% and 12 % of children with blunt injury to the abdomen and carry an associated mortality of as high as 20%.[47] The direct injury of the pancreas does not commonly cause massive hemorrhage like the spleen and liver and initially may not cause any significant physiologic or functional problems at all. Injury most commonly occurs from direct trauma to the abdomen anteriorly which causes the pancreas to be compressed against the spine and "bruise" or rupture. Any disruption of the normal pancreatic ductal system allows the contents of the ducts to become exposed to the normal pH of the body (7.4) and activate. This activation causes injury to exposed tissue and a severe inflammatory response. The inflammatory response causes damage to surrounding tissue in variable degrees and that damage is what causes the creation of pancreatic ascites, a pseudocyst or other collection of enzymes. Depending on where this occurs in the abdomen the child may suffer saponification of the surrounding lipid tissue, or potentially erosion into surrounding tissue such as the intestine or adjacent blood vessels. This can cause significant morbidity and mortality if unchecked. Direct blows anteriorly more commonly create injuries to the head or body of the pancreas whereas blows sustained laterally from the flanks have been reported to more commonly cause injury to the tail or head depending on which side they occur.[48] The retroperitoneal location of the pancreas and the common association of other adjacent organs often makes the diagnosis of pancreatic injury difficult.[49] Because of this these injuries are often under diagnosed or missed entirely causing increased morbidity and mortality.[50]

Physical Exam

As stated physical examination and the initial diagnosis of pancreatic injury is often difficult and relying on it potentially causes delay. Mid epigastric pain and tenderness can be present and the history of a direct blow to the abdomen is common. Often, the child presents with a significant delay from the initial injury complaining of vague mid abdominal pain and early satiety or anorexia. Examination may reveal a large abdominal mass which when imaged reveals a pancreatic pseudocyst that may cause gastric compression.

Laboratory Evaluation

Serum enzyme evaluation of pancreatic injury in trauma patients is not precise. Although amylase and lipase are relatively sensitive markers of pancreatitis in nontrauma patients, they are neither specific nor sensitive in trauma patients.[51,52] The initial serum amylase level has been reported to be 50% to 90% sensitive for these injuries.[46,50,53,54] Most authors agree that hyperamylasemia may be normal in the first 48hrs after traumatic abdominal injury, and that serial investigation showing a rising level is of more value than a single initial sample.[48,49,55,56] Some authors feel that very high initial amylase and lipase levels rather than only slightly elevated measurements signify a significant requirement for operative intervention. This was associated in at least some investigations with a ductal transection rather than simply a parenchymal lesion. Others however have not validated this assertion finding that elevation of amylase and lipase were more closely associated with length of hospitalization and not severity of injury or need for operative intervention.[56,57] Recent publications have found lipase to be a more sensitive indicator of injury than amylase. It also appears that serial enzyme measurements increased over initial evaluations in more severe injuries.[58]

Radiology

As with other solid organ injuries CT imaging of the pancreas is considered the "gold" standard for visualization of injuries.[54,55,59] The use of ERCP and magnetic resonance cholangiopancreatography (MRCP) have also been advocated by some centers as these have been used extensively in imaging chronic or medical pancreatitis. These modalities require a general anesthetic in most children and have not been used extensively in the trauma patient.[46,60] Recent publications have also demonstrated that early CT scan (prior to 12 hrs after injury) carries with it a high degree of inaccuracy in the determination of injury to the pancreas as well as accuracy in the determination of stage of injury.[58]

Associated Injuries

The anatomic location of the pancreas in the retroperitoneum and its proximity to other organs make it prone to association with other injuries. Commonly, injuries to the duodenum, intestinal vascular injury and injury to the liver and biliary tract are encountered with blunt pancreatic injury.[50] Concomitantly, because of its relatively protected position behind the inferior ribs, severe impact causing blunt injury to the pancreas is also associated with closed head trauma, major orthopedic injury, other gastrointestinal injuries and urinary tract injuries which dramatically increase the morbidity and mortality of this injury over isolated injuries.[50]

Management

As with other solid organs in children blunt injury to the pancreas has undergone a significant metamorphosis of therapy. Most surgeons agree that minor pancreatic injuries (grade I–II) can be safely managed without laparotomy or even percutaneous interventions.[60–65] In general these low grade lesions appear to heal spontaneously and rarely develop

Table 3. Pancreatic injury stages.[74]

Grade	Injury
I	Minor contusion or laceration without ductal injury
II	Major contusion or laceration without ductal injury or tissue loss
III	Distal injury with ductal injury
IV	Proximal injury involving the ampulla
V	Massive disruption of the pancreatic head

complications. There is also fairly universal agreement that grade V lesions all require immediate intervention when identified, and even with aggressive treatment have an extremely high associated mortality and morbidity.[58] Controversy exists however over the optimal management of grade III and IV injuries. Some authors feel that all pancreatic injuries should initially be managed expectantly without any intervention at all.[48,66,67] Data indicates that expectant observation however carries with it a fairly robust morbidity rate. Development of pancreatic pseudocysts is a common complication which may require extended hospitalization and additional surgical intervention.[48,53,54,57,65,68] Others feel as strongly that early surgical intervention of varying approaches offers the best outcomes, particularly if intervention is carried out within 48 hrs of injury.[55,65,69,70] These authors feel that hospitalization is shortened with early intervention. Authors favoring expectant observation state that observation in general allows for preservation of more functional pancreatic tissue. Approaches are varied regarding operative intervention. Spleen sparing pancreatectomy is recommended for the obvious immunologic advantage of retaining the spleen, however this may be difficult, particularly in the less acute setting. Placement of stents by ERCP has also been advocated, however has not gained significant support and demonstrated varied success.[57,58,71,72] Recently early intervention for drainage of grade III and IV injuries has been advocated without surgical resection.[58] This has at least the theoretical advantage of maintaining pancreatic tissue and avoidance of complications encountered with expectant observation.

The lack of consensus regarding management of these lesions is multifactoral. Low volumes seen at each institution and the high complication rates that all of these approaches carry, make analysis of which is preferable difficult.

Nonoperative Management

Nonoperative management of pancreatic injuries is the agreed upon approach to grade I and II injuries.[58] The nonoperative approach to grade III and IV lesions is not clear. In general when these lesions are observed the treating physician can expect a fairly high rate of pseudocyst development which may or may not resolve spontaneously.[73] Small pseudocysts appear to have a high likelihood of spontaneous resolution where larger ones may require later surgical resection or drainage.[53,63,65] In general nonoperative intervention for these lesions carries a low probability of later pancreatic dysfunction.[46,48] ERCP with placement of a stent to facilitate drainage in pancreatic injury has been proposed to lessen the development of pseudocysts. This has not gained widespread acceptance in children given the difficulty, widespread availability, equipment issues, and lack of demonstrable benefit.[58,60,69] Given the location and associated injuries of grade V injuries to the pancreas nonoperative intervention is not appropriate.

In general there are no specific guidelines for protracted bed rest or limitations of physical activity for nonoperatively managed pancreatic injuries. Introduction of an oral diet is usually begun when the child is pain free and when the serum enzymes are decreasing. The use of nasogastric drainage in the acute period may be warranted until an associated intestinal injury can be ruled out but has not been shown to affect long term outcomes. Withholding oral intake until serum enzymes are completely normal does not improve outcomes.[58]

Operative Management

As previously stated operative management for pancreatic injuries is controversial. In general early intervention allows for more options in surgical intervention and a greater potential for their success.[55,58,70] Spleen sparing distal pancreatectomy is indicated where applicable, however is difficult due to inflammation and saponification in injuries when delayed intervention is undertaken. Whipple pancreatic resections may be indicated in very proximal injuries, and in all cases attempts at preserving as much pancreatic tissue as possible is mandated to prevent late pancreatic failure and its associated complications. In very distal injuries simple distal pancreatectomy has the best results. In more proximal injuries Roux-en-Y resections and reconstructions seem most appropriate, but a compelling advantage over distal pancreatectomy has not been shown. For grade V injuries pyloric exclusion, Whipple duodenopancreatectomy and total pancreatectomy have all been proposed depending on exactly what injury is encountered. This severe injury of the pancreas is often accompanied by other injuries and outcomes are extremely poor.[58]

For children who develop pancreatic pseudocysts, operative intervention is usually delayed until the lesion can mature. This has historically been described as about 3 wks from injury. Cystgastrostomy or Roux-en-Y cyst enterostomy have excellent results for resolution of these pseudocysts in children. Selection of operation is dependent on location of the cyst. Small pseudocysts have been shown to resolve spontaneously and observation is probably the best approach if they are otherwise asymptomatic.

Early intervention for grade III and IV injuries for placement of drains appears promising for maintenance of pancreatic function and lessening complications, however larger studies verifying this approach are necessary to confirm initial observations.[58]

Complications

Complications of pancreatic injuries can be devastating. Chronic pain may require total or subtotal pancreatectomy. Pancreatic fistula has been described, however in most cases these resolve spontaneously over time. Control of the fistula output is important however as the drainage is extremely irritating to the skin and can cause significant breakdown. Chronic fistulae that do not resolve spontaneously indicate an obstruction in the ductal system which may need to be addressed. Roux-en-Y pancreatico–enterostomy may be indicated or even distal pancreatectomy for control and closure.

Endocrine and exocrine pancreatic insufficiency is a devastating complication of some pancreatic injuries. These are usually grade V injuries or grade IV injuries with associated complications. This requires enzyme supplementation and often results in malabsorption, growth abnormalities and potentially severe diabetes. These complications may have a significantly delayed onset and not appear until the child has reached adult stature. This has pushed surgeons to try to save as much pancreatic tissue as possible after injury.

Posthospitalization Care

Most surgeons do not limit physical activity for children after isolated pancreatic injury. Diets are started when the child is pain free and initiation of an oral diet is not based on normalization of serum enzyme levels.[58] Enzyme deficiencies are treated with appropriate replacement if necessary to allow normalization of growth and endocrine function. Placement of children on a low fat diet until enzymes have normalized after pancreatic injury has been recommended and is commonly practiced, but no data is available indicating that this practice improves outcomes.

REFERENCES

1. Cotton BA, Nance ML. (2004) Penetrating trauma in children. *Semin Pediat Surg* **13**:87–97.
2. Beaver BL, Moore VL, Peclat M, *et al.* (1990) Characteristics of pediatric firearm fatalities. *J Pediatr Surg* **25**:97–100.
3. Lelly IP, Attwood SA, Quilan W, *et al.* (1995) The management of impalement injury. *Injury* **26**:191–193.
4. Coley BD, Mutabagani KH, Martin LC. (2000) Focused abdominal sonography for trauma (FAST) in children with blunt abdominal trauma. *J Trauma* **48**:902–906.
5. Dicker RA, Sartorelli KH, McBride WJ, *et al.* (1996) Penetrating hepatic trauma in children: Operating room or not? *J Pediatr Surg* **31**:1189–1191.
6. Leppaniemi AK, Elliott DC. (1996) The role of laparoscopy in blunt abdominal trauma. *Ann Med* **28**:483–489.
7. Feliz A, Shultz B, McKenna C, *et al.* (2006) Diagnostic and therapeutic laparoscopy in pediatric abdominal trauma. *J Pediatr Surg* **41**:72–77.
8. Cigdem MK, Onen A, Siga M, *et al.* (2009) Selective nonoperative management of penetrating abdominal injuries in children. *J Trauma* **67**:124–187.
9. Gaines BA, Ford HR. (2002) Abdominal and pelvic trauma in children. *Crit Care Med* **30**:s416–s423.
10. Moore EE, Cogbill TH, Jurkovich CT, *et al.* (1994) Organ injury scaling: Spleen and liver (1994 Revision). *J Trauma* **38**:323–324.
11. Keller MA. (2004) Blunt injury to solid organs. *Semin Pediat Surg* **13**:106–111.
12. Frumiento C, Vane DW. (2000) Changing patterns of treatment for blunt splenic injuries: An 11 year experience in a rural state. *J Pediatr Surg* **35**:985–989.
13. Rumiento C, Sartorelli KH, Vane DW. (2000) Complications of splenic injuries: Expansion of the nonoperative theorem. *J Pediatr Surg* **35**:788–791.
14. Malangoni MA, Grosfeld JL. (1980) Blunt splenic trauma: A reassessment of surgical therapy based on laboratory and clinical observations. *Surg Annu* **12**:123–138.
15. Kiankhooy A, Sartorelli KH, Vane DW, *et al.* (2010) Angiographic embolization is safe and effective therapy for blunt abdominal solid organ injury in children. *J Trauma* in press.
16. Deluca JA, Maxwell DR, Flaherty SK, *et al.* (2007) Injuries associated with pediatric liver trauma. *Am Surgeon* **73**(1):37–41.

17. Gross M, Lynch F, Canty T, Sr., *et al.* (1999) Management of pediatric liver injuries: A 13-year experience at a pediatric trauma center. *J Pediatr Surg* **34**(5):811–816; discussion 816–817.
18. Tataria M, Nance ML, Holmes JHT, *et al.* (2007) Pediatric blunt abdominal injury: age is irrelevant and delayed operation is not detrimental. *J Trauma* **63**(3):608–614.
19. Feliciano DV, Tuggle DW, Garza J. (2008) Trauma. *Pediatr Trauma* **46**:987–1001.
20. Holmes JHT, Wiebe DJ, Tataria M, *et al.* (2005) The failure of nonoperative management in pediatric solid organ injury: A multi-institutional experience. *J Trauma* **59**(6):1309–1313.
21. Stylianos S. (2005) Outcomes from pediatric solid organ injury: Role of standardized care guidelines. *Curr Opin Pediatr* **17**(3):402–406.
22. Giss SR, Dobrilovic N, Brown RL, Garcia VF. (2006) Complications of nonoperative management of pediatric blunt hepatic injury: Diagnosis, management, and outcomes. *J Trauma* **61**(2):334–339.
23. Luchtman M, Alfici R, Sternberg A, *et al.* (2004) Mesh wrap in severe pediatric liver trauma. *J Pediatr Surg* **39**(10):1485–1489.
24. Coburn MC, Pfeifer J, DeLuca FG. (1995) Nonoperative management of splenic and hepatic trauma in the multiply injured pediatric and adolescent patient. *Arch Surg* **130**(3):332–338.
25. Bond SJ, Eichelberger MR, Gotschall CS, *et al.* (1996) Nonoperative management of blunt hepatic and splenic injury in children. *Ann Surg* **223**(3):286–289.
26. Hackam DJ, Potoka D, Meza M, *et al.* (2002) Utility of radiographic hepatic injury grade in predicting outcome for children after blunt abdominal trauma. *J Pediatr Surg* **37**(3):386–389.
27. Mooney DP. (2002) Multiple trauma: Liver and spleen injury. *Curr Opin Pediatr* **14**(4):482–485.
28. Touloukian RJ, Cooney DR, Billmire DF. (1990) Hepatic, biliary tree, and pancreatic injury. In: DE Wesson, S Stylianos, R Pearl, P Babyn (eds.), *Pediatric Trauma: Pathophysiology, Diagnosis, and Treatment*, pp. 312–332. Taylor and Francis, New York.
29. Pryor JP, Stafford PW, Nance ML. (2001) Severe blunt hepatic trauma in children. *J Pediatr Surg* **36**(7):974–979.
30. Hennes HM, Smith DS, Schneider K, *et al.* (1990) Elevated liver transaminase levels in children with blunt abdominal trauma: A predictor of liver injury. *Pediatrics* **86**(1):87–90.

31. Oldham KT, Guice KS, Kaufman RA, *et al.* (1984) Blunt hepatic injury and elevated hepatic enzymes: A clinical correlation in children. *J Pediatr Surg* **19**(4):457–461.
32. St Peter SD, Keckler SJ, Spilde TL, *et al.* (2008) Justification for an abbreviated protocol in the management of blunt spleen and liver injury in children. *J Pediatr Surg* **43**(1):191–193; discussion 193–194.
33. Mehall JR, Ennis JS, Saltzman DA, *et al.* (2001) Prospective results of a standardized algorithm based on hemodynamic status for managing pediatric solid organ injury. *J Am Coll Surgeons* **193**(4):347–353.
34. Moore EE, Cogbill TH, Jurkovich GJ, *et al.* (1995) Organ injury scaling: Spleen and liver (1994 revision). *J Trauma* **38**(3):323–324.
35. Keller MS, Sartorelli KH, Vane DW. (1996) Associated head injury should not prevent nonoperative management of spleen or liver injury in children. *J Trauma* **41**(3):471–475.
36. (2006) Abdominal trauma in children. In: DE Wesson, S Stylianos, R Pearl, P Babyn (eds.), *Pediatric Trauma: Pathophysiology, Diagnosis, and Treatment*, pp. 267–301. Taylor and Francis, New York.
37. Upadhyaya P, Simpson JS. (1968) Splenic trauma in children. *Surg Gynecol Obstet* **126**(4):781–790.
38. Leinwand MJ, Atkinson CC, Mooney DP. (2004) Application of the APSA evidence-based guidelines for isolated liver or spleen injuries: A single institution experience. *J Pediatr Surg* **39**(3):487–490.
39. Stylianos S. (2002) Compliance with evidence-based guidelines in children with isolated spleen or liver injury: A prospective study. *J Pediatr Surg* **37**(3):453–645.
40. Stylianos S. (2000) Evidence-based guidelines for resource utilization in children with isolated spleen or liver injury. The APSA Trauma Committee. *J Pediatr Surg* **35**(2):164–167.
41. Sweed Y, Engel A, Halberthal M. (1997) Effectiveness of selective hepatic artery embolization in a child after blunt hepatic trauma. *Harefuah* **132**(4):252–254.
42. Puapong D, Brown CV, Katz M, *et al.* (2006) Angiography and the pediatric trauma patient: A 10-year review. *J Pediatr Surg* **41**(11):1859–1863.
43. Ohtsuka Y, Iwasaki K, Okazumi S, *et al.* (2003) Management of blunt hepatic injury in children: Usefulness of emergency transcatheter arterial embolization. *Pediatr Surg Int* **19**(1–2):29–34.
44. Fisher JC, Moulton SL. (2004) Nonoperative management and delayed hemorrhage after pediatric liver injury: New issues to consider. *J Pediatr Surg* **39**(4):619–622.

45. Ford EG, Andrassy RJ, Hallow KD. (1994) *Pediatric Trauma: Initial Assessment and Management.* **7**:201–222.
46. Jacombs ASW, Wines M, *et al.* (2004) Pancreatic trauma in children. *J Pediatr Surg* **39**:96–99.
47. Jurkovich GJ, Carrico CJ. (1994) Pancreatic trauma. *Surg Clin North Am* **70**:575–593.
48. Shilyanksy J, Sena LM, *et al.* (1998) Nonoperative management of pancreatic injuries in children. *J Pediatr Surg* **33**:343–349.
49. Firstenberg MS, Volsko TA, *et al.* (1999) Selective management of pediatric pancreatic injuries. *J Pediatr Surg* **34**:1142–1147.
50. Adamson WT, Herba A, *et al.* (2003) Serum amylase and lipase alone are not cost-effective screening methods for pediatric pancreatic trauma. *J Pediatr Surg* **38**:354–357.
51. Bouwman DL, *et al.* (1984) Serum amylase and its isoenzymes: A clarification of their implication in trauma. *J Trauma* **24**:573–578.
52. Takahashi M, *et al.* (1980) Hyperamylasemia in critically injured patients. *J Trauma* **20**:951–955
53. Burnweit C, Wesson D, *et al.* (1990) Percutaneous drainage of traumatic pancreatic pseudocysts in children. *J Trauma* **30**:1273–1277.
54. Gorenstein A, O'Halpin D, *et al.* (1987) Blunt injury to the pancreas in children. *J Pediatric Surg* **22**:1110–1116.
55. Smith SD, Nakayama Dk, *et al.* (1988) Pancreatic injuries in childhood due to blunt trauma. *J Pediatr Surg* **23**:610–614.
56. Arkovitz MS, Johnson N, *et al.* (1997) Pancreatic trauma in children: Mechanism of injury. *J Trauma* **42**:49–53.
57. Jobst M, Canty T, *et al.* (1999) Management of pancreatic injury in pediatric blunt abdominal trauma. *J Pediatr Surg* **34**:818–824.
58. Vane DW, Kiankhooy A, Sartorelli KH. (2009) Initial resection of potentially viable tissue is not optimal treatment for grades II–IV pancreatic injuries. World *J Surg* **33**(2):220–227.
59. Bosboom D, Braam AWE, *et al.* (2006) The role of imaging studies in pancreatic injury due to blunt abdominal trauma. Eur *J Radiol* **59**:3–7.
60. Canty TG, Weinman D. (2001) Treatment of pancreatic duct disruption in children by an endoscopically paced stent. *J Pediatr Surg* **36**:345–348.
61. Akhrass R, Yaffe MB, *et al.* (1997) Pancreatic trauma: A ten-year multi-institutional experience. *Am Surg* **63**:598–604.
62. Meier DE, Coln CD, *et al.* (2001) Early operation in children with pancreas transection. *J Pediatr Surg* **36**:341–344

63. Rescorla FJ, Cory D, Vane DW, *et al.* (1990) Failure of percutaneous drainage in children with traumatic pancreatic pseudocysts. *J Pediatr Surg* **25**:1038–1042.
64. Graham CA, O'Toole SJ, *et al.* (2000) Pancreatic trauma in Scottish children. *J R Coll Surg* Edinb **45**:223–226.
65. Keller MS, Stafford PW, Vane DW. (1997) Conservative management of pancreatic trauma in children. *J Trauma* **42**:1097–1100.
66. Kouchi K, Tanabe M, *et al.* (1999) Nonoperative management of blunt pancreatic injury in childhood. *J Pediatr Surg* **34**:1736–1739.
67. Wales PW, Shuckett B, *et al.* (2001) Long-term outcome after non-operative management of complete traumatic pancreatic transaction in children. *J Pediatr Surg* **36**:823–827.
68. Mattix KD, Tataria M, Holmes J, *et al.* (2007) Pediatric pancreatic trauma: Predictors of nonoperative management failure and associated outcomes. *J Pediatr Surg* **42**:340–344.
69. Hall RI, Lavelle MI, *et al.* (1986) Use of ERCP to identify the site of traumatic injuries of the main pancreatic duct in children. *Br J Surg* **73**:411–412.
70. McGahren Ed, Magnuson D, *et al.* (1995) Management of transected pancreas in children. *Aust NZ J Surg* **65**:242–246.
71. Wind P, Tiret E, *et al.* (1999) Contribution of endoscopic retrograde pancreatography in management of complications following distal pancreatic trauma. *Am Surg* **65**:777–783.
72. Kim HS, Lee DK, *et al.* (2001) The role of endoscopic retrograde pancreatography in the treatment of traumatic pancreatic duct injury. *Gastrointest Endosc* **54**:49–55.
73. Stringer MD. (2005) Pancreatic trauma in children. Brit *J Surg* **92**:467–470.
74. Moore EE, Cogbill TH, Malangoni MA, *et al.* (1990) Organ injury scaling, II: pancreas, duodenum, small bowel, colon, and rectum. *J Trauma* **30**: 1427–1429.

RENAL AND GENITOURINARY TRAUMA 15

Dennis Vane and Tres Scherer

RENAL AND COLLECTING SYSTEM TRAUMA

Approximately 5% of all children sustaining abdominal trauma have involvement of the genitourinary system.[1] The majority of these injuries are blunt in nature but penetrating mechanisms are seen more commonly in older children.

Motor vehicle collision, auto vs. pedestrian, falls, and mechanisms of rapid deceleration are the leading causes of renal injuries. Renal injuries occur more frequently in boys than girls by a ratio of 2–3:1.[1–3] Children are thought to be at higher risk for renal injury than adults due to several anatomical factors. The kidneys are seated lower in the abdomen (thus, less protected from the lower ribs), are proportionally larger with less perinephric fat, and are more mobile in younger patients.[4]

The diagnosis of renal injury requires a high index of suspicion as often details of the injury can be vague or unknown and children may have difficulty describing their symptoms.

PHYSICAL EXAMINATION

Hallmark signs of renal injury during examination of the abdomen include upper abdominal or flank tenderness, nausea, or vomiting. Additionally, flank ecchymosis or a palpable mass from extravasated blood or urine may be present. Children may present in a shock state if significant hemorrhage occurs due to the injury.[1] Any of these signs, particularly when seen together, added to a high degree of suspicion due to the mechanism of injury carrying a significant association with renal injury.

LABORATORY EVALUATION

Urinalysis is the primary screening tool for the evaluation of renal injury. Some authors have found that approximately 88–90% of children with renal injury will present with hematuria.[1,2] However, others have found that renal injury can exist in the absence of hematuria.[4] Historically, the presence of any degree of hematuria has warranted imaging to evaluate the presence of a renal injury. Recent concern about the amount of radiation sustained by children during the evaluation of traumatic injury has prompted some changes in these recommendations by creating new criteria for radiographic evaluation in order to increase the positive detection of injuries without compromising patient care. The data seems to support the recommendation that children with less than 100 red blood cells per high power field do not require emergent radiologic evaluation.[1,5–7] Using these criteria would diagnose the majority of injuries while reducing the number of radiologic studies ordered. Conversely however, Stein *et al.* and others have shown that significant injury can exist without hematuria and these injuries would be missed with these new imaging algorithms.[8] Until more data is available, the clinician should use appropriate judgment when employing diagnostic imaging. Elevations of serum BUN and creatinine are late signs of renal injury indicating urinary tract leak and intracavitary urine collection.

RADIOLOGIC DIAGNOSIS

Often plain pelvic and abdominal films are the first radiologic diagnostic images obtained on children with abdominal trauma. These studies may show fractures of the lower ribs, blunting of the renal outline or scoliosis toward the injured side, but typically are not specific.[1] Renal injuries can often be diagnosed with abdominal ultrasonography. The retroperitoneal location of the kidney and its surrounding *fascia* make it amenable to this diagnostic modality. Children sustaining abdominal trauma, however, often require broader diagnostic imaging and ultrasound is often not initially undertaken. Computerized tomography (CT), magnetic resonance (MR) and angiography have been the most favored and perhaps most accurate diagnostic tools. CT scan is usually the primary method of evaluation that is used for a complete evaluation of the abdomen and its contents. It is rapid, and today's equipment often requires no sedation for the child. It allows detection of parenchymal damage, vascular extravasation and urinary leakage. Its utility is in its widespread acceptance as the gold standard for evaluation of other intraabdominal injuries.

Ultrasound has been used in screening for perinephric fluid and although helpful in defining anatomic variations of the kidney, lacks sufficient definition to accurately grade injuries. Additionally, this modality introduces potential bias as the results are operator dependent. Wessel *et al.* found that only 70% of injuries were detected using ultrasound as a single diagnostic modality.[9] Ultrasound is perhaps most useful as a diagnostic evaluation for follow-up of renal injuries to ascertain exacerbation or amelioration of the lesion.

Intravenous pyelogram (IVP) is also useful in the evaluation of renal and urinary tract injury. IVP is especially useful for patients that require immediate operative intervention because of hemodynamic instability or other reason. A one-shot IVP can be used to assess renal function and determine level of injury or obstruction during a laparotomy being performed for other indications. However, the accuracy of IVP compared to CT scan has elicited some discussion. Studies have indicated that IVP may demonstrate as much as a 42% false–negative injury identification rate when compared to CT scan.[9]

CLASSIFICATION

Renal imaging, typically using CT, allows the practitioner to grade injuries according to the American Association for the Surgery of Trauma's criteria for grading renal injuries. These Organ Injury Scaling Guidelines are correlated against clinical outcomes to assist in treatment algorithms.[10] This system assists the clinician in determining intensity of surveillance, potential need for immediate intervention, and likelihood of successful nonoperative management. The classification system separates injuries into five grades as described in Table 1. If bilateral injuries are present, the grade is advanced by one grade.[10]

Table 1. Renal injuries.

Grade	Injury
I	Microscopic or gross hematuria with normal urologic studies. Subcapsular nonexpanding hematoma without parenchymal laceration.
II	Nonexpanding perirenal hematoma confined to renal retroperitoneum. <1 cm laceration of renal cortex without extravasation.
III	>1 cm laceration of renal cortex without extravasation or collecting system rupture.
IV	Parenchymal laceration extending through the renal cortex, medulla, and collecting system. Renal artery or vein injury with contained hemorrhage.
V	Shattered kidney. Avulsion of the renal hilum.

Note: Advance stage I level for bilateral injuries up to stage III.

This determination also allows the clinician to employ a common system when describing outcomes and therapy alternatives. Minor injuries (grades I–III) are usually managed nonoperatively. Major injuries (grades IV and V) which require more diligent monitoring are more likely to require operative intervention and critical injuries which are associated with hypotension or massive hemorrhage may require immediate surgical intervention.[1]

TREATMENT

As with all trauma patients, a systematic approach is required to manage renal trauma. After initial evaluation of an injured child and accurate diagnosis of injuries is obtained appropriate monitoring and treatment can be undertaken.

A majority of low-grade renal injuries can be treated with careful observation. Children without gross hematuria and who have sustained a grade I injury can be discharged home safely with reduced activity levels. They are followed with repeat urinalysis and imaging only if problems arise. A single follow-up urinalysis is usually obtained one or two weeks after the injury to assure healing. Children with gross hematuria and imaging demonstrating a grade I to III injury are generally admitted to the hospital for a minimum of 24 hrs in order to assure that bleeding will stop or decrease. Patients are kept on bed rest until hematuria resolves.[11] The mean duration of hematuria was 1.6 days for grade I injuries, 3.5 days for grade II and over 10 days for more severe injuries. Patients then begin ambulation and can be discharged home if hematuria does not recur. Children are followed on an outpatient basis and typically undergo ultrasound or functional nuclear imaging study.[9]

Hemodynamically stable grade IV and V injuries rarely require emergent exploration. Stable hematomas, urinary extravasation, or symptomatic urinomas in the retroperitoneum are usually managed expectantly. 7–10% may require delayed operative or endourological management with percutaneous drainage or placement of urinary tract stents.[1,2] Patients with massive hemorrhage and/or hemodynamic instability require operative intervention or possibly interventional angioembolization.[1,12] Multiple studies have found that penetrating injuries often require operative intervention and usually result in more severe injuries.[4,11] However, in most cases even high-grade renal injuries can be managed with renal sparing procedures.[13] Additionally, a child whose associated injuries warrant exploration should have a major renal injury evaluated only when a perinephric hematoma is expanding.

When exploration is required, it is essential to initially obtain control of the renal vascular pedicle prior to opening Gerota's *fascia*.[11] This allows for better control of hemorrhage while exploring and repairing the kidney. This lessens the potential for nephrectomy from uncontrolled bleeding. Accessing the renal vessels via transperitoneal approach at the base of the mesentery allows for access to both renal pedicles. During the operation, nonviable tissue is usually debrided, bleeding vessels ligated, and clots evacuated. Parenchymal lacerations can be repaired using vertical mattress sutures over fat or pledgets. Collecting system injuries should be repaired with absorbable suture. The patency of the ureter must always be confirmed. Finally, after adequate hemostasis is obtained, drainage of the retroperitoneum is recommended to prevent fluid collection (urine or blood) in the operative area.[1]

Vascular injuries should be repaired at the time of exploration. Arterial intimal tears may be tacked flat, excised with end-to-end anastomosis or undergo patch angioplasty. A renal vein injury must be repaired on the right side to maintain function due to paucity of collaterals on that side. On the left, the primary vein can be ligated if necessary as there is usually adequate collateral drainage via the adrenal, gonadal, and urethral veins. Segmental renal veins may be ligated without concern, again due to abundant collateralization. It must be noted, however, that when surgical intervention is necessitated on a renal injury, salvage of that kidney in children is far lower than with adults.[1] For this reason, the management of major renal injuries in hemodynamically stable children has undergone a paradigm shift to favor nonoperative management.

OUTCOMES

Traditionally, it was felt that conservative management would lead to a late intervention rate of 70% and a renal loss rate of up to 40%, added to an initial predicted renal loss rate of 11%.[14] Proponents of early intervention assent that significant morbidity and mortality could be avoided with repair of major cortical lacerations, ruptured poles, or collecting system tears. Recently, data indicates the opposite, with renal salvage rates far better with nonoperative management protocols in stable children.[2–4,15–17]

Buckley and McAninch found that only 4% of children sustaining blunt abdominal trauma had a grade IV or V renal injury and their overall rate of operative intervention for these children was less than 2%.[11] Henderson *et al.* found a higher interventional rate for these high-grade injuries of 16%.[17] However, their overall operative rate exclusively for renal trauma across all grades remained low at 6%. Interestingly, almost 40% of injuries were high grade in this series. The overall renal salvage rate is consistently excellent with initial nonoperative management ranging from 97 to over 99% in multiple studies.[2,3,11] Keller *et al.* demonstrated that nonoperatively managed kidneys retain excellent renal function. Their study indicated that only 31% of high-grade injuries resulted in poor function on the injured side.[18]

COMPLICATIONS

Often complications of renal trauma occur with nonoperative management. These include retroperitoneal hematoma, urinoma, and clot retention requiring continuous bladder irrigation, culture negative fever, urinary tract infection, sepsis, and recurrent gross hematuria. These occur in less than 5% of children.[2] Later complications may include hydronephrosis, chronic pyelonephritis, calculus formation, and renal artery stenosis. Hypertension and renal atrophy may also occur and cause a late change in renal function. The true incidence of late hypertension complication is unclear however due to generally short follow-up and the concomitant appearance of this disease later in life in uninsured patients. Henderson *et al.* found that only 3% of patients with grade IV and V injuries developed hypertension.[17] The incidence of late complications and decreased renal function in the affected kidney still make nonoperative management of this injury preferable to surgical intervention where initial loss of the kidney is more prevalent.[2–4,15–17]

Renal trauma may significantly contribute to the morbidity and mortality of the injured child. Correct diagnosis requires a systematic approach to children involved in trauma. Urinalysis is an excellent screening mechanism when coupled with appropriate imaging. As with other nonoperatively managed solid organs, further investigation is needed to produce clear guidelines for the need of follow-up diagnostic imaging, and return to activity in these children. Although nonoperative management of children with blunt solid organ abdominal injury has become the "gold standard", use of these algorithms mandates close observation of these children to avoid serious complications. Surgeons must understand that exploration in any hemodynamically unstable patient is mandated if an intraabdominal etiology is suspected.

Ureteral injuries are uncommon; there is a paucity of evidence-based data on management and outcomes of ureteral trauma.[19] These are rare injuries in blunt or penetrating trauma and are associated with injuries to adjacent structures. Penetrating injuries of the ureters are twice as common as blunt. Diagnosis is often delayed and requires a high index of suspicion. Repair often requires operation or endourological technique.

URINARY BLADDER TRAUMA

Bladder rupture or laceration is the most common injury of the pelvis in children. It is important to differentiate between extraperitoneal and intraperitoneal injuries. Blunt injury associated with lapbelt injury or pelvic fractures are the most common mechanisms. Since most injured children now undergo abdominal CT scanning, CT cystography should be considered on every such child to evaluate for bladder injury. When there is gross hematuria or blood at the meatus in boys, the bladder must be distended prior to performing CT cystography in association with CT of the abdomen and pelvis.[20] The majority of bladder injuries (extraperitoneal) can be treated successfully with urethral catheter, without the need for additional suprapubic drainage. Some authors recommend surgical repair of extraperitoneal bladder injuries, classically treated conservatively with bladder drainage, especially when these were associated with pelvic fractures requiring orthopedic intervention. This approach was used in up to 64% of such patients in one reported series.[21] Intraperitoneal injury requires surgical repair.

URETHRAL INJURIES

Approximately 4–14% pelvic fractures cause a posterior urethral injury. Pelvic fractures associated with straddle injuries or large trauma accidents are frequently associated with this kind of lesion. Primary open repair of the urethral injury is discouraged in the acute setting. Three to six months after urinary diversion, a formal open reconstruction can be safely attempted. This gives time for scar maturation, reabsorption of pelvic hematomas, and relative restoration of anatomical fascial layers. A retrospective study[22] reviewed 75 post-traumatic, pediatric, urethral strictures involving bulbar or posterior urethral injuries were treated by conventional urethroplasty techniques. The primary success rate was 69% and the secondary success rate, this improved to 93%. Other reports focusing on urethroplasty for pediatric posterior urethral injuries have shown similar excellent success rates.[23] Urethroplasty by experienced urethral surgeons must be available to these injured children.

MALE EXTERNAL GENITALIA INJURIES

Injuries in the preschool age group occur mostly from falls or from toilet seats.[24] Injuries of the male genitals in preschool age predominantly involve the penis due to the small size of the scrotum. A child voiding independently while standing in front of the commode puts the penis in harm's way from the accidental fall of the toilet seat. Zipper injuries are another common cause of penis injury in both the preschool age and the school age group. Boys that present with zipper injuries often experience severe pain and stress from the incident. Release of the entrapped penis should be undertaken under general anesthesia or with sedation. In school age boys, the injury pattern changes as the play environment changes. Bites, falls, kicks, sport activities, and bicycle are responsible for the majority of injuries. School age injuries account for nearly half of the injuries in childhood and adolescence.[24] Injuries of the scrotum are more frequent in the school age group. The various injuries documented include, scrotal skin lacerations and testicular contusions (causing severe pain). Those may require surgical or conservative management. In the pediatric population, testicular rupture may occur as a result of blunt trauma during athletic events. A conservative approach consisting of rest, scrotal support, antibiotics, and serial ultrasound can be utilized in most children without testicular loss or atrophy.[25] Surgical intervention may expedite the return to physical activity but at the expense of volume loss due to extensive debridement. Patients who have an expanding hydrocele, hematocele or worsening symptoms should undergo exploration. Injuries of the penis in this age group are predominantly lacerations which were mainly the result of direct trauma or falls. Injuries to the penis were less frequent than scrotal injuries but the majority of these penile injuries required surgical management.

REFERENCES

1. Fitzgerald CL, Tran P, Burnell J, Broghammer JA, Santucci R. (2011) Instituting a conservative management protocol for pediatric blunt renal trauma: Evaluation of a prospectively maintained patient registry. *J Urol* **185**(3):1058–1064.
2. Broghammer JA, Langenburg SE, Smith SJ, Santucci RA. (2006) Pediatric blunt renal trauma: Its conservative management and patterns of associated injuries. *Urology* **67**(4):823–827.
3. Nance ML, Lutz N, Carr MC, Canning DA, Stafford PW. (2004) Blunt renal injuries in children can be managed nonoperatively: Outcome in a consecutive series of patients. *J Trauma* **57**(3):474–478.
4. Nguyen MM, Das S. (2002) Pediatric renal trauma. *Pediatr Urol* **59**(5):762–766.
5. Morey AF, Bruce JE, McAninch JW. (2006) Efficacy of radiographic imaging in pediatric blunt renal trauma. *J Urol* **156**:2014–2018.
6. Herschorn S, Radomski SB, Shoskes DA, Mahoney J, Hirshberg E, Klotz L. (1991) Evaluation and treatment of blunt renal trauma. *J Urol* **146**(2):274–277.
7. Perez-Brayfield MR, Gatti JM, Smith EA, Broecker B, Massad C, Scherz H, *et al.* (2002) Blunt traumatic hematuria in children: Is a simplified algorithm justified? *J Urol* **167**:2543–2547.
8. Stein JP, Kaji DM, Eastham J, Freeman JA, Esrig D, Hardy BE. (1994) Blunt renal trauma in the pediatric population: Indications for radiographic evaluation. *Urology* **44**(3):406–410.
9. Wessel LM, Scholz S, Jester I, Arnold R, Lorenz C, Hosie S, *et al.* (2000) Management of kidney injuries in children with blunt abdominal trauma. *J Pediatr Surg* **35**(9):1326–1330.
10. Moore EE, Shackford SR, Pachter HL, McAninch JW, Browner BD, Champion HR, *et al.* (1989) Organ injury scaling: Spleen, liver, kidney. *J Trauma* **29**(12):1664–1666.
11. Buckley JC, McAninch JW. (2004) Pediatric renal injuries: Management guidelines from a 25-year experience. *J Urol* **172**:687–690.

12. Kiankhooy A, Sartorelli KH, Vane DW, Bahve AD. (2010) Angiographic embolization is safe and effective therapy for blunt abdominal solid organ injury in children. *J Trauma* **68**:526–531.
13. Angus LD, Tachmes L, Kahn S, Gulmi F, Gintautas J, Shaftan GW. (1993) Surgical management of pediatric renal trauma: An urban experience. *Am Surg* **59**(6):388–394.
14. Cass, AS. (1983) Blunt renal trauma in children. *J Trauma* **23**(2):123–127.
15. Gill B, Palmer LS, Reda E, Franco I, Kogan SJ, Levitt SB. (1994) Optimal renal preservation with timely percutaneous intervention: A changing concept in the management of blunt renal trauma in children in the 1990s. Br *J Urol* **74**(3):370–374.
16. Levy JB, Baskin LS, Ewalt DH, Zderic SA, Bellah R, Snyder HM III, *et al.* (1993) Nonoperative management of blunt pediatric major renal trauma. *Urology* **42**(4):418–424.
17. Henderson CG, Sedberry-Ross S, Pickard R, Bulas DI, Duffy BJ, Tsung D, *et al.* (2007) Management of high-grade renal trauma: 20-year experience at a Pediatric Level I Trauma Center. *J Urol* **178**:246–250.
18. Keller MS, Coln CE, Garza JJ, Sartorelli KS, Green MC, Weber TR. (2004) Functional outcome of nonoperatively managed renal injuries in children. *J Trauma* **57**(1):108–110.
19. Shenfeld OZ, Gnessin E. (2011) Management of urogenital trauma: State of the art. *Curr Opin Urol* **21**(6):449–454.
20. Lawson CM, Daley BJ, Ormsby CB, Enderson B. (2011) Missed injuries in the era of the trauma scan. *J Trauma* **70**:452–456.
21. Wirth GJ, Peter R, Poletti PA, Iselin CE. (2010) Advances in the management of blunt traumatic bladder rupture: Experience with 36 cases. *BJU Int* **106**:1344–1349.
22. Sunay M, Karabulut A, Dadal M, *et al.* (2011) Single-institution outcomes of open reconstruction techniques for management of pediatric and adolescent posttraumatic urethral strictures. *Urology* **77**:706–710.
23. Orabi S, Badawy H, Saad A, *et al.* (2008) Posttraumatic posterior urethral stricture in children: how to achieve a successful repair. *J Pediatr Urol* **4**:290–294.
24. Widni EE, Höllwarth ME, Saxena AK. (2011) Analysis of nonsexual injuries of the male genitals in children and adolescents. *Acta Pediatr* **100**:590–593.
25. Cubillos J, Reda EF, Gitlin J, Zelkovic P, Palmer LS. (2010) A conservative approach to testicular rupture in adolescent boys. *J Urol* **184**:1733–1738.

CENTRAL NERVOUS SYSTEM TRAUMA 16

Jodi L. Smith

INTRODUCTION

Head injury, a leading cause of death and acquired disability in the pediatric population, affects one million infants, children, and young adults each year in the United States and contributes nearly 20 billion dollars annually to health care costs. This chapter presents current concepts in the evaluation and management of pediatric patients with severe traumatic brain injury, with emphasis on the prehospital, emergency department, and intensive care management of such patients. Management strategies described herein are based on available scientific evidence and include recommendations from the existing pediatric guidelines.[1,2] In this chapter, pediatric patients are those who are 17 yrs of age or younger, severe head injury is defined using the Glasgow Coma Scale (GCS)[3] with a score equal to eight or less (Tables 1 and 2), and head injury comprises both accidental and nonaccidental causes.

PATHOPHYSIOLOGY OF HEAD INJURY

The pathophysiology of traumatic brain injury guides treatment. Severe pediatric head injury involves two types of injury — primary and secondary. Primary injury occurs at the time of the traumatic event — i.e. at the moment of impact. Examples include scalp lacerations, skull fractures (e.g. base of skull — Table 3), epidural and subdural hematomas,

Table 1. Modified Glasgow Coma Scale (GCS) for pediatric patients.[4]

Assessed Response	**Score**
Best eye response	
Spontaneously	4
To verbal stimulation or touch	3
To pain	2
No response	1
Best verbal response	
Smiles, oriented to sounds, follows objects, interacts	5
Cries but is consolable, inappropriate interactions	4
Inconsistently consolable, moaning	3
Inconsolable, agitated	2
No vocal response	1
Motor	
Normal spontaneous movement	6
Withdraws to touch	5
Withdraws to pain	4
Flexion abnormal	3
Extension, either spontaneous or to painful stimuli	2
Flaccid	1

Table 2. Presenting GCS and degree of head injury.[4]

GCS 3–8	Severe
GCS 9–12	Moderate
GCS 13–15	Mild

intraparenchymal hemorrhage, cortical contusions, diffuse axonal injury, and brain stem injury. In contrast, secondary injury evolves during the hours and days that follow the initial trauma and produces additional progressive cellular damage and dysfunction resulting from degenerative biochemical processes initiated both by the primary injury and by additional systemic insults. For example, secondary injury occurs as a result of brain swelling (from acute cerebral arterial vasodilatation and associated increased cerebral blood volume), diffuse cerebral edema (from increased cerebral water content), elevated intracranial pressure (ICP), cerebral herniation, traumatic ischemia and/or infarction, secondary hemorrhage,

Table 3. Basilar skull fracture — clinical and radiographic findings, management.

Exam
battle sign, raccoon eyes
hemotympanum or blood in external auditory canal
CSF leak — rhinorrhea, otorrhea

Head CT
pneumocephalus, fracture involving skull base

Management
elevate head of bed 45–60°
give prevnar/pneumovax vaccine series
may give dose of prophylactic antibiotics
lumbar drain for CSF diversion if CSF leak persists
direct surgical repair of fracture/dural tear

risk of meningitis — if fever and elevated WBC present, perform lumbar puncture and start antibiotics

Table 4. Major causes of secondary brain injury.[4]

Hypoxia	Hypotension
Hyperthermia	Hyperglycemia/hypoglycemia
Intracranial hypertension	Hypocapnia/hypercapnia
Anemia	Cerebral edema
Vasospasm	Seizures
Cerebral herniation	Infection

hypotension, and hypoxia (Table 4). It is the leading cause of death in the hospital after a traumatic brain injury; however, its intensity, duration, and ultimate effect on neurologic outcome can be decreased by early, aggressive, comprehensive care.[4] Hypotension and hypoxia, which commonly occur in pediatric patients with severe head injury, have the greatest negative impact on patient outcome, increasing both morbidity and mortality. For example, in a prospective study of 200 pediatric patients the mortality rate was significantly higher in the presence of hypotension, hypoxia, or hypercarbia than it was in their absence (i.e. 55% vs. 7.7%, $p<0.01$).[5] In another study analyzing the influence of hypoxia and hypotension on mortality in severely head-injured children, hypotension on admission was associated with a mortality rate of 61%; this increased to 85% when both hypotension and hypoxia were present, compared with only 22% when patients were normotensive on admission.[6] Finally, in a prospective analysis of severe head injury in 6908 adults and 1906 children younger than 15 yrs of age at 41 trauma centers, hypotension was associated with significantly higher mortality rates in children and had a more harmful effect in children than in adults.[7] Hypotension in children is defined as systolic blood pressure below the fifth percentile for age or by clinical signs of shock. The lower limit of systolic blood pressure for age (i.e. the fifth percentile) can be estimated by multiplying the patient's age in years by two, and then by adding this number to 70 mm Hg. Hypoxia in children is defined as PaO_2 <60–65 mm Hg, oxygen saturation <90%, apnea, or cyanosis. Hypoventilation, which results in hypercarbia, is defined as ineffective respiratory rate for age, shallow or irregular respirations, frequent episodes of apnea, or measured hypercarbia.

The injured brain is exquisitely sensitive to secondary systemic and local intracranial insults. The main goal of acute management of severe head trauma is to minimize the progression or the effects of secondary injury and thereby maximize the child's potential for recovery. Successful management of severe pediatric head injury requires complete and rapid physiologic resuscitation, prevention of hypotension and hypoxia, treatment of elevated ICP, and maintenance of cerebral perfusion to facilitate adequate delivery of oxygen and metabolic substrates to the brain. The remainder of this chapter provides evidence-based management strategies for the treatment of severe pediatric head injury.

PREHOSPITAL MANAGEMENT

Prehospital management (i.e. speed of access to definitive care and timing of intervention relative to the initial insult) is paramount to the survival and eventual outcome of pediatric patients with severe head injury. The pediatric guidelines recommend transporting such patients directly to a pediatric level I trauma center if available or to an adult trauma center staffed with qualified, pediatric-trained caregivers and pediatric-sized equipment if not.[1]

Essential to the prehospital care of head-injured pediatric patients is the expedited assessment and management of airway, breathing, and circulation (i.e. the ABC's of resuscitation). The goal of such management is to prevent secondary brain injury by obtaining early airway control and restoring normal physiologic age-appropriate parameters of oxygenation, ventilation, circulating blood volume, and blood pressure. Because hypotension and hypoxia commonly occur in the prehospital setting and are associated with poorer functional outcomes, they must be avoided or corrected immediately. Patients should undergo prompt fluid resuscitation with intravenous normal saline, and blood loss from all extracranial injuries should be evaluated and treated.[1,2] At present, there is no role for inducing supranormal blood pressures in the treatment of severe pediatric head injury.

Hypoxia must also be recognized and treated promptly by administering supplemental oxygen, performing bag-valve-mask ventilation, or performing rapid sequence intubation with sedation and paralysis by if care providers are trained in pediatric intubation.[1] Early airway control is essential for patients with GCS less than or equal to eight. Moreover, because pediatric patients with severe head injury are also at risk for associated cervical spine injuries due to their relatively larger heads and underdeveloped neck muscles, in-line cervical spine immobilization must be maintained during intubation to prevent additional injury.

Other key prehospital brain-directed interventions include the use of sedation, analgesia, and neuromuscular blockade to optimize transport to a pediatric trauma center, and the administration of a loading dose of Phenytoin (15–20 mg/kg) and/or Phenobarbital (15–20 mg/kg) if two or more seizures are observed. The prehospital prophylactic use of brain-directed therapies, such as mannitol, hypertonic saline, and hyperventilation, is not recommended because these treatment modalities can exacerbate intracranial ischemia and interfere with resuscitation. A mannitol bolus (0.25 g/kg IV) is warranted only if signs of herniation or acute neurological deterioration (Table 5) are present and volume resuscitation is adequate (i.e. patient is euvolemic and normotensive). Hyperventilation (i.e. 25 breaths/min in a child and 30 breaths/min in an infant), which causes cerebral vasoconstriction and reduced cerebral blood flow (CBF) and is associated with worsened neurological outcomes, should be avoided unless the patient shows signs of impending cerebral herniation (Table 5).

MANAGEMENT IN THE EMERGENCY DEPARTMENT

In the emergency department, airway, breathing, and circulation must be reevaluated and the clinical examination should be repeated to evaluate for signs and symptoms of herniation and increased ICP (Table 5).

Table 5. Signs of cerebral herniation.

Extensor posturing (GCS 4)
Motor asymmetry
Pupillary asymmetry (uncal herniation)
Bulging fontanelle
Cushing's triad — bradycardia, hypertension, erratic respirations

A noncontrasted head computed Tomography (CT) should be obtained as soon as vital signs are stabilized to evaluate for a mass lesion with associated mass effect and midline shift, focal vs. diffuse injury, and patency of the basilar cisterns. An intracranial mass lesion, if found should be promptly surgically evacuated.

MANAGEMENT IN THE INTENSIVE CARE UNIT

Meticulous management in an intensive care unit (ICU) setting with continuous monitoring of physiologic parameters has significantly reduced the mortality and morbidity of pediatric patients with severe head injury. This should include continuous invasive arterial blood pressure monitoring, pulse oximetry, and monitoring of ICP, central venous pressure, temperature, end-tidal carbon dioxide, and urine output. The primary goal of intensive management is to improve mortality rates and functional recovery by preventing secondary injury to the brain resulting from systemic hypotension, hypoxia, elevated ICP, and/or reduced cerebral perfusion pressure (CPP). To avoid secondary brain injury, normal, age-appropriate physiologic parameters must be maintained and prompt intervention must occur if deviations in these parameters arise.

Cerebral Perfusion Pressure (CPP)

The CPP, defined as the mean arterial blood pressure (MAP) minus ICP, is the physiologic variable that represents the pressure gradient driving CBF and metabolite/oxygen delivery and, therefore, is related to cerebral ischemia. A low CPP correlates with poor outcome in traumatic brain injury patients. Based on the pediatric guidelines, CPP should be maintained above a minimum of 40 mm Hg to prevent regional or global cerebral ischemia.[1,2]

Intracranial Hypertension

The harmful consequences of elevated ICP stem from its effect on regional and global CBF. Pediatric patients with severe traumatic brain injury, especially those with subdural hematomas, large multifocal contusions, hypoxic injury, and/or gunshot wounds to the head, frequently develop significant brain swelling and/or diffuse cerebral edema, which, in turn, produce intracranial hypertension (i.e. pathologically elevated ICP) and a reduction in CBF (i.e. cerebral ischemia). Because intracranial hypertension is associated with decreased survival and poor functional outcome, pediatric patients with severe head injury require aggressive ICP monitoring and ICP-directed therapies to enable rapid detection and correction of neurologic deterioration.

ICP Monitoring

An ICP monitor should be placed for continuous ICP monitoring and treatment of elevated ICP in patients with GSC less than or equal to eight (including infants), especially in the face of diffuse brain swelling, cisternal effacement, midline shift, and/or multiple contusions on the admitting head CT scan. In addition, an ICP monitor may be placed in patients with a GCS > 8 if a mass lesion is present or if serial neurologic examinations cannot be performed because of sedation, neuromuscular blockade, or anesthesia for management of extracranial injuries.[1,2] With regard to the recommended ICP level for which treatment should be initiated, there are no absolute treatment thresholds.[1,2] However, 20 mm Hg is typically chosen as the arbitrary upper limit beyond which treatment is required. Regardless of the threshold chosen, interpretation and treatment of ICP should be validated by frequent clinical examination, cranial imaging, and monitoring of physiologic variables, such as CPP and MAP. Finally, to ensure the best possible outcome related to ICP management, one must pay strict attention to details, repeatedly assessing changes in ICP and ongoing responses to therapy.

Accurate and reliable methods for monitoring ICP in pediatric patients with severe head injury include intraparenchymal fiberoptic catheter tip pressure transducer devices, a ventricular catheter connected to an external strain gauge, and external strain gauge transducers. To achieve accurate, reliable and continuous monitoring of ICP concomitant with therapeutic cerebrospinal fluid (CSF) drainage, one should place both an intraparenchymal catheter tip pressure transducer device for continuous monitoring of ICP and a ventriculostomy catheter for CSF drainage. In addition to enabling simultaneous ICP monitoring and therapeutic CSF drainage, this technique permits periodic measuring of ICP by the ventriculostomy catheter, which can then be compared to the ICP measured by the intraparenchymal catheter tip pressure transducer device to evaluate for measurement differences and drift.

Evidence-based treatment strategies

The effect of ICP in children is related to its absolute peak and duration of elevation. During the process of treating intracranial hypertension, one should always consider the possibility that a surgical mass or an unexpected intracranial lesion may have developed, necessitating a repeat head CT. When ICP is greater than 20 mm Hg and the head CT shows no surgical mass lesion, several evidence-based treatment strategies can be employed. Most importantly, all physiologic parameters must be optimized. For example, PaO_2 should be maintained greater than 80 mm Hg and $PaCO_2$ should be maintained around 35–38 mm Hg since hypoxia and hypercarbia cause cerebral vasodilatation, leading to increased cerebral blood volume and elevated ICP. In conjunction with this, blood transfusions should be administered as needed to keep the hemoglobin greater than 11 mg/dL. Fluid restriction should be avoided to prevent hypovolemia. Instead, intravenous isotonic or hypertonic crystalloid solutions should be administered in sufficient volumes to maintain a normal or slightly increased intravascular volume. Hyperthermia, defined as a core body temperature greater than 38.5°C, should be avoided, as a role for therapeutic hypothermia has not yet been established. The patient's head should be kept in a neutral position since head rotation or neck flexion can impede jugular venous outflow and increase ICP. Moreover, the endotracheal tube tape and the cervical spine collar should be sufficiently loose to avoid constricting jugular venous outflow. Finally, as long as the patient is euvolemic and normotensive, the head of the bed can be elevated 15–30° to reduce venous outflow pressure, which is an effective way to reduce ICP without compromising CPP and CBF.

Sedatives, analgesics, and neuromuscular blocking agents

Elevated ICP in children with severe head injury who have with a secure airway and are on mechanical ventilatory support can be treated with sedatives (e.g. benzodiazepines and barbiturates, but not propofol which can cause a lethal metabolic acidosis), analgesics (e.g. narcotics), and neuromuscular blocking agents. These medications aid in the management of intracranial hypertension by ameliorating agitation; reducing pain and stress; preventing coughing, straining, and shivering; minimizing movement; facilitating assisted ventilation; and facilitating patient transport to radiology or the operating room. However, care must be taken to avoid hypotension when using these agents.

CSF drainage

Elevated ICP can also be treated with CSF drainage providing a ventricular drainage catheter can be placed. If a ventricular drain is in place and ICP continues to be elevated in the face of the aforementioned maneuvers, the drain may be opened at 10–15 cm above the external auditory canal for CSF drainage, which lowers ICP by reducing intracranial fluid volume.

Hyperosmolar therapy

If ICP is still elevated after ventricular CSF drainage, hyperosmolar therapy should be instituted in the form of intermittent intravenous hypertonic saline (e.g., 3%) boluses (in doses ranging from 6.5 to 10 ml/Kg of body weight) and/or continuous intravenous infusions of hypertonic (e.g. 3%) saline (at a rate of 0.1–1.0 mL/kg of body weight/hr).[2] When treating elevated ICP with hyperosmolar therapy it is necessary to maintain the patient in a euvolemic or slightly hypervolemic state. It is also necessary to assess serum electrolytes and serum osmolarity frequently (e.g. every 4–6 hrs) in order to prevent acute renal failure when administering hyperosmolar therapy in head-injured patients. When treating elevated ICP with hypertonic saline, the serum osmolarity should not exceed 360 mOsm/L. Finally, prophylactic use of hyperosmolar agents is not recommended; such agents should only be used in conjunction with an ICP monitor and documented intracranial hypertension.[1,2] However, mannitol may be given empirically for signs of brain herniation[1], including an acute mental status decline and a pupil that is dilated and unresponsive pupil (Table 5).

Barbiturate coma

If intracranial hypertension remains refractory despite implementation of the aforementioned management strategies and there is no identifiable cause for ICP intractability noted on repeat head CT, therapy with high-dose barbiturates such as pentobarbital should be considered.[1,2] High-dose barbiturates reduce ICP by suppressing brain metabolism and reducing CBF and cerebral blood volume. Serum levels of barbiturates do not correlate well with electrical activity; therefore, patients on high-dose barbiturate therapy require continuous EEG monitoring for burst suppression ("barbiturate coma"), since this reflects a near-maximum reduction in brain metabolism and CBF. To institute therapy with pentobarbital, a loading dose of 10 mg/kg of body weight is given over a period of 30 mins. After the loading dose, a 5 mg/kg bolus of pentobarbital is given every hour for three doses, followed by a maintenance dose of 1 mg/kg body weight/hr. The maintenance dose is continued as long as the ICP remains elevated, with the goal of maintaining burst suppression on the EEG. Once the ICP has been well controlled for at least 24 hrs, the patient is weaned from the barbiturates. Because barbiturates can cause severe myocardial depression, patients on high-dose barbiturates must be monitored carefully for hemodynamic instability. If hypotension is observed, intravenous fluids and pressors must be administered immediately to provide blood pressure support, with the goal of maintaining the blood pressure within a normal, age-appropriate range.

Decompressive craniectomy

Another option for treating elevated ICP refractory to medical management is decompressive craniectomy.[1,2] This procedure has been shown to decrease ICP and have a beneficial effect on neurologic outcome. Operative techniques most commonly employed include a unilateral frontal-temporal-parietal-occipital craniectomy with expansion duraplasty for cerebral swelling localized to one side of the brain and a bilateral frontal craniectomy with expansion duraplasty for diffuse bilateral cerebral swelling. To achieve the best possible outcome from this procedure, decompressive craniectomy should be performed on salvageable patients with diffuse cerebral swelling on head CT with secondary clinical deterioration or evolving cerebral herniation syndrome who are within 48 hrs of their injury, have a GCS greater than three, and have not had any prolonged episodes of ICP elevation greater than 40 mm Hg.[1,2]

Temperature Control

In the face of persistently elevated ICP, moderate hypothermia (32–33°C) may be effective as long as it starts within eight hours after the head injury and continues for 48 hrs.[2] Pediatric patients undergoing treatment with moderate hypothermia should undergo slow re-warming at a rate of 0.5-1.0°C every 3 to 4 hours, and moderate hypothermia for 24 hrs or less should be avoided.[2]

Hyperventilation

If ICP is still elevated after employing the aforementioned management strategies, hyperventilation may be used. However, because of the risk of secondary brain injury and worsened neurologic outcome from ischemia due to hyperventilation-induced vasoconstriction, the following recommendations are made in the pediatric guidelines regarding the use of hyperventilation.[1,2] First, prophylactic severe hyperventilation (i.e. $PaCO_2$ less than 30 mm Hg) should be avoided. Second, mild hyperventilation (i.e. $PaCO_2$ 30–35 mm Hg) may be employed to treat intracranial hypertension that fails to respond to other ICP-reducing therapies. Finally, brief periods of aggressive hyperventilation (i.e. $PaCO_2$ less than 30 mm Hg) can be used to treat medically and surgically intractable intracranial hypertension as well as signs/symptoms of cerebral herniation or acute neurologic deterioration.

Anticonvulsant

The prophylactic use of anticonvulsants has not been shown to be effective in preventing late posttraumatic seizures or in improving outcome in pediatric patients with severe traumatic brain injury. Consequently, the pediatric guidelines recommend against the prophylactic use of seizure medications in such patients.[1] However, anticonvulsants should be used to treat early posttraumatic seizures since they can occur in up to 40% of pediatric patients with severe head injury and can cause secondary brain injury by generating increased ICP, hypoxia, hypercarbia, and increased cerebral metabolic demand.[2]

Corticosteroid

There is no role for corticosteroids in improving outcome or reducing ICP in the treatment of pediatric patients with severe traumatic brain injury, even in the face of severe refractory intracranial hypertension.[1,2]

Nutrition

Because the metabolic rate is significantly increased in pediatric patients with severe head injury, the pediatric guidelines recommend that feedings commence, either by parenteral or enteral formulas, by 72 hrs and should be at full replacement (i.e. 130–160% of resting energy expenditure) by seven days.[1] However, the exact role of nutritional supplementation on functional outcome has not yet been adequately investigated. Nevertheless, it is absolutely essential that blood glucose levels be monitored closely and tightly controlled during feedings to prevent hyperglycemia, which can worsen outcome from head injury by exacerbating secondary brain injury.

CONCLUSION

To maximize the potential for functional recovery in pediatric patients with severe traumatic brain injury, the progression or the effects of secondary brain injury must be minimized. Significant reductions in morbidity and mortality in pediatric patients with severe traumatic brain injury can be achieved by (1) early intubation, (2) rapid transport to an appropriate trauma care facility, (3) prompt resuscitation with avoidance of hypotension and hypoxia, (4) early CT scanning, (5) immediate evacuation of intracranial mass lesions, and (6) meticulous management in an ICU setting, including aggressive treatment of intracranial hypertension guided by ICP monitoring and maintenance of normal physiologic parameters to facilitate adequate delivery of oxygen and metabolic substrates to the brain.

REFERENCES

1. Adelson PD, Bratton SL, Carney NA, Chesnut RM, du Coudray HE, Goldstein B, Kochanck PM, Miller HC, Partington MP, Selden NR, Warden CR, Wright DW. (2003) American Association for Surgery of Trauma; Child

Neurology Society; International Society for Pediatric Neurosurgery; International Trauma Anesthesia and Critical Care Society; Society of Critical Care Medicine; World Federation of Pediatric Intensive and Critical Care Societies Guidelines for the acute medical management of severe traumatic brain injury in infants, children, and adolescents. *Pediatr Crit Care Med* **4**(3):S1–S71.

2. Kochanek PM, Carney N, Adelson PD, Ashwal S, Bell M, Bratton S, Carson S, Chcsnut RM, Ghajar J, Goldstein B, Grant GA, Kissoon N, Peterson K, Selden N, Tong KA, Tasker RC, Vavilala MS, Wainwright MS, Warden CR. (2012) Guidelines for the acute medical management of severe traumatic brain injury in infants, children, and adolescents. *Pediatr Crit Care Med* **13**(1):S1–S82.
3. Teasdale G, Jennett B. (1974) Assessment of coma and impaired consciousness. A practical scale. *Lancet* **2**:81–84.
4. Swaminathan A, Levy P, Legome E. (2009) Evaluation and management of moderate to severe pediatric head trauma. *J. Emerg Med* **37**:63–68.
5. Mayer TA, Walker ML. (1985) Pediatric head injury: The critical role of the emergency physician. *Ann Emerg Med* **14**:1178–1184.
6. Pigula FA, Wald SL, Shackford SR, Vane DW. (1993) The effect of hypotension and hypoxia on children with severe head injuries. *J Pediatr Surg* **28**:310–314.
7. Luerssen TG, Klauber MR, Marshall LF. (1988) Outcome from head injury related to patient's age. *J Neurosurg* **68**:409–416.

PEDIATRIC VASCULAR INJURIES

17

Jenny Cho and Michael Dalsing

INTRODUCTION

Pediatric vascular trauma is rare and accounts for approximately 1% of trauma admissions in children age 1–18.[1] Although uncommon, vascular injuries may have devastating outcomes if missed during the initial evaluation. Penetrating trauma is more likely to result in a vascular injury (55–68%) than blunt trauma (31–45%).[1,2] Penetrating injuries are most commonly from sharp objects, gunshot wounds and animal bites. Blunt injuries include falls, collisions with moving objects, bicycle accidents, and motor vehicle accidents.

PRESENTATION AND EXAMINATION

A complete history is invaluable in making an accurate diagnosis but often must be obtained from the child's parent or caregiver. Particular attention should be paid to the mechanism of injury (e.g. speed of the collision, height of the fall) and timing of the event.

Nearly half of all vascular injuries occur in the upper or lower extremities. The most common vessel involved is the brachial artery in the upper extremity and the femoral artery in the lower extremity.

Abdominal trauma may result in injury to major vascular structures based on the location of injury. The artery/vein involved often correlates with the zone of injury within the retroperitoneum of the abdomen. The central portion, zone 1, includes the aorta, mesenteric vessels, proximal renal vessels, vena cava and portal vein. The lateral quadrants, zone 2, has the distal renal vessels. Finally the pelvis, zone 3, involves the iliac vessels.[3]

Physical examination should start with a full body examination; inspection of entrance and exit wounds, lacerations, bone fractures, joint dislocations (particularly the knee), bruising or hematomas, pulsatile masses or active bleeding. A vascular examination includes; visual inspection of the skin, palpation and Doppler ultrasound for pulses, auscultation over the vascular bed for bruits, ankle over brachial systolic blood pressure index, as well as motor and sensory examination of affected extremity. If there is a visible injury it is important to examine pulses proximal and distal to the affected artery.

Clinical Signs of Ischemia

Clinical signs of acute limb ischemia include the "five Ps"; absent pulses, paresthesia, paralysis, paleness, and poikilothermia.[4] Paresthesia and paralysis may be difficult to assess in neonates and young children who lack communication skills.

The classic "hard" and "soft" signs of vascular injury must be modified in neonates/children from adult guidelines (Table 1).[5] This is multifactorial but is primarily due to the difficulty in assessing signs of distal ischemia because the child lacks the ability to tell what is painful or lacks appropriate feeling. This population also suffers from severe arterial vasospasm in response to injury and, therefore, immediate surgical intervention for absent pulses may not be warranted. In 80% of normothermic and normotensive children, the vasospastic response to injury resolves within 1 hr.[5] Therefore, in some cases, medical therapy or even observation may be the treatment of choice in neonates/children with soft signs of ischemia.

The degree of ischemia may be categorized based on the Rutherford criteria for acute limb ischemia (Table 2). Category I and IIa limbs are not immediately threatened, however, require prompt evaluation and serial observation with semi-urgent repair as needed. Category IIb symptomatic limbs require immediate intervention for limb salvage and III often are nonsalvageable and may require amputation.[6]

Table 1. Hard and soft signs of vascular injury (adult vs. neonate/child).

	Adult	Neonate/Child
Hard Signs	Active arterial bleeding	Active arterial bleeding
	Expanding hematoma	Expanding hematoma
	Absent pulses	
	Distal ischemia	
	Bruit/thrill over wound	
Soft Signs	Nonexpanding hematoma	Nonexpanding hematoma
	Hypotension	Hypotension
	Peripheral nerve deficit	Peripheral nerve deficit
	History of bleeding	History of bleeding
		Bruit/thrill over wound
		Absent pulse
		Distal ischemia

Table 2. Rutherford criteria of acute limb ischemia.[6]

Category	Description	Capillary refill	Muscle weakness	Sensory loss	Arterial Doppler	Venous Doppler
I	Viable	Intact	None	None	Audible	Audible
IIa	Marginally threatened	Intact, slow	None	Minimal (toes)	Often audible	Audible
IIb	Immediately threatened	Very slow, absent	Mild, moderate	More than toes	Usually inaudible	Audible
III	Irreversible	Absent	Profound	profound	Inaudible	Inaudible

DIAGNOSTIC STUDIES

Ankle–Brachial Index

The ankle–brachial index (ABI) is an important part of the examination. The ABI is calculated by dividing the highest systolic blood pressure at the ankle (dorsalis pedis or posterior tibial artery) by the arm brachial artery systolic pressure. In children older than 1 yr of age an ABI less than 0.9 is considered abnormal. A study of 200 healthy full-term newborns (less than 2 weeks old) found an average ABI of 0.88 +/− 0.11 in normal, asymptomatic extremities. Most infants will normalize their ABI to greater than 1.0 by the first year of life.[7] Therefore, a low ABI may be normal in infants, however, by 1 yr of life an ABI less than 0.9 is abnormal and an arterial injury should be considered.

Color Flow Duplex Studies

Color flow Doppler studies are particularly helpful in children because they are noninvasive. There are three components of the study to evaluate: audible Doppler pulse, blood flow spectral waveform analysis, and duplex imaging. It is best to have an experienced technician perform the duplex in order to improve the quality of the study.

The first component is an audible Doppler examination of the pulse, which may be done with a handheld devise by the technician or member of the medical team. There are three phases of the audible pulse to listen for:

(1) The first sound is high velocity, forward-flow during early systole
(2) The second sound is reverse-flow during early diastole
(3) The third sound is low-velocity, forward-flow in late diastole

These three phases make up a normal triphasic Doppler signal of an arterial pulse. When arterial stenosis is present the signal becomes monophasic. An arterial occlusion will produce a "water-hammer" signal proximal to the occlusion and an absent signal distally.

Arterial spectral waveform analysis is the second component and adds further information about blood flow. The peak systolic velocity and end-diastolic velocity are noted and any localized increase in peak systolic velocity, especially if double or triple the velocity noted in the normal proximal artery, may indicate a significant stenosis.

Lastly, duplex imaging provides a black/white picture of the underlying vessel and surrounding structures. As such it can detect abnormalities including thrombus, dissections, intimal tears, pseudoaneurysms, arterial to venous fistulas and adjacent hematomas. The introduction of color to the picture may provide some indication of vascular narrowing but is not as precise as the peak systolic velocity findings.

NonInvasive Imaging Studies

Plain radiographs are often useful in diagnosing concomitant injuries, such as bony fractures or joint dislocations. Computed Tomography (CT) angiography has significantly advanced with high quality images and three-dimensional (3D) reconstructions. The adult literature shows high sensitivity and specificity for diagnosing arterial injuries when compared with conventional angiography.[8,9,10] Currently, insufficient data specific to the pediatric population exists nevertheless it is often used to confirm the clinical impression in our practice. The benefit of shorter test time and minimal sedation needed with CT imaging makes it superior to Magnetic Resonance (MR) imaging.

Invasive Imaging Studies

Angiography may be used for diagnostic and occasionally therapeutic purposes. Due to the complication potential in the pediatric age group, angiography should only be used in select cases where other diagnostic tools are insufficient.

SPECIFIC TYPES OF ARTERIAL INJURY

Iatrogenic Injury

A large subset of vascular trauma is iatrogenic injuries. The majority are secondary to percutaneous venous or arterial access for diagnostic or therapeutic procedures. The femoral artery is the most common vessel used for percutaneous access and, therefore, is the most commonly injured. Vascular assess complications include hemorrhage, acute thrombosis, dissection, pseudoaneurysm, embolization and arterial to venous fistula. The risk of injury increases with decreasing age, number of catheterizations and increasing catheter size.[4,11] A study of 65 femoral artery catheterizations in children 5 yrs old or younger were reimaged 5 to 14yrs following their initial procedure. It was found that 37% had femoral artery occlusion and a mean ABI of 0.79.[12]

A thorough history including prior vascular interventions, bleeding disorder, blood thinning medications, coagulopathies, and vascular anomalies is essential prior to an intervention. Also, the use of ultrasound guided puncture may help decrease access site complications. A study of 87 consecutive femoral vein access procedures in children, with a median age 2 yrs old, showed inadvertent femoral artery puncture in 7% of patients while using ultrasound guidance compared to 31.8% without ultrasound.[13]

Bone Fractures and Joint Dislocation

Many arterial injuries in children are associated with a bone fracture or joint dislocation. Supracondylar humerus fractures are the most common fracture to involve a vascular injury in children.[2] Limbs with displaced bone fractures should be placed into traction and dislocated joints reduced immediately. Alignment of these structures often alleviates compression on an adjacent artery and restores blood flow to the limb. This may resolve the acutely ischemic limb, however, it is still important to evaluate for vascular injury. Often injuries such as arterial intimal tears or dissections are asymptomatic but diagnosis is essential for appropriate management and good long term outcome.

TREATMENT

As with all trauma patients initial control of airway and breathing is essential. Obvious external sources of bleeding need to be controlled with compression or a tourniquet device to minimize blood loss. This often has been accomplished at the seen of the accident by the medical responders. Hypovolemic shock from blood loss in large vascular injuries requires aggressive resuscitation and rapid vascular control. All infants and children presenting with active hemorrhage or an expanding hematoma require immediate surgical intervention to control bleeding and allow vascular repair. Treatment of an arterial injury with distal ischemia varies based on the severity of ischemia, age of the child, risk of intervention and the overall condition of the individual.

Neonates and Infants

Neonates and infants younger than 2 yrs of age present a unique population with regards to treating lower extremity arterial injuries. They have very small arteries that tend to develop rapid collateral vessels when occluded. Trauma causes intense vasospasm in this population with or without a true arterial injury. Because of this phenomenon the treatment of arterial occlusion differs in neonates and infants compared to older children. With a nonthreatened ischemic limb (Rutherford class I and IIa) the best treatment is often medical therapy with anticoagulation, warming and correction of hypotension.[14] With this treatment the majority of lower extremities show an improvement in color, temperature and pulse exam within 24 to 36 hrs. In comparison, a collective analysis of 28 children less than 2.5 yrs of age treated with surgical repair, found only 48% regained pulses, 25% mortality rate and 15% of the survivors had limb discrepancy.[15] If clinical signs are not improved with unfractionated heparin anticoagulation, catheter directed thrombolysis has shown benefit or operative intervention may be required.[14,15]

Children Two to Thirteen Years of Age

Arterial injury with severe distal ischemia requires surgical intervention in all children. Children greater than 6 yrs with mild symptoms may still benefit from an operative repair to prevent future complications with growth retardation. However, younger children from 2 to 6 yrs old may do worse with surgical repair. These children could benefit from delayed arterial repair or future limb lengthening procedures.[5,16]

During operative repair of arterial or venous injuries several principles should be followed. A preoperative dose of antibiotic is given and sterile technique is used to prepare the surgical site. Proximal and distal control of the artery is gained to control hemorrhage and prepare for repair. Full anticoagulation is given after arterial exposure is achieved and ideally prior to cross clamping the vessel. The injured area of the vessel must be excised to healthy proximal and distal tissue. Balloon embolectomy catheters are used to remove associated thrombus from inflow or runoff vessels but this must be preformed very gently in the vessels which are prone to spasm and injury. When reestablishing the continuity of injured vessel, a tension-free repair is essential. This may be accomplished by primary suture repair, patch angioplasty, interposition graft or bypass grafting. When grafting is needed, autogenous material is preferred to prosthetic material. The contralateral greater saphenous vein is the ideal vessel to use for most bypass grafts.

In addition, fasciotomies of the extremity should be considered for prolonged ischemia greater than 6 hrs, concurrent arterial and venous injuries or elevated compartment pressures (> 30 mm Hg). If this is not done, close evaluation of the extremity in the postoperative period must be undertaken to identify signs of developing compartment syndrome.

OUTCOMES AND FOLLOW-UP

Limb Length Disparity

Arterial insufficiency in children can lead to hindered growth of the affected extremity. Limb length discrepancy in the lower extremity affects ambulation, hip and spine stability, and posture.[1] Shortening of the upper extremity is better tolerated by the individual. Taylor reports an inverse relationship between ABI and severity of leg growth retardation.[12]

Follow-up Evaluation

Follow-up of a child suffering from an arterial injury is essential to detect future problems with arterial stenosis, bypass failure, venous occlusive disease, and limb length disparity. During each evaluation assessment of the patient's symptoms, ABIs and graft surveillance duplex scan when indicated should be performed. Patients who required extremity bypass surgery should have a graft surveillance duplex study at 1, 3, 6, 9, and 12 mths evaluation in the first year, followed by every 6 mths for 2 yrs, than every year for life. Those patients with isolated primary arterial repair need evaluation at 1, 6, and 12 mths than yearly thereafter. Early detection and intervention of arterial compromise will improve long term patency.

REFERENCES

1. Klinkner DB, Arca MJ, Lewis BD, Oldham KT, Sato TT. (2007) Pediatric vascular injuries: Patterns of injury, morbidity, and mortality. *J Pediatr Surg* **42**:178–183.
2. Shah SR, Wearden PD, Gaines BA. (2008) Pediatric peripheral vascular injuries: A review of our experience. *J Surg Res* **153**: 162–166.
3. Brautigam RT, Sheppard R, Robinson KJ, Jacobs LM. (2008) Evaluation and treatment of multiple trauma patients. *Skeletal Trauma*, 4th edition. W.B. Saunders Company, Philadelphia.

4. Rutherford RB, Cronenwett JL, Gloviczki P, Johnston KW, Krupski WC, Ouriel K, Sidawy AN. (2005) *Vascular Surgery*, 6th edition. Elsevier Saunders, Philadelphia.
5. Dalsing M. (2006) Lower extremity vascular injury in children younger than 13 years of age. In: W Pearce, J Matsumura, J Yao (eds.), *Trends in Vascular Surgery*, pp. 215–229. Greenwood Academic, Illinois.
6. Rasmussen TE, Clouse WD, Tonnessen BH. (2008) Lower extremity ischemia. *Handbook of Patient Care in Vascular Diseases*, pp. 200–202. Lippincott Williams and Wilkins.
7. Katz S, Globerman A, Azitzour M, Dolfin T. (1997) The ankle–brachial index in normal neonates and infants is significantly lower than in older children and adults. *J Pediatr Surg* **32**:269–271.
8. Siegel MJ. (2005) Pediatric CT angiography. *Eur Radiol* **4**:D32–D36.
9. Busquets AR, Acosta JA, Colon E, Alejandro KV, Rodriguez P. (2004) Helical computed tomographic angiography for the diagnosis of traumatic arterial injuries of the extremities. *J Trauma* **56**(3):625–628.
10. Peng PD, Spain DA, Tataria M, Hellinger JC, Rubin GD, Brundage SI. (2008) CT angiography effectively evaluates extremity vascular trauma. *Am Surg* **74**(2):103–107.
11. Lin P, Dodson T, Bush R, Weiss V, Conklin B, Chen C, Chaikof E, Lumsden A. (2001) Surgical intervention for complications caused by femoral artery catheterization in pediatric patients. *J Vasc Surg* **34**(6):1071–1078.
12. Taylor L, Troutman R, Feliciano P, Menashe V, Sunderland C, Porter J. (1990) Late complications after femoral artery catheterization in children less than five years of age. *J Vasc Surg* **11**(2):297–304.
13. Iwashima S, Ishikawa T, Ohzeki T. (2007) Ultrasound-guided versus landmark-guided femoral vein access in pediatric cardiac catheterization. *Pediatr Cardiol* **29**:339–342.
14. Saxena A, Gupta R, Kumar RK, Wasir HS. (1997) Predictors of arterial thrombosis after diagnostic catheterization in infants and children randomized to two heparin dosages. *Catheter Cardio Diag* **41**:400–403.
15. Wang M, Hays T, Balasa V, *et al.* (2003) Low-dose tissue plasminogen activator thrombolysis in children. *J Pediat Hematol Onc* **25**(5):379–386.
16. Lazarides MK, Georgiadis GS, Papas TT, *et al.* (2002) Operative and nonoperative management of children aged 13 years or younger with arterial trauma of the extremities. *J Vasc Surg* **43**(1):72–76.
17. Peter SD, Ostlie DJ. (2007) A review of vascular surgery in the pediatric population. *Pediatric Surg Int* **23**:1–10.

PEDIATRIC BURN 18

John J. Coleman III

EPIDEMIOLOGY

Of an overall trauma all injury death rate of 54.36 per 100,000 in the USA in 1998, the burn death rates varied widely geographically from 0.12 per 100,000 to 3.69 per 100,000 with an average of 1.41 per 100,000. House fires are the most common cause of death in burn injury and are much more frequent in the eastern United States particularly the southeast than in the west. The average annualized death rate of children and the elderly is five to six times that of the remainder of the population. Children are vulnerable to injury from playing with matches and other devices particularly in environments where alcohol, drugs, nonparental childcare and low income are present. In children less than 4 yrs, scald injuries predominate and often are secondary to spills while preparing food in the kitchen. Although the total number of burn injuries in the US is unknown estimates of 1.4 to 2 million with 75,000 hospitalizations have been put forth with incidence peaks in the groups less than 5 yrs, 25 to 39 yrs and greater than 65 yrs.[1]

PATHOPHYSIOLOGY

It is intuitive and there is some experimental data that demonstrates the duration of exposure and the temperature of the burning substance are directly proportional to the damage to the skin and subjacent tissues. There are, however, other variables involved such as the thickness of the skin which varies greatly over the body from an epidermis of 0.05 to 1 mm and a dermis from

0.5 to 2 to 3 mm. Skin thickness also varies with age with children and the elderly having thin skin and adults' thicker skin. The thickness of the underlying fat may impair conduction as a mechanism of heat dispersion thus making a burn more severe in a child with thin skin and a thick layer of baby fat.

Locally the burn injury impairs cellular function particularly the sodium potassium pump creating protein necrosis. The burn wound is a dynamic injury, the central area with the longest contact with the burning agent demonstrates tissue necrosis and is known as the zone of coagulation surrounding this in three dimensions, protein denaturation and loss of membrane integrity interferes with the normal flow of intravascular fluid and erythrocyte function resulting in increased platelet and neutrophil adherence and other disorders. This is, however, potentially reversible with proper care and creates a dynamic zone of stasis which may be improved by proper hydration and restoration of homeostasis with damage by hypotension or other effects of injury and shock. Enveloping this is an area where the effects of acute inflammation are demonstrated upon relatively undamaged cells and where increased blood flow, vasodilatation, and increased capillary permeability result in the zone of hyperemia (Figure 1).

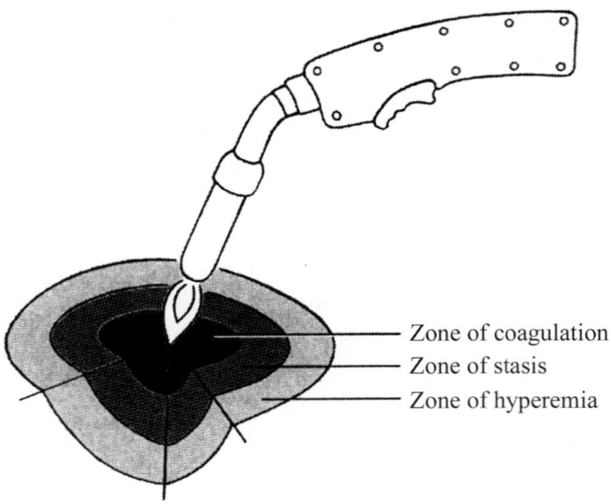

Figure 1. Burns are dynamic injuries. Outside the zone of coagulation, the area of cell death, the zones of stasis and hyperemia may shrink or enlarge depending on local or systemic conditions.

Systemic improvement or deterioration can result in changes in the zones of stasis and hyperemia creating a dynamic injury which will improve or deteriorate depending on systemic or local interventions.

In the early burn injury the presence of edema is a major consideration directing care. Burn wound edema affects the body surface area burned but may in large burns be a systemic issue involving uninjured skin mucous membranes and viscera as well. Local tissue necrosis and vasoactive cytokines released in the inflammatory response increase capillary permeability. Histamine and possibly other substances increase in the intravascular compartment driving up the hydrostatic pressure. Changes in collagen and other proteins decrease the hydrostatic pressure in the interstitial fluid. All of these changes result in a dramatic efflux of fluid and small proteins from the intravascular to the extravascular compartments. Burn edema is usually at its maximum in 12–48 hrs and depending on subsequent care of the patient may take a week to ten days to disperse. Because of its high protein content it is an excellent medium for bacterial growth in the skin lung and other areas and therapy aimed at reversing the edema is critical to the successful care of the patient.[2]

A significant size burn (greater than 10% in children and 20% in adults) creates a multifaceted systemic effect. Loss of homeostasis in the burn skin can result in hypothermia, hypotension and decreased barrier function to infectious agents. A consumption coagulopathy can occur secondary to loss of clotting factors into the injured tissue. Cytokines, prostanoids, and other inflammatory mediators can cause myocardial depression, pulmonary hypertension, bowel hypoperfusion, and many other harmful effects. Myoglobin from burned muscle and other burn wound products can impair renal function. The acute burn creates a hyper-metabolic response resulting in rapid depletion of energy stores particularly glucose and glycogen. The trauma corticosteroid response in addition to other less well defined humoral influences and inflammatory cell consumption may result in a profoundly immunosuppressed state increasing the risk of systemic infection. Moreover, the obligate large amounts of resuscitation fluid necessary to maintain intravascular volume and perfusion pressure cause additional problems as much is lost into the interstitium of the skin, lungs, intestines, etc., resulting in swelling and possible compartment syndrome, pulmonary edema, ileus, etc. The burn injury is a model of the body's response to trauma and requires the full range of physiologic management inherent in that systemic problem.

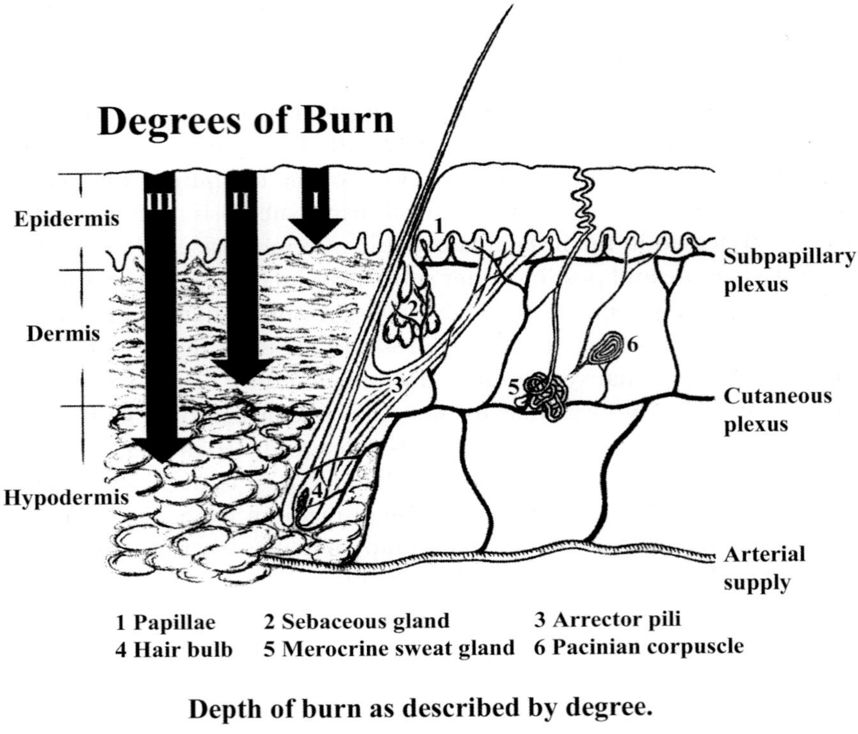

Figure 2. Depth of burn as described by degree.

Burn depth is the determinate of the likelihood of healing and the variable that defines whether surgical or nonsurgical therapy will be successful (Figure 2).

First degree burns are confined to the epidermis and are manifest by erythema from the underlying hyperemia provoked by the inflammatory response and also sometimes by desquamation of the upper layer of epithelial cells. These usually heal without scarring within 4–7 days by regrowth of epithelial cells from the basal layer. Partial thickness or second degree burns involve the epidermis and varying levels of the dermis. Second degree burns heal by reestablishing an epidermis by migration of basal cells from the skin appendages located in the dermis. Keratinocytes released from contact inhibition by the death of overlying epidermis migrate from the sebaceous glands and hair follicles to resurface the dermis with an epidermis. Concentration of these is greater in the superficial dermis than in the deeper dermis so the migration is shorter and the time to healing faster. In deeper second degree burns there are fewer epithelial appendages to repopulate the burns so granulation tissue, fibroblast capillary buds and fibrin fill in the area. The longer the duration of persistence of granulation tissue without healing the more likely hypertrophic scarring will occur. Therefore, deep second degree burns are often best treated by excision and autografting.

MANAGEMENT

Prehospital

Care of the burn patient is consistent with care of all trauma patients with several special considerations and can be divided into four stages. (1) Prehospital, (2) Emergency room, (3) Acute resuscitation, (4) Subacute and chronic.

Prehospital care in the field consists of removing the burning agent and any objects that might retain heat. Clothing, jewelry and other items should be removed. The patient should be transported in a warm environment covered with clean sheet and blankets. Sterile coverings are not necessary. Patients should not be hosed down after removing the heated agent and ice packs etc. are contraindicated since vasoconstriction can result in aggravation of the burn injury and systemic hypothermia is certainly a risk in a patient with impaired homeostasis secondary to skin injury.

Burn injuries are often associated with other injuries so full Advanced Trauma Life Support (ATLS) protocol should be observed with primary and secondary surveys dictating emergent care.

A history of the injury should be obtained from bystanders or those involved and particularly oriented to timing and duration of injury, confinement, burning agent, medical conditions, and associated injury.

When a burn injury occurs in a confined space it should be assumed that there has been an inhalation injury. Although there are several well known external signs such as singed nasal hairs, soot in the mouth, etc., there may be significant injury without signs or acute symptoms. Acute respiratory distress is uncommon prior to resuscitation but protection of the airway is critical. If the face and neck are burned and resuscitation is to begin in the field, endotracheal intubation should be performed, otherwise oxygen by nasal cannula is sufficient. In most cases establishment of intravenous access with maintenance fluid Ringers Lactate is appropriate for transfer and fluid resuscitation is best initiated on admission to hospital.

Emergency Room

Emergency room care is a continuation of prehospital care with added emphasis on establishing an accurate diagnosis and obtaining an accurate history. In major burns large bore intravenous access should be established and if necessary this can be done through burned skin although non-burned skin is preferable. Airway protection must be established and even in infants cuffed endotracheal tubes are preferable. Because of the narrow tracheal airway in children and because the resistance to airflow varies proportionally to the fourth power of the radius (Poiseuille's law) preemptive endotracheal intubation is appropriate in patients with facial burns or those who will require massive resuscitations even if the face is not burned since systemic edema can cause facial swelling and impair an unburned airway. The consideration for ventilation must be completely separate from the need for airway protection and should be determined by analysis of arterial blood gases. In children with facial burns secure fixation of the endotracheal tube may be difficult. In older children a circumdental 24 or 26 French stainless steel wire around a tooth with at least two roots is effective. In infants and younger children transmandibular wiring may be necessary.

In the emergency room as in the field protection from hypothermia is critical. Keeping the patient covered with clean sheets and blankets and the liberal use of heat lamps will help prevent this troublesome complication.

Repetition of the primary and secondary ATLS surveys with appropriate radiographic and chemical tests is necessary. Specific to the burn patients' complete blood count (CBC), electrolytes, BUN and creatinine, and arterial blood gasses are necessary as is a baseline chest film. In patients with profound acidosis a cyanide test may be useful. Type and screen or cross match is appropriate for major burns and urinalysis with testing for myoglobinuria and placement of a urinary catheter to monitor urine output. The diagnosis of the burn must include the total body surface area (TBSA) burned and a description of the depth of the burn in the various areas. It may be difficult to assess the patient who has been removed from a burning environment until all smoke, soot and debris has been removed but examination of the total skin surfaces is essential to accurate diagnosis. This may require shaving the head to accurately assess

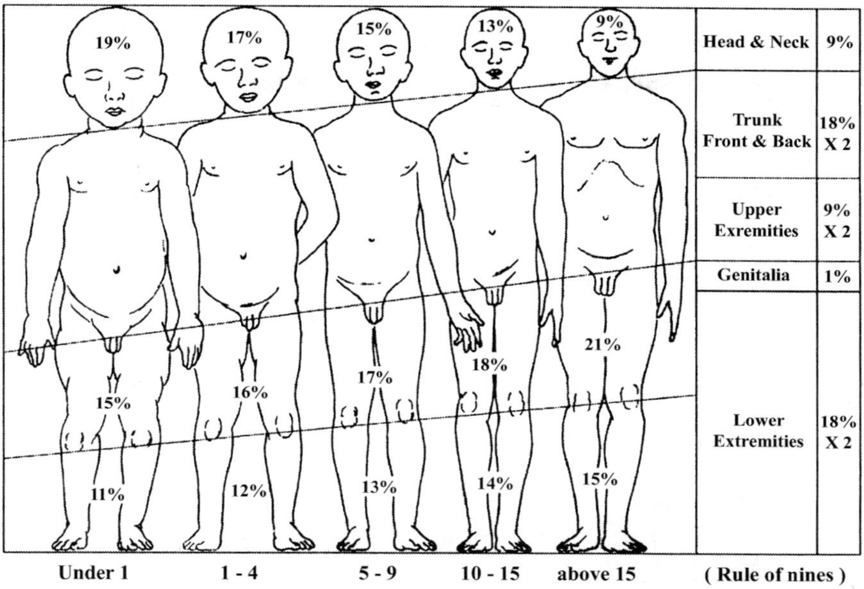

Figure 3. The rule of nines is an excellent way to estimate TBSA in the burned adult. The large heads and short limbs of babies make it less reliable at early ages.

particularly in children in whom the head makes up a larger percentage of the body surface. Exact estimation of the TBSA which ranges from roughly 0.2 to 0.3 m^2 in children to 1.5 to 2m^2 in adults is very difficult but a reasonable estimation can be made by the use of the rule of nines or by the knowledge that the surface area of the palm equals approximately 1% of the TBSA (Figure 3). Accurate measurement of the TBSA is critical since the volume of fluid resuscitation as well as the prognosis is determined by this figure.

In patients with circumferential burns of the extremities or the chest consideration of escharotomy must be made particularly if the transfer to the burn unit will be prolonged and significant fluid resuscitation will be required in transport. If the patient is to be immediately admitted escharotomy of the arm, hands, fingers, legs, chest, and rarely penis can be delayed until reaching the burn unit or operating room. Fasciotomy is rarely necessary in burns. If there has been a delay in performance of escharotomy and there is suspicion of compartment syndrome or if the

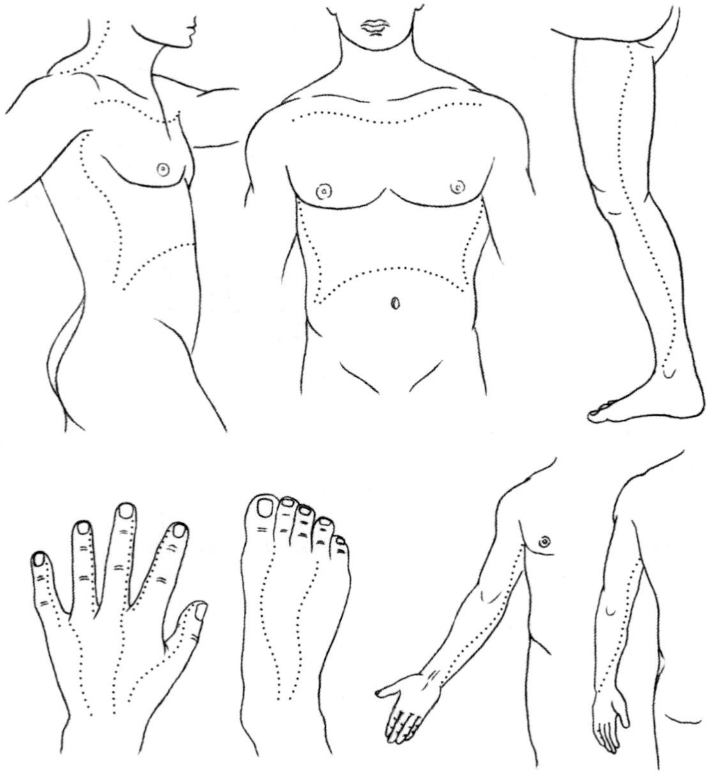

Figure 4. Location of escharotomy incision. In general these should be located medially and laterally in areas with least amount of external contact. In the arms the ulnar nerve at the elbow and the dorsal radial and ulnar nerves at the wrist must be avoided. Finger incisions should be placed on the less functionally important side. In the leg the superficial peroneal nerve near the fibula should be avoided.

muscle itself has been burned and is swelling with resuscitation, fasciotomy should be added to escharotomy (Figure 4).

The complexity of the burn injury requires that children so injured should be treated by a multidisciplinary team familiar with the problem in a surgical unit devoted to burn care. The American Burn Association (ABA) and American College of Surgeons (ACS) have developed an accreditation process for burn units similar to that of level I trauma centers.

Table 1. ABA criteria for transfer to a burn center.

Second degree burns greater than 10% TBSA
Burns to face, hands, feet, genitalia, perineum, major joints
Third degree burns
Electrical burns including lightening
Burns with serious preexisting medical conditions
Burns accompanied by trauma where burn injury poses greatest risk of morbidity or mortality
Burns in children when hospital does not have high level pediatric services
Patients with special social emotional or rehabilitative needs
Chemical burns

They have also developed a set of criteria that suggests transfer to a burn unit. When such a transfer is initiated communication regarding the transfer should occur in a physician to physician contact and be enacted only when the patient is stable enough for travel (Table 1).

Acute Resuscitative Phase

The definitive care of the burned child is begun on admission to the burn unit. Careful reassessment of the patient by the treating surgeon and the entire burn team begins and a plan of therapy is developed. The plan and its execution must not be considered as exclusive and sequential but as an integrated synthesis of immediate and future problems that addresses not only the life threatening issues but future functional and aesthetic considerations.

Consolidation of the emergency care is done by rechecking the secure fixation of the endotracheal tube and changing the tube to the optimal size and position if necessary since field of intubation of children may be imprecise. The sufficiency of IV access and urinary drainage must be assured. The patient is cleaned and minor debridement can be carried out under sedation and analgesia. A warm environment to prevent hypothermia is maintained. TBSA burn and the areas involved are reassessed and determination of depth in the various areas is repeated. These findings are carefully recorded on standard burn diagrams and included in the medical record. Whenever possible a detailed history of the event should be obtained and compared with the previously obtained histories especially when neglect or abuse is a concern (Figure 7).

Fluid resuscitation dominates this phase of burn care although many other considerations are initiated simultaneously including splinting, physical therapy, etc. All of the formulas developed for fluid resuscitation in burn care are empiric and depend on the TBSA burn. Thus accurate measurement of TBSA is critical since inaccurate calculation may result in under resuscitation with consequent hypovolemia, hypotension and its sequelae or over resuscitation with excess edema, potential congestive heart failure, compartment syndrome, etc. Since these formulas attempt to provide sodium and water empirically the adequacy of treatment is judged by the patients response especially urine output. In children the desired response is 1 to 1.5 mL/kg/hr of urine output. Base deficit, blood pressure and serum sodium are useful but less accurate measures of resuscitation and heart rate may remain elevated despite normovolemia because of inflammatory mediator release. For adults or grown children the Parkland resuscitation formula is often used which is calculated as 4 mL Ringers Lactate per percent TBSA per kilogram body weight for the first 24 hrs. One half of the calculated volume is administered over the first 8 hrs and one half over the next 16 hrs. Because children rapidly deplete their glycogen scores in the highly catabolic environment of the burn injury the Parkland formula is modified to 3–4 mL lactated Ringers per TBSA per kilogram plus maintenance fluid calculated by weight administered as D5LR. The use of colloid is usually reserved for the second 24 hrs of resuscitation and may be administered by weight and burn area as in the Brooke formula or by calculation of plasma volume deficit. In very large burns in children colloid may be necessary in early resuscitation.

Other injuries associated with the burn such as fractures or blunt trauma may greatly impact on the need for fluid resuscitation and should be dealt with as part of the overall therapy. The most problematic aspect of fluid calculation is the associated inhalation injury. The numerous toxic agents in smoke can cause direct alveolar damage and initiate an inflammatory response in the lung which results in greatly increased bronchial blood flow, capillary permeability and fluid loss into the alveoli. This increases fluid resuscitation requirements to maintain normovolemia an unknown amount even as it causes local problems in lung.

Severe inhalation injuries can double the amount of fluid necessary to be administered to obtain normovolemia but the resuscitation should be carefully monitored so as not to increase the risk of pulmonary edema.

Sequestration of fluid in the abdomen either as ascites or visceral edema may be the consequence of massive fluid resuscitation in the acute burn or later in the treatment of pulmonary or other sepsis. Increased intraabdominal pressure can impair mechanical ventilation and even cause pressure on the intraabdominal viscera, abdominal compartment syndrome. When intravesical pressure approaches 30 mm of mercury and continued fluid administration is necessary consideration must be given to decompressive laparotomy. The increased domain and decreased resulting pressure may be lifesaving in children.

Circumferential burns of the extremity and chest will become more compressive as fluid accumulates in the burned skin. Compression of underlying nerves and muscles may result in tissue death. Symptoms of pain and numbness may be present but these result when tissue damage has already occurred. If prophylactic escharotomy has not been performed distal perfusion of the extremity should be monitored with physical examination and frequent (every 1–2 hrs) Doppler ultrasound evaluation of arterial flow. Compartment pressures in the extremity should be measured and as they approach 30 mm of mercury escharotomy must be performed. In patients undergoing mechanical ventilation with progressive requirement for increasing peak airway pressure, chest escharotomy may be useful even when the burns are not completely circumferential.

Inhalation injury is usually the cause of death in early burn injury. Overwhelming exposure to smoke, carbon monoxide, hydrogen cyanide, hydrochloric acid, sulfuric acid, and other toxins result in acute respiratory failure and death. Lower exposures that are not immediately lethal result in direct toxicity to the alveolar cells and increased bronchial blood flow and capillary permeability. The obligate fluid resuscitation results in intraalveolar fluid collection and decreased ciliary function. Desquamation of injured cells in the alveoli and bronchi can result in atelectasis and bacterial overgrowth resulting in bronchopneumonia. Acute respiratory distress syndrome (ARDS) from pulmonary sepsis is the most common cause of burn mortality in the subacute therapy phase.

The clinical presentation of ventilation injury may vary but follows a somewhat predictable pattern. Diagnosis may be made by bronchoscopy but this does not necessarily predict severity. A history of confinement is almost always predictive of inhalation injury and should dictate therapy. Initially arterial blood gases and chest radiographs may be relatively normal. During 36 to 48 hrs fluid overload in the injured lung may manifest as pulmonary edema and since systemic fluid resuscitation is usually complete by this time fluid restriction, Furosemide and bronchodilators may be useful. In extreme cases pleural effusion may occur and although this is usually reversible medically in critically ill patients tube thoracostomy drainage may be required. At 72–96 hrs the accumulation of bronchial and alveolar debris may result in airway obstruction and atelectasis or bronchopneumonia. Vigorous pulmonary toilet and culture specific antibiotics should be used to treat pneumonia. Chest physiotherapy and mucolytics are particularly important in small children who are intubated because of the narrow lumen of the endotracheal tube.[3]

Endotracheal intubation to protect the airway is a function of burn site and site and fluid resuscitation is an aggravating influence on the upper airway. The need for ventilation is determined by the clinical course of the patient particularly with respect to arterial blood gases. Severe inhalation injury may progress fairly rapidly to ARDS and ventilatory techniques that avoid barotrauma, alveolar overdistention, oxygen toxicity and other harmful concomitants of ventilation are important in pediatric burn treatment. Alternative ventilatory techniques such as pressure directed ventilation (PDV) and high frequency oscillating ventilation (HFOV) have been useful in children to decrease ventilator induced lung injury (VILI). It has been our practice to initiate HFOV when conventional mechanical ventilation is being escalated and oxygenation is deteriorating such that the PAO_2/FIO_2 is less than 150 or the oxygen index is greater than 25. HFOV is based on the concept of permissive hypercapnia and seeks to maintain an arterial SAO_2 of 90–92 with a pH of 7.1 or greater while decreasing FIO_2 to less than 60% to mitigate oxygen toxicity and mean airway pressure MAP to less than 32 cm of water to decrease the risk of barotrauma.

Tracheostomy should never be performed in acute burns in children and is rarely necessary at any time during pediatric burn care. Cuffed endotracheal tubes are usually adequate and more manageable carrying less risk of tracheomalacia or tracheostenosis.

Respiratory failure in burns may be improved by decreasing the Systemic Inflammatory Response (SIRS) in the patient by treating the burn wound itself. Excision of burn tissue and reestablishment of some elements of homeostasis with application of homograft or autograft may improve oxygenation and reduce ventilatory requirements.

BURN WOUND CARE

Initial burn wound care is aimed at preventing conversion of partial thickness burn to full thickness burn and to preventing invasive infection of full thickness burns. Hydrotherapy with tanks or shower cleans and gently debrides the wound and topical antibiotics are used to suppress bacterial colonization that inevitably occurs from respiratory and fecal contamination. The most commonly employed topicals are silver containing compounds particularly silver sulfadiazine cream although recently numerous silver impregnated adherent or nonadherent dressings (Acticoat $_{\mathrm{Rx}}$, Mepilex Ag $_{\mathrm{Rx}}$, Aquacel AG $_{\mathrm{Rx}}$) have been introduced usually for more superficial burns. If the therapeutic goal is to allow the burn to heal, as in superficial or moderate partial thickness burns, the burned skin is kept in a moist environment to encourage epithelialization. Other effective agents for topical use include bacitracin, sulfamylon, and mupirocin.

Deeper burns, deep partial thickness usually are treated with early tangential excision and grafting of some sort. Full thickness burns unless very small require excision of the skin and underlying fat down to the *fascia*. Leaving a large amount of poorly vascularized fat invites bacterial invasion from the contaminated environment and will usually result in fulminant wound sepsis. Tangential excision or excision to *fascia* is carried out as soon as the patient is adequately resuscitated hopefully by postburn day four since the burden to the body of a large burn is great. If the burn is large cadaver homograft is applied to mimic some of the homeostatic properties of skin (heat preservation, barrier function, fluid loss). If the homograft engrafts it is likely that subsequent autografting will be successful. In burns of less surface area where the excised bed of the dermis or *fascia* look good autografting at the time of excision may be performed. Tangential excision alone but especially when combined with autografting has the potential for many intraoperative dangers primarily via massive blood loss. Techniques to decrease blood loss such as segmental step wise excision and infiltration of epinephrine solution into donor site area and constant communication between surgeon and anesthesiologist and surgeon and nursing staff are critical to prevent catastrophe.

In very large burns after excision has been accomplished homograft is applied. If it does not engraft further excision of the wound may be necessary. If it does engraft it can be replaced by autografting. When the donor sites are limited grafts can be meshed and expanded to heal larger areas by

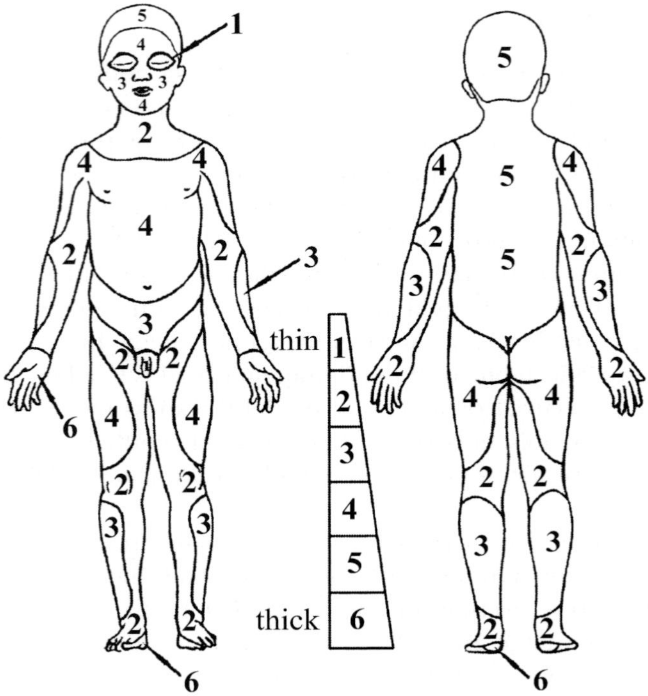

Figure 5. The priorities for skin grafting in patients with large TBSA burns. Eyes and IV sites have highest priority followed by functional and aesthetic areas.

epithelialization between the interstices of the expanded grafts. Unmeshed or sheet grafts are preferred over the hands and face. In large burns the sequence of autografting must follow the hierarchy of priorities for function in the following order. Protection of the eyes, intravenous access sites, exposed dura, major joints, hand, resurfacing of the face, resurfacing of flexor and extensor surfaces to allow motion, release of contracture, reconstruction of aesthetic deformities, reconstruction of burn alopecia should be performed in that order (Figure 5). Previously harvested donor sites in a patient who has stabilized will reepithelialize to be ready for reharvest in approximately 7 to 10 days. In some cases use of keratinocytes cultured in vitro from a sample of the patient's skin is useful. Cultured epithelial autografts can be obtained in approximately 3 wks to cover large burned areas. Coverage of the burn wound with autograft greatly improves the condition of the patient decreasing the catabolic stimulus and increasing the ability to fight associated infection.

When burned skin becomes invasively infected by colonizing bacteria burn wound sepsis occurs. This must be treated by excision of the infected skin. Systemic antibiotics are not effective in treating burn wound sepsis since penetration by the antibiotic agent of the poorly vascularized burn is minimal. Surgical excision is required when quantitative culture demonstrates ten to the fifth or more bacteria per gram of burned skin or when the clinical presentation warrants.[4]

INFECTION

Prolonged hospitalization, multiple therapeutic interventions, intratracheal intubation, and the profound immunosuppression caused by a major burn put patients at high risk of nosocomial infection of all sorts. Constant surveillance of all body sites is critical to prevent sepsis from sites other than the burn wound. Although acute septic shock warrants a shotgun antimicrobial approach, as soon as bacteriologic diagnosis is established culture specific antibiotics should be used.

Pulmonary sepsis is the most common cause of death in large burns. Multiple drug resistant bacteria, fungi and molds are seen in burn care and careful attention to hand washing and maintenance of closed circuit ventilatory systems and urinary drainage systems may decrease nosocomial infection.

Urinary tract infection commonly occurs in burned children because of prolonged indwelling urinary catheters and fecal contamination. Catheters should be removed as soon as the patient has been adequately resuscitated unless they are necessary to maintain urologic patency in the burned perineum. Ascending infection can result in pyelonephritis.

Septic thrombophlebitis and central venous catheter infection are common problems. On admission to the burn unit intravenous catheters placed in the field should be replaced under sterile conditions. Careful examination of present and past IV access sites is important when unexplainable fever and sepsis occurs. Septic thrombophlebitis often requires surgical removal of the affected segment of vein. There is some controversy over the efficacy of routine rotation of central venous catheter sites in preventing septicemia but strict hand washing, sterile insertion and daily care protocols have been shown to decrease episodes in children and adults.

Avoidance of femoral arterial and venous catheters is desirable whenever possible.

The gastrointestinal system is also a portal for systemic infection in burned children and diagnosis may be particularly difficult if the skin over the chest and abdomen is burned or grafted. Hypotension during resuscitation or delay in enteral feeding secondary to ileus or other problems can increase bacterial translocation and infection of the portal system. Antibiotic therapy can result in pseudomembranous colitis. Bile stasis and cholestasis may result in occult acute cholecystitis. Careful physical exam including rectal exam and liberal application of diagnostic ultrasound is necessary when unexplained sepsis occurs.

Valvulitis and endocarditis are also a risk in burned children because of the occurrence of septicemia and potential virulence of antibiotic resistant organisms as well as the frequent presence of long dwelling central venous catheters. Since clinical signs and symptoms may be sparse and obscured by the burn injury transesophageal echocardiography should be employed liberally.

NUTRITION

The burn in children is a classic model for the hypermetabolic state leading to profound catabolism. Some authors have advocated the use of beta blockers in resuscitation and early treatment to mitigate the disproportionate hypermetabolic response state. There are massive calorie requirements in the large burn and indirect calorimetry or other methods are useful in monitoring the state of nutrition throughout the hospital course. Early enteric feeding with milk based formula through a nasojejunal tube will possibly prevent bacterial translocation and provide essential calories. Our goal is to begin enteric feeding at 6 hrs postinjury and hopefully be at calculated amount for size and TBSA burn by 36 to 48 hrs. If rigorous attention is paid to instituting early enteric feeding, total parenteral nutrition and its attendant difficulties may be avoided. Renal failure, diarrhea, ileus or other complications may require changing the formula used. Anabolic steroids such as Oxandrolone ® have been shown to be useful in preventing or reversing some of the hypercatabolic state. In the prolonged recovery from a major burn adrenal insufficiency is not uncommon. Unexplained hypotension or electrolyte abnormalities warrant a cortisol stimulation test or other diagnostic assessment.

SUPPORTIVE CARE

Multidisciplinary care is essential to obtain good outcomes in burn care of children. From admission to the burn center throughout the course burn injury puts children at multiple repetitive risks of functional and aesthetic impairments. Splinting and physical therapy begin immediately. The hands are splinted in the position of function with wrists slightly dorsiflexed, metacarpophalangeal joints flexed to 90° and interphalangeal joints at 0° or slight flexion, elbows and knees are splinted at 0° and ankles at 90° (Figure 6). Daily physical therapy and occupational therapy puts all joints through as full a range of motion as possible and motion against resistance applied in cooperative patients or other resistive techniques may decrease loss of muscle mass. Repeated lubrication of healed burned skin and skin grafts is necessary to prevent cracking and hypertrophic scarring. Compression therapy by facemask or garment may help prevent hypertrophic scarring. Major burn injury is a devastating psychological problem for both child and family. The possibility of a loss of a child by death and the anticipation of a future clouded by deformity, dysfunction, need for multiple surgeries and a myriad of other problems can be overwhelming to the injured child and his family. It is critical to have spiritual and

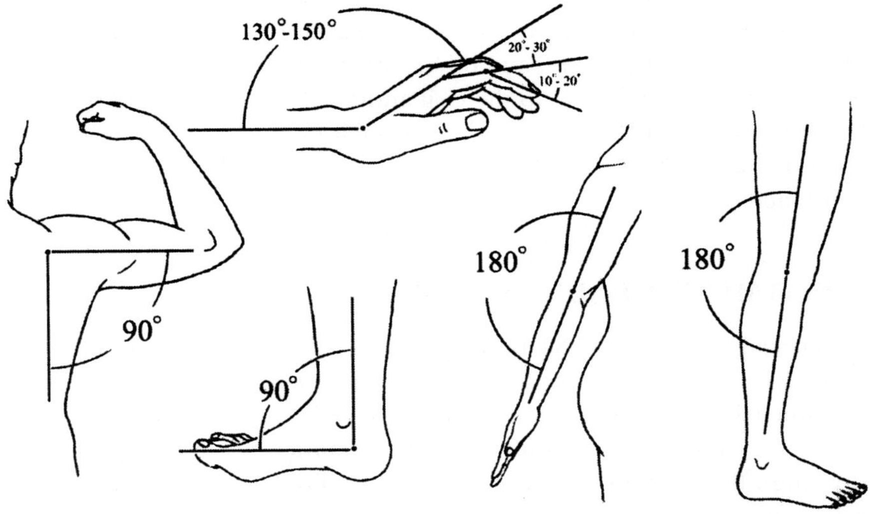

Figure 6. Positions of various joints for splinting in burned children to prevent contracture.

psychological care available at all times. Diversion by play therapy and other techniques may make the long therapy more tolerable and reduce narcotic or sedative demands. Since many serious burn injuries occur in dysfunctional family environments these adjuncts are even more important and the relationships between therapist and patient/family may also facilitate compliant long term follow up.

CHILD ABUSE

Unfortunately burning is a common method of child abuse comprising up to 30% of admissions to some burn units. Obtaining a careful history of the injury at the multiple sites of ingress to care of the burned child and comparing these histories amongst caregivers is important. Inconsistent histories and delay in presentation, previous hospitalizations for trauma are all hallmarks of child abuse. Children below 5yrs of age particularly around the age of toilet training are at highest risk. Pattern burns or scars (cigarette, curling irons, or clothes irons) a clear demarcation between burned and unburned skin particularly on the hands and arms, feet and legs and perineum known as the stocking glove burn distribution and evidence of previous trauma are all signs of abuse (Figure 7). Children presenting with such signs and symptoms require a full work up for physical and sexual abuse to obtain an accurate diagnosis and to prevent subsequent repetition of abuse. Physicians, nurses, and others are required by law in most states to report such occurrences to the civil authorities usually Child Protective Services. Early and routine reporting of such events removes the burden from the medical caregiver and creates a more favorable environment for continued care.

TREATMENT OF MINOR BURNS

Superficial burns and TBSA burns less than 5% in children can often be treated in an outpatient setting. Therapy is oriented toward promoting reepithelialization and minimizing pain. Superficial second degree burns can be covered with xenograft (pigskin) or adherent silver impregnated dressings. If successful the skin will reepithelialize beneath these dressings with minimal pain and the dressings will spontaneously separate or can be removed when fully healed. Deeper burns should be washed twice a day in a clean environment and covered with silver sulfadiazine, bacitracin,

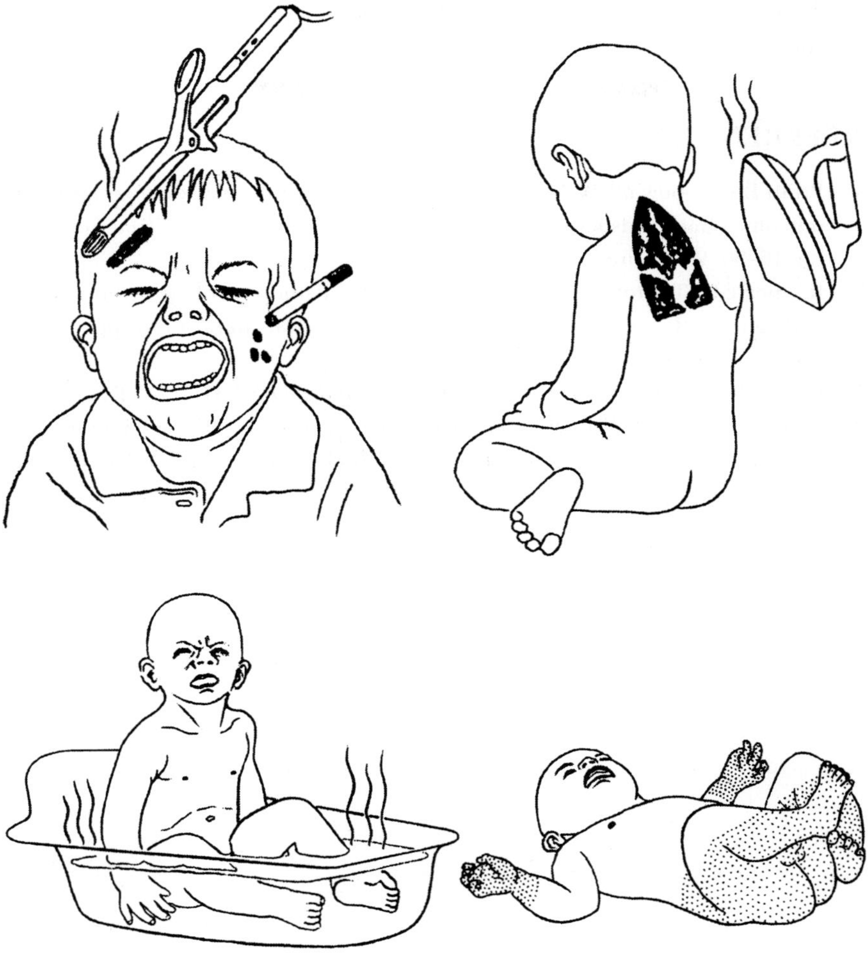

Figure 7. Child abuse by burning. Pattern burns such as cigarettes, curling iron, or clothes iron. Sharp demarcation of burn line with homogenous degree of burn and sparing of flexion creases of knees and hips suggest forced submersion in hot water.

Bactroban® or other topical antibiotics. Splinting is rarely necessary in small children. Manual debridement of loose skin and blisters should be performed prior to initiation of topical therapy. Occasionally enzymatic debridement with topical collagenase and polymixin powder is useful to prepare the wound for more rapid epithelialization and healing. Systemic antibiotics are rarely necessary and should be reserved for episodes of cellulitis.

REFERENCES

1. Pruitt BA, Goodwin CW, Mason AD. (2002) Epidemiological, demographic and outcome characteristics of burn injury. In: DN Herndon (ed.), *Total Burn Care*, pp. 16–30. WB Saunders, New York.
2. Kramer GC, Tjostolv L, Herndon DN. (2002) Pathophysiology of burn shock and burn edema. In: DN Herndon (ed.), *Total Burn Care*, pp. 78–87. WB Saunders, New York.
3. Ruddy, RM. (1994) Smoke inhalation injury. *Ped Clin NA* **41**:317–325.
4. Coleman JJ. (2006) Principles of burn reconstruction. In: BM Achauer, R Sood (eds.), *Burn Surgery: Reconstruction and Rehabilitation*, pp. 3–16. Elsevier, Philadelphia.

CHILD ABUSE 19

Dennis W. Vane and Ann DiMaio

INTRODUCTION

In most societies it is an accepted premise that parents have the authority and responsibility to provide for their children. This is based on the assumption that parents have the best interests of their children in mind when making these decisions. Unfortunately, not all parents are willing nor are some capable of basing their care decisions on their children's best interests, rather making these decisions in a more self centered manner. As a result, these children may become victims of abuse and neglect through actions or the lack of actions by these parents.

Child abuse and neglect is prevalent worldwide. It exists among all cultures, religions and all socio-economic groups. In 2007 in the United States, Children's Protective Services investigated 3.5 million reports of child abuse. Of these investigations, 794,000 children were found to be victims of abuse; 30% of all the children were less than the age of four, 20% were between the ages of 4 and 7, and 20% between 8 and 11 yrs.[1] The highest incidence of abuse occurred among children less than 2 yrs of age. This group also had the highest mortality rate from these injuries. Both male and female children were equally represented in all age groups. In 75% of cases, the investigation was the first report of suspected abuse.[1]

In order to be consistent in the discussion of abusive injuries, it is necessary to clearly define child abuse and neglect. The United States Government defines abuse as any recent act or failure to act on the part of the parent or caretaker which results in death or serious physical or emotional harm, sexual abuse or exploitation or an act or failure to act which presents imminent risk of serious harm.[1] It is important to note that no actual harm need occur to a child for abuse to exist. When there is a concern that a parent or caregiver is abusing a child, in the United States, society has the right and the obligation to intervene on behalf of that child. In all States this is mandated for certain individuals including medical and educational personnel, although the individual statutes vary from one jurisdiction to another. It is important as mandated reporters that we become familiar with the individual statutes in our local and regional areas as they pertain to abuse. In most jurisdictions mandatory reporting indicates injury or a situation which is consistent with potential or real abuse, and not actually an accusation that abuse has occurred. Proving abuse is in general the responsibility of official organizations tasked with that responsibility.

Abuse and neglect can exist in many forms. Physical and sexual abuse is the most commonly described and reported in the media and literature. Neglect, however, is actually the most common form of abuse and often accompanies all of the other forms. Neglect includes an entire spectrum of conditions encompassing emotional or physical neglect, lack of appropriate hygiene, living conditions, medical care and education.

RISK FACTORS FOR ABUSE

There is no single cause for abuse. There are, however, multiple factors that place a child at high risk to be abused that have been described. Commonly, more than one risk factor is present in a family at one time. It is important to remember that the presence of risk factors in a child's environment do not necessarily indicate that abuse has or will occur. It is equally important to identify these situations where risk factors for child abuse exist. Local family services can often provide assistance to these high risk homes to aid families that may be in crisis. These early interventions potentially reduce or eliminate the risk of abuse.[1]

Risk factors for abuse are generally classified into four broad categories. The first is the character and personality traits of the caregiver or parent, second the individual characteristics of the child, third the family dynamics and finally the environment in which the family is living.

Caregiver or Parent

Approximately 80% of all abusers are the parents.[1] Often the abuser is described as having poor impulse control, antisocial behavior, and low self esteem. Commonly, they were victims of abuse or witnessed domestic violence in the home. Often the abuser will have substance abuse problems. In many cases the parent's or caregiver's perception of the child is negative and associated with unrealistic expectations of the child's abilities. Age of the parent is another risk factor, the younger the parent or caregiver the greater the risk of abuse.

The Child

The role the victim has on abuse rates has been studied in great depth.[1] The age of the child clearly impacts the risk with children under three having the highest rates of abuse. These children require constant care and attention. They are small in stature compared to the adult and clearly are unable to adequately defend themselves. The child may be in a learning phase, such as toilet training, and may not be responding as the caregiver expects. Additionally, children with cognitive, physical or emotional disabilities are at significant greater risk to suffer abuse. This higher risk holds true for premature and low birth weight infants as well. Some authors suggest that these factors interfere with appropriate parental bonding early in the child's life.

Family Dynamics

The existing family structure clearly impacts the risk for abuse.[1] A single parent household significantly increases the risk for abuse particularly when the father is absent. Households where there are large numbers of individuals living together including family and nonfamily members compounds the potential risk for abuse as well. In families where domestic violence has been documented, reports indicate that children suffer a 30% to 60% risk of abuse.

Environment

Environmental factors such as poverty, unemployment, lack of education and living in high crime areas have all been identified as predisposing to potential child abuse. These factors often coupled with the fact that available social services to aid these families are scarce in these areas all provide added stress to the dynamics fostering the environment for abuse.[1]

INJURIES

When evaluating any child who has sustained an injury, it is important to assess whether this injury was the result of an abusive or neglectful act. While almost any injury is potentially the result of abuse, a thorough and systematic approach to evaluate the child will often identify those children who were victims of abuse. It is critical to start by obtaining a complete history surrounding the events of the "accident". How did it happen? Who was there? What did you do when the injury occurred? These are all important facts to assess when attempting to determine if abuse occurred. The physician must critically analyze if the description of the event could actually have resulted in the injury encountered. The clinician must also be familiar with the developmental abilities of children. He must ask himself is this child capable of this act. A complete history also includes a past medical history of the child and a family medical history. The clinician must exclude any underlying medical cause for the injury.

Physical abuse is defined as any physical injury deliberately inflicted on the child.[2] It includes hitting, punching, kicking, biting, burning, shaking or beating with objects such as belts, cords, paddles, etc. While cutaneous manifestations of abuse are the most obvious, these injuries are not limited to the skin. Fractures account for anywhere from 11% to 55% of abusive injuries.[3–5] Fractures may represent an isolated injury or be part of a constellation of injuries. Orthopedic injuries are commonly seen among infants, toddlers and school age children.

Abusive head trauma is the most common cause of mortality among abused infants. It is also responsible for the highest incidence of morbidity. Abusive head trauma is often not an isolated injury but is accompanied by skeletal injuries including rib fractures and metaphyseal fractures and retinal hemorrhages. Intraabdominal injuries account for less than 1% of reported cases of abuse. Intraabdominal injuries however, are the second most common cause of mortality in these children. The liver, pancreas and small bowel are the organs most commonly injured. The highest incidence of abdominal injuries is among children 6 mths to 3 yrs of age, who again are too small to protect themselves from an abusive adult.

ORTHOPEDIC INJURIES

As previously stated, skeletal injuries account for 11% to 55% of all abusive injuries.[3,6,7] A fracture may represent an isolated injury or be one of a constellation of injuries including multiple fractures in various stages of healing. These may be accompanied by evidence of nonskeletal injuries of varying ages as well.[8] Fifty five percent to seventy percent of all abusive fractures occur in children under one year of age.[3–5] In comparison, only 2% of all accidental fractures occur in this age group.[9]

Many orthopedic injuries are clinically unsuspected. Others may be missed because of inadequate evaluations. While orthopedic injuries are rarely fatal, they account for a significant portion of pain, disability, and deformity suffered by abused children.

When evaluating a child with a fracture, the clinician must decide if the fracture is the result of an unintentional or an abusive incident. Analyzing the number, type and location of the fractures, and the age and developmental abilities of the child will aid the clinician in identifying potential abuse. The physician should start with a complete history for the event. It is important to conclude if the event described could result in the fracture pattern observed. Spiral fractures are the result of torsional forces applied to the bone. Buckle or cortical fractures are the result of axial loading. Transverse fractures result from a direct blow to or bending of the extremity. Finally, oblique fractures result from a combination of forces.[10] One must also be familiar with the developmental abilities of the child to ensure he is capable of performing the act that resulted in the fracture. A thorough past medical and family medical history should be obtained to exclude a metabolic or any other medical cause for the fracture. Multiple fractures of varying etiologies are always highly suspicious.

Supportive medical studies can often be helpful to aid the clinician trying to determine whether an injury was the result of abuse. While specific tests should be obtained on a case by case basis, it is recommended that all children under the age of two, who have sustained a fracture, should have an accompanying Skeletal Survey performed. Children in this age group are rarely involved in play or activity of a sufficient force to sustain a fracture.[11,12] A skeletal survey involves a series X-rays including a skull series, frontal, and lateral projections of all the extremities including the hands and feet, chest X-ray with frontal, lateral and oblique projections, and frontal and lateral views of the spine and pelvis. After 2 yrs of age, X-rays should be obtained as a result of the physical examination.[11] When abuse is contemplated some routine screening laboratory studies including Calcium, Phosphate, and Alkaline Phosphate are recommended. This eliminates underlying medical causes of fractures which may cloud the history. If any more extensive testing is contemplated, for example testing for Osteogenisis Imperfecta, it is suggested that tests be performed in conjunction with an expert in pediatric genetic diseases.

When looking at specific fractures, it is important to remember that no one fracture is pathognomic for abuse. There are however several fractures that should arouse a high degree of suspicion.

Rib fractures are a rare skeletal injury in the pediatric population. The compliance and mobility of the thoracic cage of children prevents the ribs from fracturing in minor accidents. Rib fractures are encountered during massive vehicular accidents or other major trauma. When rib fractures are seen in children without the history of a massive trauma, child abuse is likely.

Rib fractures account for between 5% and 27% of all skeletal injuries in abused children.[3] Ninety percent occur in children under the age of two.[3] Eighty percent of the fractures occur at the posterior portion of the rib at the costo–vertebral articulation.[3] It is postulated that the infant is held facing the perpetrator. The thumbs are over the anterior chest, the fingers on the posterior thorax and the palms placed laterally. The chest is squeezed in an anterior to posterior manner causing the rib to lever over the fulcrum of the transverse process of the spine. If the force is continued or increased, fractures at the lateral aspect of the rib will occur as well. These fractures may be difficult to ascertain or be asymptomatic at initial evaluation. Caretakers may report crepitance when lifting their infants or fussiness when the infant is handled. When abusive parents are confronted with the discovery of rib fractures, they usually cannot provide an adequate explanation. They try to attribute the fractures to normal childcare activity or behavior. Sometimes the fractures are attributed to other children holding the child or a dog jumping on the infant.

Skull fractures are the second most common skeletal injury in children who have been physically abused.[13,14] They may present as a simple linear fracture or a more complex fracture. In order to sustain a skull fracture a significant direct force must be delivered to the skull. This force can result from a fall, being thrown or swung into a hard surface or from a direct impact. Most abusive skull fractures are the result of throwing the infant.

To determine whether a skull fracture is the result of an accident or abusive act it is critical to obtain a detailed history of the incident. Commonly, parents will report the infant fell or was dropped. It is essential to know the height of the fall and the surface on which the infant fell. Studies indicate that infants must fall at least three feet onto a hard surface to sustain a skull fracture.[15–18] Hard surfaces include wood floors, tile or cement. Falls onto carpeted floors, mattresses, etc. provide a cushion to the direct blow and skull fractures are extremely unlikely. Exact timing of when a skull fracture occurred can be difficult. Swelling may not appear for 24 hrs and may last for a few days. The history must include information as to where the child was for a significant time preceding presentation and the discovery of the injury.

Throwing an infant may or may not be preceded by a shaking episode. Retinal hemorrhages, subdural hemorrhages and rib fractures are usually associated injuries found with shaking. The clinician must be cognizant of this injury association and evaluate for them when examining an infant with even a simple linear skull fracture. The presence of one of these associated injuries may be the only evidence suggesting the fracture was the result of abusive act and not simply an unintentional fall.

While long bone fractures in children are common childhood injuries their occurrence in an infant is very rare. Only 2% of unintentional fractures are seen in children less than 18 mths of age however 80% of all fractures resulting from abuse occur in this group.[3–5,9] The most common long bones fractured in abused children are the middle and distal third of the humerus, the distal third of the ulna and radius and the shaft of the femur.[8] It is important to remember any fracture can be the result of abuse. The explanation provided by the care taker must be scrutinized and compared against the age and development of the child.

Metaphyseal fractures represent the one fracture pattern that could be deemed pathognomic for abuse.[19] These are usually seen at the distal aspects of the femurs and the proximal and distal aspects of the tibia. These fractures result from shearing forces seen with shaking or violent traction of the extremity.

BURN INJURIES

Burn injuries in children account for over 100,000 visits nationally to Emergency Departments.[20] Of these injuries, 10% to 20% are the result of abuse or neglect.[20] Abusive burn injuries occur most often in children less than 2 yrs of age. They are more severe, require longer hospitalizations, and have a higher fatality rate when compared with accidental burns. The most common form of inflicted burns is scald burns. Scald burns are often associated with toilet training issues.[21]

Scalding water may be straight out of the tap or may actually be heated by the abuser. The child or just extremities are immersed in the water. Occasionally, the water or other hot liquid like oil is thrown at them. These injuries leave characteristic patterns often making them easy to recognize. In addition, the depth of the burn is another clue as to whether the injury is intentional or not. The majority of unintentional burns leave irregular edges with burns of multiple depths. They are usually not greater than second degree. Inflicted burns are more often third degree with clear lines of demarcation between burned and unburned skin. Critically examining the location of the burn, aids the clinician in arriving at a conclusion as to the nature of the injury. A burn on the palm of a child's hand is not suspicious for abuse. Children explore with an open hand. A burn on the dorsum of the hand is more suggestive of an inflicted injury. If a child accidently pulls a cup or bowl of hot liquid onto himself, it classically takes on the pattern of an arrow head. It starts wide at the shoulder and then narrows as it flows down their chest. The burn at the top is deeper than the burn on the lower chest as the liquid cooled. When a hot liquid is thrown at a child, it does not create this pattern. There is usually a larger burned area and it is predominantly all of the same depth. Genital burns are always highly suspicious.

As previously stressed, one must also be sure the injury pattern is consistent with the explanation provided by the caretaker and the child is developmentally capable of acting in the manner described.

The following are a few classic burns that one must be familiar with if treating burned children.

(1) The "*donut burn*" is an example of an immersion burn. The child is cradled in the perpetrators arms and immersed into the scalding water. The burn takes on a characteristic appearance where the feet and ankles are burned but there is sparing of the popliteal fossa. The center of the buttocks is pushed against the porcelain and is spared but is surrounded by a ring of burned skin. The depth of the burn is uniform and usually deep second or third degree.

(2) The *stocking glove* distribution is another classic immersion burn. It results when a child's hand or foot is often immersed forcibly into scalding water and held there. The burned skin creates an appearance of a sock or a glove. Again, there is a clear line of demarcation between the burned and unburned skin. In addition, the depth of the burn is usually third degree and uniform throughout the hand or foot. A child testing the liquid for temperature will retract the extremity with first contact. They will not immerse an entire hand or foot and sustain a well demarcated injury.

3) *Flame burns* are usually not the result of an abusive event but more often the result of neglect on the part of the caretaker. Classically young children are left alone. A fire erupts and the children are unable to escape. They sustain severe third degree burns, smoke inhalation or may even perish.

Punishing children by burning them with a hot object is also a well recognized form of abuse. The common objects used are cigarettes, irons, and curling irons. These burns leave a characteristic pattern that is easily recognized. These injuries can be distinguished from an accidental injury by location of the burn and its depth. When a child touches a hot object they do so with the palmar surface of their hand and withdraw immediately. This results in a second degree burn. When a contact burn is inflicted it may be on any part of the body. Presence on the dorsum of the hand, which is not a primary exploring surface, is suspicious. Intentional contact burns are commonly third degree because the object is held in place not allowing the child to withdraw.

INTRATHORACIC AND INTRAABDOMINAL INJURIES

Intraabdominal and intrathoracic injuries are uncommon in children and are equally infrequent among physically abused children accounting for only 1% of injuries seen.[22] Although uncommon, they represent the second most frequent cause of death in this group, following head injuries. It is estimated that up to 20% of all pediatric abdominal injuries are the result of abuse.[23] Children between 6 mths and 3 yrs are at highest risk. This is a younger group than children who are the victims of unintentional torso injuries.[22] Intentional abdominal trauma differs from unintentional injury in that both solid organ and hollow viscera injuries frequently occur simultaneously.[24] Additionally, intentional injury carries with it a significantly higher mortality for these children than that reported for unintentional injury.[25]

The increased mortality rate seen among these victims is multifactoral. It has been attributed to a combination of the age of the child, the severity of the abuse, continuing hemorrhage, and the lack of seeking timely medical intervention.[24] These young children are not permitted or unable to defend themselves against an adult assault. The mechanism of injury is usually punching or kicking by the adult. The child is unprotected from direct impact and clearly is at an age of development where they are not actively participating in high risk behavior. As with unintentional injury, penetrating injuries are rare.

As with all children in this age group, the abdominal organs are proportionally larger and are not well protected by the thoracic cage or the child's relatively weak abdominal musculature. The energy of the assault is transmitted directly to the organs. As with unintentional injury such as a seat belt injury, the abdominal organs may be crushed against the spine during the assault.

As with unintentional injury the most commonly organs injured are the liver, spleen, pancreas and the small bowel. As stated multiple injuries are frequent. Delay in seeking medical attention contributes dramatically to the increased morbidity and mortality as often caregivers attempt to mask the injury and provide misleading information in an attempt to protect the perpetrator.

In intentional injury the liver is the most frequently injured organ and potentially the most life threatening. Usually there are no external signs of bruising to suggest an assault. Liver injuries include lacerations, hematomas and free intraperitoneal bleeding. They are usually the result of direct blunt trauma to the upper abdomen from being kicked or punched. Injury is usually confirmed by Computed Tomography (CT) scan of the abdomen done as part of the work up of the child.

The pancreas is also vulnerable to intentional injury secondary to its location in the center of the abdomen lying against the spine. Reports suggest that up to 18% of all pancreatic injuries in children are the result of abuse.[27,28] This is far higher than the incidence of pancreatic injury from unintentional etiologies. As with unintentional injury, children suffering abusive pancreatic injury often present late. Common symptoms are abdominal pain, emesis, and abdominal distention often with an abdominal mass. Often these injuries can be mistaken for acute gastroenteritis or viral pancreatitis. Pancreatic injury in an abused child carries with it a high incidence of concomitant hollow viscous injury mimicking the seat belt injury of automobile crashes.[29] Pancreatic pseudocyst may be the first presentation often developing 3 to 4 wks after the initial event.

Abuse victims sustain hollow viscous injuries far more commonly than victims of unintentional injury.[30] Most commonly the duodenum and jejunum are involved. As with the pancreas, the duodenum is particularly at risk because of its fixed location traversing the spine. As with unintentional injury, children suffering a duodenal perforation may present with relatively subtle, nonspecific initial findings. This is often clouded by a misleading history making diagnosis extremely difficult. Intraluminal duodenal hematoma usually present with emesis and findings of a proximal intestinal obstruction, often somewhat remote from the initial injury due to progressive expansion of the hematoma.

Hemorrhage due to lacerations of the liver, spleen, or vascular injury is the most common cause of death in intentionally injured children prior to arrival to the hospital. Autopsy studies indicate these children often have over a 50% blood volume loss.[7,18,40] For those children who arrive at the hospital with intraabdominal bleeding, presentation is consistent with the signs and symptoms of hemorrhagic shock.

Thoracic injuries occur in 12.5% of abused children compared with only 4.5% of unintentional trauma patients.[31] Injuries are often associated with rib fractures and include hemothorax, pneumonthorax, and pulmonary contusions. When these injuries present they suggest that a severe assault has taken place.

ANO-GENITAL INJURIES

Unintentional injuries to the genital area although not uncommon are usually minor in nature. When they occur, children usually alert their parents quickly to their injury. In general then parents bring their children quickly to a medical professional for care. The most common injuries seen in girls are straddle injuries. The soft tissues of the perineum are crushed between the pelvic bone and a hard object such as a bicycle bar or playground equipment when the child slips and falls. The resulting injuries are usually unilateral involving anterior genital tissues including the labia, clitoris, and the periurethral tissues. Rarely are injuries to the hymen and vagina encountered. If injuries to the hymen and vagina are identified the health care provider must scrutinize the history of the injury to assure that it is consistent with the physical examination.

In males, minor injury to the tip of the penis can occur when the glans is inadvertently caught in a zipper or from a falling toilet seat. Bruising on the scrotum can be seen with sport injuries or during rough play. In these situations, the explanation provided by the patient or family should appropriately explain the injuries seen.

Unfortunately, sexual assaults are also a common source of anogenital injuries in children. In girls, these injuries can present as anything from minor bruising, abrasions or erythema of the labia majora or minora, and the periurethral tissues to more significant lacerations and frank tears. These injuries commonly are the result of fondling and touching or rubbing the penis against the genitalia (vulvar coitus).[32] With actual penetration more significant injuries result including transections of the hymen, laceration of the lateral walls and floor of the vagina, laceration of the fossa navicularis, posterior forchette and at its worst perforation into the peritoneum.[33,34] In male children, injuries to the penis include abrasions, bruises, bite marks and tears to the frenulum of the glans. Injuries to the buttocks are seen in both girls and boys and consist of bruises and abrasions from being held or from rubbing the penis on the anal cleft. Injuries from penetration of the anus are dependent on the object used. Digital penetration usually does not leave any acute or permanent injury. Penile penetration on the other hand may result acutely in fissures, lacerations, and hematomas and may occur high into the rectum. Late and chronic injury often produces skin tags, scarring and laxity of rectal tone.

Assaults perpetrated by strangers tend to be more violent and result in more serious injuries to the child. As a result, they may come to medical attention sooner. These attacks are often associated with extra-genital injuries such as bite mark, bruising on the arms or legs from being held and even ligature marks on the extremities. Tearing of the anterior frenulum of the upper lip can be seen with forced fellatio.

When evaluating a child, who has been the victim of a sexual assault, it is important to remember that the majority of victims will not present with acute injuries. This does not imply that an assault did not occur. Sexual predators who target children intentionally try not to cause visible injury to their victims for fear of being discovered. They usually know their victims and have easy access to them.[35,36] Their desire is to continue abusing the child and as a result are careful not to cause an obvious injury that would provoke further investigation or interrogation of their victim. Children will often not disclose the initial assault. The perpetrator is commonly known to them and is usually someone that they trust such as a relative, family friend, teacher, or coach etc. These children often are conflicted by the actions. The perpetrator uses his or her power or authority over the child forcing secrecy of their actions and perpetrating the ongoing abuse.[35,36] Children are often threatened, told they will not be believed or intimidated to fear the consequences of their disclosure. Eventually the child wants the abuse to stop and may disclose the actions, usually to someone they trust.

ABUSIVE HEAD INJURY

Head trauma is the most devastating injury an abused infant can suffer. It has the highest fatality rate of all forms of physical abuse and is responsible for significant morbidity. Infants under 1 yr of age are at the highest risk.[37–42] The mortality rate from intentional head injuries in children is significantly higher than that found in children with unintentional injuries.[41] The most common perpetrator identified for this injury pattern is the father followed by the mother's boyfriend. The clinical presentation of an infant who has sustained abusive head trauma is variable. The symptoms may be mild and nonspecific and include vomiting, irritability, or lethargy. Symptoms may present as medical or metabolic in nature such as seizures, signs of increased intracranial pressure or unresponsiveness, and the clinician may not suspect abuse at all. In extreme circumstances presentation may be frank apnea or cardiopulmonary arrest.[43–47] In some cases, the head injury may not be the presenting concern of the family. These children may be brought to the ED for evaluation of another injury and the head trauma is discovered as part of the child's evaluation.[48,49] It is important that in any child under the age of two, who has sustained a suspicious injury, an evaluation for a potential head injury be included in the work up.

The specific medical evaluation of the infant will be determined by their clinical presentation. If the infant presents with acute neurological signs or symptoms then a head CT is the most appropriate radiological examination. If the presentation is not primarily neurological Magnetic Resonance Imaging (MRI) of the brain should be considered. While an MRI is not the modality of choice for the first 24 hours after injury, it is valuable in delineating multiple injuries or injuries that may be more chronic in nature and can provide assistance in dating injuries. An MRI should be considered in any infant who had a CT performed that suggests multiple subdural hemorrhages or other brain abnormalities. If the child is less than 2 yrs of age, and abuse is suspected a skeletal survey should be performed as well. Any other radiological studies should be dictated by the clinical exam or history. Laboratory studies should include a CBC and PT/PTT. If seizures are part of the presentation, a metabolic panel is recommended to exclude any electrolyte dyscrasias as a potential etiology. Once the infant is stabilized, a retinal exam by a pediatric ophthalmologist is essential. Retinal hemorrhages in abusive head trauma are numerous in number, are throughout the layers of the retina and extend out into the periphery of the retina. This presentation is unique to abusive head trauma and massive head injury sustained in high impact motor vehicle crashes. It is not seen with CPR, birth, minor accidental head trauma, increased intracranial pressure or seizures as has been suggested in some defense cases for suspected abuse.[50–55]

The most common intracranial injury seen in infants who have sustained abusive head trauma is a subdural hemorrhage. This injury is more frequently associated with abuse than unintentional injury. Its presence warrants further investigation into the etiology of the injury when it occurs.[47–49] Subarachnoid hemorrhage is the next most common form of brain hemorrhage encountered in intentional injury victims. Epidural hematomas, whether arterial or venous, are rarely the result of abusive injury. Parenchymal injuries to the brain may also be present and are often associated with hemorrhage as well. Subdural and subarachnoid hemorrhages are seen in other settings in infants including unintentional trauma, metabolic disorders, intracranial vascular anomalies and hematological diseases.

Skull fractures are the second most common skeletal injury found in abused children.[3,13] They are also common unintentional accidental injuries as well. They may occur anywhere on the skull but parietal fractures are the most frequently encountered. The pattern of abusive skull fractures is varied and is determined by the mechanism. Infants may present with a simple linear fracture or a complex fracture which consists of multiple skull fractures. A complex or multiple fractures are considered more indicative of abuse.[56] Depressed skull fractures are rarely the result of abuse.[13,57]

Fractures may be accompanied by bruising or swelling of the scalp or there may be no external evidence of injury. There may be associated intracranial lesions including subdural or subarachnoid hemorrhages or parenchymal injury.

Extracranial injuries may also accompany abusive head trauma including posterior rib fractures and retinal hemorrhages.[58,59] Long bone fractures especially metaphyseal fractures and intraabdominal injuries can be associated as well. All children under 2 yrs of age who have sustained a suspicious head injury should have a trauma consult, skeletal survey, and retinal exam included in their evaluation to detect potential additional injuries.[60]

The history surrounding the injury is as important as the physical examination and medical studies in abused children. The treating physicians must scrutinize the history and determine whether the explanation provided by the caretaker is consistent with the nature of the injuries observed.

The explanation for an injured infant is necessarily provided by a caregiver. The most common description is that of a fall. Someone may have accidentally dropped the baby or it may have fallen off the bed or couch. Falls are common in childhood and account for the largest number of injury visits to the Emergency Department.[61,62] One must obtain the details surrounding the "fall". Nonmobile babies cannot easily "fall", and lack of attention to a child in a potentially dangerous situation indicates neglect at least. The clinician needs to ask about the height the baby fell from and the surface onto which he fell. It is well established that short falls of approximately three feet in the home are not associated with major or fatal intracranial injuries.[62–71] Any time the explanation for a life threatening head injury is a short fall, the physician should be alerted to the fact this injury probably represents an intentional injury pattern. It is also helpful knowing how the baby was acting prior to and after the accident. It is of course critical to evaluate if the child has sustained other injuries in the past. Multiple studies have shown that many of these infants have sustained more than one documented episode of abusive head injury.[72–74]

There are of course medical conditions that can be mistaken for abusive head trauma. A complete past medical history and review of systems of the infant and a thorough family medical history is usually sufficient to exclude these etiologies.

REFERENCES

1. Office on Child Abuse and Neglect (HHS). Child Welfare Information Gateway. 2010. Ref Type: Report.
2. Keenan H, Leventhal J. (2009) The evolution of child abuse research. In: Reece RM, Christian CW, (eds.) *Child Abuse Medical Diagnosis and Management.* pp. 1–18. American Academy of Pediatrics.
3. Merten DF, Radkowski MA, Leonidas JC. (1983) The abused child: A radiological reappraisal. *Radiology* **146**:377–81.

4. Krishnan J, Barbour PJ, Foster BK. (1990) Patterns of osseous injuries and psychosocial factors affecting victims of child abuse. *Aust N Z J Surg* **60**:447–450.
5. Gross RH, Stranger M. (1983) Causative factors responsible for femoral fractures in infants and young children. *J Pediatr Orthop* **3**:341–343.
6. Anderson WA. (1982) The significance of femoral fractures in children. *Ann Emerg Med* **11**:174–177.
7. Arnholz D, Hymel KP, Hay TC, Jenny C. (1998) Bilateral pediatric skull fractures: Accident or abuse? *J Trauma* **45**:172–174.
8. Akbarnia B, Torg JS, Kirkpatrick J, Sussman S. (1974) Manifestations of the battered-child syndrome. *J Bone Joint Surg Am* **56**:1159–1166.
9. Worlock P, Stower M, Barbor P. (1986) Patterns of fractures in accidental and non-accidental injury in children: A comparative study. *Br Med J (Clin Res Ed)* **293**:100–102.
10. Pierce MC, Bertocci GE, Vogeley E, Moreland MS. (2004) Evaluating long bone fractures in children: A biomechanical approach with illustrative cases. *Child Abuse Negl* **28**:505–524.
11. Diagnostic imaging of child abuse. (2000) *Pediatrics* **105**:1345–1348.
12. Merten DF, Carpenter BL. (1990) Radiologic imaging of inflicted injury in the child abuse syndrome. *Pediatr Clin North Am* **37**:815–837.
13. Merten DF, Osborne DR, Radkowski MA, Leonidas JC. (1984) Craniocerebral trauma in the child abuse syndrome: Radiological observations. *Pediatr Radiol* **14**:272–277.
14. Merten DF, Osborne DR. (1983) Craniocerebral trauma in the child abuse syndrome. *Pediatr Ann* **12**:882–887.
15. Coats B, Margulies SS. (2008) Potential for head injuries in infants from low-height falls. *J Neurosurg Pediatr* **2**:321–330.
16. Tarantino CA, Dowd MD, Murdock TC. (1999) Short vertical falls in infants. *Pediatr Emerg Care* **15**:5–8.
17. Williams RA. (1991) Injuries in infants and small children resulting from witnessed and corroborated free falls. *J Trauma* **31**:1350–1352.
18. Kravitz H, Driessen G, Gomberg R, Korach A. (1969) Accidental falls from elevated surfaces in infants from birth to one year of age. *Pediatrics* **44**(Suppl):76.
19. Kempe CH, Silverman FN, Steele BF, Droegemueller W, Silver HK. (1962) The battered-child syndrome. *JAMA* **181**:17–24.
20. Burn Injuries in Child Abuse. 2nd. (2001). US Department of Justice: Office of Justice Programs: Office of Juvinile Justice and Delinquency. Ref Type: Pamphlet.

21. Jenny C, Reece RM. (2009) Cutaneous manifestations of Child Abuse. In: Reece RM, Christian CW (eds.), *Child Abuse Medical Diagnosis and Management*, pp. 19–51. American Academy of Pediatrics.
22. Cooper A, Floyd T, Barlow B, Niemirska M, Ludwig S, Seidl T, *et al.* (1988) Major blunt abdominal trauma due to child abuse. *J Trauma* **28**:1483–1487.
23. Trokel M, DiScala C, Terrin NC, Sege RD. (2004) Blunt abdominal injury in the young pediatric patient: Child abuse and patient outcomes. *Child Maltreat* **9**:111–711.
24. Ledbetter DJ, Hatch EI, Jr., Feldman KW, Fligner CL, Tapper D. (1988) Diagnostic and surgical implications of child abuse. *Arch Surg* **123**:1101–1105.
25. Wood J, Rubin DM, Nance ML, Christian CW. (2005) Distinguishing inflicted versus accidental abdominal injuries in young children. *J Trauma* **59**:1203–1208.
26. Nance ML, Cooper A. (2009) Visceral manifestations of child physical abuse. In: Reece RM, Christian CW (eds.), *Child Abuse Medical Diagnosis and Management*, pp. 167–187. American Academy of Pediatrics.
27. Jobst MA, Canty TG, Sr., Lynch FP. (1999) Management of pancreatic injury in pediatric blunt abdominal trauma. *J Pediatr Surg* **34**:818–823.
28. Arkovitz MS, Johnson N, Garcia VF. (1997) Pancreatic trauma in children: Mechanisms of injury. *J Trauma* **42**:49–53.
29. Nance ML, Keller MS, Stafford PW. (2000) Predicting hollow visceral injury in the pediatric blunt trauma patient with solid visceral injury. *J Pediatr Surg* **35**:1300–1303.
30. Mccort J, vaudagna J. (1964) Visceral injuries in battered children. *Radiology* **82**:424–428.
31. DiScala C, Sege R, Li G, Reece RM. (2000) Child abuse and unintentional injuries: A 10–year retrospective. *Arch Pediatr Adolesc Med* **154**:16–22.
32. Finkel MA. (2009) Medical aspects of prepubertal sexual assault. In: Reece RM, Christian CW, (eds.), *Child Abuse Medical Diagnosis and Management*, pp. 269–319. American Academy of Pediatrics.
33. Paul DM. (1977) The medical examination in sexual offences against children. *Med Sci Law* **17**:251–258.
34. Paul DM. (1986) 'What really did happen to Baby Jane?'—The medical aspects of the investigation of alleged sexual abuse of children. *Med Sci Law* **26**:85–102.
35. Summit RC. (1983) The child sexual abuse accommodation syndrome. *Child Abuse Negl* **7**:177–193.
36. Finkelhor D, Browne A. (1985) The traumatic impact of child sexual abuse: A conceptualization. *Am J Orthopsychiatry* **55**:530–541.
37. Barlow KM, Minns RA. (2000) Annual incidence of shaken impact syndrome in young children. *Lancet* **356**:1571–1572.

38. Jayawant S, Rawlinson A, Gibbon F, Price J, Schulte J, Sharples P, *et al.* (1998) Subdural haemorrhages in infants: Population based study. *Brit Med Jour* **317**:1558–1561.
39. Keenan HT, Runyan DK, Marshall SW, Nocera MA, Merten DF, Sinal SH. (2003) A population–based study of inflicted traumatic brain injury in young children. *JAMA* **290**:621–626.
40. Hobbs C, Childs AM, Wynne J, Livingston J, Seal A. (2005) Subdural haematoma and effusion in infancy: An epidemiological study. *Arch Dis Child* **90**:952–955.
41. Sills MR, Libby AM, Orton HD. (2005) Prehospital and in–hospital mortality: A comparison of intentional and unintentional traumatic brain injuries in Colorado children. *Arch Pediatr Adolesc Med* **159**:665–670.
42. Sun DT, Zhu XL, Poon WS. (2006) Non–accidental subdural haemorrhage in Hong Kong: incidence, clinical features, management and outcome. *Childs Nerv Syst* **22**:593–598.
43. Ludwig S, Warman M. (1984) Shaken baby syndrome: A review of 20 cases. *Ann Emerg Med* **13**:104–107.
44. Duhaime AC, Gennarelli TA, Thibault LE, Bruce DA, Margulies SS, Wiser R. (1987) The shaken baby syndrome. A clinical, pathological, and biomechanical study. *J Neurosurg* **66**:409–415.
45. Meservy CJ, Towbin R, McLaurin RL, Myers PA, Ball W. (1987) Radiographic characteristics of skull fractures resulting from child abuse. *AJR Am J Roentgenol* **149**:173–175.
46. Hettler J, Greenes DS. (2003) Can the initial history predict whether a child with a head injury has been abused? *Pediatrics* **111**:602–607.
47. Johnson DL, Boal D, Baule R. (1995) Role of apnea in nonaccidental head injury. *Pediatr Neurosurg* **23**:305–310.
48. Rubin DM, Christian CW, Bilaniuk LT, Zazyczny KA, Durbin DR. (2003) Occult head injury in high–risk abused children. *Pediatrics* **111**:1382–386.
49. Laskey AL, Holsti M, Runyan DK, Socolar RR. (2004) Occult head trauma in young suspected victims of physical abuse. *J Pediatr* **144**:719–722.
50. Duhaime AC, Alario AJ, Lewander WJ, Schut L, Sutton LN, Seidl TS, *et al.* (1992) Head injury in very young children: Mechanisms, injury types, and ophthalmologic findings in 100 hospitalized patients younger than 2 years of age. *Pediatrics* **90**:179–185.
51. Bechtel K, Stoessel K, Leventhal JM, Ogle E, Teague B, Lavietes S, *et al.* (2004) Characteristics that distinguish accidental from abusive injury in hospitalized young children with head trauma. *Pediatrics* **114**:165–168.

52. Vinchon M, Defoort–Dhellemmes S, Desurmont M, Dhellemmes P. (2005) Accidental and nonaccidental head injuries in infants: A prospective study. *J Neurosurg* **102**:380–384.
53. Johnson DL, Braun D, Friendly D. (1993) Accidental head trauma and retinal hemorrhage. *Neurosurgery* **33**:231–234.
54. Goetting MG, Sowa B. (1990) Retinal hemorrhage after cardiopulmonary resuscitation in children: An etiologic reevaluation. *Pediatrics* **85**:585–588.
55. Kanter RK. (1986) Retinal hemorrhage after cardiopulmonary resuscitation or child abuse. *J Pediatr* **108**:430–432.
56. Hobbs CJ. (1984) Skull fracture and the diagnosis of abuse. *Arch Dis Child* **59**:246–252.
57. Kleinman PK, Schlesinger AE. (1997) Mechanical factors associated with posterior rib fractures: Laboratory and case studies. *Pediatr Radiol* **27**:87–91.
58. Harcourt B, Hopkins D. (1971) Ophthalmic manifestations of the battered–baby syndrome. *Br Med J* **3**:398–401.
59. Gilles EE, McGregor ML, Levy–Clarke G. (2003) Retinal hemorrhage asymmetry in inflicted head injury: A clue to pathogenesis? *J Pediatr* **143**:494–499.
60. Rorke–Adams L, Duhaime C, Jenny C, Smith WL. Head Trauma. (2009) In: Reece RM, Christian CW (eds.), *Child Abuse Medical Diagnosis and Management*, pp. 53–119. American Academy of Pediatrics.
61. Rivara FP, Alexander B, Johnston B, Soderberg R. (1993) Population–based study of fall injuries in children and adolescents resulting in hospitalization or death. *Pediatrics* **92**:61–63.
62. Tarantino CA, Dowd MD, Murdock TC. (1999) Short vertical falls in infants. *Pediatr Emerg Care* **15**:5–8.
63. Helfer RE, Slovis TL, Black M. (1977) Injuries resulting when small children fall out of bed. *Pediatrics* **60**:533–535.
64. Nimityongskul P, Anderson LD. (1987) The likelihood of injuries when children fall out of bed. *J Pediatr Orthop* **7**:184–186.
65. Hall JR, Reyes HM, Horvat M, Meller JL, Stein R. (1989) The mortality of childhood falls. *J Trauma* **29**:1273–1275.
66. Musemeche CA, Barthel M, Cosentino C, Reynolds M. Pediatric falls from heights. *J Trauma* **31**:1347–1349.
67. Reiber GD. (1993) Fatal falls in childhood. How far must children fall to sustain fatal head injury? Report of cases and review of the literature. *Am J Forensic Med Pathol* **14**:201–207.
68. Chiaviello CT, Christoph RA, Bond GR. (1004) Stairway–related injuries in children. *Pediatrics* **94**:679–681.

69. Plunkett J. (2001) Fatal pediatric head injuries caused by short-distance falls. *Am J Forensic Med Pathol* **22**:1–12.
70. Johnson K, Fischer T, Chapman S, Wilson B. (2005) Accidental head injuries in children under 5 years of age. *Clin Radiol* **60**:464–468.
71. Shugerman RP, Paez A, Grossman DC, Feldman KW, Grady MS. (1996) Epidural hemorrhage: Is it abuse? *Pediatrics* **97**:664–668.
72. Ricci L, Giantris A, Merriam P, Hodge S, Doyle T. (2003) Abusive head trauma in Maine infants: Medical, child protective, and law enforcement analysis. *Child Abuse Negl* **27**:271–283.
73. Alexander R, Crabbe L, Sato Y, Smith W, Bennett T. (1990) Serial abuse in children who are shaken. *Am J Dis Child* **144**:58–60.
74. Jenny C, Hymel KP, Ritzen A, Reinert SE, Hay TC. (1999) Analysis of missed cases of abusive head trauma. *JAMA* **281**:621–626.

Section 3:
Tumors (The Abdominal Mass)

WILMS' TUMOR 20

Thomas R. Weber

CLINICAL PRESENTATION

Wilms' tumor is the most common renal tumor in childhood and the second most common abdominal tumor after neuroblastoma. There are approximately 400–500 new cases in the United States every year. This translates to one per every 10,000 infants. Wilms' tumor is felt to be more common in black children, and there is no sexual predilection known. The peak age for presentation is 2–4 yrs.

The most common presentation is an asymptomatic abdominal mass, frequently found by caregivers during activities such as bathing. These tumors can become alarmingly large before they are discovered, presumably because of the slow growth characteristics of most Wilms' tumors. Other clinical presentations include hematuria (12–14%), anorexia (5–8%), weight loss (4–8%), and hypertension (16–20%). An occasional child will have several symptoms. Males with left renal tumors may also show spermatic vein obstruction. Very rarely, children can present with catastrophic intraabdominal hemorrhage secondary to tumor capsule rupture. This can occur spontaneously as the tumor outgrows the capsule, or as a result of blunt abdominal trauma. When large tumors are involved, even minor trauma might result in hematuria or tumor rupture with subsequent anemia or even hypovolemic hypotension.

Wilms' tumor is also associated with several syndromes, and therefore children with these syndromes must be monitored carefully for the development of renal and other tumors. The Dennys–Drash syndrome is male pseudohermaphroditism and nephropathy leading to early renal failure. Ninety percent or more children with this syndrome develop Wilms' tumor. The Beckwith–Wiedemann syndrome includes organomegaly; macroglossia; omphalocele and hypoglycemia; and the risk of the development of Wilms' tumor is 5–8%. The WAGR syndrome (Wilms' tumor, aniridia, genital abnormalities, and mental retardation) has a Wilms' tumor association of 30–40%. It should also be noted that sporadic, nonfamilial and therefore, nonsyndromic aniridia is also associated with increased risk of Wilms' tumor. In addition, isolated hemihypertrophy has increased risk for Wilms' tumor.

The other renal tumors of childhood, clear cell sarcoma, rhabdoid tumor, mesoblastic nephroma, and nephroblastomatosis are much rarer and frequently present differently. Mesoblastic nephroma is a tumor found primarily in newborns as a firm flank mass. It is felt to be benign. Children with rhabdoid tumors present at ages generally younger than Wilms' tumor (18 mths) and are associated with brain tumors (10%). Clear cell tumors are usually highly malignant and often metastasize early. Bone pain from metastatic lesions, and seizures or altered mental status secondary to brain metastases is the usual presentation in these unfortunate children.

Several chromosome deletions have been found in many Wilms' tumor patients and tissue, and also in children with associated syndromes. The 11p13 gene is deleted in virtually all patients with Dennys–Drash syndrome, and has been termed Wilms' tumor 1 (WT 1). Patients with Beckwith–Wiedemann syndrome have abnormalities of the 11p15 gene (WT 2). The abnormality is variously described as deletion, duplication or over-expression in different reports. The WAGR syndrome patients show deletion of WT 1. The presence of WT 1 or WT 2 abnormality does not have prognostic significance in Wilms' tumor patients.

CLASSIFICATION AND PATHOLOGY

From a clinical standpoint, Wilms' tumor can be divided into five stages (Table 1). The different stages have prognostic importance, with the higher stages showing a lower survival. Because of this, the stages are used to direct additional therapy in terms of agents used, the need for radiation, the duration of treatment, and risk of recurrence. Each patient is carefully staged using preoperative studies and intraoperative characteristics. Great care must be taken during resectioning as accidental rupture of the mass can result in upstaging, necessitating more aggressive therapy.

Table 1. Wilms' tumor staging.

Stage	Description
I	Tumor contained within the kidney with completely intact capsule. Tumor completely removed without rupture or biopsy.
II	Tumor extends through capsule but is completely removed without gross or microscopic residual or margin involvement. Can also include tumors biopsied preoperatively or limited tumor spill in bed, but not in the peritoneal cavity. The renal vein may have tumor.
III	Tumor is not completely excised but no hematogenous spread is present. Local lymph nodes may be involved. Also includes gross peritoneal spillage or implants.
IV	Hematogenous spread to lungs, brain or any site.
IV	Bilateral renal tumors

Pathologically, Wilms' tumor is divided into favorable and unfavorable categories. Favorable histology is present in 90% of tumors, and has three components: Blastema, epithelial, and stroma. Tumors with unfavorable histology show either focal or diffuse anaplasia. At one time, clear cell and rhabdoid tumors were included in the unfavorable group but are now considered entirely different tumors that behave differently and require more aggressive therapy.

The term nephroblastomatosis refers to the presence of nephrogenic rests in the kidney after 36 weeks' gestation. One percent of kidneys in children under 3 mths of age have nephrognic rests, but the majority of these children will not develop Wilms' tumor. Forty-four percent of unilateral Wilms' tumors have nephrogenic rests, while 99% of bilateral Wilms' tumors are associated with nephrogenic rests. Increased rates of nephrogenic rests are also seen in children with the syndromes associated with Wilms' tumor.

DIAGNOSIS

Most children with Wilms' tumor present with an asymptomatic abdominal mass. Physical examination confirms the presence of a smooth, nontender abdominal or flank mass. Hematuria is occasionally seen, but it is frequently microscopic. Weight loss or anorexia doesn't usually occur unless the tumor is massive.

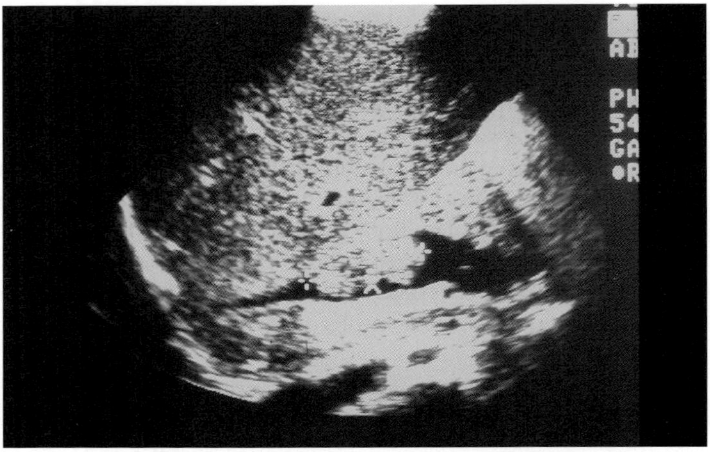

Figure 1. Ultrasound of the inferior vena cava in a child with Wilms' tumor with tumor extension into the renal vein. Note the tumor mass (markers) within the vena cava.

The initial radiologic studies should include chest computed tomography (CT) and abdominal ultrasound. The chest CT may reveal large pulmonary metastases, while the ultrasound gives valuable information confirming the kidney as the organ of origin, as well as the size and consistency of the tumor mass, the status of the opposite kidney, and extension of tumor through the renal vein and into the inferior vena cava (Figure 1). An abdominal X-ray adds little useful information.

Abdominal CT with intravenous contrast demonstrates the extent of the tumor, contralateral kidney (Figures 2 and 3) and may demonstrate enlarged lymph nodes. However, the latter determination should never be a substitute for thorough operative evaluation of the regional lymph nodes and excisional sampling. Generally the chest is included to evaluate the presence of pulmonary metastases. Magnetic resonance and arteriography examinations are rarely needed.

TREATMENT

All children with a solid renal mass should undergo operative abdominal exploration through a generous upper abdominal incision. The only exception

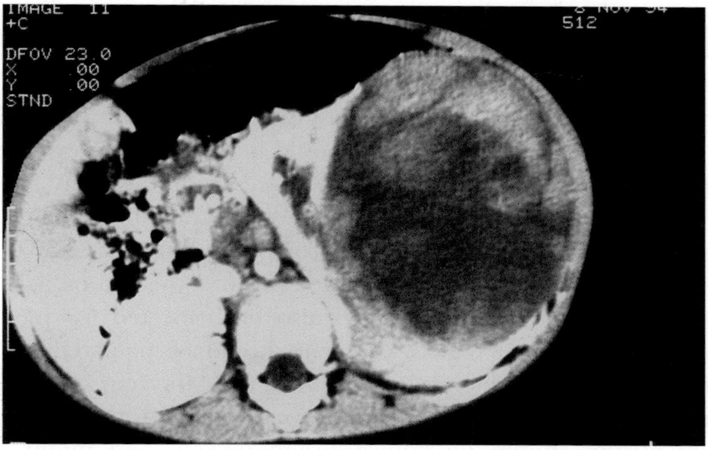

Figure 2. Abdominal computed tomography scan in a child with a large left-sided Wilms' tumor.

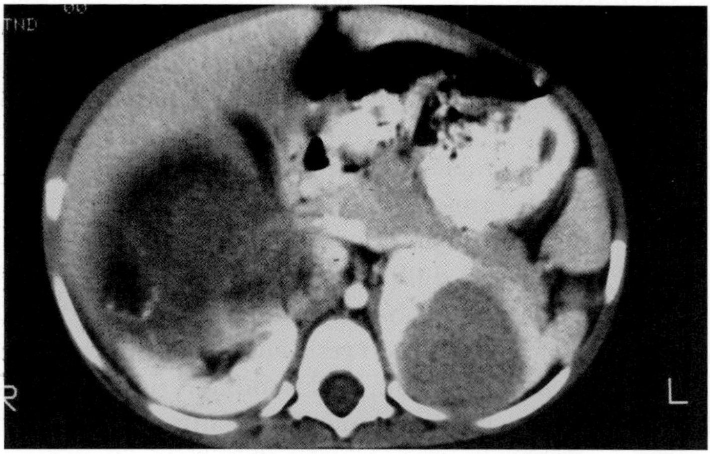

Figure 3. Abdominal computed tomography in a child with bilateral Wilms' tumor. There is a very large right kidney tumor and a smaller but significant left kidney mass. Chemotherapy resulted in tumor shrinkage in both tumors allowing complete resection and survival.

would be in cases of large bilateral tumors where excision of both tumors would leave the patient essentially anephric. In these latter cases, percutaneous needle biopsy, followed by chemotherapy is an acceptable practice.

Exploration in all assumed unilateral cases must be thorough. Bloody ascites suggest tumor rupture and it should be sampled for cytology. The contralateral kidney is preoperatively assessed by CT and any suspicious lesions are biopsied. If the exploration shows no other abnormality, radical nephrectomy is carried out, with generous sampling of regional lymph nodes. Great care must be taken to not rupture the tumor as this will change the staging. The liver should also be inspected for metastases. When ligating the renal vessels, the vein should be palpated for tumor extension. If the tumor extends into the vena cava, the vein can be opened and the tumor is carefully pulled from the cava. Extension of the tumor to the right atrium should be known preoperatively, and might require upfront chemotherapy prior to exploration. Rarely cardiopulmonary bypass is needed. Finally, the ureter should be excised to the bladder because of the possibility of tumor extension through that organ.

Advances in postoperative adjuvant therapy have been accomplished from the extensive study by the National Wilms tumor Study Group in the USA and the Société Internationale d'Oncologie Pédiatrique in Europe. Based on the results of their various randomized trials, the following are the contemporary recommendations from these groups:

(1) Stages I and II, favorable histology: Actinomycin D and Vincristine.
(2) Stages III and IV, favorable histology, and stages I, II, or III, focal anaplasia: Adriamycin and postoperative radiation are added.
(3) Stages II, III, IV with diffuse anaplasia, and clear cell sarcoma: Cyclophosphamide, etoposide, and radiation are added.
(4) Rhabdoid tumors have been resistant to most chemotherapeutic therapies and radiation, and complete surgical excision is the most efficacious treatment. Infants with mesoblastic nephroma do not require therapy after surgical excision.

TREATMENT COMPLICATIONS

Postoperative complications include adhesive bowel obstruction, infection, bleeding, and injury to adjacent organs. Patients with retroperitoneal operations are also susceptible to bowel obstruction secondary to small bowel intussusception. Analysis of data from both Wilms' tumor study groups has shown complication rates of 8–12%. Important risk factors that increase complications include flank or paramedian incision, tumor diameter greater than 10 cm, and operations performed by general surgeons instead of pediatric surgeons.

Chemotherapy and radiation therapies also have numerous potential complications. The most serious of these is cardiac toxicity, which affects 2–4% of patients receiving doxorubicin. The risk was increased in females and those receiving lung and left abdominal radiation. Secondary malignancy occurs in 2% of patients at 15 yrs post therapy, and includes both leukemia and other solid tumors. Finally, growth retardation and infertility are both rare complications of radiation therapy.

OUTCOMES

The survival rates in children with Wilms' tumor have been extremely gratifying, and are directly attributable to the multiple trials through the years, conducted in both the United States and Europe. Overall, children with favorable histology have a survival over 90%, ranging from 97% for stage I to 62% for stage IV. For children with unfavorable histology, survival in stage I is 89%, which falls to 15–50% in other stages. Two-year survival with recurrent disease is 43%. Negative prognostic signs include advanced stage of disease, unfavorable histology, and recurrence. Genetic markers and growth factors are areas of active investigation with regard to prognosis. Prognosis for clear cell sarcoma is slightly lower than for Wilms' tumor with stage I survival 100%; II, 87%; III, 74%; and IV, 36%. Rhabdoid tumor survival is poor, with rates of 24% at 4 yrs. Younger patients with rhabdoid tumor (birth–5 mths) had the lowest survival. Mesoblastic nephroma has survival rates approaching 100%.

REFERENCES

1. Shamberger RC. (2010) Renal tumors. In: GW Holcomb, JP Murphy (eds.), *Aschraft's Pediatric Surgery*, pp. 953–871. Saunders Elsevier, Philadelphia.
2. Tagge EP, Thomas PB, Othersan HG. (2006) Wilms' Tumor. In: JL Grosfeld, J O'Neil, A Coran, *et al.* (eds.), *Pediatric Surgery*, pp. 445–466. Mosby Elsevier, Philadelphia.

NEUROBLASTOMA 21

Jay L. Grosfeld

INTRODUCTION

Neuroblastoma (NB) is the most common solid tumor of infancy and childhood. The incidence is approximately 1 in 7500 to 10,000 children with 700 cases seen annually in the US. It accounts for 10% of childhood tumors and 15% of cancer deaths. The exact etiology remains unknown. NB is slightly more common in boys than girls (ratio of 1.2:1.0) and 40% of cases are diagnosed by age 1 yr, 75% by 7 yrs and 98% by age 10 yrs.[1–3]

NB is an embryonal tumor of neural crest origin that can occur anywhere in the sympathetic nervous system. The lesion can be detected on prenatal ultrasound. Neuroblasts are noted in fetal adrenal glands starting at 16 wks gestation and instances of placental invasion have been observed. NB *in situ* in the adrenal glands is seen at autopsy in 1:30 infants dying of other causes in the first 3 months of life NB may occur in infants with Beckwith–Wiedemann syndrome (BWS), Neurofibromatosis (von Recklinghausen's disease), Hirschsprung disease, Central hypoventilation syndrome (Ondine's curse), MEN-2a, and the fetal alcohol syndrome.[1] The tumor is characterized by bizarre behavior and heterogeneity. The tumor arises from primitive neuroblasts which may follow three potential clinical pathways: (1) spontaneous regression, (2) differentiation and maturation to a benign ganglioneuroma, and (3) progression to a highly undifferentiated neuroblastic malignant tumor. The tumor behavior is likely dependent on the biological factors and genetic alterations noted in each case.[3–5]

CLINICAL PRESENTATION

The primary tumor arises in the adrenal medulla in 50%, paraaortic sympathetic ganglia in 25%, posterior mediastinum in 20%, and 5% in the neck and pelvis (organ of Zuckerkandl). Patients with NB manifest varied signs and symptoms based on the location of the primary tumor, presence of metastases and secretion of biochemical products from the tumor (catecholamines and byproducts, vasoactive intestinal polypeptide [VIP]). Rarely cystic, multifocal or bilateral tumors are observed (Table 1).

Differential Diagnosis

The differential diagnosis includes other retroperitoneal tumors (Wilms' tumor, rhabdomyosarcoma, primitive neuroectodermal tumor [PNET] germ cell), mediastinal lesions (teratomas, lymphoma), pelvic tumors (rhabdomyosarcoma, anterior meningocele, teratoma) and in addition, other small round blue cell tumors (Ewing's family of tumors, PNET, rhabdomyosarcoma lymphoma, desmoplastic tumor).

DIAGNOSIS

Although some tumors can be detected on a prenatal sonogram, in most cases the diagnosis is usually achieved by radiologic imaging and isotopic studies including plain radiographs, Computed Tomography (CT), Magnetic Resonance Imaging (MRI) and MIBG scintigraphy. In the CT, the tumor appears as a solid lesion that is often (>50%) calcified, and may show central areas of necrosis (Figure 1). Adrenal tumors usually displace the ipsilateral kidney inferiorly and laterally and do not distort the collecting system. The tumor has a propensity to cross the midline, involve adjacent organs and surround major blood vessels. Thoracic NB occurs in the posterior mediastinum. Pelvic lesions arise from the organ of Zuckerkandl and are located in proximity of the sacral promontory. MRI is useful in detecting intraspinal (extradural) extension. Scintigraphy aids in determining the presence of bone metastases most commonly seen in the ribs, skull, vertebrae, pelvis and metaphyses of long bones (i.e. red marrow producing areas of bone) (Figure 2). A bone marrow aspirate is obtained to rule out marrow involvement (tumor cell rosettes). A 24-hr urinary collection for catecholamines and byproducts (VMA. HVA, metnephrines) may be diagnostic. Unlike Wilms' tumor, lung metastases in NB is uncommon (4%). Serum values are

Table 1.

Primary tumor location	Signs and symptoms
Clinical presentation	
Cervical	Neck mass, Horner's syndrome Swallowing difficulty
Mediastinal	Respiratory distress, cough Wheezing,
	Neurological deficit
	Dysphagia
Abdominal	Abdominal mass
	Abdominal distension, pain,
	Early satiety
Pelvic	Urinary tract obstruction
	Bladder compression
	Constipation,
	Neurologic deficit
Systemic effects	
Catecholeamine release	Hypertension
	Flushing, tachycardia
VIP release	Watery Diarrhea syndrome
Dancing-eye syndrome	Opsoclonus-nystagmus
	Attention deficit
	Learning disability
Metastatic disease	Panda eyes-(orbital metastases)
	Proptosis
	Bone pain, refusal to walk
	Pathologic fractures
	Anemia (bone marrow mets)
Stage IV-S	Hepatomegaly
	Respiratory distress
	Abdominal compartment syndrome
	Renal failure
	Skin nodules

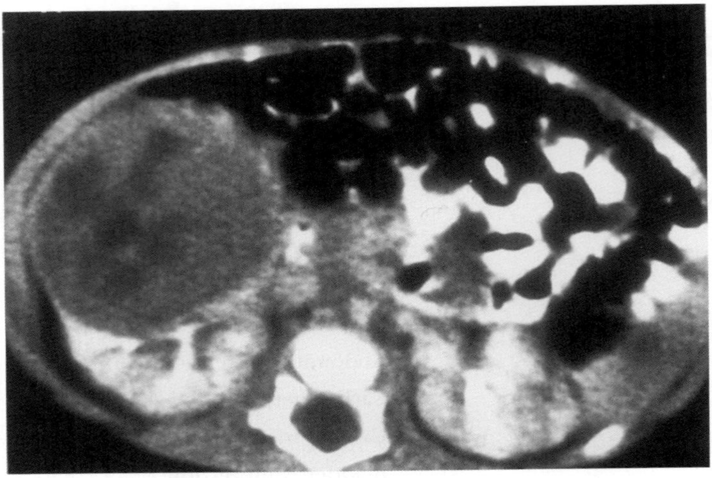

Figure 1. Computed tomography image of a neuroblastoma.

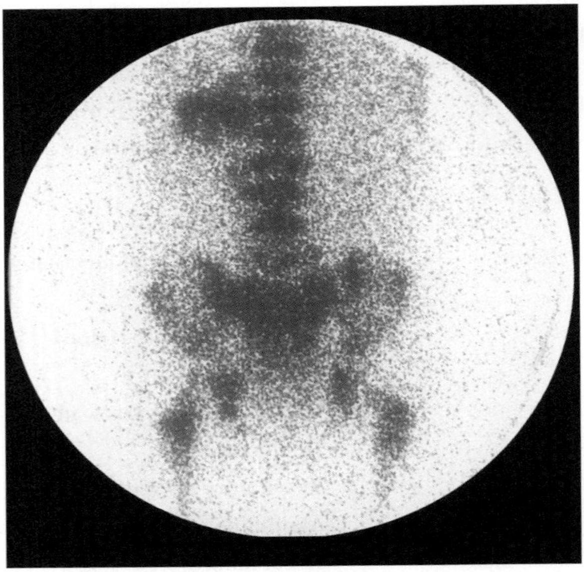

Figure 2. Scintigraphy illustrating a right-sided lesion with uptake of tracer.

absent →Ganglioneuroma Maturing subtype FH

absent→microscopic neuroblastic foci

\> 50% ↑ Macroscopically visible nodules

present →Ganglioneurobalstoma intermixed FH

Schwannian Development

present--------------------→Ganglioneuroblastoma nodular classic* UH/FH

↓

0 or <50%--→GNBn variant(with or without macroscopic visible nodule(s)* UH/FH

		%MKCells	Age	Histology
	Undifferentiated	any MKI	any age	Undifferentiated UH
		> 4%	any age	UH
Neuroblastoma----------- >	Poorly Differentiated	any MKI	> 1.5 yrs	UH
		< 4%	< 1.5 yrs	FH
		any MKI	> 5 yrs	UH
		< 4%	< 1.5 yrs	FH
	Differentiating	> 4%	< 1.5 yrs	UH
		< 2%	1.5–5.0 yrs	FH
		> 2%	1.5–5.0 yrs	UH

any

Note: FH = favorable histology; UH=unfavorable histology; GNBn = ganglioneuroblastoma nodular %MKC = mitotic and karryorectic cells; MKI = mitotic karryorexis index
*classical GNBn (single,macroscopically visible usually hemorrhagic nodule in stromarich stroma dominant tissue background **MKC 2% 100 of 5000 cells; MKC 4% 200 of 5000 cells Peuchmaur, M*etal*.

Figure 3a. International Neuroblastoma Pathology Classification.[6–8]

obtained for NSE, LDH, ferritin, telomerase, and CEA. In patients with diarrhea, a serum VIP level should be obtained.

The diagnosis is confirmed by histological studies of tumor tissue (Figures 3a and 3b). Genetic evaluation of tumor tissue for ploidy, MYCN-proto-oncogene, Trk a-c, 1p, 11q, 17q, and others provides vital prognostic information that along with age, tumor stage and histology (favorable or unfavorable) assists the clinician in determining the tumor risk stratification and selection of treatment.[6]

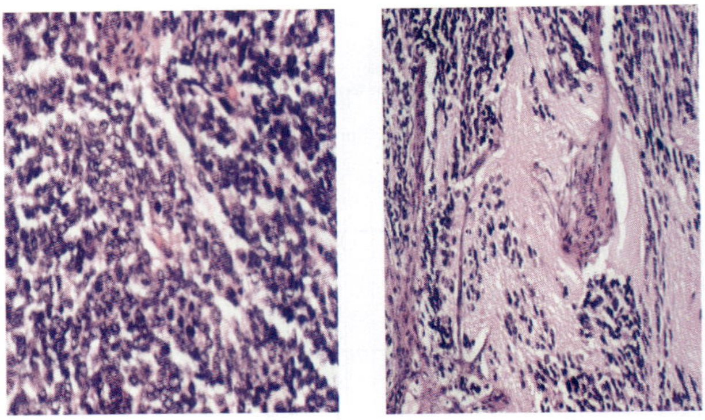

Figure 3b. Neuroblastoma histology.

Staging

Tumor stage has been an important prognostic consideration in patients with NB. The International Neuroblastoma Staging System (INSS) is dependent on operative findings in each case (Table 2).[9] While this has been a very useful method of staging and is still currently used for most COG protocols, it requires an operation to determine the stage and limits the opportunity for observational studies for patients that are stratified as low risk such as those diagnosed by prenatal ultrasonography, with cystic tumors, multifocal tumors, and localized tumors in early infancy. More recently, a new International Neuroblastoma Risk Group Staging System (INRGSS) has been developed (Table 3). The INRGSS differs from INSS in that it is based on preoperative imaging and image-defined risk factors that establishes a pretreatment classification (Table 4).[10,11] This system is neither dependent on surgical or pathological findings nor considers the vagaries of the "midline" tumor noted in INSS. INRGSS also does not include lymph node status in the staging system for stages L1 or 2 nor does it classify ascites or pleural effusion positive or negative for tumor cells as a risk factor. While INSS stage IV-S has an upper age limit of 12 months, the INRGSS extends the age group for stage MS to 18 months.

Table 2. Stages (INSS)

I	Localized tumor, complete gross excision, LN negative.
IIA	Localized tumor, gross residual disease, with either ipsilateral LN negative or LN sought and none found (mentioned specifically in op note).
IIB	Localized tumor, +/− gross residual disease, with either ipsilateral LN positive or No LN sought (including no mention in op note).
III	Unresectable unilateral tumor +/− LN | Localized tumor with contralateral LN (+) Midline tumor (If gross resection and LN (−) or LN sought/none found, then stage I; if gross resection and no LN sought, then stage III).
IV	Any primary tumor with metastases to distant LN, bone, bone marrow, liver, skin, etc.
IV-S	Localized tumor (I, IIA, IIB) mets to skin, liver, and/or bone marrow, < 1 yr of age.

1. Multifocal primary tumors (e.g. bilateral adrenal primary tumors) should be staged according to the greatest extent of disease, as defined above, and followed by a subscript "M" (e.g. 3M).
2. The midline is defined as the vertebral column. Tumors originating on one side and crossing the midline must infiltrate to or beyond the opposite side of the vertebral column.
3. Marrow involvement in stage IV-S should be minimal, i.e. less than 10% of total nucleated cells identified as malignant on bone marrow biopsy or marrow aspirate. More extensive marrow involvement would be considered to be stage IV. The MIBG scan (if performed) should be negative in the marrow.
4. Proven malignant effusion within the thoracic cavity if it is bilateral or the abdominal cavity upstages the patient to INSS.

MANAGEMENT

Perinatal Period or Early Infancy Observation-Low Risk

Based on information acquired from screening studies that identified NB in babies in the first 6 months of life, and outcomes for instances of NB detected on prenatal ultrasound where in a significant number of cases the tumor would regress spontaneously and/or the survival following resection was >95%, an *observational program* was established for low risk

Table 3. International Neuroblastoma Risk Group Staging System (INRGSS)

Stage L1 — Localized tumor not involving vital structures as defined by Image Defined Risk Factors and confined to one body compartment_
Stage L2 — Locoregional tumor with presence of one or more Image Defined Risk Factors The tumor could be ipsilaterally contiguous within body compartments i.e. left sided abdominal NB with left sided chest involvement still L2
Stage M — Distant metastatic disease (except MS)
Stage MS — Patients < 18 mths old with either an L1 or L2 tumor with metastatic disease confined to skin, liver and/or bone marrow (limited to < 10% of cells on biopsy) Bone and bone marrow should be MIBG scintigraphy negative.

cases.[8] The intent is to identify infants who are likely to have INSS stage I NB. Eligible patients are infants <3 months of age when an adrenal mass is first identified and confirmed on ultrasonography and has a tumor volume <16 mL if solid, or <65 mL if at least 25% cystic, and does not cross the midline. Bone marrow aspirate and biopsy, bone scan (+/− MIBG scan) and abdominal CT or MRI scan, are all negative for evidence of disease outside the adrenal gland, including positive contra- or ipsilateral-lymph nodes. Sonograms are analyzed to determine the tumor volume. Urine is collected for catecholamine analysis (VMA and HVA in *ug*/mg creatinine). Infants are followed closely with periodic surveillance sonograms and catecholamine levels. Surgical intervention is required if there is an increase in tumor volume or catecholamine secretion; if progressive disease or recurrence is identified or if there is secondary malignancy. Stage I cases that are completely resected in this age group may not require adjunctive therapy.

Intermediate Risk

The surgical goal in intermediate-risk patients is resection of as much of the tumor as possible that is consistent with preserving organs (spleen, kidney, bowel etc.), major blood vessels and nerves. This may leave residual disease adherent to these anatomical structures. As intermediate risk patients will have either localized or loco-regional disease, preoperative assessment of resectability is essential. A preoperative staging system using International Neuroblastoma Risk Groups (INRG) criteria (Table 3) employs imaged-defined risk factors related to location of the primary

Table 4. INRG image-defined risk factors

Risk factors related to localization

(1) Neck
   i. Tumor encasing carotid and/or vertebral artery and/or internal jugular vein
   ii. Tumor extending to base of skull
   iii. Tumor compressing the trachea

(2) Cervico-thoracic junction
   i. Tumor encasing brachial plexus roots
   ii. Tumor encasing subclavian vessels and/or vertebral and/or carotid artery
   iii. Tumor compressing the trachea

(3) Thorax
   i. Tumor encasing the aorta and/or major branches
   ii. Tumor compressing the trachea or principal bronchi
   iii. Lower left mediastinal tumor, infiltrating the costo-vertebral junction between T9 and T12

(4) Thoraco-abdominal
   i. Tumor encasing the aorta and/or vena cava

(5) Abdomen
   i. Tumor infiltrating the porta hepatic and/or the hepatoduodenal ligament
   ii. Tumor encasing branches of the superior mesenteric artery at the mesenteric root
   iii. Tumor encasing the origin of the celiac axis, and/or of the superior mesenteric artery
   iv. Tumor invading one or both renal pedicles
   v. Tumor encasing the aorta and/or vena cava
   vi. Tumor encasing the iliac vessels
   vii. Pelvic tumor crossing the sciatic notch

(6) Dumbbell tumors with symptoms of spinal cord compression
   i. Whatever the localization

(7) Infiltration of adjacent organs/structures
   i. Pericardium, diaphragm, kidney, liver, duodeno-pancreatic block, and mesentery

tumor (listed in Table 4) during the initial assessment. Analysis of MYCN amplification, ploidy, molecular genetics (1p, 11q) and histology (favorable or unfavorable) (Figure 3b) of the tumor tissue and age of the patient is essential for determining the treatment group. If the primary tumor is considered unresectable, a diagnostic biopsy (preferably open) must be obtained (>1 cm^3) and chemotherapy administered according to protocol guidelines. Delayed surgery is performed with the goal of achieving the most complete tumor resection consistent with preservation of full organ and neurologic function. Timing of delayed surgery depends on the treatment group. For example, group 2 patients will undergo resection after two cycles of chemotherapy, group 3 after four cycles, and group 4 after four or eight cycles. The intermediate risk groups are determined by how many adverse biological factors are noted in the tumor (i.e. all are MYCN negative but may have other risk factors such as age >1 yr, a diploid tumor, LOH of 1p and/or unbalanced 11q LOH and unfavorable histology) Those with higher risk receive more chemotherapy (Table 5). The INRG image-defined risk criteria are only used for the initial assessment and are not reassessed for tumors treated with chemotherapy.[13,14]

For tumors considered resectable at diagnosis, the operative approach varies according to the site of the primary tumor (cervical, thoracic inlet, mediastinum, adrenal, paraaortic, pelvic, etc.,) maintaining the principles of adjacent organ, major vessel and nerve preservation. Minimally invasive techniques (thoracoscopic and laparoscopic resection) may be feasible for small primary tumors of the mediastinum, adrenal gland and pelvis respectively or for biopsy. Extensive tumors or those with significant vascular encasement, or locoregional nodal spread can be more completely resected using an open approach. Residual tumor should be marked with titanium clips.

The reader is referred to the selected references for further details regarding the operative procedures in the various sites of primary tumor.

4S Neuroblastoma

The primary tumor in patients with 4S NB (as defined in Table 2) should not be routinely resected. An adequate amount of tissue can usually be obtained from biopsy of metastatic sites (liver or skin nodules). Adequate biologic information cannot be obtained from bone marrow alone in patients with 4S disease. If an operative biopsy is done the surgeon should acquire an adequate amount of tissue (1–2 cm^3) that is sent to appropriate laboratories. In patients with stage IV-S disease who are very ill

Table 5. Intermediate-risk neuroblastoma treatment assignment.

INSS stage	Legacy rick group & treatment	Age	Biologic features	ANBL0531 baseline treatment
Group 1				ANBL00B1 Registry
I	Low: Observation	0 ≤ 30 yr	Any	
IIA/IIB < 50% resected	Low: Observation	0 ≤ 30 yr	MYCN-NA, any histo/ploidy	
IV-S	Low: Observation	< 365 days	MYCN-NA, FH, DI > 1	
Group 2				ANBL0531: Z cycles
IIA/IIB < 50% resected or Bx only	Low: 4 cycles	0–12 yrs	MYCN-NA, any histo/ploidy normal 1p & 11q	
III	Intermediate: 4 cycles	< 365 days	MYCN-NA, FH, DI > 1 normal 1p & 11q	
III	Intermediate: 4 cycles	≥ 365 days – 12 yrs	MYCN-NA, FH normal 1p & 11q	
IV-S Symptomatic	Low: 2–4 cycles	< 365 days	MYCN-NA, FH, DI > 1 normal 1p & 11q	
Group 3				ANBL0531: 4 cycles
IIA/IIB < 50% resected or Bx only	Low: 4 cycles	0–12 yrs	MYCN-NA, any histo/ploidy 1p LOH and/or unb11q LOH or data missing for either	
III	Intermediate: 4 cycles	< 365 days	MYCN-NA, FH, DI > 1 1p LOH and/or unb11q LOH or data missing for either	
III	Intermediate: 8 cycles	< 365 days	MYCN-NA, either DI = 1 &/or UH normal 1p & 11q	
III	Intermediate: 4 cycles	≥ 365 days – 12 yrs	MYCN-NA, FH 1p LOH and/or unb11q LOH or data missing for either	

(*Continued*)

Table 5. (*Continued*)

INSS stage	Legacy rick group & treatment	Age	Biologic features	ANBL0531 baseline treatment
IV	Intermediate: 4 cycles	< 365 days	MYCN-NA, FH, DI > 1 normal 1p & 11q	
IV-S	Intermediate: 8 cycles	< 365 days	MYCN-NA, either UH & any ploidy, or FH & DI = 1 normal 1p & 11q	
IV-S symptomatic	Low: 2–4 cycles	< 365 days	MYCN-NA, FH, DI > 1 1p LOH and/or unb11q LOH or data missing for either	
IV-S	Unknown	< 365 days	Unknown biologic features	
Group 4				ANBL0531: 8 cycles
III	Intermediate: 8 cycles	< 365 days	MYCN-NA, either DI = 1 &/or UH 1p LOH and/or unb11q LOH or data missing for either	
III	High: A3973	365 ≤ 547 days	MYCN-NA, UH, any ploidy, any 1p/11q	
IV	Intermediate: 8 cycles	< 365 days	MYCN-NA, either DI = 1 &/or UH, any 1p/11q	
IV	Intermediate: 4 cycles	< 365 days	MYCN-NA, FH, DI > 1 1p LOH and/or unb11q LOH or data missing for either	
IV	High: A3973	365 ≤ 547 days	MYCN-NA, FH, DI > 1 any 1p/11q	
IV-S	Intermediate: 8 cycles	< 365 days	MYCN-NA, either UH & any ploidy, or FH & DI = 1 1p LOH and/ or unb11q LOH or data missing for either	

(i.e. respiratory distress, renal failure) and an open biopsy is considered contraindicated, tumor tissue may be obtained by fine needle aspiration of a metastatic site for determination of MYCN and 1p/11q status. Many patients with stage IV-S will have spontaneous regression of their disease. Very few (<8%) have unfavorable biologic characteristics (i.e. MYCN amplification). In many instances, survival is achieved without resection of the primary tumor. Stage IV-S patients with unfavorable biological characteristics (MYCN amplification) require more aggressive treatment. Overall survival for stage IV-S is >88%.

Intraspinal Tumor Extension

Tumor extension into the extradural space/spinal canal on imaging requires a careful neurological examination to document the degree of neurologic dysfunction at diagnosis, during and post-therapy. Laminectomy should not be performed in neurologically asymptomatic patients. Those with symptomatic spinal cord compression secondary to epidural extension of NB through neural foramina may require laminectomy, or osteoplastic laminotomy at diagnosis to prevent permanent paralysis. However, treatment with chemotherapy alone or chemotherapy and radiation therapy will often promptly reverse symptoms of cord compression. Patients should receive neoadjuvant chemotherapy. Neurologic deterioration that occurs during chemotherapy administration may require operative decompression according to the degree of neurological impairment. An osteoplastic laminotomy is preferred with replacement of the laminae after decompression. Neurological function is assessed prior to each cycle of chemotherapy. Neurologic and orthopedic evaluations are required during follow-up to evaluate patients for neurologic impairment, scoliosis and extremity deformities.

High Risk Neuroblastoma

Patients with unresectable stage tumors and those with metastatic disease at diagnosis (stage IV) are considered high risk patients. The latter have traditionally had the worst prognosis with event free survival (EFS) noted in only 30–35% of cases. These patients require the most intense treatment regimens including numerous courses of multiagent chemotherapy, myoablative agents, radiation therapy and bone marrow transplantation. Despite intensive therapy, tumor relapse is >43% and long-term survival remains poor.[15]

Resection of the primary tumor and bulky metastatic disease is usually necessary to achieve a complete response (CR), very good partial response (VGPR), or PR after induction chemotherapy. A retrospective analysis of high risk NB patients (CCG 3891) demonstrated improved resectability after initial chemotherapy and a trend toward improved survival for patients with gross total resection of the primary tumor.[16] However, almost 20% of the patients required ipsilateral nephrectomy to achieve gross total resection. Patients enrolled in the recent studies underwent delayed surgical resection of the primary tumor after five cycles of chemotherapy. Current protocols attempt to prospectively evaluate if complete primary tumor resection is predictive of local control and EFS in high-risk NB patients. Studies also attempt to evaluate early and late postoperative complications such as adhesive bowel obstruction, chylous leak, ipsilateral renal injury (atrophy or loss), and chronic diarrhea.[17]

Adequate preoperative imaging of the primary tumor and sites of regional spread is accomplished by either CT or MRI or both of these modalities. Sites of distant metastases are evaluated by clinical and bone marrow assessment as well as bone scan and MIBG scans. Patients with paraspinal or epidural lesions should have preoperative neurosurgical consultation and a baseline neurologic assessment as noted above in the discussion of intermediate risk cases.

In high-risk patients with NB the surgical goal is to achieve the most complete tumor resection possible compatible with preservation of full organ and neurologic function. The main purpose of the initial surgical procedure is to obtain enough tissue to establish a diagnosis, determine stage, and secure enough tumor for biological studies. The great majority of high-risk patients will undergo initial diagnostic biopsy without resection. Biopsy of the primary tumor or an accessible metastatic site is acceptable. The biopsy (at least 1 cm^3 of viable tumor tissue) is necessary for a histopathological diagnosis, MYCN determination, cytogenetics, and other biological studies. Complete primary excision of the tumor can occasionally be performed if the tumor is easily resectable without requiring a lengthy procedure or extensive dissection. Resection should not be attempted if it might result in significant morbidity or delay the start chemotherapy. In some instances of stage IV disease, the diagnosis is established by finding NB in bone marrow specimens in conjunction with elevated urinary catecholamines. A central venous access line is also placed at the time of biopsy.

The majority of patients will undergo resection of the primary tumor after initial induction chemotherapy. Induction therapy includes two courses of cyclophosphamide and topotecan followed by peripheral stem cell harvest. A course of cisplatin and etoposide, is then followed by a course of cyclophosphamide, doxorubicin and vincristine. The glomerular filtration rate (GFR) is evaluated after the fourth course. A fifth cycle of cisplatin and etoposide is administered and the primary tumor is imaged by CT and MRI before embarking on surgery. Cycles are administered 6 wks apart.[18]

Surgical resection should be performed after cycle 5 of induction when the absolute neutrophile count (ANC) is 500/μL and the patient is medically stable. This usually allows maximum tumor reduction by chemotherapy and decreases tumor vascularity prior to the resection. Surgical resection may be performed later in induction, (i.e. after the sixth course of chemotherapy with cyclophosphamide, doxorubicin and vincristine) if necessary, but must occur prior to the consolidation phase of therapy.

The goal of delayed surgery is gross total resection of residual tumor in the primary site and any regional spread (usually lymph nodes). Achieving a microscopic negative margin may not be feasible because of proximity of the tumor to major vessels and the spine. The tumor should be removed as completely as possible (i.e. all gross disease). It may be necessary, to incise the tumor and remove it in a segmental fashion. Titanium clips are used to mark areas of residual disease as a guide for possible radiation therapy. Attempts should be made to preserve adjacent organs especially the kidney. Rarely, nephrectomy may be necessary for complete tumor removal but this should only be done if the involved kidney has greatly diminished function. If nephrectomy is being considered a differential, GFR should be obtained preoperatively to determine renal function in the contralateral kidney. Carboplatin is used for consolidation therapy and toxicity may be greater for patients with a GFR <100. Kidney preservation when feasible is recommended.

Radiation therapy has been used to control local disease when residual tumor is present, reduce the tumor burden in preparation for bone marrow transplantation and manage pain from extensive bony metastases.

Usually the sixth cycle of induction therapy is given after surgical resection. An assessment of disease extent is then made including, CT. MRI, 24-hr urine collection for VMA, HVA, etc.) and patients are randomized for consolidation therapy which may include, autologous bone marrow transplantation (ABMT) vs. stem cell transplantation, and myeloablative therapy with thiotepa, cyclophosphamide and radiation or alternatively carboplatin, etoposide and melphalan and radiation followed by administration of a retinoid as a differentiating agent in patients without disease progression.[19–21]

SURVIVAL

The overall survival for patients with NB is approximately 50–60%. Low risk patients have the best outlook with survival rates of 90%. Intermediate risk survival is 70% and high risk patients continue to have a guarded prognosis with long-term survival of 30–35%. Key predictors of outcome include age, INSS-stage, INPC (International Neuroblastoma Pathology Classification), MYCN status, ploidy and allelic loss (1p36) 11q and 17q gain.

A more favorable prognosis is observed in patients with stages I, II, and IV-S tumors, infants < 1 yr, those with favorable histology and a near triploid karyotype, nonamplified MYCN, tumors identified prenatally, infants with high Trk-A expression, and those with cystic, multifocal, and bilateral tumors. Patients with primary tumors in the pelvis, neck and mediastinum, and those with VIP secreting tumors and opsoclonus/nystagmus ("dancing eye-syndrome") also have an improved outcome. Of interest is that infants < 1 yr of age have a significantly better outcome (80%) than children > 1 yr (35%) in all stages.

A poor prognosis is noted in patients with stages III and IV, children > 1 yr of age, those with unfavorable histology, and structural genetic alterations characterized by deletions of 1p, unbalanced 11q, 17q gain, MYCN amplification, Trk B expression (with BDNF), increased Bcl-2 expression (inhibits apoptosis), and a diploid or near tetraploid karyotype.The use of intense treatment programs including multiagent chemotherapy, radiation therapy, bone marrow transplantation, and myeloablative management in growing children has resulted in a number of early and late complications related to treatment including: radiation damage, immunosuppression/infection, catheter sepsis, cardiac and renal toxicities, inhibition of growth and development, scoliosis, endocrine problems, learning disabilities, and the occurrence of second tumors (EBV associated LPD, bone, renal, thyroid cancer).[22,23] More dose intense induction chemotherapy for maximum cell kill has resulted in a slightly improved EFS (better remission) but does not improve overall survival. Treatment with ABMT has slightly improved event-free survival in children with high-risk NB. Post-transplant isotretinoin therapy is beneficial in patients without progressive disease when used following chemotherapy or transplantation. High-dose therapy with tandem autologous peripheral-blood stem cell rescue has been effective in some patients with high-risk NB. As the survival in advanced disease (very high risk cases) has not improved significantly despite aggressive treatment, use of more novel, less toxic therapies such as differentiating agents (retinoids:cis-13 retinoic acid and fenretinide), antiangiogenic agents (thalidomide, VEGF and VEGF-R antibodies, imitinab mesylate, trk-A), apoptosis regulation (Bcl-2 and survivin inhibitors, caspase enhancers), immunotherapy (IL-2, IL-12, dendritic cell vaccines, GD-2 monoclonal antibodies), targeted therapies with radionucleides (I^{131} MIBG), and proteosomic inhibitors that affect gene transcription are being studied as therapeutic adjuncts.[21] The goal is to improve the outlook of patients with NB at high risk (age >1 yr, stages III and IV, unfavorable histology, diploid karyotype and tumors expressing genetic instability) while at the same time reduce the incidence of untoward complications associated with intense programs of treatment in patients with low and intermediate risk tumors that require either no or minimal adjunctive therapy and improve the quality of life among survivors. The thrust of COG protocols is to reduce cytotoxic therapy in low-risk and intermediate-risk patients and those with stages III and IV disease with favorable histology, nonamplified MYCN and hyperdiplody.

REFERENCES

1. Grosfeld JL. (2006) Neuroblastoma. In: JL Grosfeld, JA O'Neill, Jr, EW Fonkalsrud, *et al.* (eds.), *Pediatric Surgery*, 6th edition, pp. 467–494. Mosby-Elsevier Philadelphia.
2. La Quaglia MP, Rutigliano DN. (2008) Neuroblastoma and other adrenal tumors. In: R Carachi, JL Grosfeld, A Azmy (eds.), *The Surgery of Childhood Tumors*, 2nd edition, pp. 201–226. Springer-Verlag, Berlin.
3. Maris JM. (2010) Recent advances in neuroblastoma. *N Engl J Med* **362**: 2202–2211.
4. Ishihara H, Toyoda y, Tanaka Y, *et al.* (2004) Natural course of neuroblastoma detected by mass screening: a 5 year prospective study at a single institution. *J Clin Oncol* **18**:3012–3017.
5. Tanaka M, Kigasawa H, Kato K, *et al.* (2010) A prospective study of a long-term follow up of an observation program for neuroblastoma detected by mass screening. *Pediatr Blood Cancer* **54**:573–578.
6. Shimada H, Umehara S, Monobe Y, *et al.* (2001) International neuroblastoma pathology classification for prognostic evaluation of patients with peripheral

neuroblastic tumors: A report from the Children's Cancer Group. *Cancer* **92**:2451–2461.

7. Peuchmaur M, d'Amore ES, Joshi VV, *et al.* (2003) Revision of the international neuroblastoma pathology classification: Confirmation of favorable and unfavorable prognostic subsets in ganglioneuroma, nodular. *Cancer* **98**: 274–2281.
8. Hero B, Simon T, Spitz R, *et al.* (2008) Localized infant neuroblastoma often show spontaneous regression: Results of the prospective trials NB95-S and NB97. *J Clin Oncol* **26**:1504–1510.
9. Brodeur GM, Pritchard J, Berthold F, *et al.* (1993) Revision of the international criteria for neuroblastoma diagnosis, staging and response to treatment. *J Clin Oncol* **11**:1466–1477.
10. Monclair T, Brodeur GM, Ambros HJ, *et al.* (2009) The International Neuroblastoma Risk Group (INRG) staging system: An INRG Task Force report. *J Clin Oncol* **27**:298–303.
11. Cohn SL, Pearson AD, London WB, *et al.* (2009) The International Neuroblastoma Risk Group (INRG) classification system: An INRG Task Force report. *J Clin Oncol* **27**:289–297.
12. Ceccheto G, Masseri V, De Bernardi B, *et al.* (2005) Surgical risk factors in primary surgery for localized neuroblastoma: The LNESG1 Study of the European International Society of pediatric oncology Neuroblastoma Group. *J Clin Oncol* **23**:8483–8489.
13. Bagatell R, Rumcheva P, London WB, *et al.* (2005) Outcomes of children with intermediate risk neuroblastoma after treatment stratified by MYCN status and tumor cell ploidy. *J Clin Oncol* **23**:881–8827.
14. Schneiderman J, London WB, Brodeur GM, *et al.* (2008) Clinical significance of MYCN amplification and ploidy in favorable-stage neuroblastoma: A report from the Children's Oncology Group. *J Clin Oncol* **26**:913–918.
15. Adkins ES, Sawin R, Gerbing RB, *et al.* (2004) Efficacy of complete resection for high risk neuroblastoma: a Children's Cancer Group Study. *J Pediatr Surg* **39**:931–936.
16. La Quaglia MP, Kushner BH, Su W, *et al.* (2004) The impact of gross total resection on local control and survival in high risk neuroblastoma. *J Pediatr Surg* **39**:412–417.
17. Escobar MA, Grosfeld JL, Powell RL, *et al.* (2006) Long-term outcomes in stage IV Neuroblastoma. *J Pediatr Surg* **41**:377–381.
18. Matthay KK, Villablanca JG, Seeger RC, *et al.* (1999) Treatment of high-risk neuroblastoma with intensive chemotherapy, radiotherapy, autologous bone marrow transplantation, and 13-cis-retinoic acid. *N Engl J Med* **341**:1165–1173.

19. George RE, Li S, Medeiros-Nancarrow C, *et al.* (2006) High-risk neuroblastoma treated with tandem autologous peripheral-blood stem cell-supported transplantation: long-term survival update. *J Clin Oncol* **24**:2891–2896.
20. Kreissman SG, Villablanca JG, Diller L, *et al.* (2007) Response and toxicity to a dose-intensive multi-agent chemotherapy induction regimen for high risk neuroblastoma (HR-NB): a Children's Oncology Group (COG A3973) study. *J Clin Oncol* **25** (Suppl 18), A-9505, 527s.
21. Cheung NK, Sowers R, Vickers AJ, *et al.* (2006) FCGRA polymorphism is correlated with clinical outcome after immunotherapy of neuroblastoma with anti-GD2 antibody and granulocyte macrophage colony-stimulating factor. *J Clin Oncol* **24**:2885–2889.
22. Bassal M, Mertens AC, Taylor L, *et al.* (2006) Risk of selected subsequent carcinomas in survivors of childhood cancer: A report from the Childhood Cancer Survivor group. *J Clin Oncol* **24**:476–483.
23. Meadows AT, Friedman DL, Neglia JP, *et al.* (2009) Second neoplasms in survivors of childhood cancer: Findings from the Childhood Cancer Survivors Group cohort. *J Clin Oncol*(epub) **27**:2356–2362.

LIVER TUMORS 22

Frederick J. Rescorla

Liver tumors are relatively rare in children[1] accounting for approximately 1–4% of all solid tumors in children. Malignant liver tumors occur in approximately 1–1.5 per million children per year, resulting in approximately 150 malignant liver tumors per year in the United States. Hepatoblastoma is the most common malignant tumor in children followed by hepatocellular carcinoma (HCC). Benign lesions include hemangioendothelioma, mesenchymal hamartoma, focal nodular hyperplasia (FNH) and adenoma.

HEPATOBLASTOMA

Most hepatoblastomas occur in children 3 yrs or younger with a median age of 18 mths. The incidence of hepatoblastoma is increasing primarily due to the increased survivorship among premature infants. There is a relationship between hepatoblastoma and extreme prematurity, that being less than 1000 g, with risk factors also including maternal age younger than 20 yrs and maternal smoking. The risk of hepatoblastoma also increases with longer duration of oxygen therapy. Hepatoblastoma is also noted with increased frequency in children with Beckwith–Wiedemann syndrome and familial adenomatous polyposis.[2] Children with Beckwith–Wiedemann syndrome should undergo screening for Wilm's tumor, as well as hepatoblastoma with serial alpha fetoprotein (AFP) levels every 3 mths until age 4 yrs of life and abdominal ultrasounds every 3 mths until 8 yrs of life.

Clinical Presentation

The most common clinical presentation is that of an asymptomatic right upper quadrant abdominal mass that is noted by a parent or the child's physician. Fifty percent of these tumors are within the right lobe, 15% in the left lobe and 27% located centrally in both lobes. Anemia and thrombocytosis are frequently noted. Elevation of the serum AFP is almost uniformly noted and occurs in 90% of affected children. The AFP often exceeds 1 million ng/mL. AFP has a half life of 4 to 5 days and can be normally elevated in children up to 8 mths of age, however usually at levels below 50,000 ng/mL. It is a useful marker for response to chemotherapy as well as surgical resection and potential development of recurrence.

Although an abdominal ultrasound is often the first diagnostic test, an abdominal Computed Tomography (CT) scan is usually performed to determine the organ of origin as renal tumors can present in a very similar fashion. Magnetic Resonance Imaging (MRI) is being used with increased frequency as it is very useful in determining the relation of the tumor to the arterial and venous supply of the liver.

Staging

The Children's Oncology Group (COG) staging system defines stage I as a complete resection with clear margins, stage II as a gross total resection with microscopic residual or perioperative rupture, stage III as unresectable or resection with gross residual or lymph node involvement and stage IV as metastatic disease. Most tumors are also classified by the pretreatment extent of disease (PRETEXT) group system from the International Society of Pediatric Oncology (SIOP). In this staging system the right lobe of liver is divided into the anterior and posterior sector and the left lobe into the medial and lateral. PRETEXT I is tumor in one sector with three adjoining sectors free of tumor. PRETEXT II has two sectors involved with two adjoining sectors free. PRETEXT III occurs when only one sector is free or two nonadjoining sectors are free and PRETEXT IV is when no sector is free of tumor.

Treatment

Although surgical resection is the mainstay of treatment of hepatoblastomas many of these tumors require neoadjuvant therapy in order to prepare the patient for resection. The approach of COG has generally been to assess the ability of resection with an open technique whereas the SIOPEL approach has been more towards initial treatment with chemotherapy followed by delayed resection. Chemotherapy usually consists of cisplatin, vincristine, and 5-fluorouracil. Doxorubicin is also occasionally utilized. Standard resections include segmental resections as well as right and left lobectomy and right and left trisegmentectomy. If complete resection cannot be performed at presentation and there is no evidence of extra hepatic disease, consideration should be given to liver transplantation. If metastatic disease is noted at presentation, chemotherapy should be given and the absence of extra hepatic disease or resection of metastatsis should be performed prior to consideration of a transplant.[3]

The treatment of hepatoblastoma is risk based. Children with very low risk tumors, defined as stage I pure fetal histology tumors with complete resection require no further treatment and have excellent survivorship of 100%. Low risk tumors include those resected at the time of diagnosis consisting of nonpure fetal histology and nonsmall cell histology stage I and II tumors. These children receive cisplantin, vincristine and 5-FU. Intermediate risk tumors include those tumors not resected at diagnosis. These children generally receive 4–6 cycles of chemotherapy followed by surgical resection and then two cycles postoperatively. An alternate plan is to perform resection or transplant after four cycles. High risk tumors include stage IV tumors or any stage with an AFP less than 100 ng/mL. These children receive a combination of chemotherapy and surgical resection with potential consideration of transplant if there is no evidence of extra hepatic disease at the time of surgical resection.

Outcome

Survivorship of hepatoblastoma has improved significantly. The current survival for stage I pure fetal histology is 100%. In the most recent COG study, the 3-yr event free survival was 90% for stage I and II tumors, 50% for stage III tumors and 20% for stage IV tumors. Comparative data of the COG and PRETEXT system survival by the stage in each system demonstrated stage I tumors 100% for PRETEXT and COG survival of 100% for COG stage II and 95% for PRETEXT II; survival 64% COG stage III and 84% PRETEXT III; and, stage IV COG 37% and stage IV PRETEXT 61%.[4]

The outcome for liver transplantation from resectable hepatoblastoma has demonstrated a recurrence free survival rate of between 79% and 92%.

There is obviously some selection bias in this data as some of the transplants are performed for incidentally detected tumors. It should be noted that liver transplantation for local tumor recurrence is associated with a very poor prognosis which includes a post-transplant recurrence rate of 30%. A recent study from Vanderbilt of a database with children with hepatoblastoma undergoing transplant demonstrated 1-, 5-, and 10-yr survival of 79%, 69%, and 69%, respectively.[5]

HEPATOCELLULAR CARCINOMA

HCC is a very rare but highly malignant tumor that is much more commonly seen in adults than children. It is the second most common pediatric malignant liver tumor, but accounts for less than 1% of all pediatric cancers. Predisposing factors for HCCs include cirrhosis and multiple conditions including α1-antitrypsin deficiency, Alagille syndrome, biliary atresia, hepatic adenoma, hepatitis B and C infection, hereditary tyrosinemia, hyperalimentation and familial intrahepatic cholestasis. Although cirrhosis is often not part of the process in children, the association with metabolic, familial and infectious disorders is still significant. The relationship between HCCs and biliary atresia include some tumors that are found at autopsy or incidentally at the time of liver transplant for biliary atresia. Some have suggested a screening protocol for children with biliary atresia that includes a hepatic ultrasound every 6 mths, as well as AFP levels to check for development of HCC.

Clinical Presentation

The most common clinical presentation of HCC is that of an abdominal mass or pain. Other symptoms can include vomiting, anorexia, and weight loss. Greater than one-third of HCC involve multiple tumors rather than a single tumor. AFP elevation is noted in about 85% of patients and is only mildly elevated with the fibrolamellar variant. Both CT and MRI are useful in identifying the mass, as well as the relationship to the vascular supply.

Treatment

The treatment of HCC is surgical resection. Unfortunately, primary resection is often not possible due to the extensive involvement of the tumor in multiple sectors.[6] In addition in patients with cirrhosis, there is the potential that the resection may leave the child without sufficient residual functioning liver. Complete resection is only possible in approximately 10% of children. In the rare child who can undergo a complete resection with microscopic free margins, the prognosis includes survival of approximately 80%. The overall survival for all children with HCC is approximately 20% at 5 yrs as chemotherapy is relatively ineffective for this tumor. Clemoembolization has been utilized but has not been proven effective. Fibrolamellar histology is a favorable variant which occurs in adolescents and young adults. Although adults have a more favorable survivorship of approximately 50% at 5 yrs with the fibrolamellar variant, studies in children have not shown this to be a beneficial histology.

Liver Transplantation for Hepatocellular Carcinoma

In patients with unresectable tumors and lack of extrahepatic disease, liver transplantation can yield a good result. Extrahepatic spread and vascular invasion are two contraindications to liver transplantation. Various criteria have been used to determine eligibility for transplantation. The Milan criteria includes a single tumor with maximum diameter of less than 5 cm or with a maximum number of three tumors with the largest being less than 3 cm. The University of California San Francisco criteria allow a larger tumor of up to 6.5 cm as a single lesion and allows up to three separate tumors all being less than 4.5 cm. These criteria have found to be very useful in adults and are excellent predictors of low recurrence after transplantation, however they have not been validated in pediatric patients. A study of liver transplantation in children with HCC demonstrated a patient survival at 1, 5, and 10 yrs of 86%, 63%, and 58%, respectively. Some children have had a significant response to chemotherapy pretransplant, although at the time of transplant nearly all tumors still have viable tumor cells.

BENIGN HEPATIC TUMORS

Hemangioendothelioma

Infantile hemangioendothelioma is the most common benign hepatic tumor in children, generally presenting during the first few months of life. They may be asymptomatic but can also present with a large mass and abdominal distention. Occasionally these can lead to hepatomegaly and high output heart failure, as well as severe abdominal distention with subsequent respiratory distress. Hemangioendotheliomas can also develop a consumptive coagulopathy termed the Kasabach–Merritt Syndrome. They can have a very aggressive course with rapid growth.

Associated hemangiomas can be identified in the skin and lung. AFP can be elevated although this can be somewhat difficult to determine as AFP can normally be elevated up to 8 to 9 mths of age. Ultrasound evaluation is useful as an initial screen, however MRI is the most useful test to identify the location, as well as the flow characteristics.

Treatment

The natural history of these lesions is generally growth for the first 6–12 mths of life and they then frequently regress spontaneously. It should be noted that all of these patients should be screened for associated hypothyroidism. Patients with congestive heart failure require intervention with initial diuresis. If there is significant hemodynamic or respiratory compromise, treatment with steroids or interfereon alpha can utilized. Interfereon alpha has also been utilized in the presence of the Kasabach–Merritt Syndrome. Embolization may be useful if the lesion does not respond to initial medical therapy. Liver transplantation has also been utilized for extensive lesions causing heart failure in which there is inadequate response to medical management.

Mesenchymal Hamartoma

Mesenchymal hamartoma, although still very rare, is the third most common hepatic tumor and the second most common benign liver tumor. These can also be detected prenatally. They can be both solid and cystic in appearance and can occasionally cause cardiac failure in neonates. The clinical presentation in the older age child is frequently an abdominal mass. These lesions are typically large circumscribed tumors.

Treatment

Early surgical resection with a margin of normal liver is the optimal treatment. Resection is necessary as this has been reported to degenerate into an undifferentiated embryonal sarcoma.

Focal Nodular Hyerplasia

FNH is relatively rare in children and most are identified incidentally. These can be associated with other conditions including hemochromatosis, Klinefelter's syndrome and smoking. Oral contraceptive use is a significant risk factor in development of FNH. These lesions may be congenital vascular abnormalities and are characterized by a feeding artery with absence of bile ducts in the lesion. Most of these are asymptomatic but some can present with abdominal pain or anorexia and weight loss.

Diagnosis

CT findings are that of early enhancement of the lesion and the presence of a central scar. Use of hepatoiminodiacetic acid (HIDA) or sulfur colloid imaging can demonstrate increased vascularity with increased tumor uptake and a central cold area. A technetium 99M sulfur colloid scan can help to differentiate between FNH and hepatic adenoma with the colloid taken up by the Kupffer cells in most FNH lesions but not in hepatic adenomas.

Treatment

If the diagnosis is certain and the patient is asymptomatic they can be followed with serial ultrasounds to ensure that no progression occurs. Malignant transformation or association with malignancy is rare, but has been reported. If the diagnosis is uncertain a percutaneous biopsy can be considered. If the patient is symptomatic and there are lesions greater than 5 cm or if progression has occurred a biopsy or resection should be performed. A regression rate up to 40–50% have been reported.

Hepatic Adenoma

Hepatic adenoma is also a very rare lesion occurring most commonly in women in their 20's associated with use of oral contraceptives. In children they are usually asymptomatic and discovered as an incidental finding. The incidence of adenomas has increased significantly with increased use of oral contraceptives. These have also occurred in association with Fanconi's anemia, galactosemia, as well as use of anabolic steroids. They have also been reported in patients with type IA glycogen storage disease. HCC can occur in association with adenomas and thus these merit very careful follow-up.

Treatment

In patients on oral contraceptives or steroids, discontinuing the medication is the preferred management option. If a lesion has ruptured and the patient is stable, nonoperative management can be utilized. After the patient is stabilized, elective resection should be performed. In patients with ruptured adenomas with bleeding, hepatic arterial embolization should be performed with resection at a later date.

REFERENCES

1. Dabari A, Sabin KM, Shapiro CN, Schwarz KB. (2003) Epidemiology of primary hepatic malignancies in U.S. children. *Hepatology* **38**(3):560–566.
2. Aretz S, *et al.* (2006) Should children at risk for FAP be screened for HB and children with apparently sporadic HB be screened for APC germ line mutations? *Pediatr Blood Cancer* **47**(6):811–818.
3. Rana AN, *et al.* (2006) Successful treatment of multifocal unresectable hepatoblastoma with chemotherapy only. *Pediatr Hematol Oncol* **23**(2):153–158.
4. Perilongo G, Shafford E, Maibach R, *et al.* (2004) Risk-adapted treatment for childhood hepatoblastoma: final report of the second study of the international Society of Paediatric Oncology-SIOPEL 2. *Euro J Cancer* **40**:411–421.
5. Austin MT, *et al.* (2006) Liver transplantation for childhood hepatic malignancy: a review of the United Network for Organ Sharing (UNOS) database. *J Pediatr Surg* **41**:182–186.
6. Pawlik TM, *et al.* (2005) Tumor size predicts vascular invasion and histologic grade: Implications for selection of surgical treatment for hepatocellular carcinoma. *Liver Transpl* **11**(9):1086–1092.

GASTROINTESTINAL TUMORS

23

Alan P. Ladd

CLINICAL PRESENTATION

Recognizing the scarcity of primary gastrointestinal (GI) tumors within the alimentary tract, meaningful comments as to the natural presentation of these masses are limited. Clinical presentation of these tumors that arise anywhere from the level of the esophagus to the rectum is on either an incidental basis or based on symptoms related to the mass or mass-effect of the tumor. Tumors, then, may present as an incidental abdominal mass, as occult GI bleeding, or with signs of intestinal obstruction. A portion of these tumors may lead to intestinal obstruction by comprising the pathologic lead-point of an intussusception process. Site of origin of this heterogenic population of tumors plays as much a role in their presenting complaints, as the pathology involved with the tumor.

INCIDENCE/EPIDEMIOLOGY

Malignancy of the alimentary tract is quite rare in children and adolescents. Primary malignances of the GI tract account for as few as 1.2% of all pediatric cancers.[1] Including primary GI lymphomas in these estimates, this estimate may be as great as 5% of all childhood malignancies.[2] The average age for these malignances has been reported to be between 13.8–14.4 yrs of age.[3]

Based on a SEER database review of over 30 yrs, primary malignancies of the GI tract (excluding the colon) are derived from the stomach in 64%, the small bowel in 32% and the esophagus in 9%. In this review by Zhuge *et al.*, the annual incidence of pediatric foregut and small bowel solid tumors was approximately 0.027 cases per million in 2005. These tumors have a nearly equal distribution among carcinomas (43%) and sarcomas (46%), with neuroendocrine tumors comprising the remaining 11%.[3]

TUMOR PATHOPHYSIOLOGY

Non-Hodgkin's Lymphomas

Non-Hodgkin's lymphoma is the most common malignancy of the GI tract in children. These tumors, including Burkitt's lymphoma, currently comprise 50% of the reported GI malignancies.[4] Burkitt's lymphoma is the most common tumor of the small intestine and comprises the second most common malignancy of the colon, behind adenocarcinoma. Gastrointesinal lymphomas usually occur in the region of the terminal ileum and ileocecal valve; however, they may occur anywhere along the GI tract.[1,4] Presentation and impetus for evaluation often comes from the identification of an idiopathic, intraabdominal mass of apparent intestinal origin or from the presence of intestinal obstruction. Obstructive symptoms are either from their involvement in an intussusception process or from direct mass-effect. Surgical management of these lesions is directed at either complete resection or palliative intervention for relief of associated signs of obstruction.

Isolated gastric lymphomas in children are similar in apparent etiology to those noted in adults, with an association to *Helicobacter pylori* infection. The mucosa-associated lymphoid tissue lymphoma (MALToma) results from the malignant degeneration of the stomach wall mucosa, with rare cases of metastasis. Specific treatment for the MALToma relies on the focused treatment of the infectious *H. pylori* organism, with the use of systemic chemotherapy in the treatment of recurrent or metastatic disease.[5,6]

Colorectal Carcinoma

Colorectal carcinoma is the second-most common solid malignancy of the GI tract in children, behind primary liver malignancies. Though it is the most common GI malignancy in adults, only 1% of cases are noted in patients under 30 yrs of age.[8] However, this malignancy has been reported in children as young as 9 mths.[9] In contrast to notable survival rates of this malignancy in adults, its presence in children is usually fatal with 5-yr survival rates less than 12%. This poorer prognosis is believed to be related to the often advanced stage of disease at time of diagnosis. Greater than 60% of children with this malignancy will have evidence of metastasis to local lymph nodes and beyond.[10,11]

Though the majority of cases of colorectal adenocarcinomas in children occur sporadically, predisposing factors for this malignancy have been noted in up to 10% of patients in reported series. Predisposing conditions include the presence of familial polyposis and other polyposis syndromes, ulcerative colitis, familial cancer syndromes, and familial variants of colorectal cancer.[12]

As in the adult disease, surgical resection remains the mainstay of treatment for colorectal carcinoma in adolescent patients. Complete surgical excision along with the associated lymph node basins confers the best prognostic outcomes. The use of adjuvant chemotherapy in the treatment of metastatic colon cancer in children has not shown true success or benefit in the treatment of this malignancy, mostly related to the scarcity of cases treated by standard regimens and possibly related to the higher stage of disease at time of diagnosis. However, 5-fluorouracil and leucovorin-based chemotherapy regimens are routinely applied to the treatment of these children with metastatic disease.[4,10]

Gastrointestinal Stromal Tumor/Sarcoma

Defined as a distinct neoplasm since 1990, this tumor may have been previously defined within the categories of leiomyoblastoma or leiomyosarcoma, for lack of better distinction. Thus the true incidence for this tumor is unclear, but in adults, GISTs are the most common nonlymphoid mesenchymal tumors of the GI tract.[13] The occurrence of GIST tumors in children is quite rare, with their prevalence only noted cumulatively through review of case reports. Characteristics of these tumors in children include a predominance in girls (94%), a majority with occurrence in the stomach (88%) and often of a multifocal distribution. Unique to their presence in children, the prevalence of metastasis at time of diagnosis is over 50% in patients less than 18 yrs of age.[14]

Based upon their ultrastructural similarity, GIST tumors are felt to arise from interstitial cells of Cajal or their precursor cells, noting their shared expression of the KIT receptor tyrosine kinase. Histologically these tumors have an epithelioid predominant morphology or a mixed-cellular makeup with variable mitotic rates. Diagnosis is often made through immunohistochemical analysis for their strong staining for vimentin (CD-117) a *c-kit* proto-oncogene protein and CD-34, but not for smooth muscle actin.[13,15]

GISTs present as either an incidental abdominal mass, a diathesis of occult GI bleeding, or as an intestinal obstruction from mass-effect or possibly intussusception. These lesions most often occur within the wall of the GI tract, but may also be noted within the mesentery of the intestine or omentum. En bloc resection is the treatment of choice, as well as regional lymph node assessment for involvement and assessment of the liver for potential metastatic lesions. Postoperative assessment by way of CT and PET scans are used to evaluate for intraabdominal recurrence, which can occur within 24 mths of resection.[4] Those lesions with either residual disease following resection, unresectable lesions or potential resection that would lead to significant morbidity, or lesions with concurrent metastatic disease are often enrolled on adjuvant study protocols that utilize kinase inhibitors imatinib mesylate (Glevac®) or sunitinib (Sutent®).[14,16]

As noted the majority of tumors occur sporadically. Rarely these tumors may occur as a familial tumor of autosomal dominant inheritance. Concurrent association with neurofibromatosis type I has also been noted. Rare syndromic presentations occur in association with gastric leiomyosarcoma, extra-adrenal paraganglioma and pulmonary chondroma — Carney's Triad.[16]

Juvenile Polyps

Juvenile polyps are hamartomatous lesions the can occur in both children and adults with an overall mean age of presentation of 18 yrs. Polypoid processes often occur as single lesions and diffuse juvenile polyposes are rare. Presentation for either of these occurrences often involves concurrent anemia or findings of GI hemorrhage, prolapse or intussusceptions.[18] GI endoscopy is often the modality of diagnosis in cases not presenting with evidence of bowel obstruction, which often requires more immediate surgical intervention and direct diagnosis.

Though the occurrence of malignancy is rare for these lesions in children, reports in adolescents have noted the occasional presence of concurrent dysplasia within elements of the polypoid lesions.[19,20] The risk is amplified in patient with polyposis syndromes with an 18% to 35% risk of malignancy by 35 yrs, on average. A family history of polyposis or polypoid disease is often present in 50% of these children or adolescents.[4,21]

The treatment of the more common single or sparse polypoid involvement of the GI tract is endoscopic polypectomy or local intestinal resection. This intervention is often dictated by the technique of diagnosis of the anomaly. Those patients with diffuse juvenile polyposis will require both upper and lower endoscopic surveillance and polyp excision. Given the potential risk of malignancy for each polypoid lesion, treatment of significant polyposis often mirrors that of familial adenomatous polyposis syndrome with the use of prophylactic proctocolectomy and ileoanal reconstruction by the second or third decade of life.[4] Regardless of the timing of resectional therapy, surveillance must be maintained for the potential involvement of the foregut and small intestine in these individuals with extensive polyposis.

Gastrointestinal Carcinoid Tumors

Carcinoid tumors comprise 16% of alimentary tract malignancies and represent 0.1% of all pediatric cancer. Though more prevalent in the second decade of life, they have been reported in children as young as 3 yrs, with an observed female-to-male ratio of 3:1. Though carcinoid tumors are most prevalent in the appendix and small intestine, cases have been described in all portions of the GI tract from the stomach to the rectum.[1,22]

The diagnosis of these lesions is often made through their incidental occurrence in appendix specimens or within Meckel's diverticulum specimens. Cases may also present with clinical signs of hematochezia or occult anemia, from chronic GI blood loss, or vomiting associated with a small bowel obstruction from intussusception or local mass-effect.[22,23]

Few cases of malignant carcinoid tumors have been described in children. The great majority of tumors are benign, with only the occasional tumor showing evidence of local tumor invasion. Only rare anecdotal reports of metastatic disease to the liver, lung or bone, or of carcinoid syndrome, have been reported in children.[24]

The treatment for carcinoid tumors remains local resection. In cases where additional workup has shown no evidence for local extension or regional metastasis, no adjuvant treatment is needed. Verification of adequate margins of resection and thorough evaluation for local invasion through the serosal surface must be performed on each specimen. Evidence of full-thickness penetration of the intestinal wall or extension of tumor growth into the local mesentery must be followed with intestinal or colonic resection with associated mesenteric resection for eradication of locoregional disease, as well as abdominal surveillance for metastatic disease. Similar assessment is required for tumors exceeding 2 cm in size, as well as evaluations for distant metastasis to the liver, lung, and bone.[22]

A poor response is noted in the adjuvant treatment of metastatic disease with cytotoxic chemotherapy, similar to results seen in adults with metastatic disease. Occasional reports denote symptomatic relief of metastatic lesions through administration of octreotide.[22]

Inflammatory Myofibroblastic Tumors

Inflammatory myofibroblastic tumors of the GI tract originally were labeled as inflammatory pseudotumors. These tumors are defined histologically as a spindle cell proliferation with an inflammatory component of plasma cells, lymphocytes and occasional histiocytes. This tumor is differentiated from the histologic findings of sarcomas through noted cellular heterogeneity and absent mitosis.[25–27]

Similar to reports in adults depicting this tumor to occur in a variety of organs, especially the lung and throughout the body, the occurrence of these tumors in children remains mostly anecdotal. The greatest occurrence of these tumors within the GI tract lies in the stomach.[28] Nondescript abdominal pain is the most common symptom, with additional symptoms of dysphagia, intestinal obstruction, and chronic anemia also reported.

The management of these tumors lies in complete surgical excision. These tumors demonstrate a variety of biologic behaviors from local mass-effect without infiltration to locally infiltrative cases or the presence of distant metastases. Recurrence often only follows incomplete resection and ranges from 18% to 40%. The finding of an associated marker of anaplastic lymphoma kinase is often associated with an improved prognosis, when complete resection is successful. Adjuvant treatment for unresectable masses has often incorporated nonsteroidal and steroidal anti-inflammatory medications with variable success.[29,30]

REFERENCES

1. Bethel CAI, Bhattacharyya N, Hutchinson, *et al.* (1997) Alimentary tract malignancies in children. *J Pediatr Surg* **32**:1004–1009.
2. Pickett LK, Briggs HC. (1967) Cancer of the gastrointestinal tract in childhood. *Pediatr Clin North Am* **14**:223–234.
3. Zhuge Y, Cheung MC, Yang R, *et al.* (2009) Pediatric intestinal foregut and small bowel solid tumors: a review of 105 cases. *J Surg Res* **156**:95–102.
4. Ladd AP, Grosfeld JL. (2006) Gastrointestinal tumors in children and adolescents. *Semin Pediatr Surg* **15**:37–47.
5. Wu TC, Chen LK, Lai CR. (2001) Primary gastric lymphoma associated with Helicobacter pylori in a child. *J Pediatr Gastroent Nutr* **32**:608–610.
6. Horstmann M, Ertmann R, Winkler K. (1994) Relapse of MALT lymphoma associated with Helicobacter pylori after antibiotic treatment. *Lancet* **343**:1098–1099.
7. Rao BN, Pratt CB, Fleming ID, *et al.* (1985) Colon carcinoma in children and adolescents. A review of 30 cases. *Cancer* **55**:1322–1326.
8. Hardin WJ. (1972) Unusual manifestations of malignant disease of the large intestine. *Surg Clin North Am* **52**:287–297.
9. Kern WH, White WC. (1958) Adenocarcinoma of the colon in a nine-month-old infant. *Cancer* **1**:855–857.
10. Karnak I, Ciftci AO, Senocak ME, Buyukpamukcu N. (1999) Colorectal carcinoma in children. *J Pediatr Surg* **34**:1499–1504.
11. Shahrudin MD, Noori SM. (1997) Cancer of the colon and rectum in the first three decades of life. *Hepato-Gastroent* **44**:441–444.
12. O'Neill JA. (1986) Colorectal tumors. In: KJ Welch, JG Randolph, MM Ravitch, *et al.* (eds.), *Pediatric Surgery*, pp. 1020–1022. Year Book Medical Publishers, Chicago, IL.
13. Haider N, Kader M, McDermott M, *et al.* (2004) Gastric stromal tumors in children. *Pediatr Blood Cancer* **42**:186–189.
14. Prakash S, Sarran L, Socci N, *et al.* (2005) Gastrointestinal stromal tumors in children and young adults. *J Pediatr Hematol Oncol* **27**:179–187.
15. Trupiano JK, Stewart RE, Misick C, *et al.* (2002) Gastric stromal tumours. *Am J Surg Pathol* **26**:705–714.
16. Pappo AS, Janeway KA. (2009) Pediatric gastrointestinal stromal tumors. *Hematol Oncol Clin N Am* **23**:15–34.
17. Cobern MC, Pricolo VE, Deluca FG, Bland KI. (1995) Malignant potential in intestinal juvenile polyposis syndromes. *Ann Surg Oncol* **2**:386–391.
18. Sachatello CR, Hahn IS, Carrington CB. (1974) Juvenile gastrointestinal polyposis in a female infant: Report of a case and review of the literature of a recently recognized syndrome. *Surgery* **75**:107–114.

19. Desai DC, Neale KF, Talbot IC, *et al.* (1995) Juvenile polyposis. *Brit J Surg* **82**:14–17.
20. Liu TH, Chen MC, Tseng HC. (1978) Malignant change of juvenile polyp of colon. A case report. *Chin Med J* **4**:434–439.
21. Howe JR, Mitros FA, Summers RW. (1998) The risk of gastrointestinal carcinoma in familial juvenile polyposis. *Ann Surg Oncol* **5**:751–756.
22. Spunt, SL, Pratt CB, Rao BN, *et al.* (2000) Childhood carcinoid tumors: The St. Jude children's research hospital experience. *J Pediatr Surg* **35**:1282–1286.
23. Goldthorn JF, Canizaro PC. (1986) Gastrointestinal malignancies in infancy, childhood, and adolescence. *Surg Clin North Am* **66**:845–861.
24. Chow CW, Sane S, Campbell PE, Carter RF. (1982) Malignant carcinoid tumors in children. *Cancer* **49**:802–811.
25. Curtis JL, Burns RC, Wang L, Mahour GH, Ford HR. (2008) Primary gastric tumors of infancy and childhood: 54-year experience at a single institution. *J Pediatr Surg* **43**:1487–1493.
26. Karnak I, Senocak ME, Ciftci AO, *et al.* (2001) Inflammatory myofibroblastic tumor in children: Diagnosis and treatment. *J Pediatr Surg* **36**:908–912.
27. Kovach SJ, Fiacher AC, Katzman PJ, *et al.* (2006) Inflammatory myofibroblastic tumors. *J Surg Oncol* **94**:385–391.
28. Riedel DB, Wong RC, Ey EH. (1996) Gastric inflammatory myofibroblastic tumor(inflammatory pseudotumor) in infancy: Case report and review of the literature. *J Pediatr Gastroenterol Nutr* **2**:437–443.
29. Williams E, Longmaid HE, Trey G, *et al.* (1998) Renal failure resulting from infiltration by inflammatory myofibroblastic tumor responsive to corticosteroid therapy. *Am J Kidney Dis* **31**:E5.
30. Chun YS, Wang L, Nascimento AF, *et al.* (2005). Pediatric inflammatory myofibroblastic tumor: Anaplastic lymphoma kinase (ALD) expression and prognosis. *Pediatr Blood Cancer* **45**:796–801.

TESTICULAR TUMORS 24

Deborah F. Billmire

INTRODUCTION

Testicular tumors are rare in children and have an incidence of approximately 0.5–2.0 per 100,000.[1] Although there has been an increase in the incidence of testicular tumors in adult males in recent years, the incidence in children has remained stable according to the Surveillance, Epidemiology and End Results (SEER) program of the National Cancer Institute.[2] The development of the Prepubertal Testis Tumor Registry by the urologic section of the American Academy of Pediatrics (AAP) in 1980 has been instrumental in providing a helpful database to study these rare tumors.[3] This work has led to the recognition that testis tumors in prepubertal boys have a different pathology distribution, clinical behavior and management strategy compared to adults.

CLINICAL PRESENTATION

Testicular tumors are seen throughout childhood and classically present as a painless scrotal mass. The most important physical feature is the finding of asymmetry on scrotal examination. Scrotal asymmetry should always be evaluated and most differential diagnoses can be discriminated by careful physical examination. The most common causes of asymmetry are inguinal hernia and hydrocele. These are easily distinguished in most cases. It should be noted that 7–22% of testicular tumors have an accompanying hydrocele and are occasionally discovered unexpectedly during routine hydrocele repair.[4,5] This lack of preoperative diagnosis can be avoided by careful preoperative physical examination. If a large tense hydrocele prevents distinct palpation of the testis on exam, transillumination to define the testis size and the possibility of testicular ultrasound should be considered preoperatively.

The majority of true scrotal masses arise in the testis. In a retrospective series of boys 1 to 16 yrs of age with scrotal masses by Aragona *et al.*, 86% arose from the testis and 14% were paratesticular.[6] In this series, only 46% of the scrotal masses were due to testicular neoplasia with the remaining testicular lesions due to congenital malformations or torsion. The testes should be symmetric in size and little growth occurs prior to puberty. Nonsurgical causes of testicular enlargement include McCune–Albright syndrome, Fragile X syndrome, Beckwith Weidemann syndrome, sarcoidosis, and idiopathic benign macro-orchidism.[7,8,9] In most cases of benign testicular hypertrophy, the condition is bilateral, but unilateral or asynchronous presentation may raise concern regarding a tumor.[7] The finding of a testicular mass should also prompt a careful general physical examination with review of systems, assessment of pubertal status, and attention to the regional lymph nodes for enlargement.

PATHOPHYSIOLOGY

Testis tumors are generally considered in two categories based on age. Prepubertal boys are more likely to have benign tumors and have been studied extensively.[10,11] Most tumors in this age group are seen within the first 3 yrs of life. The prepubertal testis tumor registry developed in 1980 by the pediatric urology section of the AAP has provided a large body of data on incidence and behavior of these tumors.[12] Adolescents have not been given adequate attention and are often presumed to follow adult patterns of incidence and tumor behavior although little specific data is available to support this view. The risk of malignancy is markedly increased in adolescents compared to prepubertal boys with one series from Finland reporting benign tumors in 77% of prepubertal patients and only 38% of adolescents.[13]

The testis is formed from three primordial cell lines.[14] Each of these cell lines gives rise to a different spectrum of tumors within the testis and has characteristic features, clinical behavior, and age range.

Epithelial Tumors

The celomic epithelium is the origin of the seminiferous tubules, rete testis, sertoli cells, and tunica. This cell line provides the origin for epididymal cysts and sertoli cell tumors. Sertoli cell tumors are seen at a mean age of 52.5 mths in prepubertal boys and may be associated with gynecomastia.[15,16] They usually behave in a benign fashion although malignancy may occur in rare cases. Sertoli cell tumor in adults has a malignancy rate of approximately 10%.

Mesenchymal Tumors

The mesenchyme is the origin of the Leydig cells and is the cell of origin for Leydig cell tumors. These tumors secrete 17 ketosteroids and may be associated with precocious puberty or gynecomastia. They occur with a mean age of 70 mths in prepubertal boys and behave in a benign fashion.[15] In adult males, Leydig tumors have a 10% malignancy rate. Juvenile granulosa cell tumors also arise from the mesenchyme and are seen in prepubertal boys in early infancy with mean age of 1.5 mths.[17] They also behave in a benign fashion.

Undifferentiated stromal tumors occur in a small number of prepubertal boys. In eight mixed or undifferentiated stromal tumors in the pediatric prepubertal testis tumor registry, five exhibited malignant features.[15]

Germ Cell Tumors

The primary germ cells are the origin of the spermatogonia. Tumors of germ cells include teratoma, germinoma, choriocarcinoma, yolk sac tumor, and embryonal carcinoma. Mixed tumors containing more than one of these germ cell types may also be seen. The distribution of the various histologic cell types varies by age and there are two distinct age peaks, one in infancy and one in adolescence.

Prior to puberty, benign teratoma is most common and accounts for 48% of testis tumors.[18] The malignant germ cell tumors of the testis prior to puberty are almost all yolk sac histology.

Teratoma in postpubertal boys is considered to have malignant potential similar to adults. In adults, testicular teratoma is known to have the potential for metastatic spread. The finding of intratubular germ cell neoplasia (ITGCN), also called carcinoma in situ of the testis (CIS), is common in adult teratoma and other germ cell tumors. These cells are felt to be the precursors of germ cell tumors in the testis and are not seen prior to puberty. They are felt to be hormonally sensitive and replicate in response to raised sex hormone levels after puberty.[19] As a consequence, orchiectomy is recommended for postpubertal boys with testicular teratoma.[12,20] Adolescents are more likely to have mixed tumors and embryonal carcinoma is a frequent component.[21]

Some germ cell tumor subtypes secrete serum markers that may be helpful in diagnosis and in follow-up for evidence of recurrence. Tumors with yolk sac histology secrete alpha fetoprotein (AFP). AFP is also secreted by the fetal liver and serum levels are more difficult to interpret in the first year of life. Tumors with choriocarcinoma secrete beta human chorionogonadotrophin (βHCG) and may be associated with precocious puberty.

The scrotum may also be the site of a paratesticular tumor arising from either normal or ectopic tissue such as rhabdomyosarcoma, neuroblastoma or extra-renal Wilms' tumor.[22,23] Generalized infiltration of the testis from leukemia may also occur.[24]

DIAGNOSIS

Initial history and physical examination should include attention to potential causes of testicular enlargement that are not due to neoplasia. General health status, evidence of precocious puberty and developmental or learning difficulties should particularly be sought. Testicular hypertrophy is associated with Fragile X syndrome and Beckwith Weidemann Syndrome. In McCune–Albright syndrome, peripheral precocious puberty is usually present with the testicular hypertrophy.

Scrotal ultrasound is the primary imaging modality for evaluation of the scrotal mass and will direct the subsequent imaging and serological work-up (Figures 1 and 2). The finding of testicular enlargement with normal echogenicity is seen in benign hypertrophy. Boys with McCune–Albright syndrome may have testicular microlithiasis.

Unlike adults, all abnormal echo patterns may be seen in both benign and malignant pathologies. Decreased echogenicity may be seen with orchitis, granuloma, hematoma, and malignant infiltration (most often due to leukemia). Mixed echogenicity occurs in both malignant tumors and hematocele. A diffuse, uniform hyper-echoic pattern may be seen with teratoma.

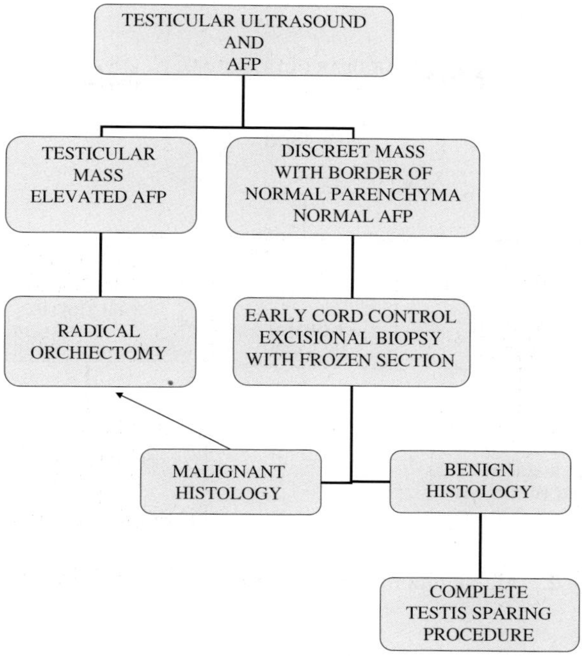

Figure 1. Management algorithm for prepubertal testis tumors, Adapted from Metcalfe.[11]

Confirmation of an abnormal pattern of testicular echogenicity should lead to determination of serum AFP and βHCG to evaluate for germ cell tumors. Determination of testosterone and androstenediol is needed for Leydig cell tumors. Luteinizing hormone (LH) and follicle-stimulating hormone (FSH) are normal or low with Leydig cell tumors in contrast to true precocious puberty where these are elevated and are the stimulus for testosterone secretion.

The confirmation of a testicular tumor by ultrasound should also lead to a preoperative Computed Tomography (CT) scan of the abdomen and pelvis to evaluate the retroperitoneum for lymph node enlargement.

SURGICAL MANAGEMENT

Testicular tumors should always be approached from an inguinal incision with early vascular control. In prepubertal boys with normal serum markers

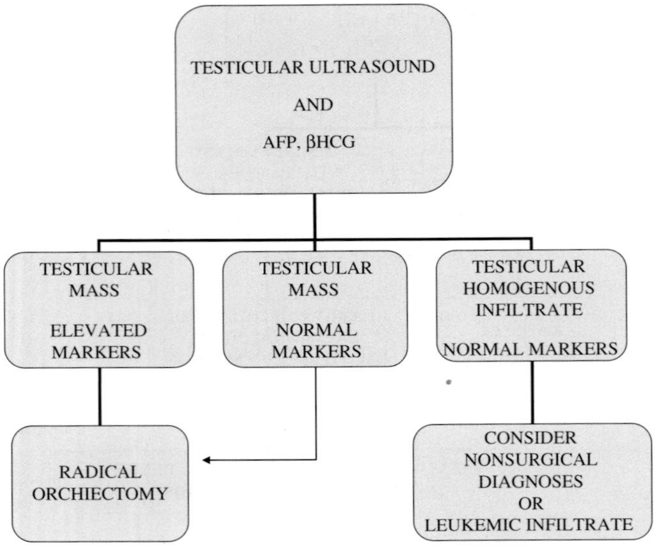

Figure 2. Management algorithm for postpubertal testis tumors.

and a focal lesion on ultrasound, simple enucleation of the tumor may be considered. In all postpubertal boys and in prepubertal boys with elevated serum markers or diffuse involvement of the testis, radical orchiectomy is required.

A standard incision overlying the inguinal canal is made. The external ring is opened to expose the entire inguinal canal. The cremaster fibers are separated and the cord components are identified at the level of the internal ring. The vessels are occluded with a noncrushing clamp. The testis is then mobilized from the scrotum for inspection. For large tumors, the incision may need to be extended down in a hockey stick configuration onto the upper scrotum. The tunica vaginalis is opened and the confirmation of a testis tumor then proceeds with either orchiectomy or enucleation as planned. For cases of enucleation, the tumor capsule should not be violated in situ and frozen section to confirm a benign lesion should be done. For radical orchiectomy, the vessels and vas deferens should be ligated at the internal ring. If the preoperative CT scan shows normal inguinal and iliac nodes, no biopsy is required. If the nodes are borderline enlarged (2–4 cm), a biopsy will be required for staging. If there is obvious pathologic adenopathy, no biopsy is required. It is preferable to obtain the

CT prior to orchiectomy since there may be some reactive adenopathy related to the procedure which will impact on lymph node size.

In boys with a known diagnosis of leukemia in whom testicular relapse is suspected and tissue confirmation is desired, a trans-scrotal biopsy is acceptable.[24] In all cases of suspected primary testis neoplasia or uncertain diagnosis, an inguinal approach is required. Trans-scrotal biopsy is known to predispose to local relapse for certain tumor types and will upstage a tumor and increase chemotherapy requirements.[5]

Retroperitoneal lymph node dissection (RPLND) is not recommended for prepubertal testis tumors.[12,25] Adolescents are often treated with adult management algorhythms and may be recommended to have RPLND depending on local institution preference. The dissection should be undertaken using a nerve sparing technique to reduce the risk of retrograde ejaculation.[21]

CHEMOTHERAPY

The Children's Oncology Group uses a simplified staging system as shown in Figure 3. In adults, a more detailed staging system is employed that was

Stage I

Limited to testis, completely resected by high inguinal orchiectomy; no clinical, radiologic, or histologic evidence of disease beyond the testis; tumor markers normal after resection.

StageII

Trans-scrotal orchiectomy; microscopic disease in scrotum or high in spermatic cord; retroperitoneal node involvement (< 2 cm)and /or increased tumor markers after resection.

StageII

Gross residual disease, retroperitoneal lymph node involvement (> 2 cm), or malignant cells in pleural or peritoneal fluid.

Stage IV

Distant metastases involving lung, liver, brain, bone, distant nodes, or other sites.

Figure 3. Children's Oncology Group staging system for malignant germ cell tumors of the testis.[29]

developed by the International Germ Cell Cancer Collaborative Group (IGCCC) with further stratification into good, intermediate and poor risk groups.

Stage I Germ Cell Tumors

For boys less than 15 yrs of age, radical orchiectomy is undertaken with close follow-up. Evaluation for metastatic disease is done at diagnosis and tumor markers and imaging are followed closely. Failure of tumor markers to normalize is suggestive of persistent occult disease and a rise in tumor markers or evidence of new mass on imaging is suggestive of recurrence. In the intergroup study by the Children's Cancer Study Group and the Pediatric Oncology Group reported in 2003, this regimen resulted in an overall survival of 100%.[5] These boys were all less than 10 yrs of age and all malignant tumors had yolk sac histology providing a useful serum marker for recurrence. Thirteen of sixty three patients had recurrence, but all were salvaged with chemotherapy. This approach allowed almost 80% of boys to be spared chemotherapy. Similar results have been seen in series from England, Germany, and Italy.[25–28]

Stage II–IV Germ Cell Tumors

Chemotherapy is indicated for malignant germ cell tumors stage II and above. Platinum based regimens are employed with the addition of etoposide and bleomycin. The intergroup study by the Children's Cancer Study Group and the Pediatric Oncology Group for stage III to IV malignant germ cell tumors of the testis included 44 boys who presented with advanced disease. The majority of the boys were older than 13 yrs and most had mixed germ cell tumors. Surgical management recommended radical orchiectomy at diagnosis with second look surgery for residual masses. The overall survival was 93.3%.[29]

LONG-TERM FOLLOW-UP

Patients with testicular tumors are at risk for metachronous contralateral tumor. Long-term follow-up with periodic ultrasound in addition to physical examination is recommended to detect tumors at an early stage.[19]

REFERENCES

1. Coppes M, Rackley R, Kay R. (1994) Primary testicular and paratesticular tumors of childhood. *Med Pediatr Oncol* **22**:329–340.
2. Walsh TJ, Grady RW, Porter MP, Lin DW, Weiss NS. (2006) Incidence of testicular germ cell cancers in U.S. children: Seer program experience 1973 to 2000. *J Urol* **68**(2):402–405.
3. Ross JH. (2009) Prepubertal testicular tumors. *J Urol* **74**(1):94–99.
4. Ciftci AO, Bingol-Kologlu M, Senocak ME, Tanyel FC, Buyukpamukcu M, Buyukpamakcu N. (2001) Testicular tumors in children. *J Pediatr Surg* **36**(12): 1796–1801.
5. Schlatter M, Rescorla F, Giller R, Cushing B, Vinocur C, Colombani P, Cullen J, London W, Davis M, Lauer S, Olson T. (2003) Excellent outcome in patients with stage I germ cell tumors of the testes: a study of the children's cancer group/pediatric oncology group. *J Pediatr Surg* **38**(3):319–324.
6. Aragona F, Pescatori E, Talenti E, Toma P, Malena S, Passerini Glazel G. (1996) Painless scrotal masses in the pediatric population: Prevalence and age distribution of different pathological conditions — A 10-year retrospective multicenter study. *J Urol* **155**:1424–1426.
7. Wasniewska M, Matarazzo P, Weber G, Russo G, Zampolli M, Salzano G, Zirilli G, Bertelloni S. (2006) Clinical presentation of McCune–Albright syndrome in males. *J Pediatr Endocrinol Metab* **19**(2):619–622.
8. Evans S. (1997) Sarcoidosis presenting as bilateral testicular masses. *Pediatr* **100**(3):392–394.
9. Samarakkody UKS, Bruce J, Morris P, Chow CW, Woodward AA. (1993) Idiopathic unilateral benign macro-orchidism. *Pediatr Surg Int* **8**:175–176.
10. Grady RW. (2000) Current management of prepubertal yolk sac tumors of the testis. *Pediatr Urol Oncol* **27**(3):503–508.
11. Metcalfe PD, Farivar-Mohseni H, Farhat W, McLorie G, Khoury A, Bagli DJ. (2003) Pediatric testicular tumors: Contemporary incidence and efficacy of testicular preserving surgery. *J Urol* **170**:2412–2416.
12. Ross FH, Rybicki L, Kay R. (2002) Testis tumors, cryptorchidism, varicocele. *J Urol* **168**:1675–1679.
13. Taskinen S, Fagerholm R, Aronniemi J, Rintala R, Taskinen M. (2008) Testicular tumors in children and adolescents. *J Pediatr Urol* **4**(2):134–137.
14. Skandalakis JE, Gray SW, Parrott TS, Ricketts RR. (1994) The embryological basis for the treatment of congenital anomalies. In: JE Skandalkis, SW Gray (eds.), *Embryology for Surgeons*, pp. 736–772. Williams & Wilkins.

15. Thomas JC, Ross JH, Kay R. (2001) Stromal testis tumors in children: A report from the prepubertal testis tumor registry. *J Urol* **166**:2338–2340.
16. Talon I, Moog R, Kauffmann I, Grandadam S, Becmeur F. (2005) Sertoli cell tumor of the testis in children, reevaluation of a rarely encountered tumor. *J Pediatr Hematol Oncol* **27**(9):491–493.
17. Shukla AR, Huff DS, Canning DA, Filmer RB, Snyder HM, Carpintieri D, Carr MC. (2004) Juvenile granulosa cell tumor of the testis: Contemporary clinical management and pathological diagnosis. *J Urol* **171**:1900–1902.
18. Pohl HG, Shukla AR, Metcalf PD, Cilento BG, Retik AB, Bagli DJ, Huff DS, Rushton HG. (2004) Prepubertal testis tumors: Actual prevalence rate of histological types. *J Urol* **172**:2370–2372.
19. Dieckmann KP, Skakkebaek NE. (1999) Carcinoma in situ of the testis: Review of biological and clinical features. *Int J Cancer* **83**:815–822.
20. Walsh C, Rushton H. (2000) Diagnosis and management of teratomas and epidermoid cysts. *J Pediatr Hematol Oncol* **27**(3):509–517.
21. Terenziani M, Piva L, Spreafico F, Salvioni R, Massimino M, Luksch R, Cefalo G, Casanova M, Ferrari A, Polastri D, Mazza E, Bellani FF, Nicolai N. (2002) Clinical stage I nonseminomatous germ cell tumors of the testis in childhood and adolescence: An analysis of 31 cases. *Pediatr Hematol Oncol* **24**(6):454–458.
22. Encinas A, Matute JA, Gomez A, Castellano VM, Cuadros J, Berchi FJ. (1997) Primary neuroblastoma presenting as a paratesticular tumor. *J Pediatr Surg* **32**(4):624–626.
23. Arkovitz MS, Ginsburg HB, Eidelman J, Greco MA, Rauson A. (1996) Primary extrarenal Wilms' tumor in the inguinal canal: Case report and review of the literature. *J Pediatr Surg* **31**(7):957–959.
24. Agarwal PK, Palmer JS. (2006) Testicular and paratesticular neoplasms in prepubertal males. *J Urol* **176**(3):875–881.
25. Mann JR, Raafat F, Robinson K, Imeson J, Gornall P, Sokal M, Gray E, McKeever P, Hale J, Bailey S, Oakhill A. (2000) The united kingdom children's cancer study group's second germ cell tumor study: Carboplatin, etoposide, and bleomycin are effective treatment for children with malignant extracranial germ cell tumors, with acceptable toxicity. *J Clin Oncol* **22**(15):3809–3818.
26. Haas RJ, Schmidt P, Gobel U, Harms D. (1994) Treatment of malignant testicular tumors in childhood: Results of the german national study 1982–1992. *Med Pediatr Oncol* **23**:400–405.
27. Haas RJ, Schmidt P, Gobel U, Harris D. (1999) Testicular germ cell tumors, an update. Results of the german cooperative studies 1982–1997. *Klin Padiatr* **211**(4):300–304.

28. LoCurto M, Lumia F, Alaggio R, Cecchetto G, Almasio P, Indolfi P, Siracusa F, Bagnulo S, DeBernardi B, DeLaurentis, T, DiCataldo A, Tamaro P. (2003) Malignant germ cell tumors in childhood: Results of the first Italian cooperative study "TCG 91". *Med Pediatr Oncol* **41**:417–425.
29. Cushing B, Giller R, Cullen JW, Marina NM, Lauer SJ, Olson TA, Rogers PC, Colombani P, Rescorla F, Billmire DF, Vinocur CD, Hawkins EP, Davis MM, Perlman EJ, London WB, Castleberry RP. (2004) Randomized comparison of combination chemotherapy with etoposide, bleomycin, and either high-dose or standard-dose cisplatin in children and adolescents with high-risk malignant germ cell tumors: A pediatric intergroup study — Pediatric Oncology Group 9049 and Children's Cancer Group 8882. *J Clin Oncol* **22**(13):2691–2700.

OVARIAN TUMORS 25

Deborah Billmire

INTRODUCTION

Ovarian masses are uncommon in the pediatric age group. Approximately 50–65% are true neoplasms[1,2] and the remainder are nonneoplastic cysts of follicular or paratubal origin. In the neonate, follicular cysts account for virtually all ovarian masses and the majority are managed nonoperatively. Beyond the neonatal period, nonneoplastic cysts account for approximately 50% of ovarian masses and most of these are managed nonoperatively as well. Ultrasound can distinguish nonneoplastic cysts from true neoplasm in most cases and serial studies are useful for monitoring. Nonneoplastic cysts will not be further discussed in this chapter.

The risk of malignancy in pediatric ovarian neoplasm is approximately 20% and surgical approach should always be undertaken with concern for malignancy in mind. Some series report malignancy rates as high as 30% to 55%.[3]

The vast majority of malignant ovarian tumors in children should be managed with fertility preserving surgery. Total hysterectomy with bilateral oophorectomy should rarely occur. The role of the surgeon should emphasize conservative resection and careful staging at diagnosis. Unlike adult women in whom epithelial tumors with poor prognosis are predominant, the majority of malignant ovarian tumors in children and adolescents are of germ cell origin and are successfully treated with limited surgery and chemotherapy. In the past, adult staging guidelines for ovarian tumors were applied to girls without evidence based data. More recently, guidelines for malignant germ cell tumors of the ovary in girls have been provided based on data from a cooperative study by the Pediatric Oncology Group and Children's Cancer Study Group.[4] Specific guidelines for the rare malignant epithelial based ovarian neoplasms in children and adolescents are lacking.

CLINICAL PRESENTATION

The presentation of ovarian tumors is quite variable and is dependent on the size of the tumor and whether hormone secretion is present. Tumors that secrete estradiol may cause pseudo-precocious puberty in young girls. This generally includes both breast bud enlargement and vaginal bleeding. Usually a palpable mass is also present. Rupture may occur and cause an acute abdomen with generalized peritoneal signs.

Pain from an ovarian neoplasm may be chronic and low grade due to mass effect, or acute and severe secondary to torsion. Most large tumors have some degree of chronic torsion at laparotomy but do not cause severe pain or ischemia. Urinary symptoms may also occur with urgency and frequency due to bladder compression. Constipation is seen less commonly. A gradual increase in abdominal girth without other symptoms may also be seen. In most series of pediatric ovarian tumors, approximately 11% present with an acute abdomen due to torsion.[4,5] That creates a situation in which surgical management must occur without the benefit of known marker status preoperatively.

PATHOPHYSIOLOGY

The ovary is formed from three primordial cell lines.[6] Each of these cell lines gives rise to a different spectrum of tumors and has characteristic features and clinical behavior (Table 1).

Germ Cell Tumors

The primary germ cells are the origin for the majority of ovarian tumors in children and adolescents. They account for 67% to 89%[1,2] of all neoplastic ovarian masses. Teratomas are the benign germ cell tumors and they are derived from all three cell layers including endoderm, mesoderm and ectoderm. They may have mature tissue only or contain a mixture of mature

Table 1. Overview of ovarian tumor histology in children.

Cell of origin	Benign	Uncertain	Malignant
Epithelial tumors	Mucinous cystadenoma Serous cystadenoma	Borderline mucinous cystadenoma Borderline serous cystadenoma	Adenocarcinoma
Sex cord stromal tumors	Fibroma Thecoma Gonadoblastoma		Juvenile granulosa cell tumor Sertoli–leydig cell tumor Gonadoblastoma with germ cell malignancy
Germ cell tumors	Mature teratoma Immature teratoma	High grade immature teratoma	Yolk sac tumor Choriocarcinoma Germinoma Embryonal carcinoma

and immature tissues. They may have associated glial implants that are termed "gliomatosis peritonei". These implants are composed of low grade immature glial tissue and should not be confused with malignant peritoneal implants. Malignant germ cell tumors follow a variety of pathways in differentiation from the totipotential primitive germ cell (Figure 1). The most common histology is the yolk sac tumor which secretes alpha fetoprotein (AFP). Other histologies include germinoma (also called dysgerminoma), choriocarcinoma which secretes beta human chorionogonadotrophin (βHCG) and embryonal carcinoma. Ovarian germ cell tumors often contain a mixture of benign and malignant elements. Size and appearance on imaging are not helpful in distinguishing benign from malignant tumors.

Epithelial Tumors

The celomic epithelium is the cell of origin for the spectrum of epithelial tumors. This group accounts for approximately 13–19%[1] of ovarian neoplasms in children and adolescents. CA-125 is occasionally elevated in girls with epithelial tumors but is not a consistent marker.[1,7,8] These tumors tend

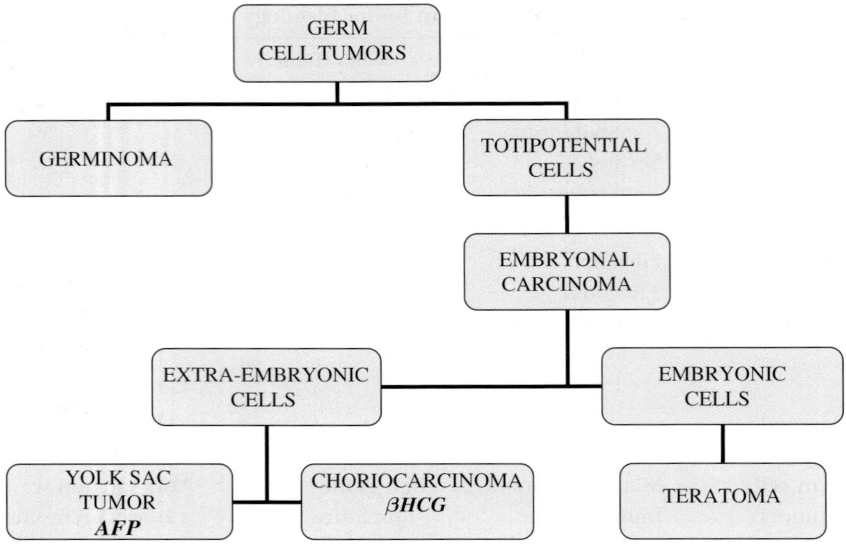

Figure 1. Differentiation pathways for ovarian germ cell tumors.

to occur more often after puberty but can also be seen in younger girls.[9,10] There are two general categories of epithelial tumors, serous and mucinous tumors. Bilateral tumors occur in 11–21% of cases.[1,11] These tumors may be benign, "borderline" or overtly malignant. Benign tumors are most common and account for 70–80% of the epithelial tumors. In some reported series, mucinous tumors predominate[7] and in other series serous tumors are more common.[11] Borderline tumors have a variable degree of nuclear atypia but lack stromal invasion[12] and are also called "tumors of low malignant potential". In some pediatric series they are grouped with malignant ovarian tumors. In both the pediatric age group and in adults, these tend to be large tumors with low stage at laparotomy. Malignant epithelial ovarian tumors in children are exceedingly rare and are adenocarcinomas similar in histology to those seen in adults.

Mesenchymal Tumors

The mesenchyme is the cell of origin for sex cord and stromal tumors. These are the least common ovarian neoplasms in childhood and tend to occur in prepubertal patients. The benign variants include fibroma, thecoma, and gonadoblastoma. Fibromas can be seen in association with basal cell nevus syndrome. They may be calcified and bilateral.[13] Thecomas produce estrogen or androgens and may present with pseudo-precocious puberty. After menarche they may present with hirsutism and irregular menses. Gonadoblastomas occur in patients with gonadal dysgenesis. They contain both stromal and germ cell elements. Karyotypes include 46XY and mosaic 45X/46XY. Bilateral gonadoblastomas are found in 40% to 75% of patients.[14]

The malignant variants of the sex cord and stromal tumors are the granulosa cell and Sertoli–Leydig tumors. Although local invasion and metastasis are seen in some adult granulosa cell tumors, these tumors generally behave in a localized fashion in children and adolescents. Juvenile granulosa cell tumors comprise 1–20% of ovarian carcinoma in the pediatric and adolescent age groups. They secrete estradiol and may present with pseudo-precocious puberty or with menstrual irregularity after menarche. Abdominal distention or a palpable mass may be noted. Sertoli–Leydig tumors are also called arrhenoblastoma. They secrete testosterone metabolites and present with symptoms of androgen excess in about 40% of cases.[12]

DIAGNOSIS

Initial history and physical examination should include attention to signs of precocious puberty or alteration of menses. If palpable, the mass may tend to sit in the midline if it has grown large enough to rise above the pelvic brim. It may be mobile on abdominal or rectal examination. Auscultation of the lungs may reveal diminished breath sounds at the bases if pleural effusion is present.

In young children, signs of precocious puberty may lead to the finding of an ovarian mass. Girls with McCune Albright syndrome may present with the acute onset of painless vaginal bleeding. These girls have autonomous, estrogen producing ovarian cysts. The cysts are most often unilateral and unilocular. They may be accompanied by uterine enlargement. These are not true neoplastic cysts but transient functional cysts that will resolve spontaneously with time. Surgical intervention is not indicated. In these girls, vaginal bleeding is often the initial presentation of the syndrome. The triad of findings for McCune Albright syndrome consists of precocious puberty, café au lait spots and fibrous dysplasia of bone. Not all features may be present at diagnosis. Serum AFP and βHCG are normal but estradiol is elevated. These children may be mistakenly diagnosed with juvenile granulosa cell tumor if McCune Albright syndrome is not considered. Juvenile granulosa tumors occasionally present in prepubertal girls and also have an elevated estradiol level. They are more likely to present with a mass and abdominal pain than with isolated vaginal bleeding. Girls presenting with apparent precocious puberty should undergo endocrine consultation prior to any surgical procedure to avoid unnecessary surgical resection.[15] If there is some uncertainty in diagnosis, a short period of observation with repeat ultrasound and estradiol levels may be helpful in distinguishing these entities.

Ultrasound is the cornerstone of imaging for girls with suspected ovarian masses. Simple cysts, hemorrhagic cysts and flow to the ovary can all be assessed. For those girls felt to have a true ovarian neoplasm, Computed Tomography (CT) scan should also be obtained. This will allow better definition of the retroperitoneal nodes as well as any suspicious areas of possible metastasis to the liver or other regions of the peritoneal cavity that will require special attention at laparotomy.

Serum markers should be obtained to include AFP and βHCG. Measurement of CA-125 is seldom helpful and can be reserved for those children found to have the occasional borderline or malignant epithelial neoplasm on pathology.

SURGICAL MANAGEMENT

All pediatric ovarian neoplasms should be approached with the possibility of a malignant tumor in mind. The staging classifications for the Children's Oncology Group (Figure 2) and the adult Federation Internationale de Gynecologie et d'Obstetrique (FIGO)/American Joint Committee on Cancer (AJCC) (Figure 3) are as shown. Preoperative elevation of AFP or βHCG will confirm the presence of some malignant germ cell element. Tumors with only germinoma or embryonal carcinoma will not have elevated markers. In some cases, neuron specific enolase will be elevated with germinoma[16] but this is an inconsistent finding. The finding of a cystic component on imaging is also not a reassuring finding since at least 57% of malignant pediatric ovarian tumors have a cystic component.[4]

An algorithm for operative approach is outlined in Figure 4. On initial exploration, fluid should be obtained for cytology prior to manipulation of the tumor. If no fluid is present, washings should be done. The tumor

Germ cell tumors
Cog tumor staging

Stage I	Limited to ovary, capsule intact
	Peritoneal cytology negative
	Nodes/omentum/peritoneal surfaces negative
Stage II	Rupture of capsule, microscopic residual
	Peritoneal cytology negative
	Nodes/omentum/peritoneal surfaces negative
Stage III	Contiguous visceral involvement or
	Peritoneal cytology showing malignant cells or
	Lymph node involvement or
	Positive peritoneal surfaces (not gliomatosis)
Stage IV	Distant metastases, including liver parenchyma

Figure 2. Children's Oncology Group staging for malignant ovarian germ cell tumors.

should next be assessed for mobility. If there is evidence of fixation or invasion of neighboring structures, only a biopsy should be done. There is no indication for radical resection without confirmation of histology. Germ cell tumors are very chemo-sensitive and postchemotherapy resection with fertility preserving surgery can be done in almost all instances. If the tumor is mobile and preoperative markers are normal, consideration may be given to cystectomy if this can be accomplished without rupture of the tumor capsule. If there is no plane of dissection from the normal ovarian parenchyma on careful inspection and/or markers are elevated, oophorectomy should be undertaken. If the fallopian tube is involved salpingo-oophorectomy is necessary. Regardless of marker status, staging for a potential malignant germ cell tumor should be completed at the initial laparotomy. A review of malignant ovarian germ cell tumors in girls and young adults revealed no relapse in completely evaluated FIGO stage Ia tumors when treated with surgery only, but relapse did occur in 5 of 13 patients that were

Epithelial tumors
Figo/ajcc staging

Stage I (Limited to the ovaries)
Ia: Tumor limited to one ovary; capsule intact, no tumor on ovarian surface. No malignant cells in ascites or peritoneal washings.
Ib: Tumor limited to both ovaries; capsules intact, no tumor on ovarian surface. No malignant cells in ascites or peritoneal washings.
Ic: Tumor limited to one or both ovaries with any of the following: capsule ruptured, tumor on ovarian surface, malignant cells in ascites or peritoneal washings.

Stage II (Involving one or both ovaries with pelvic extension and/or implants)
IIa: Extension and/or implants on the uterus and/or fallopian tubes. No malignant cells in ascites or peritoneal washings.
IIb: Extension to and/or implants on other pelvic tissues. No malignant cells in ascites or peritoneal washings.
IIc: Pelvic extension and/or implants (Stage IIa or IIb) with malignant cells in ascites or peritoneal washings.

Stage III (Involving one or both ovaries with microscopically confirmed peritoneal implants outside the pelvis. Superficial liver metastasis equals stage III. Tumor is limited to the true pelvis but with histologically verified malignant extension to small bowel or omentum.)
IIIa: Microscopic peritoneal metastasis beyond pelvis (no macroscopic tumor).
IIIb: Macroscopic peritoneal metastasis beyond pelvis 2 cm or less in greatest dimension.
IIIc: Peritoneal metastasis beyond pelvis more than 2 cm in greatest dimension and/or regional lymph node metastasis.

Stage IV (Distant metastasis)
Stage IV ovarian cancer is tumor involving one or both ovaries with distant metastasis. If pleural effusion is present, positive cytologic test results must exist to designate a case to stage IV. Parenchymal liver metastasis equals stage IV.

Figure 3. Ovarian cancer staging by FIGO/AJCC classification.

incompletely staged and followed conservatively as stage I tumors.[18] The surgeon is responsible for evaluating and documenting all components of the staging laparotomy. This requires removal of the intact tumor so that the pathologist can assess for capsular penetration or invasion, inspection of the omentum with excisional biopsy of any abnormal areas, inspection of peritoneal surfaces with biopsy of any abnormal areas, careful palpation of retroperitoneal nodes with biopsy of any enlarged or firm nodes and inspection and palpation of the opposite ovary with biopsy of any abnormal areas. Careful review of the retroperitoneum on the preoperative CT scan will be helpful in assuring that any suspicious nodal areas are carefully examined. Frozen section, once the tumor is removed intact, may be obtained to assist in further intraoperative decision making. It is not reliable to definitively conclude benign or malignant status but may be helpful

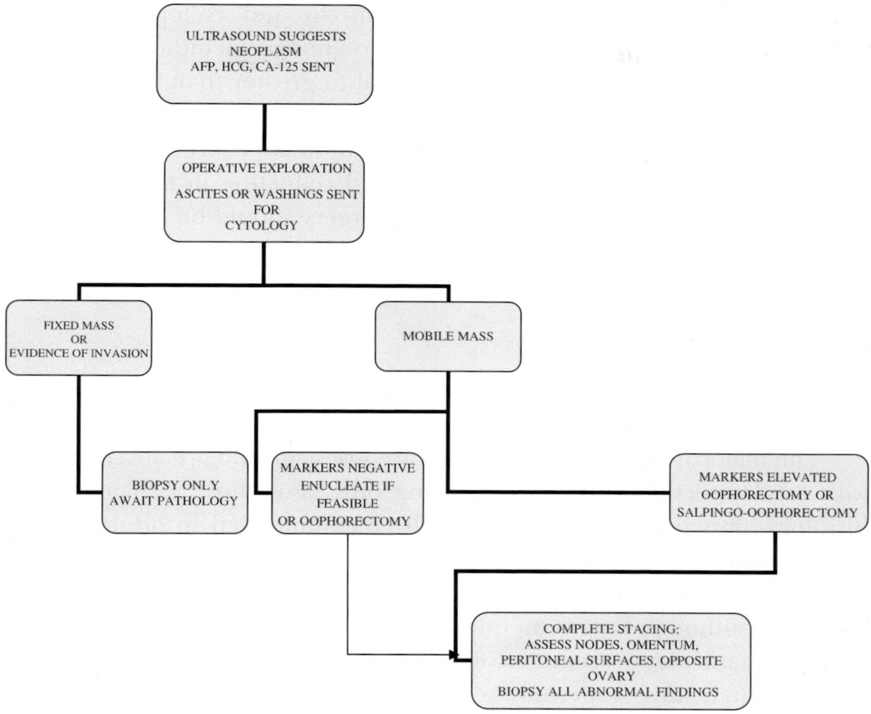

Figure 4. Algorithm for operative approach for pediatric ovarian neoplasm.

in distinguishing germ cell tumors from epithelial tumors. If an epithelial tumor is noted, additional staging would include omental biopsy even if grossly normal and consideration of appendectomy for mucinous tumors.

ADJUNCTIVE MANAGEMENT

Germ Cell Tumors

Benign teratomas and low grade immature teratomas may all be treated with surgical resection only and careful follow-up. Treatment of high grade immature teratomas is controversial. They may have evidence of spread to lymph nodes and distant sites and are often treated as malignancies.[5,19]

Malignant germ cell histologies including yolk sac, choriocarcinoma, germinoma, and embryonal carcinoma are treated with chemotherapy and have had a dramatic improvement in prognosis over time. They were initially treated with vincristine, dactinomycin and cyclophosphamide (VAC) chemotherapy. The evolution to regimens including platinum, etoposide and bleomycin has raised survival to greater than 90% for girls with malignant germ cell tumor of the ovary at all stages.[4,20–22] For girls who undergo only a biopsy at diagnosis, reexploration after three or four cycles of chemotherapy generally reveals a marked reduction in tumor burden and successful efforts for fertility sparing surgery should be anticipated in virtually all patients.

Epithelial Tumors

Benign mucinous and serous cystadenomas are successfully treated with local resection and close follow-up.

The majority of borderline tumors are low stage and are also managed with local resection and careful staging only.[7] For those with mucinous histology, appendectomy is traditionally recommended in adult women due to simultaneous or metachronous mucinous tumors in the appendix. Appendiceal tumor has not been reported in the adolescent or pediatric age group although long-term follow-up is lacking.

Malignant adenocarcinoma of the ovary in childhood and adolescence is exceedingly rare with only a handful of reported cases. In adults, complete staging followed by total abdominal hysterectomy and bilateral salpingo-oophorectomy is recommended. Unilateral salpingo-oophorectomy may be considered for low grade tumors that are localized in patients that desire fertility sparing approach with the recognition that there is increased risk of local relapse.[7] Shanker[23] reported three premenarchal girls with adenocarcinoma of the ovary. All were treated with surgical resection and chemotherapy but succumbed to malignant disease. Morowitz[1] reported three girls with mucinous adenocarcinoma including one prepubertal patient. Two had early stage disease and survived. Tsai[11] reported nine teenage girls with invasive ovarian carcinoma. Five had FIGO stage Ia disease (four treated with unilateral salpingo-oophorectomy) and survived. Four had FIGO stage III disease and two survived.

Sex Cord and Stromal Tumors

Fibroma and thecoma are effectively treated with resection and follow-up only. Gonadoblastoma should be treated with bilateral gonadectomy even if the tumor is unilateral since the dysgenetic gonad is prone to tumor development.

Juvenile granulosa cell tumor and Sertoli–Leydig tumors are localized in the vast majority of cases and are effectively treated with local fertility-preserving resection and close follow-up.[24] In advanced disease, platinum based therapy may be considered.[25]

LONG-TERM FOLLOW-UP

All ovarian neoplasms in childhood have some risk of contralateral recurrence. Regular interval ultrasounds should be planned for all patients. This will allow for early detection of tumors at a size where localized resection with salvage of residual ovarian tissue may be possible with preservation of fertility and hormonal status.

REFERENCES

1. Morowitz M, Huff D, vonAllmen, D. (2003) Epithelial ovarian tumors in children: A retrospective analysis. *J Pediatr Surg* **38**(3):331–335.
2. Cass DL, Hawkins E, Brandt ML, Chintagumpala M, Bloss RS, Milewicz AL, Minifee PK, Wesson DE, Nuchtern JG. (2001) Surgery for ovarian masses in infants, children, and adolescents: 102 consecutive patients treated in a 15-year period. *J Pediatr Surg* **36**(5):693–699.
3. Schultz KAP, Sencer SF, Messinger Y, Neglia JP, Steiner ME. (2005) Pediatric ovarian tumors: A review of 67 cases. *Pediatr Blood Cancer* **44**:167–173.
4. Billmire D, Vinocur C, Rescorla F, Cushing B, London W, Schlatter M, Davis M, Giller R, Lauer S, Olson T. (2004) Outcome and staging evaluation in malignant germ cell tumors of the ovary in children and adolescents: An intergroup study. *J Pediatr Surg* **39**(3):424–429.
5. Baranzelli MC, Bouffet E, Quintana E, Portas M, Thyss A, Patte C. (2000) Non-seminomatous ovarian germ cell tumours in children. *Eur J Cancer* **36**:376–383.
6. Skandalakis JE, Gray SW, Parrott JS, Ricketts RR. (1994) Ovary and Testes. In: JE Skandalakis and SW Gray (eds.), *Embryology for Surgeons*, pp. 736–772.
7. Aggarwal A, Lucco KL, Lacy J, Kives S, Gerstle JT, Allen L. (2009) Ovarian epithelial tumors of low malignant potential: A case series of 5 adolescent patients. *J Pediatr Surg* **44**:2023–2027.
8. Stankovic Z, Djuricic S, Djukic M, Jovanovic D, Vasiljevic M. (2006) Epithelial ovarian tumors and CA125 in premenarchal girls. *Eur J Gynaecol Oncol* **27**(6):597–599.

9. Sri Paran T, Mortell A, Devaney D, Piner A, Puri P. (2006) Mucinous cystadenoma of the ovary in perimenarchal girls. *Pediatr Surg Int* **22**(3):224–227.
10. Barton SE, Kurek KC, Laufer MR. (2010) Recurrent bilateral serous cystadenomas in a premenarchal girl: A case report and literature review. *J Pediatr Adolesc Gynecol* **23**(1):27–29.
11. Tsai JY, Saigo PE, Brown C, LaQuaglia MP. (2001) Diagnosis, pathology, staging, treatment, and outcome of epithelial ovarian neoplasia in patients age <21 years. *Cancer* **91**(11):2065–2070.
12. von Allmen, D. (2005) Malignant lesions of the ovary in childhood. *Sem Pediatr Surg* **14**:100–105.
13. Templeman CL, Fallat M. (2005) Benign ovarian masses. *Sem Pediatr Surg* **14**:93–99.
14. Zielinska D, Stanislaw Z, Rzepka-Gorska I. (2007) Tumors of dysgenetic gonads in swyer syndrome. *J Pediatr Surg* **42**:1721–1724.
15. Nabhan ZM, West KW, Eugster EA. (2007) Oophorectomy in McCune–Albright syndrome: A case of mistaken identity. *J Pediatr Surg* **42**:1578–1583.
16. Tatekawa Y, Kemmotsu H, Mouri T, Joe K, Ohkawa H. (2004) A case of pediatric ovarian dysgerminoma associated with high serum levels and positive immunohistochemical staining of neuron-specific enolase. *J Pediatr Surg* **39**(9):1437–1439.
17. National Cancer Institute. (2010) Cancer topics, ovarian epithelial cancer treatment. PDQ available at www.cancer.gov.
18. Palenzuela G, Martin E, Meunier A, Beuzeboc P, Laurence V, Orbach D, Frappaz D. (2008) Comprehensive staging allows for excellent outcome in patients with localized malignant germ cell tumor of the ovary. *Ann Surg* **248**(5):836–841.
19. Culine S, Lhomme C, Kattan J, Michel G, Duvillard P, Droz JP. (1995) Pure malignant immature teratoma of the ovary: The role of chemotherapy and second-look surgery. *Int J Gynecol Cancer* **5**(6):432–437.
20. Mann JR, Raafat F, Robinson K, Imeson J, Gornall P, Sokal M, Gray E, McKeever P, Hale J, Bailey S, Oakhill A. (2000) The United Kingdom Children's Cancer Study Group's second germ cell tumor study: Carboplatin, etoposide, and bleomycin are effective treatment for children with malignant extracranial germ cell tumors, with acceptable toxicity. *J Clin Oncol* **18**(22):3809–3818.
21. Terenziani M, Massimino M, Casanova M, Cefalo G, Ferrari A, Luksch R, Spreafico F, Polastri D, Fontanelli R, Piva L, Fossati-Bellani F. (2001) Childhood malignant ovarian germ cell tumors: A monoinstitutional experience. *Gynecol Oncol* **81**:436–440.

22. Suita S, Shono K, Tajiri T, Takamatsu T, Mizote H, Nagasaki A, Inomata Y, Hara T, Okamura J, Miyazaki S, Kawakami K, Eguchi H, Tsuneyoshi M. (2002) Malignant germ cell tumors: Clinical characteristics, treatment and outcome. A report from the study group for pediatric solid malignant tumors in the Kyushu Area, Japan. *J Pediatr Surg* **37**(12):1703–1706.
23. Shankar KR, Wakhlu A, Kokai GK, McDowell H, Jones MO. (2001) Ovarian adenocarcinoma in premenarchal girls. *J Pediatr Surg* **36**(3):511–515.
24. Bouffet E, Basset T, Chetail N, Dijoud F, Mollard P, Brunat-Mentigny M, David M. (1997) Juvenile granulosa cell tumor of the ovary in infants: A clinicopathologic study of three cases and review of the literature. *J Pediatr Surg* **32**(5):762–765.
25. Calaminus G, Wessalowski R, Harms D, Gobel U. (1997) Juvenile granulosa cell tumors of the ovary in children and adolescents: Results from 33 patients registered in a prospective cooperative study. *Gynecol Oncol* **65**:447–452.

SACROCOCCYGEAL TERATOMAS

26

Frederick J. Rescorla

INTRODUCTION

Germ cell tumors in children are a varied group of unusual tumors. At least 50% of childhood germ cell tumors present in extragonadal locations, and in infancy, over 90% present in these unusual locations with the sacrococcygeal region being the most common. This is in comparison to adults where only 10% of germ cell tumors are at extragonadal locations. In addition, the introduction of platinum-based therapy has markedly improved the survival for malignant germ cell tumors.

CLINICAL PRESENTATION

Sacrococcygeal teratomas are generally present in two distinct fashions: newborns with large predominantly external masses which are noted *in utero* or at the time of delivery and are rarely malignant; and, older infants and young children presenting with tumors predominantly confined to the pelvis with a much higher rate of malignancy. Neonatal sacrococcygeal tumors are rare occurring in approximately one in 35,000 live births. They do represent the most common extragonodal tumor in neonates and in most childhood series account for up to 70% of teratomas. Most reports have noted a 3 to 4:1 female to male ratio. Newborns generally present with the mass protruding from the sacral region and if detected prenatally should be considered for abdominal delivery if the mass is greater than

5 cm in size. In addition, some develop *in utero* high output cardiac failure resulting in fetal hydrops and may be candidates for *in utero* resection.

Older infants and children usually have no external portion noted at birth and presentation is usually related to compression of the bladder and rectum by the presacral mass. In some of these cases with small lesions noted at birth, an increased rate of malignancy has been noted. A small group of patients present with what is known as the Currarino Triad consisting of presarcal teratomas, anal stenosis, and sacral defects. This was initially described by Ashcraft and Holder who suggested the autosomal nature of the defect and subsequently Currarino suggested that the etiology may be related to adhesions between the endoderm and neuroectoderm causing the split notochord.

PATHOPHYSIOLOGY

Embryology

The blastocyst produces the primordial germ cells which originate near the allantois. These cells migrate from the yolk sac along the mesentery of the hindgut to the retroperitoneum at 4–5 wks gestation. Arrested or aberrant migration results in deposition of germ cells at extragonadal sites. These cells can undergo differentiation into embryonal carcinoma, which can then differentiate into embryonic or extraembryonic cells. The embryonic tumors are mature or immature teratoma with mature teratoma being the most common extragonadal germ cell tumor. Both mature and immature teratomas are considered benign tumors although high grade immature teratomas are often associated with malignant elements in tumors with more than one histologic type. The extraembryonic tumors include choriocarcinoma and endodermal sinus tumor, which is also known as yolk sac tumor. The yolk sac tumors are well differentiated highly malignant tumors. Of all teratomas which occur in children, approximately one half occur at the sacrococcygeal region followed by ovary and then sites such as the testes, mediastinum, retroperitoneum, neck and central nervous system.

Classification

Altman *et al.* in 1974 proposed a classification system based on a survey of the American Academy of Pediatrics (AAP) Surgical Section, which is still used today (Figure 1). In this classification system, type I is a predominantly external lesion and in the Altman series represented 47% of all cases with an 8% malignancy rate and 0% metastatic rate at presentation. Type II tumors present with both external and internal components and compromise 35% of all cases with a malignancy rate of 21% and a metastatic rate of 6%. Type III tumors are predominantly hidden in the pelvis with a very small external portion. These only represented 9% of the total cases, however, they had a malignancy rate of 34% and a metastatic rate of 20%. Type IV were entirely hidden within the pelvis and only represented 10% of the total cases, but had a malignancy rate of 38% and metastatic rate of 8%.

As noted above, neonates, infants and children generally present in two clinical scenarios; predominantly external tumors (types I and II) present in the newborn period with a malignancy rate of 6–10%, and, the types III & IV, more hidden lesions present at an older age with a higher rate of malignancy.

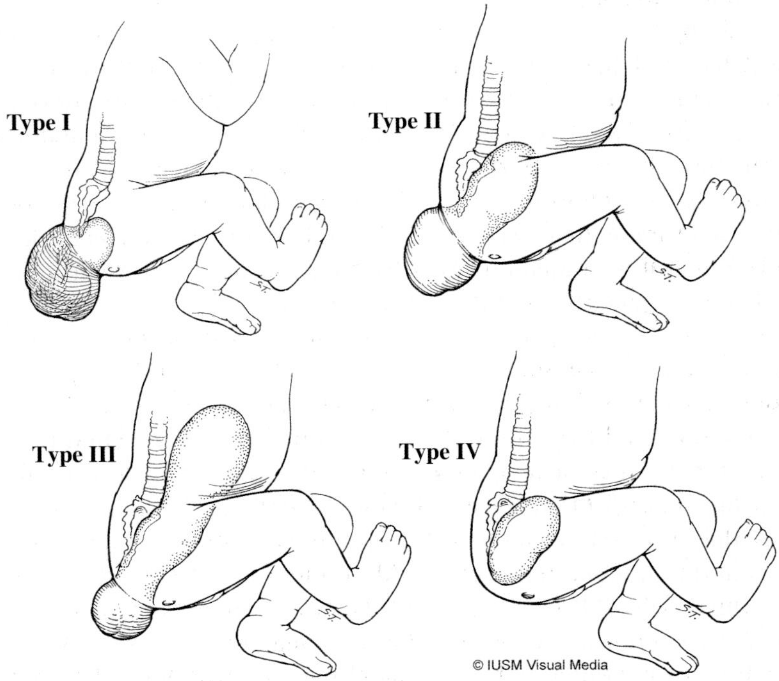

Figure 1. Altman classification of sacrococcygeal teratoma.

Pathology

Most neonatal cases have a benign pathological examination. In the CCG series of 126 children of which 111 were neonates, the pathology demonstrated mature teratomas in 69%, immature teratomas in 20%, and endodermal sinus in 11%. In the AAP survey by Altman, children younger than 2 mths of age had a 7% malignancy rate in girls and 10% in boys. Older infants had a very high rate of malignancy. Donnellan and Swenson noted that after 2 mths of age, 91.7% of these tumors were malignant. Malignancy rates in the 50–90% range in older children have been reported in many other studies.

In infants noted with lesions at birth in which no intervention occurs, there is a significant malignancy rate. In the CCG survey of 126 infants and children, six neonates had a delay in diagnosis and in these there was a 33% malignancy rate.

DIAGNOSIS

In newborns, the large external appearance generally makes the diagnosis quite easy by simple external inspection. In some cases, however, a neural tube defect may have a very similar appearance. If a definitive diagnosis cannot be determined by inspection and a neural defect is considered possible, an MRI is the most useful diagnostic modality. A careful abdominal examination should be performed in all affected neonates to determine any abdominal extension. An ultrasound examination is useful preoperatively to determine the intraabdominal extent as this may not be obvious by simple physical examination. This can also be useful to determine the blood flow characteristics of the pelvic portion.

In the less obvious cases, particularly in older children, a lipoma or perirectal abscess has sometimes been the initial clinical diagnosis. An abdominal examination along with a rectal examination is useful to determine the presacral location of the mass. In most cases, the child presents with symptoms related to bladder or rectal compression leading to the diagnostic work-up. On rectal examination, the finger is deviated anteriorly due to the presacral mass. CT or MRI is the diagnostic modality of choice and in addition alpha fetoprotein (AFP) and beta HCG levels should be determined. The AFP level is generally elevated in the neonatal period and does not reach normal levels until 9 mths of age. Elevated AFP levels in an older infant or toddler with a presacral mass is suggestive of the highly malignant yolk sac tumor.

Over half of the older children with malignant sacrococcygeal tumors have metastatic disease at initial diagnosis with the lung being the most common site, and thus a chest CT is usually obtained preoperatively to determine the presence of metastatic disease. The female predominance has also been noted in the older children presenting with malignant sacrococcygeal tumors with the Pediatric Oncology Group/Children's Cancer Group (POG/CCG) study observing 62 girls among a total of 74 children. The average age in this series was 21 mths and the initial AFP averaged 35,500 ng/mL. The oldest child was 37 mths of age.

MANAGEMENT

Many neonatal sacrococcygeal teratomas are detected prenatally by ultrasound. Lesions greater than 5 cm in size should be considered for abdominal delivery to avoid dystocia and tumor rupture. In some fetal cases, high output cardiac failure occurs leading to shunting and fetal hydrops. The involvement of this early in gestation, prior to 30 wks is ominous with a high percentage of these resulting in fetal demise. Some of these neonates may benefit from fetal resection or intervention. Adzick *et al.* reported the first successful fetal resection in a fetus diagnosed at 20 wks by routine ultrasound. At 25 wks, the fetus developed placentomegaly and polyhydramnios and underwent resection of a 400 g immature teratoma. The child was delivered at 29 wks and at 2 mths of life underwent exploration at which time no tumor was identified.

Consideration for fetal resection should only occur in children developing hydrops early in gestation, that being prior to 30 wks. Makin reported 41 antenatally diagnosed sacrococcygeal teratomas and performed fetal intervention in 12 of these with nonresection therapy including cyst drainage to facilitate delivery or alleviate bladder obstruction as well as laser ablation or alcohol sclerosis. The overall survival for antenatal diagnosis was 77%, however the survival for those undergoing fetal intervention was only 50%, and was only 14% if the fetal intervention was for hydrops. A review of the University of California San Francisco experience with fetal resection noted a survival rate of 20%. One study noted that the survival for prenatally detected lesion was highest for lesions smaller than 10 cm in size or predominantly cystic tumors which had a 100% survival. Survival is lowest at 48% in tumors greater than 10 cm in size or those with increased vascularity, vascular steal syndrome or rapid growth.

Operative Management

In cases with pelvic or intraabdominal extension or lesions with high flow, consideration of an abdominal approach, either open or laparoscopic to mobilize the pelvic component and divide the middle sacral artery and other feeding vessels should be considered. In cases with high flow, it may also be useful to gain control of the distal aorta. In these cases, a vascular tape can be passed around the aorta and a ramel clamp used which can be tightened while the child is in the prone position should bleeding be encountered thus allowing occlusion of the aorta on a selective basis. Several large series in the 1970's, 80's and 90's noted operative mortality rates between 5–10% based primarily on hemorrhage.

In selected cases, a staged approach may be useful and Robertson reported a 26-wk old child with a birth weight of 1800 g with a giant tumor who underwent initial ligation of the internal iliac artery and a small middle sacral artery along with a diverting colostomy. At 36 hrs of age, they resected the external component and at 111 days of life excised the internal component.

A small degree of pelvic tumor can be excised through the sacral incision, however, if the lesion is up towards the sacral prominence, consideration may be given to an initial abdominal approach. In any event, the child should be prepped circumferentially to allow movement from prone to supine position during the procedure. In general, the operative resection can wait until the child is a few days of age and allow work-up and stabilization. In occasional cases with rupture at the time of delivery, the surgeon may be forced to perform an urgent resection.

With the child in the prone position, an inverted V-type incision is marked out. The tip of the anterior V is just below the rectum which is displaced anteriorly due to the tumor. The posterior V-incision is inverted and has the base up near the sacrum. The use of a Hegar dilator within the rectum is useful to allow identification of the rectal musculature during the dissection and resection of the tumor.

Resection of the coccyx from the sacrum is an essential component of the operation and Gross noted a higher recurrence rate in cases in which the coccyx was not excised. Once this is excised the surgeon also has access to the middle sacral artery which should be carefully divided. Should hemorrhage occur, consideration should be given to occlusion of the aorta. The dissection continues and the presacral space can be entered as the tumor is traced up into this region. After resection of the tumor, the apex of the two

V's is lined up to prepare for closure. This puts the rectum back to a more normal posterior location and careful repair is of utmost importance. Fishman described a buttocks contouring incision in which the more anterior lateral portions are brought back to the posterior transverse portion creating two vertical closure lines in the mid portion of each buttock which join the transverse incision close to the sacrum. A drain is usually placed to evacuate fluid and blood which may accumulate postoperatively.

In older infants presenting with sacrococcygeal tumors, over 50% have metastatic disease and many of these tumors are very large, encasing the rectum or spine. Data from the POG/CCG study, including 74 children with malignant sacrococcygeal tumors noted that of the 74 patients, only 29 had an initial resection and 42 had a delayed resection. There was no difference in the event free survival between the two groups, thus supporting an initial approach with biopsy and neoadjuvant chemotherapy. In the POG/CCG study, all the tumors were yolk sac tumors and response to chemotherapy was usually excellent. After shrinkage with chemotherapy, an approach similar to that of a newborn can be utilized to enter the presacral region sometimes with an abdominal approach. In this study of older infants, surgeons utilized a sacral approach in 45 infants, a combined abdominal sacral approach in 25 and an abdominal approach in one patient. In many of these cases, the postchemotherapy tumor volume is quite small and a limited smaller incision is possible to remove the tumor. It should be noted that the coccyx should also be excised with this procedure.

In a large series from CCG involving primarily newborns, there were 126 children of which 111 were diagnosed either prenatally or at birth. In these, resection was by a sacral approach in 96 and was an abdominal sacral in 28 indicating the higher likelihood of accomplishing this procedure with a sacral only incision in the neonatal period.

POSTOPERATIVE MANAGEMENT

Neonates and infants with benign lesions (mature and immature teratomas) require no further therapy. Unfortunately, even in neonates undergoing complete resection of benign lesions such as mature or immature teratomas, there is a significant recurrence rate. In the CCG study, the recurrence rate for immature teratomas was 4% and for mature teratomas was 11%. Other series have documented recurrence rates between 3–23%. In general, a recurrence rate of 10–20% should be considered for these children. The time to recurrence has not exceeded 36 mths in these series, thus supporting the rationale for follow-up including rectal examinations and AFP determinations. We recommend quarterly determinations of both until the AFP level is normal and then ongoing rectal examinations every quarter until the child is 3 yrs of age.

The reported malignancy rate for recurrent tumors varies between zero and 75%, with the average around 50%. Thus, any evidence of recurrence merits immediate work-up with consideration for resection. A recurrence which is malignant requires postoperative chemotherapy or if the lesion is not amenable to initial resection, neoadjuvant therapy followed by a delayed resection. The AFP elevation in neonates should return to normal by 8–9 mths of age. Recurrence after resection of a benign tumor such as a mature teratoma can occur from various possible etiologies. A small area of a yolk sac tumor could have been overlooked in the original specimen, thus missing the initial malignancy. In addition, tumor could be left behind in the presacral space which may be malignant or may with time degenerate from benign to malignant thus leading to a malignant recurrence. A review from the POG/CCG Pathology Committee demonstrated that six initial mature/immature teratomas that developed a malignant tumor had on further review of the original slides microscopic yolk sac tumor in four or five patients, thus emphasizing the need for close examination of the entire specimen. In the current standard Children's Oncology Group (COG) protocol these children would have received chemotherapy.

The current COG study recommends postoperative chemotherapy for all malignant lesions even those which are stage I. The management of newborns with malignant components in a predominantly benign lesion is somewhat controversial. In the CCG study, six children with endodermal sinus tumor diagnosed at birth received no chemotherapy and recurrence disease developed in two of the six children. Both of these were treated with chemotherapy and surgery and survived long term. Older children with malignant lesions should be treated on a COG protocol including chemotherapy with a long term follow-up plan. Many of these will have initially unresectable lesions and will undergo neoadjuvant chemotherapy followed by delayed resection. The pathology in older children is nearly uniformly yolk sac tumor. If an older child with a recurrence has a mature teratoma or immature teratoma, simple observation should be performed for a 3-yr period.

Outcome

The survivorship in infant and neonates on the CCG study for mature teratomas was an 89% relapse free survival and overall survival of 98.7%. For immature teratomas, the relapse free survival is 95.8% with the survival of 100%. The survival for older children with malignant tumors formerly was dismal, however with the introduction of platinum based therapy in the late 70's and early 80's the survivorship markedly improved. In one large series, the survivorship before 1978 was 11% and after 1978 it was 86% with the introduction of platinum based chemotherapy. The POG/CCG trial of malignant sacrococcygeal tumors reported an overall event free survival rate of 84% with a survival rate of 90%. There was no statistical difference between children who presented with or without metastatic disease. In addition, there was no difference in survival based on initial resection vs. delayed, postchemotherapy resection.

Long-term Sequelae

Long-term studies have demonstrated significant postoperative functional complications in these children. Constipation rates in the 30–36% range have been reported. In addition, some have noted a soiling rate of 27–40% with some of these having a decreased anal resting pressure. Urinary incontinence has been reported in 19–22% and neurogenic bladder in up to 12% with most of these occurring with the type IV lesions. This emphasizes the need for postoperative follow-up during the first several years of life as the children go through potty training to ensure that bowel and bladder function are normal.

REFERENCES

1. Ashcraft KW, Holder TM. (1974) Hereditary presacral teratoma. *J Pediatr Surg* **9**:691–697.
2. Currarino G, Coln D, Votteler T. (1981) Triad of anorectal, sacral, and presacral anomalies. *Am J Roentgenol* **137**:395–398.
3. Altman RP, Randolph JG, Lilly JR. (1974) Sacrococcygeal teratoma: American Academy of Pediatric Surgical Section Survey — 1973. *J Pediatr Surg* **9**:389–398.
4. Fishman SJ, Jennings RW, Johnson SM, *et al.* (2004) Contouring buttock reconstruction after sacrococcygeal teratoma resection. *J Pediatr Surg* **39**:439–441.

5. Rescorla F, Billmire D, Stolar C, *et al.* (2001) The effect of cisplatin dose and surgical resection in children with malignant germ cell tumors at the sacrococcygeal region: A pediatric intergroup trial (POG 9049/CCG8882). *J Pediatr Surg* **36**:12–17.
6. Bilik R, Shandling B, Pope M, *et al.* (1993) Malignant benign neonatal sacrococcygeal teratoma. *J Pediatr Surg* **28**:1158–1160.

PEDIATRIC BONE TUMORS 27

Daniel Wurtz

INTRODUCTION

Lesions of bone found in childhood age groups are common. Many of these are nonneoplastic and may result from inflammatory, metabolic, or developmental conditions. Of the true neoplasms of the bone, the vast majority are benign. Once detected, however, bone tumors often cause diagnostic difficulty for many clinicians. This uncertainty of diagnosis then adds to the level of fear and anxiety in these patients and their families. This chapter will discuss the recognition and management of the most common benign and malignant bone tumors of skeletally immature patients. The optimal evaluation of patients with bone tumors requires a multidisciplinary team approach.

Evaluation and Staging

The work-up of a patient with a bone lesion should proceed in a systematic way to ultimately secure an accurate diagnosis and then proceed to treatment, if indicated. Clinicians who first encounter a patient with a bone abnormality will initiate the evaluation. This initial assessment should always begin with a carefully taken history and physical examination. The history is extremely important and should include questions regarding symptoms (if any), injuries, fever and chills, etc. The pattern and quality of pain as well as measures useful to relieve it are important historical items to obtain. The physical examination should include the presence or absence of fever, erythema, a mass or lump, tenderness, lymphadenopathy, muscle atrophy, joint effusion, and neurovascular abnormalities. Decisions for appropriate imaging should come only after a thorough history and physical exam have been completed.

Imaging modalities for bone tumors include plain radiographs, technetium bone scans, Computed Tomography (CT), and Magnetic Resonance Imaging (MRI). Good quality, plain radiographs taken recently are mandatory to evaluate a patient with a bone tumor. In fact, the plain radiograph is the most underused but most helpful modality for diagnosis of bone tumors. Plain radiographs are often the only image needed particularly if the underlying diagnosis is an asymptomatic, incidental finding. Old radiographs may be useful for comparison to those films taken recently to assess changes in the tumor. Radiographs should be reviewed carefully paying particular attention to the location of the tumor within a given bone. Some tumors have a predilection for specific anatomic areas within the bone. Radiographic features of bone lesions such as narrow vs. wide peripheral zones of transition and bone destruction vs. surrounding sclerosis are helpful to assess the biologic activity of the lesion. Many bone tumors have easily identifiable matrix characteristics on plain radiographs such as the stippled calcification of chondroid tumors (e.g. enchondromas) or ground (frosted) glass appearance of fibrous dysplasia. Additional imaging may be helpful after the plain radiograph is assessed. These additional modalities should be used to add diagnostic clues and ultimately to further investigate the extent of the local disease both inside and outside of the bone. To that end CT scans may be useful to define osseous architecture and, to a lesser extent, any soft tissue extension or component. It is ideal for small intracortical or cortex based bone lesions such as an osteoid osteoma and osteochondroma, respectively. For very young pediatric patients, CT scanning can be completed quickly often without the need for general anesthesia that is often required for longer (MRI) scans. MRI, however, has been the cross-sectional image of choice in most circumstances of patients with bone lesions that have some level of aggressive features on plain radiograph. It has been useful to identify cortical destruction, bone lesional edema, fluid-fluid levels, and any associated soft tissue mass. This modality is superior to the CT scan when reviewing the proximity of the tumor to the surrounding bone and soft tissue anatomy. Lastly, the technetium bone scan is a useful and sensitive imaging modality to evaluate the activity or ongoing new bone turnover of osseous lesions. Positive uptake of the radiopharmaceutical however is common among benign and often incidental bone lesions (e.g. enchondroma and fibrous dysplasia) and care must be taken not to over interpret a positive scan. Unfortunately bone scans are occasionally cold (little or no uptake) for some bone lesions (e.g. Langerhans cell histiocytosis [LCH]). Bone scans are extremely useful for systemic staging for metastatic disease and as a screening tool to help identify a subtle or elusive bone tumor in a large anatomic area such as the spine or pelvis.

After a careful history and physical exam are performed and appropriate imaging studies are reviewed, the clinician needs to make a decision regarding the nature of the bone lesion. Often this decision comes after careful review of all the available information and often after consultation with skilled musculoskeletal radiologists. At this time in the early management of these patients, surgeons with little experience in caring for patients with bone tumors should consider referring these patients to a trained clinician to better recognize and treat the problem to optimize the patient outcome. Not all bone lesions can or even need to be assigned an accurate diagnosis based on the above steps of initial evaluation. Importantly, however, the treating physician should have at this point an understanding of the aggressive behavior or nature of the bone lesion in question. This assessment may conclude that the lesion generally falls into the broad categories of latent benign (inactive, quiescent, likely incidental), active benign (growing, some aggressive features, symptomatic), or malignant (aggressive). Most patients with nonactive or latent benign bone lesions need no further surgical treatment. Patients with either active benign or aggressive (possibly malignant) bone tumors should have a biopsy to establish or confirm a histologic diagnosis, assess the grade of the lesion if malignant, and complete the staging of the patient.[1]

Biopsy of a bone tumor is technically easy, but this procedure requires a significant amount of thought and preparation. The biopsy should be done by the surgeon who will ultimately provide the definitive surgical care for the patient (or only after consultation with this person). A badly performed or placed biopsy will often jeopardize the successful treatment of an aggressive, possibly malignant bone tumor and unfortunately can lead to an amputation over a limb salvage result.[2] Biopsies of the bone may be done with either a needle or an incision (open). Those with a needle are commonly done under image guidance such as CT scan using a core cutting needle for adequate tissue samples. Intraosseous tumors are biopsied with trephine needles to enter the bone. Fine needle aspiration is not recommended due to frequent problems of inadequate tissue sampling. Most if not all primary malignant bone tumors should undergo incisional biopsy to ensure sufficient representative tissue acquisition. Incisional biopsy tracts should be longitudinally oriented on the limb and have meticulous hemostasis before wound closure.

BENIGN BONE TUMORS

The majority of pediatric bone tumors are benign. Bacterial osteomyelitis appears rather commonly in this age group mostly because of the bone environment in skeletally immature patients. Radiographic features may be radiolytic, blastic, or mixed depending upon the type of organism, the host, and the duration of involvement. Suffice it to say that osteomyelitis should always be considered in the differential diagnosis when evaluating a child. The topic of bone infection is complex and is discussed in another chapter of this book.

Table 1 lists common benign neoplasms of bone. Note that some of these tumors such as nonossifying fibroma (NOF), fibrous dysplasia, and enchondroma may be completely asymptomatic and present as incidental findings. Others such as osteochondroma, osteoid osteoma, aneurismal bone cyst, chondroblastoma, and osteoblastoma may be symptomatic. Important clinical information combined with a careful review of plain

Table 1.

	0–5 yrs	6–20 yrs
Benign	Osteomyelitis Eosinophilic Granuloma	Nonossifying fibroma Aneurysmal bone cyst Chondroblastoma Osteoblastoma Enchondroma Osteomyelitis Osteoid osteoma Eosinophilic granuloma
Malignant	Metastatic Neuroblastoma	Osteosarcoma Ewing's sarcoma Lymphoma

radiographs and other imaging is most useful to create a differential diagnosis. The radiographs should be reviewed by those with diagnostic experience such as musculoskeletal radiologists and musculoskeletal surgeons. Patients without symptoms often have benign, inactive bone lesions. Occasionally patients may have symptoms caused by a common musculoskeletal condition and found to have an incidental bone lesion on further work-up. These situations occasionally present some diagnostic difficulty, but it is incumbent upon the treating physician to prove the benign nature of the bone lesion. Lesions such as enchondromas, bone islands, NOFs, and fibrous dysplasia may be diagnosed in most cases on the basis of plain radiographs alone. Further imaging is usually unnecessary and biopsy in these situations is rarely indicated. Patients with active and aggressive benign lesions will have plain radiographic features that reveal ongoing bone changes such as cortical destruction, periosteal changes such as reactive bone formation, and a soft tissue mass in some cases. These lesions often need a biopsy to complete an accurate diagnostic work-up and staging. Biopsy in many of these cases may be done at the time of definitive management as long as an experienced musculoskeletal pathologist is available to review a frozen section of the lesion. If the material sampled during a biopsy is insufficient or the diagnosis cannot be made with certainty on the frozen section, then the treating surgeon should delay definitive surgical management and wait for permanent histopathology review before proceeding to treat a misdiagnosed malignant bone tumor improperly. These misadventures often lead to inadequately treated bone tumors and occasionally an unfortunate need for amputation.

Treatment Rational and Technique

The need for surgical treatment of a benign bone tumor depends upon the inherent biologic activity and expected behavior of the lesion. Those that are inactive, asymptomatic, and do not compromise bone strength are included in group I stage. These lesions need limited observation and no treatment. Those lesions that are active, but self-limited, grow slowly, and generally remain intracompartmental are included in the group II stage. These lesions may need surgical treatment if symptomatic or cause mechanical weakness of the host bone. Curettage or intralesional excision of these lesions is frequently needed to remove gross tumor. This technique is generally done with the aid of fluoroscopy through a formal incisional approach, creation of a bone window, and mechanical removal of tumor with curettes or a motorized burr. In children, the bone cavity is filled with bone graft or a bone substitute. Those in group III are active and aggressive. These tumors all eventually cause symptoms and continue to grow and destroy bone. These tumors require excision or curettage performed in a similar fashion to those of group II however particular diligence should be made to accomplish an extended curettage. This procedure should be done with meticulous mechanical removal of the bone tumor with a high speed burr and irrigation with repetition. Adjuvant modalities have been included such as use of phenol, liquid nitrogen, hydrogen peroxide, and argon beam coagulator. These additional modalities have not been proven to lessen local recurrence rates and may add significant risk of local tissue injury, bone necrosis and pathologic fracture. The tumor cavity may be filled with bone graft or bone substitutes. Internal fixation is usually not necessary in children unless significant bone weakness and increased fracture risk is anticipated.[3]

Benign bone tumors are generally divided into three categories based on the predominant histology of the tumor matrix. These are cystic, bone-forming, chondroid or cartilage, and fibrous tumors. The most common examples of each category of benign tumor are discussed briefly below.

BENIGN CYSTIC TUMORS

Benign cystic lesions of bone include unicameral or solitary bone cysts and aneurysmal bone cysts (ABC). Unicameral bone cysts (UBC) are common fluid-filled bone cysts and most commonly found in the proximal metaphysic of the humerus followed by the proximal femur. These lesions may have a vascular etiology and are generally asymptomatic until the patient sustains a pathologic fracture through the weak bone often during sports activities. These cysts have a characteristic appearance on plain radiographs in that they are geographic, centrally located, and may have partial septations. There is usually a thin adjacent bone cortex without bone erosion. Occasionally the radiograph will show a "fallen leaf" sign cause by a fracture and displacement of a cortical bone fragment within or to the bottom of the cyst. Recommended treatment of UBCs varies depending upon location, cyst activity, and patient age. Generally, a patient with an acute fracture should be treated with immobilization to allow for bone healing. Because most UBCs occur in the humerus, a sling or splint is recommended initially to support the extremity for 4–6 wks. Since curettage and bone grafting procedures have historically resulted in high recurrence rates for active cysts, treatment has evolved to less invasive methods such as injection with corticosteroids and other bone fillers such as demineralized bone matrix available commercially. Occasionally, refractory cysts will need internal fixation. Cysts in older children may heal or consolidate after a fracture. They will ultimately fill in with bone healing when the child reaches skeletal maturity. Active cysts or those in young patients less than 10 yrs of age tend to be more problematic. Most in this age group will persist or grow and require treatment.

ABC are aggressive, benign bone lesions that cause increasing pain and swelling. They may arise as de novo lesions or as part of another benign or malignant bone lesion. The etiology is still unclear, but is related to a vascular phenomenon within the bone. These lesions can cause considerable bone destruction that is usually apparent on plane radiographs. Radiographic features also typically include a radiolucent destructive lesion frequently with multiple septae and an expansive periphery made of periosteal reactive bone. MRI is useful to demonstrate fluid-fluid levels within the lesion. This feature helps to differentiate it from a UBC. These tumors belong to a group III stage and require a confirmatory biopsy and treatment with a meticulous, extended curettage to remove all grossly visible tumor. A thorough mechanical curettage of the tumor cavity is usually followed with insertion of bone graft to fill the tumor void with allograft or autograft. Because of inherent significant risk of local recurrence, these patients require continued periodic radiographic surveillance for at least 2 yrs.

BENIGN BONE-FORMING TUMORS

Benign lesions of bone with a predominate appearance of bone formation include osteoid osteoma, bone island, and osteoblastoma. Osteoid osteoma is a benign, painful, osteoblastic bone lesion of uncertain etiology. These tumors may arise in any bone but most commonly arise in the femur and tibia. Symptoms include a dull ache unrelieved with rest and often worse at night. Those in the posterior elements of the spine typically cause a painful scoliosis. Pain is characteristically relieved quickly and effectively with aspirin and other nonsteroidal anti-inflammatory agents. This tumor may often be seen on plain radiographs as a small, 1 cm radiolucency or nidus surrounded by dense, sclerotic bone. The may be difficult to visualize however in the axial skeleton. Technetium bone scan is a very helpful tool for diagnostic screening as these tumors are reliably focally positive. Further cross sectional imaging with CT scanning will ideally demonstrate the nidus within the abundant surrounding dense bone. Treatment includes the routine use of anti-inflammatory medication until spontaneous healing occurs over 3–5 yrs or invasive methods of either surgical curettage of the nidus and radiofrequency ablation of the tumor under CT guidance.

A bone island is a dense collection of lamellar bone often found within cancellous bone. It is an asymptomatic, incidental finding on plain radiographs. They can occur in any bone and are usually of no consequence. The technetium bone scan typically shows no uptake as the lesion is quiescent. Treatment is usually not needed.

Osteoblastomas are rare, aggressive, benign bone tumors of a group III stage. There are no characteristic radiographic features as these lesions can present as radiolytic, blastic, or mixed. They are usually painful and can appear in nearly any bone location, but about 40% occur in the posterior elements of the spine. They may have ABC-like elements within them. MRI may show an associated soft tissue mass. The radiographic appearance and the histologic features may be confused with low-grade osteosarcoma. An experienced pathologist is therefore required for accurate interpretation of biopsy material. An extended surgical curettage is the treatment of choice. Close postoperative surveillance is recommended periodically for at least 2 yrs because the local recurrence rate is reported at 10–20%.

CARTILAGINOUS TUMORS

Benign tumors with chondroid or cartilage matrix are the most frequently encountered in the pediatric population. Specific diagnoses include osteochondroma, enchondroma, chondroblastoma, and chondromyxoid fibroma.

Osteochondromas or exostoses are the most common benign bone tumor in children. They result from an abnormality of the growth plate resulting in an aberrant growth of a "new" bone or exostosis through enchondral ossification. Most of these lesions are asymptomatic but they often result in a lump or pain due to mechanical irritation of the surrounding soft tissues. They may be pedunculated or broadbased (sessile). Plain radiographs are usually diagnostic but CT scan can be helpful to define the extent of the tumor particularly for sessile lesions. The cartilage cap is responsible for continued growth until skeletal maturity. Solitary lesions are most common but some patients present with multiple exostoses as a result of an autosomal dominant condition called multiple hereditary exostoses. Malignant transformation is very rare particularly in children. Surgical treatment usually involves removal of the prominent lesion or correction of an angular limb deformity. Surgery is best reserved for symptomatic lesions and is best done when the patient is closer in age to skeletal maturity to lessen the risk of growth plate injury or local recurrence.

Enchondromas are benign chondroid tumors that are found inside of a bone. They are caused by incomplete ossification of the cartilage produced by the growth plate. The residual hyaline cartilage remains in the medullary canal and will continue to separate from the physis with continued bone growth. These lesions are asymptomatic. Plain radiographs show the radiolucent appearance within the medullary canal of the bone metaphysis with stippled calcification. When the diagnosis of a solitary enchondroma is confirmed, continued observation is not needed. The condition of multiple enchondromas is referred to as Ollier's disease. Children with this condition have bone changes caused by multiple enchondromas earlier than those with single lesion disease. They often have unilateral extremity disease presentation resulting in short extremities. Ollier's is associated with a 10% risk of malignant transformation during the life of the patient. Continued observation is indicated. Maffucci's syndrome is a very rare variant of enchondromatosis with extensive skeletal involvement, soft tissue vascular malformations, dwarf-like features, and severe limb deformity. Malignant transformation occurs in nearly 100% of these patients.

Chondroblastoma is a rare benign but locally aggressive bone tumor. It always occurs in an epiphyseal or apophyseal location within the bone. Most occur in the proximal humerus followed by the distal femur and proximal tibia. Patients complain of moderate pain and occasionally swelling. Radiographs typically show a radiolucent area with the bone epiphysis with subtle stippled calcification. The mineralization of the tumor matrix can be confirmed with CT scanning. These are group III tumors and cause continued bone destruction and surgical treatment in the form of extended curettage with bone grafting is indicated. Local recurrence rates have been reported as high as 10%. Therefore periodic radiographic follow-up should continue for at least 2 yrs after treatment.

Chondromyxoid fibroma is a very rare benign but locally aggressive tumor containing chondroid, myxoid, and fibrous tissue. Pain is the most common presenting symptom. These tumors have a varied radiolucent appearance and most occur in the metaphyseal region of bone. The radiographs often show a lobulated appearance within the bone. Additional features may appear aggressive with cortical destruction, but some lesions may have a narrow zone of transition and resemble NOF. Surgical treatment for group III lesions is indicated with this tumor to lessen local recurrence risk. Continued periodic radiographic follow-up for at least 2 yrs is recommended.

FIBROUS TUMORS

Tumors with a predominance of fibrous stroma include NOF, fibrous dysplasia, and osteofibrous dysplasia.

NOF or fibrous cortical defect is a relatively common fibrous proliferation of bone resulting from a developmental aberration of normal remodeling during bone growth. These lesions are usually asymptomatic, self-limited, and have a characteristic radiographic appearance. The most common location for involvement is the distal femur and proximal tibia. NOFs are often multiple and bilateral. Characteristic radiographic features include a lobulated or soap-bubble appearance, eccentric and metaphyseal location, thin overlying cortex, and sclerotic intraosseous borders. The technetium bone scan shows mild activity. MRI has a characteristic low signal on T1 and T2 weighted sequences indicative of fibrous tissue. Jaffe–Campanacci syndrome is characterized by multiple large NOF's, *café-au-lait* spots, and increase incidence of associated mental retardation and cardiovascular abnormalities. Symptoms related to NOF's are mechanical due to weakened bone. Affected children occasionally present with a pathologic fracture though the lesion. Larger lesions fall into a group II state and treatment is indicated in patients with mechanical symptoms. Curettage and bone grafting the tumor void is occasionally indicated. NOF's spontaneously regress or mineralized after skeletal maturity is reached.

Fibrous dysplasia is a fibroosseous proliferation of bone resulting from the mutation of the GNAS gene. Patients with fibrous dysplasia will fall into a clinical spectrum of this disease ranging from monostotic disease (30%) to polyostotic involvement (70%), and the severe form of presentation called McCune–Albright syndrome. Patients with this syndrome present at an early age and characteristically have polyostotic bone involvement, *café-au-lait* spots, and endocrine abnormalities such as precocious puberty.

Patients with extensive bone disease often present with pain, limp, and fractures. Plain radiographic features are usually diagnostic and include the findings of widened bone diameter, thin cortices, frosted or ground glass appearance, and bone deformity. The proximal femur is a preferred sight of involvement of fibrous dysplasia and sometimes results in a profound varus deformity of the femoral neck into a "shepherds crook" deformity. Fibrous dysplasia may also contain cystic components much like ABC. Histologic features include areas of immature trabecular bone resembling alphabet soup without osteoblastic rimming in a fibrous stroma background. Treatment may be observational in patients with minor disease involvement. Monostotic disease may present purely as an incidental finding. Moderate to severe bone involvement causing pain and deformity may require surgical stabilization. Curettage and bone grafting procedures are usually ineffective. Patients with McCune–Albright syndrome should be evaluated by an endocrinologist. Bisphosphonate drugs are often prescribed for patients with severe skeletal involvement but have had only modest success.

Osteofibrous dysplasia is a rare fibroosseous condition with a predilection for the anterior tibial diaphysis in young children, usually less than 5 yrs of age. Clinical features include painless bowing deformity of the involved bone. Plain radiographs are diagnostic and show an eccentric, radiolytic, bubbly bone lesion with a dense sclerotic rim. Biopsy is occasionally needed to confirm the diagnosis. Histology resembles that of fibrous dysplasia; however osteoblastic bone rimming is present. Treatment is rarely indicated. Osteofibrous dysplasia is thought to be a precursor to the rare malignancy adamantinoma. Continued observation with periodic radiographs is indicated. Adamantinoma is very uncommon in skeletally immature patients.

HISTIOCYTIC LESIONS

LCH is the accepted name given to a spectrum of a nonneoplastic condition where the skeletal lesions involve the Langerhans histiocyte. The etiology of this disease is still unclear. Most patients with LCH are skeletally immature. Symptoms include a dull achy pain particularly at night. Bone involvement is the most common manifestation of the disease with monostotic or polyostotic involvement. Radiographic features typically include radiolytic lesion with a punched-out appearance and periosteal reaction.

There may been significant bone destruction and an associated soft tissue mass. Common sites of involvement include the skull, spine, pelvis, and femur. A skeletal survey for systemic evaluation is recommended. Technetium bone scan is active in less than 50% of cases. Those in the spine may cause a flattening of the vertebral body to varying degrees called vertebrae plana. Biopsy is helpful to establish the diagnosis. The presence of the LCH is diagnostic. These lesions may also include eosinophils of varying amounts. Extraskeletal manifestations may include a skin rash, granular pulmonary infiltrates, and rarely hepatosplenomegaly. Those patients with systemic involvement may present with diabetes insipidus. Treatment of these patients varies depending upon the degree of systemic involvement. Those with an isolated bone lesion need only biopsy and possible curettage or steroid injection to affect bone healing. Systemic involvement often necessitates a referral of the patient to the oncologist for further evaluation and consideration of systemic chemotherapy.

MALIGNANT BONE TUMORS

Refer again to Table 1 for a list of the most common malignant bone tumors in the pediatric age group. Patients with malignant tumors ultimately present with symptoms most commonly a mass and/or pain. Symptoms may initially be mild and become severe over a few weeks duration. Pain may be either due to symptoms caused by mechanical problems such as irritation of adjacent soft tissues or due to secondary weakness of the bone or pain caused by bone destruction or directly by the tumor. Radiographic changes are diagnostic in most patients of an aggressive lesion. The changes may range on a spectrum of subtle to obvious. The clues to understanding the aggressive behavior of a bone tumor lie in its ability to change or destroy the host bone. In general descriptive terms, malignant bone tumors have radiographic appearances that fit one of three patterns: geographic, moth-eaten, and permeative. Look first at the periphery of the bone tumor. The tumor-host bone interface in these cases will be ill-defined in those with a geographic appearance and frequently show frank destruction of bone trabeculae and cortex. Those with a moth-eaten appearance have patchy bone destruction. Tumors that fit this appearance include osteosarcoma, and aggressive benign lesions such as ABC and chondroblastoma. Remember that osteomyelitis may have a similar appearance. Permeative lesions are often difficult to appreciate because the overall bone architecture may be preserved on plane radiographs. This appearance may be one of subtle osteopenia and is characteristic of those tumors that percolate through bony trabeculae quickly without obvious destructive changes. Look for periosteal reaction adjacent to the bone cortex or lifting of the periosteum outside of the bone in sequential layers known as onion-skinning. Tumors often demonstrating this characteristic appearance include Ewing's sarcoma, lymphoma, and metastatic neuroblastoma. The clinician should compile a short list of possible diagnoses based on the clinical information and the plain radiographs.

Additional imaging of the affected limb should be performed to complete the local staging of the disease process before biopsy is performed by the treating surgeon. MRI is the most useful cross-sectional imaging for a number of reasons. Standard MRI sequences add important clues as to the behavior and specific tumor diagnosis. These studies should be reviewed by an experienced surgeon or musculoskeletal radiologist. Particular attention should be paid to the location of the tumor and the extent of disease. The presence or absence of a soft tissue mass should be assessed. The relationship of the tumor to surrounding host tissues, especially neurovascular structures is very important. Systemic staging for primary malignant bone tumors should include a whole body technetium bone scan and a chest CT scan. Biopsy of the tumor should be performed after these studies are complete.

There are several important guidelines for biopsy of musculoskeletal lesions suspected to be malignant. Once again, the biopsy procedure should be done or at least supervised by the surgeon who will provide the definite surgical management. Open biopsies are preferred for primary malignant bone tumor to insure adequate tumor sampling. Biopsy incisions should be longitudinal so that they may be excise en bloc with the underlying tumor at a later date. Meticulous hemostasis is required prior to wound closure to prevent unnecessary tumor contamination by a hematoma. Drains are permitted as long as they exit the wound distal, close, and in line with the biopsy incision. Frozen section analysis is advisable at the time of the incisional biopsy to confirm that representative tumor tissue has been obtain for permanent and definitive analysis by the experienced musculoskeletal pathologist.

Osteosarcoma is the most common primary malignant bone tumor in skeletally immature patients. It is most common in the second decade of life. This tumor occurs most commonly in the metaphyseal region of the distal femur, proximal tibia, and proximal humerus, respectively. Typical symptoms include increasing pain and swelling or mass over a 6–8 wks period. Since most high grade osteosarcomas occur about the knee, patients may complain of pain with ambulation and loss of joint motion. Laboratory studies are usually nonspecific but there may be an elevation of alkaline phosphatase. Plain radiographs typically reveal an area of bone destruction of the medullary canal and frequently the bone cortex. As osteosarcoma is a heterogeneous malignancy, the bone changes may be radiolytic, blastic, or mixed depending upon the predominant matrix subtype. Most patients will have extraosseous or extra-compartmental extension as a visible mineralized soft tissue mass at presentation. MRI is necessary to help define the extent of local disease within the bone and the surrounding soft tissues. This sophisticated imaging is required to visualize the relationship of the tumor to vital neurovascular structures. Systemic staging studies should include a CT scan of the chest and a whole body technetium bone scan. Visible pulmonary nodules are present in 20% of patients. It is estimated that 80% of patients will have at least micrometastases at presentation. Biopsy with an incisional technique as outlined above should be performed by the surgeon who will provide the definitive care for the patient. Histologic features of osteosarcoma include evidence of osteoid production by malignant osteoblasts. Osteoid is often difficult to identify in some osteosarcoma specimens. An experience musculoskeletal pathologist is required. When the diagnosis is confirmed with biopsy and the staging is complete, care should continue with a multidisciplinary approach. Because the disease process significantly weakens the host bone, the involved limbs need to be protected. Patients with osteosarcoma of the lower extremity should be nonweightbearing to avoid pathologic fracture. Unfortunately, this complication usually leads to amputation rather than limb-salvage surgery. Optimal treatment of high grade osteosarcoma includes surgery and chemotherapy. Those with lung metastases may require metastatectomy. Neoadjuvant multidrug chemotherapy is the initial treatment and includes doxorubicin, high-dose methotrexate, cisplatin, and ifosfamide.[4] After three cycles or about 11 wks of neoadjuvant drug treatment, these patients are restaged for local and systemic disease. The musculoskeletal surgeon will then assess the patient for the most appropriate surgical resection or amputation. The majority of patients (80–90%) undergo limb sparing surgery and reconstruction. Studies have not shown a survival advantage of amputation over a properly performed limb sparing surgery.[5] Limb amputation is preferred in some cases of tumor progression on chemotherapy and/or tumor involvement of vital neurovascular structures. When opting for limb sparing surgery, the surgeon must anticipate a functional outcome as good as that expected with amputation. Most limb sparing procedures of the lower extremity will result in less oxygen consumption with ambulation that that of amputation. The patient (and family) should be aware that the acute and delayed complication rate of limb sparing surgery is greater than amputation. This surgery requires a meticulous margin-free resection of the tumor en bloc with the biopsy site while sparing neurovascular structures and sufficient muscle for adequate limb function. Reconstruction requires replacing bone loss with large endoprosthetic metal devices or large bulk allografts with metal fixation. Another reasonable surgical treatment option includes rotationplasty, but successful limb sparing procedures have had better psychological acceptance. Prognosis of patients with high-grade osteosarcoma is about 70% at 5 yrs. Patients with visible metastatic disease at presentation have less than 25% survival despite treatment. Response to chemotherapy is based on the percentage of tumor kill seen on the resected specimen after neoadjuvant treatment. Less than 95% tumor necrosis is believed to indicate a less favorable prognosis.

Ewing's sarcoma is the second most common primary malignant bone tumor. Like osteosarcoma, it occurs most frequently in the second decade of life. It rarely occurs in black children. Most patients report limb pain and a mass. Constitutional symptoms such as fever and malaise are also common complaints. This malignancy is often identified in long bones, pelvis, and spine. Laboratory studies may be useful but results may overlap those of osteomyelitis. Specifically, elevated erythrocyte sedimentation rate is common. Plane radiographs of the involved extremity typically show subtle radiolytic changes in the bone. Often there may only be osteopenia. Periosteal reaction is common however and appears as "onion skinning" or multiple laminations of periosteal reactive bone caused by tumor soft tissue extension through the bone cortex. Because plane radiographic changes are subtle, MRI is indicated to appreciate the extent of disease. This tumor often has a large soft tissue mass and may extend for a significant distance within the medullary canal. Similar to the staging of patients with osteosarcoma, a chest CT scan and a whole body technetium bone scan is required. Most oncologists advocate an iliac crest bone marrow aspiration biopsy to complete the systemic staging. Incisional biopsy should be performed to obtain adequate tissue for diagnostic studies including chromosomal analysis. Samples obtained with needle biopsies are usually inadequate.

Histologically, Ewing's sarcoma appears as a sheet of monotonous small, round blue cells on H&E slides. This appearance may be confused with that of lymphoma and metastatic neuroblastoma. Immunohistochemistry (CD99) is diagnostic of Ewing's sarcoma. Cytogenetic testing reveals the chromosomal translocation t(11:22)(q24;q12) in 90% of patients. Ewing's sarcoma responds to a multimodal treatment including chemotherapy, surgery, and radiation. Standard chemotherapy is given as a neoadjuvant program and includes doxorubicin, vincristine, cyclophosphamide, and ifosfamide. Ewing's sarcoma often presents with a large soft tissue mass and in the majority of patients with this finding, chemotherapy given before surgical resection results in a significant reduction in size of the soft tissue component of the tumor. Local control is achieved preferably with margin-free surgical resection when possible. The surgical technique is performed in a manner consistent with wide resection of any other high grade bone sarcoma. Attention should be given to a meticulous dissection around the tumor preserving as much vital tissue as possible to maximize a good functional result but removing the biopsy site and the underlying malignant tumor with uninvolved surgical margins. Reconstruction is achieved with one of several options including use of an endoprosthesis, allograft, or autograft. Patients with tumor involvement of certain anatomic areas are best treated with resection alone. These areas may include portions of the pelvic ring, the proximal fibula, and metatarsal or metacarpal. Occasionally, patients with Ewing's sarcoma have extensive local disease that is technically not possible to remove with clear surgical margins. These situations arise mostly in the pelvis and spine. Because Ewing's sarcoma is quite sensitive to radiation, local control measures may warrant either radiotherapy alone with a total dose of about 60 Gy or preferably surgical resection with positive margins combined with a radiation modality such as external beam with doses of about 60 Gy.[6] Patients with suspected pulmonary metastases may require metastatectomy in addition to chemotherapy for systemic treatment.

Lymphoma of bone in the pediatric age is very uncommon and is usually of the non-Hodgkin's, diffuse, large, B-cell type. Patients often present with a dull achy pain. Most cases in the skeletally immature patients are in the second decade of life. Plain radiographs may appear essentially early in the course of symptoms and later have only subtle abnormal features of diffuse osteopenia or a mixed radiolytic and blastic appearance. A technetium bone scan may be a useful screening tool as they are typically abnormal in the region of bone involvement. MRI is also useful to evaluate the extent of local osseous and soft tissue components. Incisional biopsy is recommended to obtain adequate tissue sampling because this tumor often causes diagnostic confusion for pathologists. Ideally, biopsy material is sent fresh without formalin preservative for flow cytometry. Treatment is based on combined modalities of systemic chemotherapy and local radiotherapy. Surgery is required only for establishing the diagnosis with biopsy and surgical stabilization of a pathologic fracture or impending fracture. Multidrug chemotherapy is recommended and includes cyclophosphamide, doxorubicin, vincristine, and prednisone.

Lastly, neuroblastoma may present as metastatic bone disease as an initial manifestation or late in the course of this malignancy. These patients are usually less than 5 yrs of age. Surgery is warranted for pathologic fracture fixation. Radiotherapy may be needed for local control.

REFERENCES

1. Simon MA, Finn HA. (1993) Diagnostic strategy for bone and soft tissue tumors. *J Bone Joint Surg Am* **75**:622.
2. Mankin HJ, Mankin CJ, Simon MA, *et al.* (1996) The hazards of the biopsy, revisited. *J Bone Joint Surg Am* **78**:656–663.
3. Gitelis S, Wilkins R, Conrad EU III. (1996) Benign bone tumors. *Instr Course Lect* **45**:425–446.
4. Link MP, Goorin AM, Horowitz M, *et al.* (1991) Adjuvant chemotherapy of high grade osteosarcoma of the extremit: Updated results of the multi-institutional osteosarcoma study. *Clin Orthop Relat Res* **270**:8–14.
5. Simon MA, Aschliman MA, Thomas N, Mankin HJ. (1986) Limb-salvage treatment versus amputation for osteosarcoma of the distal end of the femur. *J Bone Joint Surg Am* **68**:1331–1337.
6. Bacci G, Ferrari S, Longhi A, *et al.* (2003) Local and systemic control in Ewing's sarcoma of the femur treated with chemotherapy, and locally by radiotherapy and/or surgery. *J Bone Joint Surg Br* **85**:107–114.

SOFT TISSUE SARCOMAS 28

Frederick J. Rescorla

INTRODUCTION

Soft tissue sarcomas represent approximately 7% of all childhood tumors and are generally classified as rhabdomyosarcoma and nonrhabdomyosarcoma tumors. Approximately 40% of all soft tissue sarcomas in childhood are rhabdomyosarcomas, however, in children less than 9 yrs of age, rhabdomyosarcomas are more common and after 10 yrs of age, nonrhabdomyosarcomas are at least twice as common as rhabdomyosarcomas. The pediatric nonrhabdomyosarcomas are split among approximately nine histologic types accounting for between 2% and 8% of the entire group of including synovial sarcoma, dermatofibrosarcoma protuberans, malignant fibrous histocytoma, fibrosarcoma, malignant peripheral nerve sheath tumor, and several other histologic types.

RHABDOMYOSARCOMA

Rhabdomyosarcoma was first described by Weber in 1854. This tumor is derived from primitive mesenchymal cells which are destined to become skeletal muscle. There are approximately 250 to 300 new cases per year in the United States with a slight male predominance. Risk factors for rhabdomyosarcoma include the Li-Fraumeni Familial Cancer Syndrome which is a constitutional P53 mutation occurring as an autosomal dominant disorder with family members having various malignancies including rhabdomyosarcoma, adenocortical carcinoma, breast cancer, glioblastoma and lung cancer. Other risk factors include neurofibromatosis type I and Beckwith–Wiedemann syndrome. Environmental risk factors include radiation as well as parental use of marijuana and cocaine.

Clinical Presentation

The presence of a soft tissue mass is the most common presentation. Approximately 20% are noted with metastatic disease at the time of initial presentation, with approximately one half in the lung and 25% in the bone marrow.

Presentation and Initial Site

Head and neck tumors account for approximately 35% of rhabdomyosarcomas. They are divided into three sites: (1) the orbit; (2) head and neck nonparameningeal, including the oral cavity, oropharynx, parotid, cheek and neck; and, (3) head and neck parameningeal including the middle ear, nasal cavity, nasopharynx, infratemporal fossa and parapharyngeal area. Genitourinary sites account for 25% of all rhabdomyosarcomas and are divided into bladder/prostate and the better prognostic, nonbladder prostate including paratesticular, vaginal, uterus and cervical sites. Extremity sites represent approximately 15% of tumors and lymphatic spread unfortunately is common thus these tumors need lymph node sampling. Other sites including the chest and abdomen along with the paraspinal region, biliary tract and perineum account for 25% of lesions.

Classification by Histology

Rhabdomyosarcomas are small round blue cell tumors and are placed in a category which includes neuroblastoma, Ewing's sarcoma, osteogenic sarcoma and non-Hodgkin's lymphoma. Rhabdomyosarcomas are divided into embryonal and alveolar with embryonal being more common and having a better prognosis. Embryonal lesions are further divided into spindle cell; botryoid, which are often grape-like and in such favorable sites as the vagina and biliary tree; typical; and, anaplastic, which has a worse prognosis. Alveolars are divided into typical and solid histologic classifications, both of which have the same poor prognosis. Most alveolar rhabdomyosarcomas have translocation t(2;13) or t(1;13). Some embryonal rhabdomyosarcomas have loss of heterozygosity (LOH) at 11p 15.5.

Initial Evaluation

A complete physical examination with routine laboratory studies along with an assessment of regional lymph nodes is part of the initial work-up. For most extremity, body wall, or head and neck tumors, a MRI scan is the preferred imaging modality. CT scanning is preferable for intrathoracic/intraabdominal, as well as pelvic and retroperitoneal sites. Ultrasound is also used for pelvic sites including the bladder, prostate, uterus, vagina and paratesticular tumors. In view of the high (20%) metastatic rate, evaluation should include potential metastatic sites including lymph nodes along with a CT scan of the chest. In addition, bone marrow aspirates and biopsies are necessary. Additional diagnostic studies are indicated for specific sites such as endoscopy (airway, bladder, vagina), audiography or dental examinations with films.

Surgery

The initial approach should be excision of the entire tumor, if possible, and if this can be performed without compromise of function of a major organ. Adequate margins should be excised. Excision of an entire muscle or compartment is normally not necessary. If a resection is planned, care should be taken to avoid penetration of the tumor and the tumor should be marked carefully to allow complete pathologic review for margins. Separate biopsies of the margin outside of the resection are recommended to confirm the presence of a complete resection. If resection is not possible, adequate tissue should be obtained to allow molecular pathology studies. Large lymph nodes present at the time of diagnosis should be biopsied. In addition, regional lymph node sampling is required for extremity sites, as well as paratesticular sites in boys over 10 yrs of age. Sentinel lymph node biopsies may be helpful in extremity tumors that do not have enlarged lymph nodes.

For children in whom the initial resection procedure is not an adequate cancer operation with clear margins, a pretreatment reexcision (PRE) should be performed. This is a wide excision of the previous operative site, which is performed prior to chemotherapy or radiotherapy. This is not performed if an unacceptable loss of function would occur with the procedure.

In cases where an initial biopsy is performed, chemotherapy is administered with a second operation for resection at 12 wks. This may be needed to remove gross disease, to improve local control or to confirm the response of patients with a complete response. Metastatic sites require a biopsy to confirm the presence of malignancy. Most of these metastatic sites are treated with radiation therapy alone. Should residual disease be present in such sites as the lung after therapy, resection may be needed.

SURGICAL GUIDELINES FOR SPECIFIC ANATOMIC SITES

Head and Neck Parameningeal

Due to the location, gross total resection is rarely possible and virtually all of these are managed with definite radiation therapy. Regional lymph node involvement is very unusual in these tumors. They are associated with a poor prognosis as they present in hidden sites, often with a delay in diagnosis.

Extremity Sites

As mentioned above, there is a very high incidence of regional lymph node involvement and in view of this lymph node sampling should be performed. Tumor resection should usually be performed as a limb sparing technique and the plan should be to remove the entire tumor. Amputation is generally reserved for recurrence after initial treatment.

Bladder/Prostate

Initial biopsy can usually be performed by endoscopy. If there is an obstructive uropathy, this can be relieved by percutaneous or endoscopic techniques. A residual mass is common after therapy. This is rarely tumor and should be biopsied only if it is growing. Pelvic exenteration is rarely utilized.

Vagina

These tumors usually respond well to chemotherapy however, definitive local control is recommended at week 12 of therapy. Pelvic exenteration is generally reserved for tumor progression or recurrence not amenable to conservative therapy.

Paratesticular Tumor

This tumor should be removed by an inguinal orchiectomy with resection of the spermatic cord to the level of the internal ring. If a transscrotal approach is performed, a hemiscrotectomy or else hemiscrotal radiation therapy should be given. Studies have demonstrated that CT imagining underestimates the incidence of positive lymph nodes in the retroperitoneum. In view of this, the standard of care is currently ipsilateral retroperitoneal lymph node dissection for patients over 10 yrs of age.

Biliary Tree

These usually have favorable histology and most do well without aggressive therapy. The biliary obstruction usually resolves in response to chemotherapy and external drains of the biliary tree should be avoided as they are associated with a high incidence of sepsis.

CLASSIFICATION BASED ON TUMOR FACTORS AND LOCATION

Outcome for rhabdomyosarcoma depends on clinical assessment of various tumor features including primary site (unfavorable vs. favorable), histology (embryonal vs. alveolar), clinical group reflecting extent of resection, and stage, encompassing features of the size of the tumor, lymph node metastases and distant metastases. The treatment is therefore based on assessment of these risk factors.

Favorable sites include the orbit which has a 100% survival, head and neck (nonparameningeal), genitourinary (not bladder or prostate) and the biliary tract. Unfavorable sites include head and neck (parameningeal), genitourinary (bladder/prostate), extremity and other sites.

Clinical Group

Clinical group is determined by the extent of the surgical procedure. Clinical group I reflects children with no residual disease after surgery. Clinical group II represents microscopic residual disease and is further divided into IIA with margins positive and lymph nodes negative, IIB margins negative and lymph nodes positive and IIC margins positive with lymph nodes positive; however, in these later two groups all of the lymph node sites must be excised at the operative procedure. Clinical group III represents those with gross residual disease including those with biopsy only as with regional lymph nodes. Clinical group IV is defined by metastatic disease. Survival is clearly correlated to clinical group with groups I and II having very favorable outcome (over 80%), whereas group III is around 60% and group IV is less than 20%.

Stages

The stage of the tumor is classified between I and IV and takes into account the site, size, lymph nodes and presence of metastatic disease. Stage I is favorable site with any size or presence of lymph nodes, but no metastatic disease. Stage II is unfavorable site with a tumor less than 5 cm and no lymph node involvement and no metastatic disease. Stage III is also unfavorable and includes tumors less than 5 cm with positive nodes or tumors greater than 5 cm and negative nodes, both however with no metastatic disease. Stage IV represents patients with metastatic disease.

Treatment

Rhabdomyosarcoma is a systemic disease and all patients require chemotherapy. The advancements in the treatment of rhabdomyosarcoma are an example of the value of multi-center clinical trials. The Intergroup Rhabdomyosarcoma Study Group (IRSG) was formed in 1972 and there have been six major trials since that time. In 2000, with the formation of the Children's Oncology Group, it was renamed the Soft Tissue Sarcoma Committee. Prior to IRS-1 the survival for all children was around 30%. IRS-1 was conducted between 1972 and 1978 and the survival went up to over 50% and has gradually improved to survivorship of around 75% during the time of IRS-4, which was conducted between 1991 and 1997. The most recent studies which are the sixth overall study started in 2006. The chemotherapy consists of either vincristine and dactinomycin or vincristine, dactinomycin and cyclophosphamide (VAC) for 48 wks. Local therapy is also essential and consists of surgical resection of primary sites or radiotherapy at sites not amenable to primary resection although clinical group I embryonal tumors do not require radiotherapy. Survival can be stratified by risk group. Low risk group has a survival of around 90% and includes all embryonal tumors except those incompletely resected at an unfavorable primary site. Intermediate risk group has a survival of around 65% and includes all nonmetastatic alveolar tumors and embryonal tumors at unfavorable primary sites that have been incompletely resected. High risk group with a survival around 20% includes metastatic tumors.

NONRHABDOMYOSARCOMAS SOFT TISSUE SARCOMAS

As noted above, the pediatric nonrhabdomyosarcomas are distributed over nine histologic types each counting for between 2–8% of all sarcomas. Predisposing factors can include the Li-Fraumeni Syndrome, which is a constitutional P53 mutation, as well as hereditary retinoblastoma, neurofibromatosis type I and several other syndromes including HIV infection associated with leiomyosarcoma, lymphedema associated with angiosarcoma and the effect of ionizing radiation. The extremity is the most common site followed by the body wall, viscera and head and neck. Presenting symptoms are similar to that of rhabdomyosarcoma with a soft tissue mass and loss of normal function due to the mass. Metastases are present in 15% at presentation with the lung accounting for three-fourths of metastatic disease. The initial evaluation and metastatic work-up is very similar to that of rhabdomyosarcoma. Surgical guidelines are also similar to that of rhabdomyosarcoma except that the importance of adequate resection is even greater since the presence of gross residual is less well controlled with radiation therapy compared with rhabdomyosarcoma. In addition, the radiation therapy doses are higher. Enlarged lymph nodes must be sampled and regional lymph node sampling is required for the epithelioid sarcoma and clear cell sarcoma. In addition, sentinel lymph node biopsies are helpful in some large high grade tumors without clinically enlarged lymph nodes and this also allows the determination of the appropriate lymph node for biopsy. All grossly enlarged lymph nodes must be excised in children with nonrhabdomyosarcoma. Surgery on metastatic sites is also aggressive and most metastatic sites are treated with a wide excision either at diagnosis or at the conclusion of therapy.

The prognostic factors for survival include the presence or absence of metastatic disease, the histologic grade that being low or high, tumor size less than or greater than 5 cm and the extent of resection, that being grossly resected or unresected. The staging system takes into account the size or depth, the presence or absence of nodes and metastatic disease, as well as the grade of the tumor. A risk stratification system also exists for nonrhabdomyosarcomas. This is defined as low risk consisting of resected low grade tumors, as well as resected high grade tumors that are <5 cm and is associated with a survival of around 90%. Intermediate risk tumors are resected high grade tumors that are >5 cm and unresectable tumors regardless of grade and size and these have a survival of around 50%. The high risk groups are those with metastatic disease and these have a very dismal prognosis. Radiation therapy is an important component of the therapy for nonrhabdomyosarcoma tumors. Local control rates are lower than that of rhabdomyosarcoma and in the presence of gross disease have a 45% cure rate, however this is only 9% if the tumor is greater than 10 cm in diameter. If there is microscopic disease the survival is up to 85%, however higher doses of radiation are required and even for microscopic disease, 60–63 GY are administered. In patients with recurrent disease a biopsy may be needed to confirm the recurrence.

In patients with nonmetastatic disease, aggressive therapy would include amputation or pelvic exenteration. Chemotherapy for nonrhabdomyosarcomas include ifosfamide and doxorubicin. Indications for chemotherapy are an unresectable primary tumor or a >5 cm high grade tumor or a high grade metastatic tumor. The role of surgery is important for nonrhabdomyosarcoma tumors in terms of diagnosis as well as facilitating local tumor control when appropriate.

REFERENCES

1. Andrassy RJ, Corpron CA, Hays D, *et al.* (1996) Extremity sarcomas: An analysis of prognostic factors from the Intergroup Rhabdomyosarcoma Study III. *J Pediatr Surg* **31**:191–196.
2. Anderson JR, *et al.* (1998) Improved outcome for patients with embryonal histology but not alveolar histology rhabdomyosarcoma: Results from Intergroup Rhabdomyosarcoma Study IV (IRS-IV). *Proc Soc Clin Oncol* **17**:526a.
3. Andrassy RJ, *et al.* (1995) Conservative surgical management of vaginal and vulvar pediatric rhabdomyosarcoma: A report from the Intergroup Rhabdomyosarcoma Study-III. *J Pediatr Surg* **30**:1034.
4. Crist WM, *et al.* (1995) Intergroup Rhabdomyosarcoma Study (IRS) III. *J Clin Oncol* **13**:610.

5. Crist WM, *et al.* (1999) Preliminary results for patients with local/regional tumors treated on the Intergroup Rhabdomyosarcoma Study-IV (1991–1997). *Proc Am Soc Clin Oncol* **18**:18.
6. Crist WM, *et al.* (2001) Intergroup Rhabdomyosarcoma Study-IV: Results for patients with nonmetastatic disease. *J Clin Oncol* **19**:3091.
7. Keus RB, Rutgers EJ, Ho Gh, *et al.* (1994) Limb-sparing therapy of extremity: Treatment outcome and long-term functional results. *Eur J Cancer* **30A**: 1459–1463.
8. Newton WA, Jr, Soule EH, Hamoudi AB, *et al.* (1988) Histopathology of childhood sarcomas, Intergroup Rhabdomyosarcoma Studies I and II: Clinicopathologic correlation. *J Clin Oncol* **6**:67–75.
9. Pappo AS, Parham D, Lobe TE. (1999) Soft tissue sarcomas in children. *Semin Surg Oncol* **16**:121–143.
10. Wiener ES, *et al.* (1991) Retroperitoneal node biopsy in paratesticular rhabdomyosarcoma. *J Pediatr Surg* **29**:171.

Section 4: Transplantation

HISTORY OF ORGAN TRANSPLANTATION

29

Richard S. Mangus

The idea of organ transplantation in the modern era began with Dr. Alexis Carrel who pioneered the concept of sewing two individual blood vessels together with suture to establish alternative vascular flow. As this technique was refined, the possibility of removing an individual organ on a vascular pedicle with reimplantation at a remote site became a reality. It was a natural extension, then, to consider similar connections between the ureter and the bladder, the common bile duct and the intestine, and similar connections for other organs. Contemporaneously, Karl Landsteiner and Peter Medawar performed groundbreaking research of the human immune system including establishment of ABO compatibility and skin allograft rejection. These concepts eventually led to the first kidney transplant, a living donor transplant between identical twins, in the 1950s. The donor from this transplant died in 2011. Early kidney transplant success was followed by the initiation of liver transplantation in the 1960s and intestinal transplantation in the 1980s. Each of these organs progressed through a significant learning curve with frequent graft losses and patient deaths before consistent success was realized.

In 1984, cyclosporine was introduced clinically as an immunosuppressive agent and all clinical solid organ transplant outcomes immediately improved. For the first time, 1 yr graft and patient survival after liver and kidney transplant was greater than 50% as the risk of rejection could be reliably managed in most patients. Critical care management improved, along with advances in surgical technique and immunosuppression, throughout the 1980s and 1990s. One-year survival rates improved to the 80–90% range in the 1990s. With improved outcomes, competition for scarce donor organs increased. The United States congress passed important federal laws facilitating organ donation and procurement, as well as allocation and distribution. The *National Organ Transplant Act of 1984* (NOTA) strictly forbid the buying and selling of human organs, created the Organ Procurement and Transplantation Network (OPTN), and established a Scientific Registry of Transplant Recipients (SRTR) to follow outcomes. The OPTN is administered through the United Network for Organ Sharing (UNOS) which maintains the national organ waiting list, facilitates organ distribution and transplantation (including computerized donor-recipient matching), and monitors member centers for compliance with OPTN policies.

Another critical law passed at this time was the *Uniform Determination of Death Act.* This established a legal definition of death through one of two mechanisms:

(1) Permanent cessation of function of the cardiopulmonary system, or
(2) Irreversible loss of brain function.

Prior to the establishment of a legal definition of brain death, all deceased donor organs were procured only after cessation of cardiopulmonary function. This subjected all donor organs to a period of warm ischemia time, as the initiation of organ procurement could not occur until the declaration of cardiac death. This necessary period between the declaration of death and the initiation of procurement frequently resulted in irreversible injury to the donor organs which had a direct impact on clinical transplant outcomes. With the legal establishment of brain death, the potential donor could be declared legally dead with a completely intact, and clinically stable, cardiopulmonary system. Organ procurement from a donor who has been declared brain dead permits rapid exsanguination and cooling of the organs with no warm ischemia time, which improves initial and long-term function of the graft. The legislation to establish a definition for brain death has been critical to the growth of transplantation and today, 96% of all deceased donors have been declared brain dead at the time of organ procurement.

These legislative mandates had a direct impact on the ability of transplant physicians to improve clinical outcomes and save lives. Private and

Table 1. Chronologic history of liver transplantation.

Early 1900s	Alexis Carrel becomes the father of experimental organ transplantation with his pioneering work in developing vascular anastomoses.
1906 to 1912	Basic concepts of transplant immunology, including rejection, established by Karl Landsteiner (ABO compatibility), Alexis Carrel (physiologic disturbances of organs caused by biologic factors) and Peter Medawar (skin allograft rejection through the immune system).
Early 1950s	Successful renal transplantation in humans.
Late 1950s	Earliest attempts at experimental liver transplantation.
1963	Dr. Thomas Starzl attempts first human liver transplant in a child at University of Colorado — patient does not survive surgery.
	After two additional unsuccessful attempts by Dr. Starzl, and failures in Boston and Paris, there is a worldwide moratorium on liver transplantation (which lasts 3 1/2 yrs).
1967	First successful liver transplant by Dr. Starzl. Between 1967 and 1979; more than 160 patients undergo liver transplantation at the University of Colorado with marginal success.
1980	Uniform Determination of Death Act (UDDA) provides a comprehensive and medically sound basis for determining death in all situations (establishes brain death law).
1984	Cyclosporin becomes clinically available as the first effective immunosuppressant.
	National Organ Transplant Act of 1984 (NOTA) forbids buying and selling of human organs and establishes the organ procurement and transplantation network (OPTN) to administer transplantation in the United States.
1984	First reduced-size liver transplant by Bismuth.
1987	First successful intestinal transplant at the University of Pittsburgh by Dr. Starzl.
1988	Pichlmayr performs first split-liver transplant.
1989	Tacrolimus (Prograf, FK 506) introduced as an effective immunosuppressant agent and early reports suggest improved survival compared to cyclosporine.
1990	First successful living-related liver transplant by Strong in Australia.

(*Continued*)

Table 1. (*Continued*)

1996	The first lobar transplant in the U.S. from an adult to an adult was performed at Barnes Jewish Hospital.
1990s	Introduction of minimally invasive surgery and living donor nephrectomy which increases living donor renal transplant volume.
2002	Liver allograft allocation by scoring through the model for end-stage liver disease score (MELD) is instituted.

governmental payers accepted liver transplantation as an indicated procedure for the treatment of End-Stage Liver Disease (ESLD) and established reimbursement mechanisms. With adoption of these measures, there was a dramatic increase in the number of patients listed for transplantation. Broad public media campaigns were initiated to encourage organ donation to supply the burgeoning need for this resource. Soon the demand for donor organs outstripped the need, and living donor liver transplantation began to grow. The definition of an acceptable deceased donor was expanded to include liver allografts from the elderly, obese, those with known traumatic liver injury, and patients with known exposure to infectious diseases. More recently, the use of donors who have already experienced cardiac death has started to increase. Today, the bulk of research in clinical liver transplantation centers on expanding the use of available organ donors. Because of the experimental nature of early organ transplantation, the bulk of clinical and scientific advances occurred in the adult population. Fortunately, the lessons learned were quickly expanded to children, and the pediatric population today has clinical outcomes similar to, or superior, to those seen in adult transplantation for all solid abdominal organs.

PEDIATRIC KIDNEY TRANSPLANTATION

30

Richard S. Mangus

INTRODUCTION

Children account for only 1% of all patients who develop end-stage renal disease (ESRD) and require renal replacement therapy (RRT). Over the last decade, there were 1200 new cases of ESRD per year in the pediatric population, equating to an annual incidence of 15 cases per million population. This rate appears to be slowly increasing with a greater risk with increasing age.[1,2] RRT is indicated when the cumulative complications of chronic kidney disease (CKD) result in significant risk of morbidity or mortality, or impact upon the growth and development of the child (Table 1).

The causative etiologies for ESRD in the pediatric population differ by age with renal dysplasias and obstructive uropathies being more common in infants and young children, while glomerulonephritis is more frequent in older children[3] (Tables 2 and 3).

One in five children with ESRD undergo preemptive kidney transplantation prior to initiation of RRT.[4] Unfortunately, not all children have a readily available organ donor and the rate of preemptive transplantation varies by child gender, race and age group. There are 700 pediatric kidney transplants yearly, accounting for ~4% of the total in the United States. Absolute and relative contraindications to kidney transplantation generally relate to the underlying medical condition of the patient, or their immunologic status as a match to a particular donor (Table 4).

Table 1. Complications of chronic kidney disease (CKD).

Hypervolemia
Hyperkalemia
Metabolic bone disease (from renal osteodystrophy)
Failure to thrive
Delayed psychomotor development
Refractory symptoms of uremia
Recurrent catheter infections or loss of vascular access

Table 2. Common causes of pediatric chronic kidney disease (CKD).

Primary disease	Disease incidence (%)	Transplanted children (%)
Unspecified glomerulonephritis	13	4
Focal glomerulosclerosis, focal glomerulonephritis	10	11
Renal hypoplasia, dysplasia, aplasia	9	16
Congenital obstructive uropathy	6	16
Systemic lupus erythematosus	5	2
Hypertension	5	<1
Nephrolitiasis	5	<1
Alport's	3	2
Membranoproliferative glomerulonephritis	3	3
Polycystic kidneys, adult	3	n/a
Pyelonephritis or chronic interstitial nephritis	2	2
Rapidly progressive glomerulonephritis	2	
Hemolytic uremic syndrome	2	3
IgA nephropathy	1	1
Henoch-Schonlein syndrome	1	1
Medullary cystic disease	<1	3
Cystinosis	<1	2
Congenital nephrotic syndrome	<1	3
Prune belly syndrome	<1	3
Polycystic kidneys, infantile	<1	3
Wegener's granulomatosis	<1	<1

Table 3. Etiology of end-stage renal disease (ESRD) in transplanted children by age group.

Disease process	Age at transplant (yrs)				
	0 to 1 (%)	2 to 5 (%)	6 to 12 (%)	13 to 17 (%)	17 and older (%)
Renal dysplasias	28	24	17	11	10
Obstructive uropathy	19	23	17	14	8
Focal segmental glomerulosclerosis	1	8	13	12	16
Other	52	45	53	63	66

Table 4. Contraindications to kidney transplantation.

Absolute

(1) Active or untreated malignancy.

(2) Chronic HIV infection.

(3) Chronic active infection with hepatitis B.

(4) Severe multi-organ failure that precludes a combined transplant with a kidney.

(5) Positive current direct cross-match or positive direct cross-match within the previous 3 to 12 mths.

(6) Debilitating, irreversible brain injury.

Relative

(1) ABO incompatibility with the donor.

(2) Active autoimmune disease such as Systemic Lupus Erythematosus or anti-Glomerular Basement Membrane disease with high levels of Anti-GBM antibodies.

(3) Psychomotor retardation or psychiatric illness of such severity that custodial care is required.

(4) Chronic infection with hepatitis C virus.

(5) Serious long-standing noncompliance with medical management.

(6) Lack of adequate home supervision or family support of a transplant patient

Despite these listed contraindications, children almost universally have a better quality of life with kidney transplantation and every effort is made to achieve this goal. Patient survival is superior for those children who undergo kidney transplantation (5-yr survival >90%) when compared to those who remain on maintenance RRT (5-yr survival hemo or peritoneal dialysis 80–85%).[5]

Living donors are the primary source of donor kidney grafts for children, accounting for 60% of transplants, 80% of which come from parents of the child. While deceased donors account for one-third of kidney transplants in children less than 10 yrs of age, they comprise nearly 50% of those in children age 11 yrs and older. Of all children on the waitlist for a deceased donor kidney, 70% are in this older age group. Children on the kidney transplant list can wait from 6 to 18 mths, with wait time increasing with increasing age. In general, young children do not make ideal kidney donors due to the smaller graft size which equates with less functional capacity and a higher risk for transplant related complications. For pediatric deceased donor recipients, 75% receive their graft from a donor age 11 or older. There is a reasonable correlation between the blood types of donors and recipients, with half of recipients being blood type O, followed by A (36%), B (12%) and AB (4%). Donor matching carries less emphasis today than in previous years because of better immunosuppression and a desire to avoid the complications related to long-term RRT. There are six primary HLA alleles, two each for A-, B-, and DR-, with a higher number of matches related to a decreased risk of rejection and improved graft survival. In children, living donor matches result in three or more matched alleles in 75% of recipients. Nearly the exact opposite is the case for deceased donors in which only 25% of recipients match at three or more alleles. The pretransplant evaluation of the potential living donor and the recipient is extensive and may include the testing listed in the tables (Table 5).

There are known sociodemographic differences in access to care, similar to those seen with other medical therapies. Female are less likely than male children to undergo preemptive kidney transplantation and to be listed for deceased donor transplantation.[6] White children are more likely than other races to receive a kidney transplant and African-American children less likely to receive a living donor kidney. There is a higher incidence of ESRD in African- and Native-American children when compared to Whites. A large component of this disparity relates to the rapidly rising incidence of glomerulonephritis in the later teen years in African–American children leading to a 3x greater risk of ESRD compared to White children for this age group.[7]

Table 5. Living donor assessment.

Assessment	Identify donor/recipient pair Adult transplantation nephrologist, surgeon, coordinator, dietician, social services
Histocompatibility testing	ABO/Rh, HLA typing A, B, DR, MLC, ABO antibody, preliminary and final cross-match
Medical history	Complete H/P: (height, weight, allergies, blood pressure), GU exam, rectal, pelvic, pap smear, mammogram (age appropriate)
Laboratory studies	Na, K, Cl, CO_2, BUN, Cr, Ca, Mg, Phos, CBC/diff/plt, PT, PTT, Glu, Trig, Alb, Alk Phos, Bili, AST, ALT, GGT, pregnancy test, PPD with controls
Serology studies	CMV (IgG, IgM), EBV (IgG, IgM), HIV, ELISA, Western Blot, Hep A (IgG, IgM), Hep B (sAg, antibody), Hep C (IgG, IgM, PCR), VZV (IgG, IgM), HSV 1, 2, (IgG, IgM), RPR
Renal function studies	U/A, urine culture, 24-hr urine for protein and creatinine clearance
Other studies	CXR, EKG, Abd U/S angiogram vs. MRA, or spiral CT
Special studies	Cardiac/pulmonary evaluation if indicated
Standard pretransplant evaluation of pediatric kidney transplant candidates	
History and physical examination	
Laboratory tests	
— hematology	(CBC with platelets and differential)
— coagulation	(INR/PT, PTT, TT)
— chemistry	(serum electrolytes, BUN, creatinine, liver function tests, lipid panel, serum electrophoresis, N-terminal PTH)
— urine	(urinalysis, urine culture, 24-hr urine for protein)
— blood bank/ immunology	(ABO type, hepatitis profile, HIV, HLA type, antileukocyte antibody screening)
Virology (CMV, EBC, HSV, VZV, MMR titers). PPD.	
X-ray (VCUG, CXR, bone age, gallbladder ultrasound)	
EEG	
Consults	
— cardiologist	
— neurologist	
— nutritionist	
— dentist	
— psychologist	
— Social worker	
Vaccines	
— pneumococcal	
— hepatitis B	
— varicella vaccine if patient has no history of prior varicella and/or has no positive varicella titer	

SURGICAL ISSUES IN KIDNEY TRANSPLANTATION

As previously mentioned, many pediatric patients with CKD undergo preemptive kidney transplantation. Preemptive transplantation, when feasible, is preferred and is associated with superior graft and patient survival. Pretransplant evaluation of the potential recipient is critical to optimize outcomes and should begin when the patient's glomerular filtration rate is less than $30\,mL/min/1.73\,m^2$. A large percentage of CKD in younger pediatric patients is directly related to anatomic anomalies and these frequently must be remedied prior to implanting a new kidney. Additionally, native kidney nephrectomy is performed in one-fourth of recipients to prevent ongoing pathology from the presence of the diseased kidneys. Historically, splenectomy was performed at certain centers as a means of reducing graft rejection. Splenectomy has not been found to significantly reduce the risk of post-transplant rejection, but has been associated with an increased risk of post-transplant sepsis, and should not be performed routinely. Preemptive transplantation allows the pediatric patient to avoid the most common vascular complications associated with hemodialysis including loss of access and recurrent blood stream infections (BSI). Complications associated with peritoneal dialysis are also common and include peritonitis and the formation of intraperitoneal adhesions. In addition to these acute complications, both forms of dialysis impose a strain on the child's family. The time and costs associated with dialysis can also drain limited family resources and lead to lost time at work.

Approach to the surgical implantation of the donor kidney depends upon recipient size. Whereas in adults the vascular anastomoses are generally constructed to the external iliac vessels through a right lower quadrant retroperitoneal approach, these vessels are frequently too small in children. Therefore, for children these anastomoses can be performed either to the infrarenal aorta and vena cava, or to the common iliac vessels, or to some combination of these vessels. For children smaller the 10 kg, a midline incision is generally required with complete mobilization of the right colon and duodenum to provide adequate exposure to the retroperitoneum and to allow adequate space for placement of the adult size kidney. For children between 10 and 30 kg, the incision location and approach to the retroperitoneal vasculature is surgeon dependent. Once the kidney has been implanted and reperfused, ureteral reimplantation is undertaken. The ureteroneocystostomy in now performed in an extravesical manner at most centers and is similar to that used for adults. This anastomosis involves opening the wall of the bladder, anastomosis of the ureter to the bladder mucosa, followed by construction of a submucosal tunnel over the ureter as an antireflux measure. A large percentage of centers stent this anastomosis which appears to decrease risk of obstruction and stricture, but may be associated with a higher rate of post-transplant urinary infections. In cases of an ischemic or shortened donor ureter, a ureteroureterostomy can be constructed in an end-to-side or an end-to-end fashion with good outcomes. These anastomoses are also frequently stented and in both cases, ureteral stents remain in place for 6 wks prior to removal. Besides infection, stent complications can include bleeding from erosion and stent migration. All of these complications are easily reversed by simple cystoscopic removal of the stent. Perioperative and postoperative issues are listed in the tables (Tables 6 and 7).

One-third of children who require kidney transplantation have an anomaly of the urinary tract. Common findings include vesicoureteral reflux, posterior urethral valves, neurogenic bladder, outflow obstruction, bladder extrophy and Prune belly syndrome. Most children with CKD have undergone extensive testing of the urinary tract, but these studies should be reviewed by the surgeon and should include imaging such as intravenous pyelogram (IVP), ultrasound, and voiding cystourethrogram (VCUG). When anatomic anomalies have been identified, kidney transplantation should be

Table 6. Anesthesia and peri-operative considerations for pediatric kidney transplantation.

(1) on release of the aortic and inferior vena cava clamps, the ischemic lower extremities and new kidney are reperfused, which may cause hypovolemia and acidosis.

(2) the new kidney may initially sequester about 300 mL of blood which can cause severe hypotension.

(3) the new kidney may produce urine in amounts equal to the infant's blood volume every hour.

(4) washout of the cold preservation solution from the kidney into the recipient may cause life-threatening hyperkalemia and hypothermia.

(5) the infant's abdomen must accommodate a new, large organ, which in addition to receiving a large percentage of the cardiac output, may impede respiration and decrease venous return.

Table 7. Postoperative management.

(1) Nursing	
	Vital signs every 30 mins for 4 hr, then every hr for 24 hrs
	CVP and urine output every hr for 24 hrs
	Urine for glucose, abdominal girth, peripheral pulses
(2) Laboratory	
	Serum electrolytes, hematology, coagulation, and arterial blood gas immediately post operative and at 4 hrs postoperatively
	Serum electrolytes, calcium, and phosphorus every 4 hrs for 24 hrs
	Daily electrolytes and hematology, coagulation and liver function tests twice weekly; cyclosporin/tacrolimus levels daily
(3) Fluids	
	0.5 to 1 mL I.V. for 1 mL urine each hr (5% dextrose in water/45% normal saline
	± 10 mEq sodium bicarbonate/L based upon urine production
	dextrose may be changed to .25% dextrose for high volume replacement
(4) Medications	
	Trimethroprim sulfa (2–4 mg/kg/day)
	Antacid
	Nystatin four times/day, docusate, pain medication, and immunosuppression
(5) Radiology	
	CXR postoperative and on the first postoperative day

performed in close consultation with pediatric urology to minimize the negative effects of a poorly functioning urinary system on the kidney allograft. Examples of procedures that may be required prior to, or at the time of transplantation, include formation of a neobladder or bladder augmentation, vesicostomy closure, and cystoscopy with fulguration of posterior urethral valve leaflets. Additionally, the abdominal and iliac vasculature should be scrutinized to assure adequate blood inflow and outflow for the graft. Previous placement of femoral central venous or arterial access may damage small pediatric vessels. Fixed thrombus can form around long-standing catheters which will impact on the quality of the available vessels. These vessels may be assessed with contrasted imaging or Doppler ultrasound.

Dysfunction of the native kidneys may be an indication for native kidney nephrectomy either prior to, or at the time of kidney transplantation. Conditions such as severe nephrotic syndrome, recurrent infections, treatment resistant hypertension, severe polyuria with dehydration and electrolyte wasting may respond only to nephrectomy. Large polycystic kidneys can lead to poor feeding, severe reflux and respiratory compromise and resection may be indicated. Finally, some children with genetic syndromal anomalies may carry an increased risk for the development of Wilm's tumor and should undergo native nephrectomy. Though the majority of nephrectomies are performed surgically, medical options have been described such as renal artery embolization, metallic salts and the use of high dose nonsteroidal anti-inflammatory medications (NSAIDS).

The use of multiorgan transplantation in children has increased over the last decade. CKD frequently accompanies other end-organ failure such that combined transplants are often indicated. Commonly encountered multiorgan transplants include heart-kidney, liver-kidney, pancreas-kidney and intestine kidney. Some children with a bone marrow disease process develop CKD and combined bone marrow-kidney transplant from the same donor may provide an ideal match. The ability to simultaneously treat end-organ failure and avoid dialysis in these complex patients makes the consideration of kidney transplantation an important component of the surgical evaluation.

KIDNEY DONOR CONSIDERATIONS

Historically, children awaiting a deceased donor kidney were allocated grafts from other children. These transplant matches were found to have inferior outcomes. The majority of the complications were related to technical issues, primarily early graft loss from graft thrombosis. With the growth of living donor transplantation, outcomes with adult kidney grafts have demonstrated superiority and have become the rule rather than the exception. Extended criteria donors (ECD) are unlikely to be used for children given the higher risk of graft failure or shorter anticipated period of graft function. Examples of ECD kidneys include those from donors over age 50, procured using a donation after cardiac death (DCD) protocol, or with a donor history of diabetes or hypertension.

Living kidney donors must undergo extensive screening. Anatomically, the donor must have two kidneys with normal appearance and size, normal urinary drainage and normal vasculature. Laboratory testing includes measurement of serum creatinine with calculation of the GFR and analysis of the urine for protein, blood or other abnormalities. Medically, living donors must meet acceptable criteria for both physical and psychological health and require evaluation by the surgical team as well as psychiatric and social screening. The donor and recipient must have a negative T-cell crossmatch and be ABO compatible. Importantly, the donor must not be coerced in any way and must not receive remuneration outside of their medical expenses and/or lost time from work. Donors should be made fully aware that costs such as travel, lodging and lost time from work are often not covered by the recipient's insurance. Transplant tourism, traveling abroad to pay for and receive an organ transplant, is particularly prevalent in kidney transplantation. There are a large number of willing living donors in third world nations (because of their indigent circumstances) and the donor and recipient procedure is relatively straightforward when compared to transplantation of other organs. Unfortunately, transplant outcomes from this black market practice are inferior to those for nonincentivized donors and this practice is inherently coersive because of the large donor-recipient financial disparity. All major national and international transplant organizations have issued statements condemning transplant tourism.

The rapid advancement of minimally invasive surgery has been a boon to living donor kidney transplantation. The donor operation imparts minimal tissue trauma and the immediate recovery period is shortened to a 2–3 day hospital stay. Time off work may range from 2–8 wks, but most people return to work within 4 wks. Using either a transperitoneal or retroperitoneal approach, the donor operation can now be performed with a maximal incision size of 7–10 cm. The donor kidney is removed, flushed and cooled. Reimplantation is timed to minimize overall ischemia time and usually occurs within 1–2 hrs. A "mini-nephrectomy" has also been described in which the entire donor operation is performed using an open technique, but through a 7–10 cm incision making it similar to the laparoscopic approach. While the minimally invasive donor operation engenders much less morbidity than the classic open nephrectomy, it is still major surgery and carries important risks such as postoperative hemorrhage, hernia, ileus, infection, nerve damage, testicular swelling/pain, and CKD and hypertension.

PATHOLOGY OF THE TRANSPLANT KIDNEY

Early dysfunction of the kidney graft may be divided into pathology related to graft rejection or to a nonrejection process. Differentiation between these etiologies may be initially assessed from laboratory values, urine studies or imaging. Frequently, a kidney biopsy is required when these studies are inconclusive. Biopsy sampling error can lead the investigation astray and the kidney biopsy should consist of at least one core sample. A second core sample is known to improve the sensitivity of the biopsy. Obtaining a biopsy in the pediatric patient is not without risk. Standard risks of bleeding, infection and graft injury exist, but there can be added risks in smaller children. With placement of the kidney in the retroperitoneum with anastomosis to the aorta and vena cava, access to the kidney can be problematic. To avoid intestinal or vascular injury in children, guided biopsy with computed tomographic imaging may be required, whereas ultrasound guided biopsy should be adequate for larger children with pelvic placement of the kidney.

Rejection is divided into cell- and antibody-mediated rejection. Early and accurate diagnosis of rejection is critical to initiate timely intervention. A decrease in the incidence of acute rejection translates into a decreased risk of chronic rejection in children.[8] *Cell-mediated rejection* occurs through action of the T-cells and is most common in the first 2 months post-transplant. However, cell-mediated rejection can occur at any time and should always be a top consideration in any kidney graft with dysfunction. Cell-mediated rejection is described by its primary injury site: the interstitium, the artery and the glomerulus. These sites may be affected individually or in combination, but the form of the cell-mediated rejection is related directly to the areas involved. *Tubulo-interstitial rejection* is the most common cell-mediated form and is characterized by a lymphocyte infiltrate extending from the peritubular capillaries to the interstitium with edema and infiltration of the walls of the tubules (tubulitis). *Arterial rejection* is characterized by infiltration of T-cells (primarily lymphocytes) into the arterial walls where they undermine the endothelium (endothelialitis or endarteritis). Arterial rejection is present in 50% of patients with interstitial rejection and portends a prolonged course as arterial rejection is less responsive than interstitial rejection to corticosteroid therapy. *Glomerular rejection* is the least common type of cell-mediated rejection, but is considered the most severe form. Glomerular rejection is characterized by severe glomerular inflammation with cell damage from lymphocyte and monocyte infiltration. Coexistence of glomerular rejection with arterial rejection is common, but coexistence with interstitial rejection is rare.

Antibody-mediated rejection (humoral rejection) results from the presence of donor-specific antibodies (DSA) directed towards the vascular endothelium.[9,10] Three types of antibody-mediated rejection are described: hyperacute, acute and chronic. *Hyperacute rejection* occurs when preformed antibodies adhere to the endothelium causing thrombus formation, vascular thrombosis, and leading to cortical necrosis. This diagnosis is made by an acute graft thrombosis with a large concentration of neutrophils within the thrombus. The process may begin in the glomerular or peritubular capillaries but invariably results in early graft loss. *Acute antibody mediated rejection* is characterized by immune complex formation in the capillaries or arterioles. Identification of a complement breakdown product (C4d) is considered requisite for a diagnosis of humoral rejection. The complement cascade is activated by the antibody attack against the endothelium. Complement deposition occurs, including C4 fixation. C4d is a breakdown product of C4 and is covalently bound representing a persistent marker of immune complex formation at a specific site. C4d positive acute antibody mediated rejection is most commonly found in the peritubular capillaries. Most pathologists recommend the routine screening of all kidney transplant biopsies for C4d. Chronic antibody mediated rejection results in a gradual loss of kidney function over years' time. *Chronic rejection* is characterized by diffuse injury across the graft, including glomerular and arterial lesions, interstitial fibrosis, tubular atrophy, and arterial wall thickening with fibrosis. C4d deposition occurs in up to 50% of kidney grafts affected by chronic rejection.

Acute kidney injury occurs on a frequent basis in the transplant kidney and subsequent investigation attempts to identify the etiology of the injury to provide appropriate intervention. *Acute tubular necrosis* (ATN) refers to a spectrum of injury to the tubules of the kidney resulting in acute kidney failure. ATN results from a structural change to the tubule generally resulting from a period of ischemia or acute injury. Examples of inciting causes include: hypotension, sepsis, nephrotoxic agents (antibiotics, contrast dyes), transfusion reaction, and rhabdomyolysis. ATN results in oliguria and can last from a few days to several weeks, but complete recovery is expected. *Calcineurin inhibitor (CI) toxicity* is a common cause of acute injury in the transplant patient. CIs provide the basis for the majority of immunosuppressive regimens. Unfortunately, these agents are nephrotoxic and levels must be closely monitored to decrease the risk of both acute and chronic kidney damage. Acute injury is generally identified by an episode of acute kidney failure accompanied by high CI serum levels. As the levels decrease, kidney function returns to normal. Differentiation of chronic CI toxicity from chronic rejection and progressive nephrosclerosis can be difficult and these processes may coexist.[11] The term *chronic allograft* nephropathy is a "catch-all" phrase frequently used to indicate chronic graft injury without respect to the etiology.

POSTKIDNEY TRANSPLANT CLINICAL MANAGEMENT

Much of the early management of the adult kidney-to-pediatric recipient transplant relates to the size discrepancy of the graft for the recipient. The adult kidney graft may require a disproportionate percentage of the available blood flow from a small child. At the time of vascular clamp removal intraoperatively, this blood flow discrepancy can lead to hypotension for the recipient and inadequate blood flow to the kidney graft. The longer this situation persists, the higher the risk of thrombosis of the vasculature or graft ATN. Therefore, intra and peri-operative fluid management of the kidney recipient is critical. Intravascular volume repletion prior to graft reperfusion will decrease the risk of hypotension and avoid DGF. Continued meticulous fluid management will aid in establishing and maintaining consistent urine production and avoid early complications related to overdiuresis, electrolyte abnormalities and DGF. Early post-transplant fluid orders frequently replace urine output at 1 cc fluid per 1 cc output, and this may continue for some time. Frequent measurement of vital signs, central venous pressure, serum electrolytes and patient weight may provide early indication of fluid imbalance. Adequate venous access must be provided to allow the simultaneous infusion of fluids and medications along with frequent blood draws to assess electrolytes. In conjunction with fluid management is modulation of the blood pressure. Hypotension is particularly detrimental, risking ATN, DGF and graft thrombosis. Low dose dopamine has been advocated for "renal perfusion" but benefits to the use of this agent have never been proven rigorously. Hypertension can be associated with immunosuppressant administration, large volume fluid infusion, and postoperative pain and agitation. Care must be taken to actively monitor the blood pressure and provide treatment as indicated.

Some centers choose to leave the newly transplanted child intubated in the immediate post-transplant period. Rationale for this approach range from the argument that large fluid shifts can affect respiratory status, to the concern for antilymphocyte induction agents which can result in "leaky" pulmonary capillaries and pulmonary edema. The decision for the type and location of post-transplant care is center-specific and is made by the primary transplant surgeon. Certainly, continuous pulse oximetry monitoring with hourly measures of vital signs and urine production are indicated, and nurses experienced in the care of transplant patients should provide this care. Care of the urinary catheter must be meticulous as the catheter can easily become obstructed with small amounts of postoperative bleeding and thrombus. A well functioning newly transplanted kidney can produce well over 100 cc/hr of urine and this urine will rapidly fill a pediatric bladder with obstruction of the urinary catheter. High bladder pressures will then lead not only to hydroureter and hydronephrosis, but can disrupt the ureterocystostomy leading to a urinary leak which can require reoperation. Any abrupt decrease in urine production should be investigated by a physician, with most blockages resolved with gentle irrigation of the catheter with a syringe. Perioperative use of immunosuppressive agents and antibiotics is program specific and will not be addressed.

Any unexplained poor function of the newly transplanted kidney should be evaluated radiographically. Renal ultrasound with Doppler evaluation is noninvasive and will establish the presence of both arterial and venous blood flow and can assess for hydronephrosis and hydroureter and for fluid collections suggestive of abscess, urinary leak or lymphocele. A nuclear medicine renal scan (Mag3 scan) is frequently utilized to establish perfusion of the kidney with subsequent excretion of the radioactive marker through the ureters and into the bladder. For a kidney with no blood flow, there will be no activity visualized. For a kidney with blood flow but urinary obstruction, there will be filling of the kidney and urinary system to the level of the obstruction. A urinary leak will be seen as extravasation of the marker outside of the contained urinary system. A partial obstruction may be seen as slow passage of contrast.

KIDNEY TRANSPLANT COMPLICATIONS AND OUTCOMES

As previously mentioned, early post-transplant oliguria or anuria may be the earliest indication of graft dysfunction and should be thoroughly evaluated. If a bedside diagnosis is not readily available, imaging should be pursued expeditiously. Some complications, such as vascular compromise, may be amenable to correction with early reoperative intervention. If adequate blood flow is demonstrated, a step-wise approach is undertaken to rule out complications. In general, a newly transplanted kidney with good urine production and a decreasing serum creatinine level carries a lower risk of significant complication.

Delayed graft function (DGF) may result from a variety a clinical factors including prolonged warm or cold ischemia time, poor donor renal function at procurement, low recipient blood pressure, inadequacy of graft blood flow, drug toxicity, young donor age, and poor immunologic match or high recipient sensitization. Any need for dialysis in the first 7 days post-transplant constitutes DGF. Though long-term outcomes for kidney grafts that experience DGF are similar to non-DGF kidneys, there are considerable costs associated with DGF including dialysis, testing of the graft (including biopsy) and prolonged hospitalization. The rate of DGF varies for deceased (17%) and living donor (5%) grafts.[12]

Post-transplant vascular complications must be diagnosed early and dealt with definitively. Hemorrhage can lead to hemodynamic instability, and the accumulation of blood can result in compression of the kidney and the renal vein. The pressure resulting from graft or vascular compression will slow flow through the graft and can lead to thrombosis. Whereas renal vein thrombosis is more likely related to external compression, renal artery thrombosis is more likely to be technical in nature. Any thrombosis must be resolved quickly or the graft will be lost. Intervention generally entails reexploration, but anticoagulation may suffice if the thrombus is diagnosed several days after transplant and there is flow remaining in the graft. Any resulting fluid collections increase not only the risk of graft compromise, but also infection, and should generally be evacuated. The risk of vascular thrombosis ranges from 1–5% and increases with younger recipient and donor age, prolonged ischemia time, coagulation disorders, a history of peritoneal dialysis, and with the development of ATN.[13,14] Renal artery stenosis should be investigated in the transplant recipient with severe or increasing blood pressure and may be present even with normal renal function. Though Doppler ultrasound is a reasonable screen for this condition, the gold standard is renal arteriography. Percutaneous intervention is generally adequate to treat renal artery stenosis and may include balloon angioplasty or stent placement.

Urinary complications are common and include problems as diverse as obstruction, leak, and infection. Any post-transplant fluid collection adjacent to the transplant kidney or bladder should be sampled. Common etiologies for a fluid collection include hematoma, urinary leak (urinoma), lymphocele, seroma or abscess. These fluid collections can compress the transplant ureter, obstructing urinary outflow and resulting in hydroureter and/or hydronephrosis. Contained fluid collections that are not infected, and are not impacting on graft function, can be safely observed with serial ultrasound studies. If conservative management fails, percutaneous drainage is a safe and effect means of evacuating the collection. Certain fluid collections, such as a lymphocele, may require repeat percutaneous drainage with infusion of a sclerosing agent. Surgery may be indicated for a nonresolving fluid collection. The risk of infection of the fluid collection increases with the number of interventions required.

A radionuclide scan demonstrating urinary leak with any extravasation of contrast outside of the urinary system is an indication for exploration. Etiologies of urinary leak include disruption of the ureterocystostomy, necrosis of the distal ureter, and erosion of a ureteral stent. Repair may include reimplantation of the donor ureter into the native bladder or into the native ureter (ureteroureterostomy), or anastomosis of the urinary pelvis to the native ureter (pyelo-ureterostomy). Some surgeons routinely place a ureteral stent at the time of transplant. The ureteral stent extends from the renal pelvis to the urinary bladder. This stent is felt to prevent kinking of the ureter and helps to maintain urinary flow through the ureter in the presence of external compression. It may also prevent or decrease stenosis. Stent complications include erosion with bleeding or perforation, infection, and stent migration with obstruction. Ureter stents can be removed with bedside or operative cystoscopy 3–6 wks post-transplant. Stent complications such as infection, bleeding and migration generally resolve with stent removal. Late urinary complications can be much more difficult to management after severe postoperative scarring has occurred. In these cases, percutaneous nephrostomy with placement of an internal–external stent may be required to provide adequate drainage, prior to operative intervention.

Infections are common in the post-transplant period.[15,16] The newly immunosuppressed patient is at high risk for not only urinary infection, but other common postoperative sites such as the lungs and surgical incision site. Preoperative antibiotics are indicated, but postoperative antibiotics should only be initiated with the onset of fevers, leukocytosis, wound erythema or urinary infection. When signs of infection exist, broad spectrum antibiotics should be initiated pending culture results. The spectrum can then be narrowed as culture results become available. Prophylactic daily antibiotics therapy is indicated in some children with recurrent urinary infections, particularly in those with documented ureteral reflux on VCUG. Factors which predispose children to infection are found in the table (Table 8). Early infections tend to be related to bacteria more than viral or fungal origins.

Late post-transplant infections are common. Whereas early infections are related to the surgical intervention, late infections are associated more with immunosuppression levels, exposures, patient age, and the underlying disease process. Vigilant surveillance of the transplant recipient patient will minimize the complications of opportunistic infections such as cytomegalovirus, Ebstein–Barr virus, pneumocystis pneumonia, toxoplasmosis and oral/esophageal candidiasis. BK virus infection is the most common and clinically important infection of the kidney graft. Its incidence has increased significantly in recent years with increasing use of tacrolimus. Emergence of BK virus is directly related to immunosuppression level, and treatment generally involves an overall reduction in immunosuppression. Unfortunately, this treatment approach can lead to graft rejection.[17]

Table 8. Factors associated with infection risk in the post-transplant period.

Pretransplant
Primary disease process
History of immunizations
Previous infections
Patient age
Organ(s) affected by disease
Malnutrition
Intraoperative
Type of surgery
Technical surgical issues
Duration of surgery
Exposure to donor tissue/blood products
Postoperative
Immunosuppression
Technical surgical issues
Catheters (central, urinary, endotracheal)
Nosocomial/other exposures

Prior to the introduction of CI-based immunosuppression (cyclosporine and tacrolimus), the primary cause of kidney graft loss was acute and chronic rejection. As immunosuppression has improved, recurrence of the primary disease has taken an increased role in the loss of the kidney graft.[18,19] Focal segmental glomerulosclerosis (FSGS), a common cause of ESRD in children, has a recurrence rate as high as 50%. The recurrence rate for hemolytic uremic syndrome can also approach 50%.[20] For this reasons, the pediatric nephrologist takes an important role in the long-term management of the renal transplant recipient to optimize the functional life of the graft. Close surveillance of the kidney graft must include evaluation for both rejection and disease recurrence, as well an infectious and anatomic complications.

Kidney transplant outcomes are measured as graft survival (patient off dialysis) at 1-, 3- and 5-yrs post-transplant. The U.S. results for all organs are available on the internet site for the Organ Procurement and Transplantation Network. The results from 1997 to 2004 are shown in the table (Based upon OPTN data as of March 1, 2011; http://optn.transplant.hrsa.gov), (Table 9). The mean hospital length of stay after a kidney transplant has now decreased to 7 days. This is followed by close outpatient follow-up with frequent measures of kidney function. Medical management of the transplant patient is critical to minimize complications and readmissions. Patient adherence is an important issue in the pediatric

Table 9. United States kidney transplant outcomes, 1997–2004, based upon data from the Organ Procurement and Transplantation Network (OPTN).

Recipient age (yrs)	1-yr (%)	3-yr (%)	5-yr (%)
<1	*	*	*
1–5	93	88	84
6–10	95	86	82
11–17	94	82	68
Donor type			
Living	95	88	80
Deceased	89	78	66

*Numbers too small to calculate.

transplant population. It is estimated that nonadherence in the adolescent population is as high as 50%, which compares to 10–15% in adults.[21] A significant proportion of pediatric graft losses are likely due to nonadherence rather than chronic rejection, though under-reporting makes this assessment problematic.

REFERENCES

1. Benfield MR, McDonald RA, Bartosh S, Ho PL, Harmon W. (2003) Changing trends in pediatric transplantation: 2001 Annual Report of the North American Pediatric Renal Transplant Cooperative Study. *Pediatr Transplant* **7**:321–335.
2. Magee JC, Bucuvalas JC, Farmer DG, Harmon WE, Hulbert-Shearon TE, Mendeloff EN. (2004) Pediatric transplantation. *Am J Transplant* 4 Suppl **9**:54–71.
3. van der Heijden BJ, van Dijk PC, Verrier-Jones K, Jager KJ, Briggs JD. (2004) Renal replacement therapy in children: Data from 12 registries in Europe. *Pediatr Nephrol* **19**:213–221.
4. Kasiske BL, Snyder JJ, Matas AJ, Ellison MD, Gill JS, Kausz AT. (2002) Preemptive kidney transplantation: The advantage and the advantaged. *J Am Soc Nephrol* **13**:1358–1364.
5. McDonald SP, Craig JC. (2004) Australian and New Zealand paediatric nephrology A. Long-term survival of children with end-stage renal disease. *New Engl J Med* **350**:2654–2662.
6. Garg PP, Furth SL, Fivush BA, Powe NR. (2000) Impact of gender on access to the renal transplant waiting list for pediatric and adult patients. *J Am Soc Nephrol* **11**:958–964.
7. Furth SL, Garg PP, Neu AM, Hwang W, Fivush BA, Powe NR. (2000) Racial differences in access to the kidney transplant waiting list for children and adolescents with end-stage renal disease. *Pediatrics* **106**:756–761.
8. Tejani A, Ho PL, Emmett L, Stablein DM, North American Pediatric Renal Transplant Cooperative S. (2002) Reduction in acute rejections decreases chronic rejection graft failure in children: A report of the North American Pediatric Renal Transplant Cooperative Study (NAPRTCS). *Am J Transplant* **2**:142–147.
9. Mauiyyedi S, Colvin RB. (2002) Humoral rejection in kidney transplantation: New concepts in diagnosis and treatment. *Curr Opin Nephrol Hy* **11**:609–618.
10. Racusen LC, Colvin RB, Solez K, Mihatsch MJ, Halloran PF, Campbell PM, Cecka MJ, *et al.* (2003) Antibody-mediated rejection criteria — an addition to

the Banff 97 classification of renal allograft rejection. *Am J Transplant* **3**:708–714.

11. Koop K, Bakker RC, Eikmans M, Baelde HJ, de Heer E, Paul LC, Bruijn JA. (2004) Differentiation between chronic rejection and chronic cyclosporine toxicity by analysis of renal cortical mRNA. *Kidney Int* **66**:2038–2046.
12. Benfield MR, Herrin J, Feld L, Rose S, Stablein D, Tejani A. (1999) Safety of kidney biopsy in pediatric transplantation: A report of the Controlled Clinical Trials in Pediatric Transplantation Trial of Induction Therapy Study Group. *Transplantation* **67**:544–547.
13. Singh A, Stablein D, Tejani A. (1997) Risk factors for vascular thrombosis in pediatric renal transplantation: A special report of the North American Pediatric Renal Transplant Cooperative Study. *Transplantation* **63**:1263–1267.
14. Fischereder M, Gohring P, Schneeberger H, Lohse P, Von Appen K, Samtleben W, Schlondorff D, *et al.* (1998) Early loss of renal transplants in patients with thrombophilia. *Transplantation* **65**:936–939.
15. Dharnidharka VR, Stablein DM, Harmon WE. (2004) Post-transplant infections now exceed acute rejection as cause for hospitalization: A report of the NAPRTCS. *Am J Transplant* **4**:384–389.
16. Lopez MJ, Thomas S. (2003) Immunization of children after solid organ transplantation. *Pediatr Clin N Am* **50**:1435–1449.
17. Nickeleit V, Klimkait T, Binet IF, Dalquen P, Del Zenero V, Thiel G, Mihatsch MJ, *et al.* (2000) Testing for polyomavirus type BK DNA in plasma to identify renal-allograft recipients with viral nephropathy. *New Engl J Med* **342**:1309–1315.
18. Mathew TH. (1988) Recurrence of disease following renal transplantation. *Am J Kidney Dis* **12**:85–96.
19. Seikaly MG. (2004) Recurrence of primary disease in children after renal transplantation: An evidence-based update. *Pediatr Transplant* **8**:113–119.
20. Loirat C, Niaudet P. (2003) The risk of recurrence of hemolytic uremic syndrome after renal transplantation in children. *Pediatr Nephrol* **18**:1095–1101.
21. Gerson AC, Furth SL, Neu AM, Fivush BA. (2004) Assessing associations between medication adherence and potentially modifiable psychosocial variables in pediatric kidney transplant recipients and their families. *Pediatr Transplant* **8**:543–550.

PEDIATRIC LIVER TRANSPLANTATION 31

Richard S. Mangus

INTRODUCTION

Liver transplantation (LT) has experienced dramatic growth in recent years as indications for this procedure have broadened, clinical outcomes have improved, and third party payers (including Medicaid and Medicare) have become more willing to fund organ transplantation. Improvements in the transplant surgical procedure, postoperative management and immunosuppressive agents have led to thousands of lives being saved on a yearly basis. The majority of these patients return to a good functional status, including many patients who return to work and school and a high level of physical activity. Unfortunately, such progress has inevitably brought about an increased demand for LT and shortages of ideal donor organs. Current growth in the field of LT is directly proportional to expansion of the organ donor pool through the use of living donors and the use of nonideal deceased donors, so called extended criteria donors (ECD). Indications for LT have expanded to include elderly patients with co-morbidities, patients with hepatocellular carcinoma (HCC), hepatoblastoma, and other tumors, and retransplantation in patients with recurrent disease. Current research in the field of LT attempts to provide more donor organs through improvement in organ preservation and procurement techniques, expanded use of ECD organs and living donors. The pressure from this increased demand impacts directly on organ availability for the pediatric population. An increasing number of children now receive transplant allografts from adult living donors and split liver grafts from deceased adults.

HISTORY AND CURRENT TRENDS

LT was first successfully performed in the 1960s by Dr. Thomas Starzl. He worked tirelessly throughout the subsequent two decades to establish this procedure as the standard of care for patients with end-stage liver disease (ESLD). Unfortunately, LT was a complex surgical procedure undertaken for physiologically decompensated, high-risk patients. Early transplants were marked by massive blood loss, hemodynamic instability, prolonged hospital stays, and predictably poor clinical outcomes. Early survival was measured in months rather than years. The primary causes of ESLD at that time were alcoholic liver disease (ALD) and hepatitis B (HBV)-related cirrhosis. Early growth of LT was understandably slow. With improvements in immunosuppression, surgical technique and critical care management, outcomes consistently improved throughout the 1980s and 90s.

In 2007, there were 96 U.S. liver transplant centers that performed 10 or more LTs, with a total LT volume of 6,494. Overall, there were 6,941 (96%) deceased donors and 266 (4%) living donors. Pediatric LT recipients (less than 18 yrs of age) comprise 8% and 16% of the deceased and living donor transplants.

Table. United States liver transplant volume and liver allograft donations over 20 years time from 1988 to 2008.

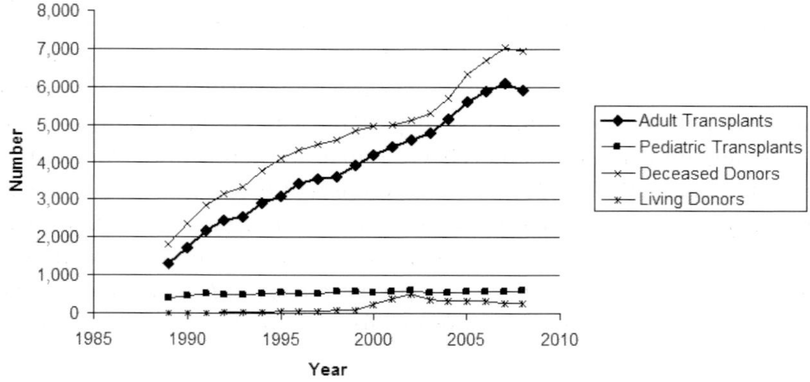

Overall LT outcomes include graft survival for deceased and living donors of 82% and 85% at 1-yr, and 67% and 68% at 5-yrs (Table 1).

Overall, LT patients enjoy a good quality of life. Many patients return to school and work, and survival more than 20 yrs is not uncommon. Many

Table 1. United States liver transplant graft survival by age of transplant recipient for deceased and living donors.

		3 mths (Tx 2004–2005)		1 yr (Tx 2004–2005)		3 yrs (Tx 2002–2005)		5 yrs (Tx 2000–2005)	
Deceased donor		N	%	N	%	N	%	N	%
Total	All	11,115	90	11,115	82	20,848	74	29,685	67
Age at Transplant	<1 yr	246	89	246	86	471	80	686	75
	1–5 yrs	286	86	286	82	579	76	850	74
	6–10 yrs	136	88	136	85	247	79	371	77
	11–17 yrs	216	92	216	88	443	81	682	73
	18–34 yrs	639	86	639	81	1,187	73	1,719	68
	35–49 yrs	2,755	90	2,755	84	5,684	75	8,636	68
	50–64 yrs	5,759	90	5,759	82	10,394	73	14,270	67
	65 + yrs	1,078	87	1,078	77	1,843	68	2,471	61

		3 mths (Tx 2004–2005)		1 yr (Tx 2004–2005)		3 yrs (Tx 2002–2005)		5 yrs (Tx 2000–2005)	
Living donor		N	%	N	%	N	%	N	%
Total	All	640	91	640	85	1,319	77	2,234	68
Age at Transplant	<1 yr	42	94	42	89	103	83	200	77
	1–5 yrs	46	96	46	92	106	80	185	75
	6–10 yrs	6	87	6	87	16	76	34	76
	11–17 yrs	11	82	11	82	18	73	51	63
	18–34 yrs	57	86	57	84	105	79	170	65
	35–49 yrs	152	93	152	90	334	82	565	71
	50–64 yrs	276	90	276	80	548	74	889	65
	65 + yrs	50	84	50	78	89	72	140	63

Note: Adapted from data from the Scientific Registry of Transplant Recipients (SRTR) at www.ustransplant.org.

female recipients have reported successful pregnancies, though not without risk of graft injury or loss.

COMMON INDICATIONS FOR PEDIATRIC LIVER TRANSPLANTATION

In pediatric kidney transplantation, the primary disease processes generally mirror those seen in the adult population. However, in pediatric LT, the primary diseases are altogether different. The primary indication for LT in children is hepatic failure. Hepatic failure can result from a chronic primary disease process, such as biliary atresia, alpha-1-antitrypsin deficiency, progressive familial intrahepatic cholestasis, primary sclerosing cholangitis, or autoimmune hepatitis. LT may also be indicated in children with a nonprogressive primary liver disease in which the symptoms or morbidity of the disease outweigh the risks of transplantation. Examples of these diseases include Alagille syndrome and inborn errors of metabolism. Cystic fibrosis is an example of secondary liver disease in which the primary disease process is systemic but results in life-threatening liver dysfunction. The decision to perform LT in a child without end-stage liver failure can result from debilitating symptoms such as pruritis which leads to chronic skin lesions, malnutrition and growth failure, or fatigue which impedes the ability to participate in school.

Another cause of secondary liver disease is related to chronic parenteral nutrition (PN) in children with short gut. PN can be especially toxic to the immature pediatric liver and progression to liver failure is more rapid at younger ages. In these children, however, consideration should be given to multivisceral transplantation (liver and intestine) to simultaneously correct the short gut and liver failure. Interestingly, isolated intestinal transplant in these short gut children, performed prior to the development of bridging liver fibrosis, can lead to complete recovery from the liver dysfunction where PN is stopped and the child is able to receive all nutrition enterally.

Finally, LT can be an effective therapy for children with primary hepatic malignancy. HCC can develop in children and, though rare, tends to occur in those patients with a metabolic liver disease. LT in these HCC patients has excellent survival if the HCC is small with few discrete nodules. For those with large or multiple nodules, post-transplant survival is poor. Hepatoblastoma can also be treated with LT. Unlike HCC, hepatoblastoma with a large tumor mass is not a contraindication to LT because these tumors are generally responsive to chemotherapy and can be controlled, or reduced in size, prior to transplantation.[1,2]

Common indications for liver transplantation in pediatrics.

Cholestatic diseases
- Biliary atresia
- Alagille syndrome
- Progressive familial intrahepatic cholestasis
- Giant cell hepatitis or neonatal hepatitis of unknown etiology
- Chronic parenteral nutrition therapy related to intestinal failure

Hepatocellular diseases
- Acute and subacute hepatic failure
  - Hepatotoxins
  - Acute Wilson's disease
- Autoimmune liver disease
- Chronic hepatitis B or C
- Polycystic liver disease

Metabolic diseases
- Alpha-1-antitrypsin deficiency
- Tyrosinemia type I
- Wilson's disease
- Neonatal hemochromatosis
- Glycogen storage disease type I
- Cystic fibrosis
- Inborn errors of metabolism
  - Crigler–Najjar Syndrome type I
  - Ornithine transcarbamylase (OTC) deficiency
  - Maple syrup liver disease (MSUD)
  - Familial hypercholesterolemia

Tumors
- Hepatoblastoma
- Hepatocellular carcinoma

Contraindications to liver transplantation in children
- Terminal nonhepatic disease
- HIV positive
- Metastatic cancer
- Lack of informed consent

ACUTE LIVER FAILURE

Acute liver failure (ALF) is a consequence of severe liver damage from a nonchronic process which results in encephalopathy and cerebral edema, acute renal failure, coagulopathy and physiologic disturbances of blood glucose and acid-base status. Depending on the amount of hepatic damage present, patients with ALF have the potential for complete recovery with return to normal liver function. Unfortunately, many affected persons progress to massive, nonreversible end-organ damage requiring LT. The primary cause of death in these critically ill patients is brain herniation related to severe cerebral edema and multiorgan failure related to severe acidosis. Patients who do recover may have persistent neurologic damage, and many have persistent renal failure which recovers over weeks' to months' time either with liver regeneration or LT. ALF accounts for 10% of all liver transplants in the U.S., Europe and Australia.

The most common etiology of ALF in Western countries is acetaminophen toxicity, most frequently related to an intentional overdose, though unintentional overdoses are common. Another important etiology is drug toxicity related to other agents such as methotrexate, antituberculosis drugs and anticonvulsants. Unintentional overdoses commonly occur when a combination of an hepatotoxic prescribed drug is combined with a high level of over-the-counter acetaminophen. In patients with moderate to heavy daily alcohol use, ALF may occur when this alcohol use is combined with otherwise acceptable levels of one or two other hepatotoxic drugs over several consecutive days or weeks. Other causes of ALF are much less common. Any virus that impacts the liver can give rise to ALF. Other infrequently seen acute immunologic or metabolic processes can lead to ALF including autoimmune hepatitis, Wilson's disease, acute fatty liver of pregnancy and the HELLP syndrome, acute Budd–Chiari syndrome, massive hepatic ischemia, and ingestion of *Amanita phalloides.*

The decision to transplant a patient with ALF is a critical juncture in clinical management. Patients who recover with supportive care only can have no long-term sequelae and resume all normal life activities. Transplanted patients can also experience a full recovery, though they will require lifelong immunosuppression, with its associated risks. Various prognostic criteria have been developed to assist the clinician in this critical decision and generally employ clinical and laboratory data such as systemic pH, severity of coagulopathy, severity of encephalopathy, period from onset of jaundice to onset of encephalopathy, serum bilirubin, factor V levels, percent necrosis on liver biopsy, acute physiology and chronic health evaluation (APACHE) score, and model for end-stage liver disease (MELD) score. Patients who do undergo transplantation for ALF have a decreased survival when compared to those patients undergoing LT for chronic liver disease. However, most of the decrease in survival for ALF occurs in the first 3-months post-transplant in which many deaths occur in relation to the acute illness and transplant procedure.

LIVER TRANSPLANT RECIPIENTS

Patient evaluation for LT is extensive and thorough. Though strict age criteria are avoided, all patients must demonstrate acceptable cardiopulmonary function and risk, be free from active infection, have no recent history of malignancy, have no recent history of substance abuse, and demonstrate sufficient coping ability to comply with a strict post-transplant health and medication regimen. The decision to list a patient for transplantation is not undertaken lightly. The listing process is multidisciplinary and includes input from hepatology, transplant surgery, social work, psychology, and financial counselors. The patient's history is formally presented at a listing meeting in which all involved services participate and contribute to the final decision. After listing, the patient maintains regular contact with a designated transplant coordinator to obtain routine follow-up testing and to notify the team if the patient has an important medical event that may require them to be inactivated or removed from the list.

ESLD is frequently accompanied by a host of co-morbidities that may impact the outcome of the transplant. Hepatorenal syndrome (HRS) is a condition in which chronic liver disease leads to renal insufficiency. The presence of renal failure is an important predictor of survival in patients with cirrhosis and in those who undergo LT. A significant proportion of liver transplant recipients develop chronic kidney disease (CKD) as a direct result of pretransplant renal injury and this frequently leads to dialysis post-transplant. Application of the National Kidney Foundation CKD classification is important in liver failure patients to determine their need for a possible combined liver/kidney transplant.

HRS is part of a spectrum of illness associated with increased pressures in the portal vein circulation, which begins with the development of ascites in the abdomen. The spectrum continues with diuretic-resistant ascites, where the kidneys are unable to excrete sufficient sodium to clear the fluid even with the use of diuretic medications. Most individuals with HRS have diuretic-resistant ascites before they develop deterioration in kidney function. The predominant theory (termed the "Underfill" theory) is that blood vessels in the renal circulation are constricted due to the dilation of blood vessels in the splanchnic circulation, which is mediated by factors released because of the liver disease. The consequence of this phenomenon is a decrease in the "effective" volume of blood sensed by the juxtaglomerular apparatus, leading to the secretion of renin and the activation of the renin-angiotensin system, which results in the vasoconstriction of vessels systemically and in the kidney specifically. However, the effect of this is insufficient to counteract the mediators of vasodilation in the splanchnic circulation, leading to persistent "underfilling" of the renal circulation and worsening renal vasoconstriction, leading to renal failure. Studies to quantify this theory have shown that there is an overall decreased systemic vascular resistance in HRS, but that the measured femoral and renal fractions of cardiac output are respectively increased and reduced, suggesting that splanchnic vasodilation is implicated in the renal failure. Though some of the effects of HRS are reversed with LT, patients do not generally return to completely normal renal function.[3]

Hepatopulmonary syndrome (HPS) also results from differences in vascular pressures related to the primary liver disease. The vasodilation resulting from liver failure results in a direct vasodilatory effect in the lungs, resulting in increased blood flow in relation to ventilation and a ventilation–perfusion mismatch. This is seen clinically as a right-to-left shunt and the patient experiences dyspnea. As with HRS, HPS is an important marker of disease severity and prognosis is poor without a timely liver transplant. Symptoms of HPS improve markedly with LT.[4–6]

Patients with ESLD have many other signs and symptoms of their liver disease. Jaundice, ascites, edema, malnutrition, fatigue, and encephalopathy are all commonly seen. Resolution of these derangements can be immediate, as with encephalopathy, or can take months to reverse, as with malnutrition. Post-transplant supportive care is critical and many of these patients require intensive physical and occupational therapy before they are able to safely return to normal activities of daily living.

Retransplantation is a complex issue in the field of LT. With a large number of children awaiting a first LT, and many others dying each year while awaiting LT, it is difficult to justify a second or third liver transplant. The most common indications for retransplant are those in which a primary liver transplant has failed in the immediate post-transplant period secondary to vascular thrombosis, PNF, or hyperacute rejection. Thereafter, retransplantation occurs in the setting of recurrence of the primary disease, chronic rejection or chronic biliary complications. In the U.S., approximately 8% of all liver transplants are performed in a patient who has had a previous transplant. Retransplantation raises many clinical, financial and ethical questions. Technically, retransplantation is significantly more complex than a primary liver transplant, resulting in increased risk of complications and prolonged post-transplant recovery with higher costs.

CLINICAL PEDIATRIC TRANSPLANTATION

LT is an effective and appropriate therapy for children with liver disease. Unfortunately, outcomes very greatly depending upon the age, size and general health status of the child at the time of transplant.[7–9] Infants undergoing LT are at high risk of mortality, both on the waitlist and in conjunction with the transplant itself. These children have limited reserve, can be very ill, and are at high risk of vascular thrombosis which is often a fatal complication. The waitlist time for a small child can be prolonged as deceased donor organs of this size are infrequently available. Many centers now offer living donor transplantation using the left lateral segment of an adult liver if it is of an appropriate size. These reduced size grafts now have survival rates in the pediatric population which are similar to or better than whole organ grafts. Children over age 3 have significantly better outcomes as they have more physiologic reserve and are often not as severely decompensated. Also, there are more viable organs available for these children simply due to increasing size of the abdomen. Older children are also less likely to develop hepatic artery thrombosis (HAT) with a larger blood vessel diameter and higher baseline blood pressure.

Work-up for LT in children is similar to that for adults. Severe cardiopulmonary disease must be ruled out. Though chronic diseases are less common, pediatric patients can experience significant decompensation from their liver disease and present with severe malnutrition, ascites, edema, portal hypertension, and hepatorenal and HPSs. Patients who become critically ill prior to transplantation, requiring mechanical ventilation or dialysis, have markedly diminished post-transplant survival. As with adults, there is a scoring system to predict waitlist mortality. The pediatric end-stage liver disease (PELD) score, however, takes into account age and growth failure, in addition to the liver factors of international normalized ratio (INR), serum bilirubin and serum creatinine seen in the adult MELD score.[10] PELD and MELD scores can be readily determined by calculators available on the internet. The most common indication for retransplantion for all children is HAT which occurs in children at a higher frequency when compared to adult LT. These retransplants may be urgent and carry a high risk of mortality because of the difficulty in finding a replacement allograft of the appropriate size. Other indications for retransplantation include disease recurrence, primary nonfunction (PNF), and chronic rejection. Chronic rejection is commonly related to noncompliance and is often seen in the teenage years.

There has been considerable discussion regarding the appropriate timing for listing a patient for transplantation. Clearly, patients with severe disease should be listed and transplanted in an expeditious fashion. Those patients with a very low PELD score, who are well compensated, may be better served to await progression of their disease prior to taking on the risks of the LT. Recent studies suggest that adult patients with a MELD score as low as 11–12 derive a better clinical outcome from LT as opposed to delaying the procedure (MELD ranges from 6 to 40).[11] All patients with cirrhosis, however, retain the underlying risks of the disease process of cirrhosis including an increased risk for gastrointestinal hemorrhage, development of HCC, encephalopathy, malnutrition and debility, and worsening hepatorenal and HPS.

Liver Transplant Donors

Though indications for organ transplantation broaden each year, and the number of listed patients consequently increases, organ donation rates have leveled off in recent years. This has resulted in an increased waitlist time at many centers. Efforts to increase donation rates and to expand the donor supply in recent years have met with limited success. Use of partial liver grafts has become more common in providing donor organs in a timely fashion to recipients in need. This approach takes advantage of the unique ability of the liver to rapidly regenerate and may provide additional organs not previously available. There are significant risks of donor morbidity and mortality from living donation and these should be fully disclosed to the potential donor. Some deceased donors are classified as ECD. This ECD term refers to donor health or organ characteristics that result in a less than optimal donor graft and may include advanced age, excess steatosis, prolonged ischemia time, trauma and a high-risk social history. The use of ECD liver grafts is surgeon-specific and the full history of the donor must be measured in relation to the acute need of the recipient and the appropriateness of the match between the donor and recipient.

With the on-going shortage of donor liver allografts, there has been an increased use of organs donors under the donation after cardiac death protocol (DCD). DCD organs are procured after cessation of cardiopulmonary function. The DCD protocol is utilized in organ donors who do not meet brain death criteria, but who have nonrecoverable illness for which medical support will be electively withdrawn. For these patients, consent can be obtained for withdrawal of life support under controlled conditions. A physician who is not affiliated with the organ procurement team independently declares death after withdrawal of support. From the time of the declaration of death, a waiting period is then observed to assure no recovery of cardiovascular function (usually 5 mins), after which the donor surgeon can begin the procurement procedure. The organ procurement proceeds rapidly with cannulation of the aorta to begin exsanguination and cold flushing of the organs, followed by rapid cooling with topical ice and, finally, removal of the organs with placement in cold preservation solution. The DCD protocol, of necessity, imposes a period of warm ischemia on the procured organs which has been shown to worsen transplant outcomes and these organs are rarely used in children. In LT, the most commonly described complication of the DCD protocol is diffuse intrahepatic biliary strictures. Though DCD organs are rarely transplanted into children, pediatric patients are frequently used successfully as DCD donors.

Matching a donor liver to a specific recipient is primarily based upon two factors: blood type and size match. However, graft/recipient matching can be much more complex than simply choosing the next person of the appropriate blood type that the liver allograft will size fit. For example, many liver recipients are also listed for additional organs such as combined liver and kidney, and all organs to be included in the transplant must be evaluated individually. With the ongoing shortage of donor organs, a greater number of ECD livers must be assessed. Critically ill patients in the intensive care unit may not tolerate transplantation with a donor liver that has little reserve or is at risk for delayed graft function. The transplant team, and the organ recipient, must remain somewhat flexible in allocating the organ to the most appropriate recipient.[12]

Partial Liver Grafts

As a consequence of the shortage of deceased donor liver allografts, the use of partial liver allografts has been developed. In countries with limited access to deceased donors, partial liver allografts from living donors may be the only option available for patients in need of transplantation. Also, splitting of a deceased donor liver can result in two viable grafts, though each split portion carries an increased risk of complications when compared to a whole organ allograft. Much of the impetus for the development of split liver transplants grew from two areas of need: pediatric LT and transplantation in countries with few deceased donor organs. A recent review of 10-yr clinical outcomes demonstrates similar outcomes for whole organ and partial liver grafts in children, but a significant decrease in survival for split liver grafts in adults.[13]

Pediatric patients have a high rate of decompensation and death on the liver transplant waitlist, as high as 25–50%. Because the death rate among healthy children is very low, there are few whole organ deceased donors of an appropriate size. For small infants, the left lateral segment (segments 2 and 3) or left lobe (segments 2, 3, and 4) of an adult size liver provides adequate hepatic function and can be obtained from either a living donor or from a deceased donor. As with a standard liver transplant, there are three requirements for a partial organ graft: vascular inflow (including both arterial and portal), venous outflow, and biliary drainage. The graft must be of adequate size to provide the hepatic mass required to support normal physiologic processes. The liver graft will then regenerate to a mass determined by both available space and functional capacity. Partial grafts for pediatric transplantation can be obtained through a variety of mechanisms. A reduced size graft is one in which the whole organ is procured for a single recipient, and the graft is reduced in size to match the recipient. This approach does not increase the number of available organs, but does shorten the waitlist time for small children. A living donor graft is when a segment of the liver, either the right lobe, left lobe or left lateral segment is procured from a healthy living donor as an elective procedure. This approach does increase the number of available organs and also decreases waitlist time. A split liver graft is taken from a deceased donor. The liver is divided into right and left portions and the two grafts are transplanted into two separate recipients, commonly an adult for the right portion and a child for the left portion (Figures 1a and 1b). The split procedure can occur either *in situ* at the time of organ procurement, or

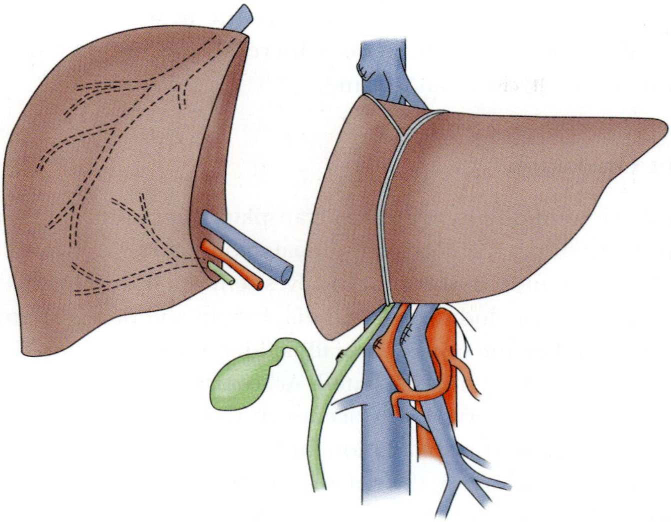

Figure 1a. Liver donor right side AP view.

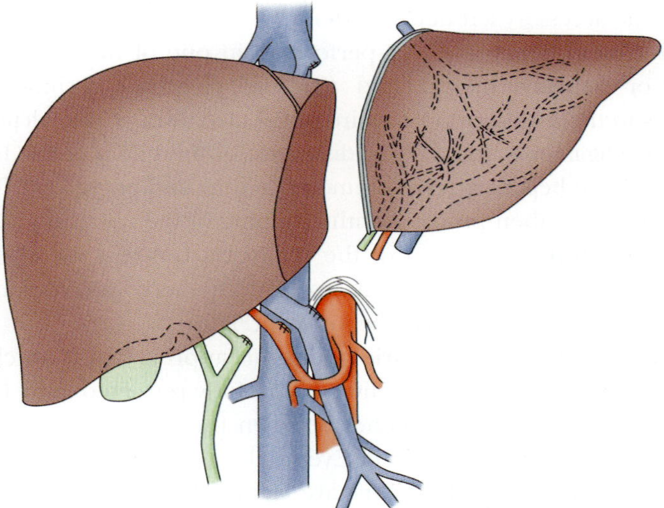

Figure 1b. Liver donor left side AP view.

ex vivo under cold ischemic conditions after the liver has been procured. Splitting a deceased donor liver does increase the number of available organs and also decreases waitlist time.

Recipient Operation

There are three components to the liver transplant operation: (1) Preparation of the transplant organ, (2) Recipient hepatectomy, and (3) Transplantation of the graft. Preparation of the graft involves removal of residual tissue from the donor operation including residual diaphragm and pericardium around the vena cava and hepatic veins. The gallbladder is always removed from the donor liver and the cystic duct is ligated. Accessory hepatic arteries are carefully dissected and preserved. An accessory right hepatic artery requires reconstruction prior to transplantation and can be reconstructed directly to the gastroduodenal artery or the splenic artery. Alternatively, the origin of the accessory right hepatic artery at the superior mesenteric artery can be preserved with the superior mesenteric artery being reconstructed to the splenic artery. In general, an accessory left hepatic artery cannot be safely reconstructed (due to small size) and is dissected and preserved *in situ* with careful ligation of small vessels, including the distal left gastric artery after the take off of the accessory left hepatic artery.

The recipient hepatectomy is performed in one of two ways: (1) Conventional or standard bicaval, and (2) The piggyback technique. Both approaches to the hepatectomy require initial takedown of the falciform and gastrohepatic ligaments, followed by dissection of the hilum of the liver with transection of the hepatic artery, common bile duct and portal vein. The conventional approach then proceeds with clamping of the vena cava above and below the liver with transection of the vena cava between the clamps and removal of the liver. This technique necessarily requires complete clamping of the vena cava, though a shunt can be formed (Figure 2).

The piggyback technique varies from this approach and no clamping of the vena cava is required. The liver is carefully retracted away from the vena cava with perforating branches between the vena cava and the liver individually ligated and transected. Eventually, the liver remains attached only by the hepatic veins. The veins are clamped and transected and the liver is removed. The piggyback technique is technically more difficult than the conventional approach, but the recipient tends to remain more hemodynamically stable as the preload to the heart from the lower body is never interrupted (Figure 3).

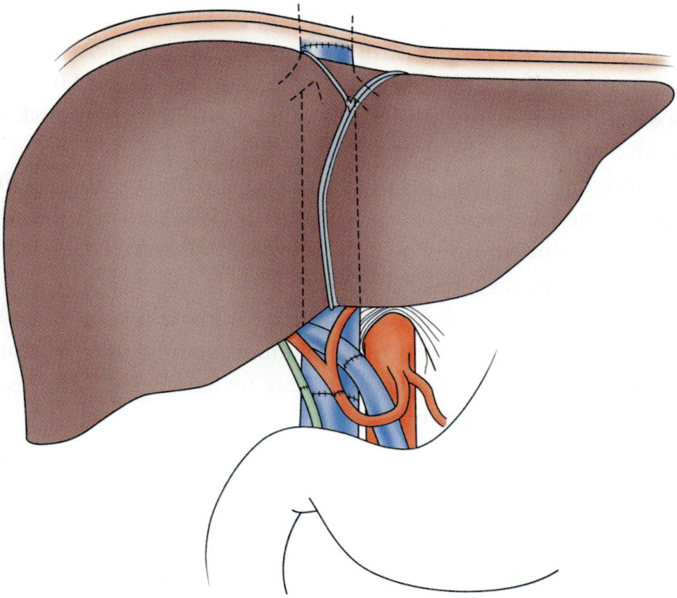

Figure 2. Bicaval anastomosis AP view.

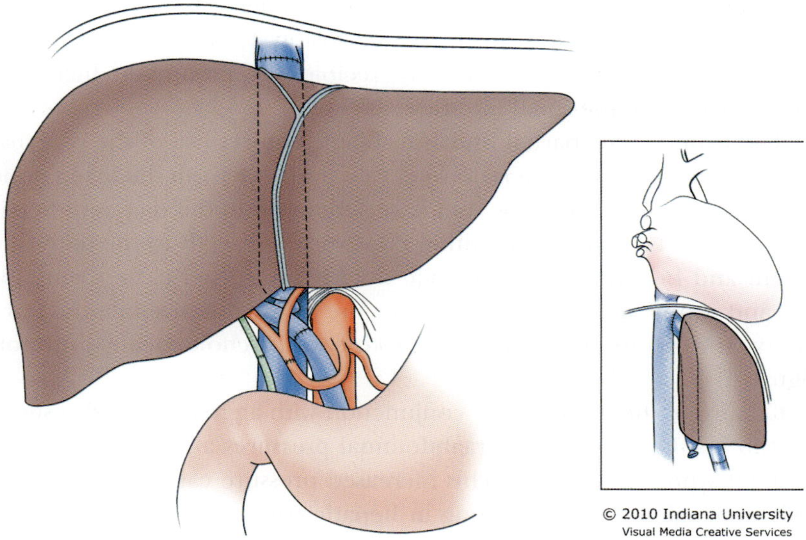

Figure 3. Piggyback anastomosis with side view.

Some surgeons who use the piggyback approach construct a temporary porto-caval shunt to decompress the portomesenteric system until the time of liver allograft reperfusion. For transplant recipients with HCC, surgeons may choose to use the conventional approach to minimize the risk of retaining the native vena cava which may have macrovascular invasion or through which hematogenous spread my occur during the hepatectomy. Our center uses the piggyback for nearly all patients with HCC and has demonstrated no difference in clinical outcomes.[14] The piggyback approach may be the preferred method in high-risk patients such as the elderly, those with poor physiologic reserve, or patients who are hemodynamically unstable. The piggyback technique tends to preserve hemodynamic and physiologic stability throughout the transplant which may be associated with less perioperative morbidity and mortality.

Finally, the transplant is performed. For the conventional approach, the vena cava must be reanastomosed both above and below the liver. An additional benefit of the piggyback hepatectomy is that one less anastomosis is required during the transplant. For the piggyback hepatectomy, the liver outflow is through the clamped hepatic veins so that a single anastomosis is required. This reduction from two to one anastomosis can decrease critical warm ischemia time by as much as 5–10 mins. Next, the portal vein and hepatic artery are anastomosed and the liver is reperfused. Again, the liver is generally flushed immediately prior to reperfusion to minimize the cardiac and hemodynamic effects of reperfusion. Finally, the common bile duct can be anastomosed either to the recipient common bile duct or to a Roux-en-Y limb of the small intestine.

The living donor partial liver transplant requires use of the piggyback hepatectomy because there is no vena cava available from the living donor. Therefore, the donor hepatic vein is anastomosed to the recipient hepatic veins, with portal and arterial inflow constructed directly to the native portal vein and hepatic artery. The bile duct is transected close to the liver graft and can be anastomosed to either the residual native bile duct or to a Roux-en-Y reconstruction to the intestine with a choledochojejunostomy (Figure 4).

Closure of the abdomen in conjunction with aggressive fluid resuscitation can result in elevated intraabdominal pressures and abdominal compartment syndrome post-LT. This increased pressure can compromise the newly transplanted liver, resulting in hepatic congestion. Additionally, systemic effects of abdominal compartment syndrome can lead to increased inspiratory pressures and slow weaning from the ventilator, as well as poor

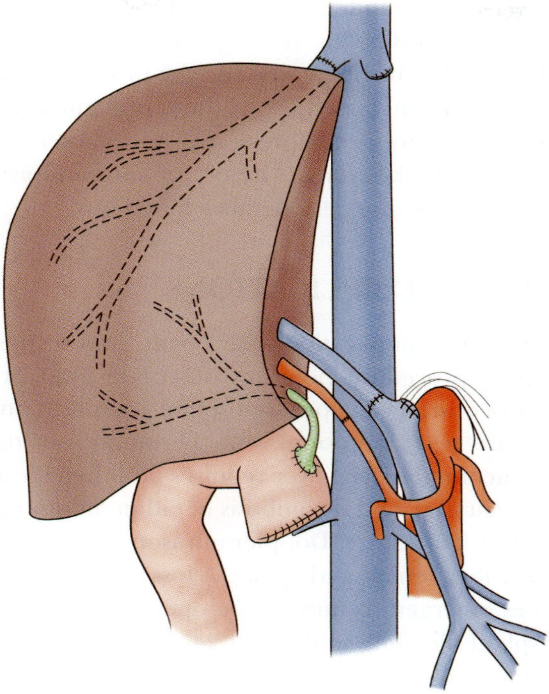

Figure 4. Liver recipient right side AP view.

renal vein outflow and compromised renal function. The decision to delay final closure of the abdomen for 24–72 hrs post-transplant is center dependent. Venous outflow for the liver is critical to avoid hepatic congestion which can lead to graft injury and vascular thrombosis. Maintaining the post-transplant patient with a low central venous pressure in the immediate post-transplant period optimizes liver allograft blood flow and may improve early function.

The role of the anesthesiologist is critical in the liver transplant procedure. Prior to initiating the procedure, large bore vascular access is generally placed to allow rapid infusion of blood products, if necessary. Two arterial catheters are placed to allow continuous monitoring of systemic blood pressure and frequent review of blood gases. LT has historically been associated with massive blood loss related to the presence of portal hypertension and varices, underlying coagulopathy and thrombocytopenia, and the overall complexity of the procedure. Patients with liver failure maintain a baseline vasodilatory status which, when added to intraoperative blood loss, can lead to significant hemodynamic instability. As surgeons have gained increasing experience with LT, blood loss has improved and the procedure has become more safe.[15] Additionally the increased use of the transjugular intrahepatic portosystemic shunt serves to decompress the portomesenteric system which lessens variceal-related bleeding. The use of antifibrinolytics varies, but may have a role in minimizing perioperative blood loss.

POST-TRANSPLANT COMPLICATIONS

Immediate post-transplant complications may result from technical issues related to the transplant procedure, poor function of the graft, or recipient health issues. The most critical early post-transplant complication is thrombosis of the hepatic artery or the portal vein. Thrombosis of the hepatic vein anastomosis is uncommon. The liver requires both hepatic artery and portal vein inflow for survival, and thrombosis of either anastomosis places the graft at imminent risk of failure. Doppler ultrasound is utilized post-LT to assure that vascular flow remains adequate. A loss of flow in either vessel generally necessitates emergent return to the operating room to reestablish flow. Post-transplant bleeding in the first 24–48 hrs is not uncommon and requires reexploration to identify and control the source.

PNF is a definition of exclusion in which there is graft failure within 7 days of the transplant with no other identifiable cause. PNF occurs in 1–5% of liver transplants and may be related to prolonged ischemia time, graft steatosis or unrecognized injury in the donor. Liver recipients who experience PNF are immediately relisted for transplantation, but they experience a high death rate, both while awaiting a second transplant and after the second transplant.[16,17] Delayed graft function is not well defined but may be manifest as prolonged elevation of the serum bilirubin level, a prolonged elevation of the INR, renal dysfunction, and persistent encephalopathy. Patients experiencing poor early graft function may have deterioration of their renal function and require continuous venovenous hemodialysis (CVVH). This therapy permits the clinician to closely modulate patient fluid status when the renal function is marginal. Small for size graft is a syndrome seen almost exclusively in partial LT. The small size of the transplant graft in relation to the recipient blood flow results in persistent portal hypertension and liver congestion as the portomesenteric flow is too great for the liver segment. This syndrome is a major cause of early graft loss in living donor transplantation.[18]

Elevation of liver function enzymes in the post-LT period is often the first indication of a late complication. Work-up starts with liver Doppler ultrasound to evaluate the vascular flow to the graft. If this study is normal, evaluation of the biliary system is next indicated. The biliary system can be visualized either through percutaneous transhepatic cholaniography (PTC) or endoscopic retrograde cholangiopancreatography (ERCP). Finally, percutaneous liver biopsy can be obtained and will often uncover the etiology when other studies are inconclusive. The liver biopsy in this scenario can frequently differentiate etiologies as diverse as drug effect, biliary obstruction, graft congestion, ischemia, rejection or recurrent disease. Serial surveillance liver biopsies are employed at many centers and may provide predictive information for long-term outcomes.[19]

Biliary complications may be seen within the first week post-transplant, but may also occur several weeks or months later.[20] There are three primary complications of the bile duct: (1) Biliary leak, (2) Anastomotic stricture, and (3) Intrahepatic strictures. Biliary leak is encountered in the perioperative period and may be technical in nature or may result from bile duct necrosis. Because the common bile duct protrudes from the liver, its blood supply lessens with increasing distance from the hilum of the liver. The recipient duct receives its blood supply from the native recipient pancreaticoduodenal complex and does not have the same blood supply issue. When duct necrosis occurs, a revision can be performed operatively with a shortening of the duct followed by reanastomosis to the recipient duct or construction of a Roux-en-Y choledochojejunostomy. Biliary complications are particularly problematic in living donor LT and are a major cause of graft loss and patient death in this population.[21]

Development of an anastomotic stricture is the most commonly encountered bile duct complication and may occur in up to 25% of patients. The anastomosis between the donor and recipient bile ducts will scar as it heals. The development of a stricture, or excessive scar, may depend in some measure on the surgical reconstruction of the duct, however, the size of the ducts and the strength of the donor blood supply to the duct are also important determinants of anastomotic narrowing. Most anastomotic strictures can be treated nonoperatively with ERCP and stent or PTC and drainage tube. Through these techniques, stents can be placed across the narrowed anastomosis to permit drainage, and these can be increased in size over time to dilate the duct.

Intrahepatic biliary strictures are rare and can be a difficult complication to diagnose and treat. Intrahepatic strictures appear as multiple diffuse strictures within a region of the liver or across the entire liver. Diffuse intrahepatic stricturing points to a systemic problem usually related to arterial blood flow. The biliary system is supplied through the arterial microcirculation of the liver. An arterial anastomotic stricture may result in this complication, and placing a vascular stent across the arterial anastomosis may improve blood flow and minimize the stricturing problem. Patients who develop diffuse intrahepatic biliary strictures have a high rate of graft loss and frequently require retransplantation within 1-yr.

Hepatic outflow obstruction is relatively rare, but is seen more frequently in patients who have undergone LT with piggyback hepatectomy. The etiology of this process is unclear, but appears to be directly involved with the anastomosis between the donor and recipient hepatic veins or with a mechanical obstruction of the outflow of this anastomosis because of the orientation of the liver. The result is a pressure gradient that results in chronic congestion of the liver. This pressure gradient can result in parenchymal damage to the liver or chronic ascites or splenomegally related to portal hypertension. Treatment can be performed using interventional radiology with balloon angioplasty to widen the outflow or placement of a stent across the hepatic vein outflow tract to reduce the pressure gradient.

Rejection of the liver allograft is less common than that seen for other solid organs. In fact, the liver appears to lessen the rejection risk of other organs when they are transplanted simultaneously. The reason for this finding is unclear. Unfortunately, the diagnosis and treatment for acute and chronic rejection in LT varies widely among liver transplant centers. This lack of standardization impedes research in this area. Individual centers report acute rejection rates ranging from less than 5% to nearly 50%. This raises the question of diagnostic criteria utilized as such disparity is unlikely to result simply from intercenter variability. The patient with rejection generally presents with elevated liver function enzymes and may have fever and abdominal pain. Commonly accepted liver biopsy criteria for acute cellular rejection in LT include: (1) Periportal inflammation, (2) Bile duct damage, and (3) Endothelialitis. Treatment may include pulse steroids and/or antibody therapy with an increase in baseline immunosuppression. Successfully treated acute rejection of the liver is not felt to impact on the long-term survival of the liver graft. Late acute rejection can occur, but chronic rejection of the liver is rare. Groups at increased risk of acute rejection include younger patients, females, patients of African descent, and those with autoimmune diseases. Ultimately, the most common etiology of rejection may be related simply to patient compliance with medications, though this is difficult to prove definitively. The rate of acute rejection is higher in older children and teens as these groups have a more active immune system. For this reason, children often receive higher dosing of immunosuppressive medications. Though children have more renal reserve and tolerate the nephrotoxicity of the calcineurin inhibitors better than adults, they still have a high rate of chronic renal dysfunction.[22] Very young children may actually develop a degree of tolerance to their graft and it is not unusual to observe teens and young adults, who were transplanted as infants, who have completely stopped their immunosuppression.[23]

Infectious complications post-LT are not uncommon but can be minimized with appropriate patient management. Because the liver transplant procedure itself is relatively clean, intraabdominal infections post-LT are rare. The most common viral infection in the liver transplant patient is cytomegalovirus (CMV) infection with a 1-yr risk of 5–20%.[24,25] Anti-CMV prophylaxis with ganciclovir and minimization of immune suppression lowers the rate of this infection. Fungal infections can occur in up to 20% of patients are most commonly seen in the mouth, esophagus and urine. These infections almost always result from candida species and respond to standard treatments.[26] Children have a much better healing capacity than adults so that wound and postoperative infections are rare. These patients are at higher risk for opportunistic infections when compared to nonimmunosuppressed children, but the rates are still lower than those seen in adults. Common infectious agents seen in pediatric transplantation include CMV, respiratory syncytial virus, rotavirus, candida species and common bacteria.[27] Post-LT prophylactic medications are the same as those used in adults. Unique to the infant population is the risk of spontaneous intestinal perforation which can also be life-threatening if not detected in a timely fashion. Spontaneous perforation may be related to perioperative steroid dosing, pressor use or surgical stress or unrecognized injury.[28]

The immune system plays a critical role in neoplasm surveillance in the human body. The chronic immune suppression required by all transplant patients places them at increased risk for the development of cancer. Unfortunately, the registries that follow post-transplant cancer are limited with voluntary reporting and incomplete follow-up. Therefore, the reported incidences by organ and tumor type vary widely.[29] The cancers found in transplant patients tend to mirror those seen in the general population, but with increased frequency. Therefore, the cancer most commonly seen in transplant patients is skin cancer (squamous and basal cell). Patients with HCC at the time of transplant have a risk of HCC recurrence post-transplant but their survival is similar to that for non-HCC patients if they are within the Milan criteria at the time of transplant. Post-transplant lymphoproliferative disorder (PTLD) is well described and appears to have increasing risk with increasing levels of immune suppression.

PTLD is a serious complication of transplant immunosuppression that may occur in children within months of immunosuppression induction. The risk of PTLD increases with increased level of immunosuppression. With increasing immunosuppression, there are less T-cells in circulation. This T-cell suppression permits the systemic propagation of Ebstein–Barr virus (EBV). EBV stimulates the clonal expansion of B-cells which leads to PTLD. As with CMV disease, the children at highest risk are those who are EBV negative but receive an EBV+ donor organ. This disease is manifest by lymphadenopathy or the presence of any mass lesion after transplant. Treatment for PTLD includes resection of mass lesions and chemotherapy including rituximab (anti-CD 20 receptor antibody).[30]

REFERENCES

1. Srinivasan P, McCall J, Pritchard J, Dhawan A, Baker A, Vergani GM, Muiesan P, *et al.* (2002) Orthotopic liver transplantation for unresectable hepatoblastoma. *Transplantation* **74**:652–655.
2. Fuchs J, Rydzynski J, Von Schweinitz D, Bode U, Hecker H, Weinel P, Burger D, *et al.* (2002) Pretreatment prognostic factors and treatment results in children with hepatoblastoma: A report from the German Cooperative Pediatric Liver Tumor Study HB 94. *Cancer* **95**:172–182.
3. Arroyo V, Fernandez J, Gines P. (2008) Pathogenesis and treatment of hepatorenal syndrome. *Semin Liver Dis* **28**:81–95.
4. Mandell MS. (2004) Hepatopulmonary syndrome and portopulmonary hypertension in the model for end-stage liver disease (MELD) era. *Liver Transplant* **10**:S54–S58.
5. Krowka MJ, Mandell MS, Ramsay MA, Kawut SM, Fallon MB, Manzarbeitia C, Pardo M, Jr, *et al.* (2004) Hepatopulmonary syndrome and portopulmonary hypertension: A report of the multicenter liver transplant database. *Liver Transplant* **10**:174–182.

6. Arguedas MR, Abrams GA, Krowka MJ, Fallon MB. (2003) Prospective evaluation of outcomes and predictors of mortality in patients with hepatopulmonary syndrome undergoing liver transplantation. *Hepatology* **37**:192–197.
7. Bucuvalas JC, Alonso E. (2008) Long-term outcomes after liver transplantation in children. *Curr Opin Organ Tran* **13**:247–251.
8. Soltys KA, Mazariegos GV, Squires RH, Sindhi RK, Anand R, Group SR. (2007) Late graft loss or death in pediatric liver transplantation: an analysis of the SPLIT database. *Am J Transplant* **7**:2165–2171.
9. Ng VL, Fecteau A, Shepherd R, Magee J, Bucuvalas J, Alonso E, McDiarmid S, *et al.* (2008) Outcomes of 5-year survivors of pediatric liver transplantation: Report on 461 children from a north american multicenter registry. *Pediatrics* **122**:e1128–e1135.
10. Barshes NR, Lee TC, Udell IW, O'Mahoney C A, Karpen SJ, Carter BA, Goss JA. (2006) The pediatric end-stage liver disease (PELD) model as a predictor of survival benefit and posttransplant survival in pediatric liver transplant recipients. *Liver Transplant* **12**:475–480.
11. Sharma P, Schaubel DE, Guidinger MK, Merion RM. (2009) Effect of pretransplant serum creatinine on the survival benefit of liver transplantation. *Liver Transplant* **5**:1808–1813.
12. Tector AJ, Mangus RS, Chestovich P, Vianna R, Fridell JA, Milgrom ML, Sanders C, *et al.* (2006) Use of extended criteria livers decreases wait time for liver transplantation without adversely impacting posttransplant survival. *Ann Surg* **244**:439–450.
13. Hong JC, Yersiz H, Farmer DG, Duffy JP, Ghobrial RM, Nonthasoot B, Collins TE, *et al.* (2009) Longterm outcomes for whole and segmental liver grafts in adult and pediatric liver transplant recipients: A 10-year comparative analysis of 2,988 cases. *J Am Coll Surgeons* **208**:682–689; discusion 689–691.
14. Mangus RS, Fridell JA, Vianna RM, Cooper AB, Jones DT, Tector AJ. (2008) Use of the piggyback hepatectomy technique in liver transplant recipients with hepatocellular carcinoma. *Transplantation* **85**:1496–1499.
15. Mangus RS, Kinsella SB, Nobari MM, Fridell JA, Vianna RM, Ward ES, Nobari R, *et al.* (2007) Predictors of blood product use in orthotopic liver transplantation using the piggyback hepatectomy technique. *Transplant Proc* **39**:3207–3213.
16. Uemura T, Randall HB, Sanchez EQ, Ikegami T, Narasimhan G, McKenna GJ, Chinnakotla S, *et al.* (2007) Liver retransplantation for primary nonfunction: Analysis of a 20-year single-center experience. *Liver Transplantation* **13**:227–233.

17. Kemmer N, Secic M, Zacharias V, Kaiser T, Neff GW. (2007) Long-term analysis of primary nonfunction in liver transplant recipients. *Transplant Proc* **39**:1477–1480.
18. Chan SC LC, Ng KKC, Fan ST. (2010) Alleviating the burden of small-for-size graft in right liver living donor liver transplantation through accumulation of experience. *Am J Transplant* **10**:859–867.
19. Ekong UD, Melin-Aldana H, Seshadri R, Lokar J, Harris D, Whitington PF, Alonso EM. (2008) Graft histology characteristics in long-term survivors of pediatric liver transplantation. *Liver Transplant* **14**:1582–1587.
20. Welling TH, Heidt DG, Englesbe MJ, Magee JC, Sung RS, Campbell DA, Punch JD, *et al.* (2008) Biliary complications following liver transplantation in the model for end-stage liver disease era: Effect of donor, recipient, and technical factors. *Liver Transplant* **14**:73–80.
21. Shah SA, Grant DR, McGilvray ID, Greig PD, Selzner M, Lilly LB, Girgrah N, *et al.* (2007) Biliary strictures in 130 consecutive right lobe living donor liver transplant recipients: Results of a Western center. *Am J Transplant* **7**:161–167.
22. Campbell KM, Yazigi N, Ryckman FC, Alonso M, Tiao G, Balistreri WF, Atherton H, *et al.* (2006) High prevalence of renal dysfunction in long-term survivors after pediatric liver transplantation. J *Pediatr* **148**:475–480.
23. Annunziato RA, Emre S, Shneider B, Barton C, Dugan CA, Shemesh E. (2007) Adherence and medical outcomes in pediatric liver transplant recipients who transition to adult services. *Pediatr Transplant* **11**:608–614.
24. Paya C, Humar A, Dominguez E, Washburn K, Blumberg E, Alexander B, Freeman R, *et al.* (2004) Efficacy and safety of valganciclovir vs. oral ganciclovir for prevention of cytomegalovirus disease in solid organ transplant recipients. *Am J Transplant* **4**:611–620.
25. Shiley KT, Gasink LB, Barton TD, Pfeiffenberger P, Olthoff KM, Blumberg EA. (2009) Increased incidence of cytomegalovirus infection in high-risk liver transplant recipients receiving valganciclovir prophylaxis versus ganciclovir prophylaxis. *Liver Transplant* **15**:963–967.
26. Reed A, Herndon JB, Ersoz N, Fujikawa T, Schain D, Lipori P, Hemming A, *et al.* (2007) Effect of prophylaxis on fungal infection and costs for high-risk liver transplant recipients. *Liver Transplant* **13**:1743–1750.
27. Hollenbeak CS, Alfrey EJ, Sheridan K, Burger TL, Dillon PW. (2003) Surgical site infections following pediatric liver transplantation: Risks and costs. Transpl Infect Dis **5**:72–78.

28. D'Alessandro AM, Knechtle SJ, Chin LT, Fernandez LA, Yagci G, Leverson G, Kalayoglu M. (2007) Liver transplantation in pediatric patients: Twenty years of experience at the University of Wisconsin. *Pediatr Transplant* **11**:661–670.
29. Gutierrez-Dalmau A, Campistol JM. (2007) Immunosuppressive therapy and malignancy in organ transplant recipients: A systematic review. *Drugs* **67**:1167–1198.
30. Newell KA, Alonso EM, Whitington PF, Bruce DS, Millis JM, Piper JB, Woodle ES, *et al.* (1996) Posttransplant lymphoproliferative disease in pediatric liver transplantation. Interplay between primary Epstein-Barr virus infection and immunosuppression. *Transplantation* **62**:370–375.

PEDIATRIC INTESTINAL AND MULTIVISCERAL TRANSPLANTATION

32

Richard S. Mangus

BACKGROUND AND HISTORY

The small intestine is one of the organs of the body most frequently in need of surgical intervention. Acute clinical episodes such as intestinal obstruction, perforation or hemorrhage can necessitate emergent intervention, and may result in decreased intestinal length when resection is necessary. A single massive resection, or multiple smaller resections, may lead to a condition classically referred to as short-gut syndrome (SGS). This syndrome is characterized by malnutrition and deficiencies of nutritional components, frequent loose stools or high ostomy output, and electrolyte abnormalities and dehydration. Additionally, these patients may suffer from chronic abdominal pain, chronic intraabdominal infections, enterocutaneous fistulas, and loss of abdominal domain. After the development of long-term parenteral nutrition (PN), additional complications of SGS arose including cholestatic liver disease, recurrent in-dwelling catheter infections and loss of vascular access. Though individual patients may survive for several years with SGS, long-term survival is rare. A classical teaching for many surgeons in training is that complete necrosis of the small intestine is a terminal event, and patients in this condition are often closed in the operating room, without resection, and allowed to expire.

Fortunately, transplantation of the intestine has now become a viable therapeutic option for many patients with SGS, and the so-called "open-and-close procedure" for massive necrosis of the intestine in no longer universally acceptable. Additionally, intestinal transplantation has been expanded to offer additional options for certain patients with nonresectable tumors, portomesenteric thrombosis and disorders of gastrointestinal dysmotility. Therefore, the option of intestinal transplantation must now be entertained for a large number of conditions, and for a large number of patients, once thought to be untreatable.

Inadequate intestinal length has been a surgical problem recognized for over a century. The field of intestinal transplantation was first explored by Alexis Carrel in 1902 when he implanted intestinal segments into the necks of dogs. Further dog studies occurred in the early 1960s by Dr. Richard Lillehei at the University of Minnesota, USA.[1,2] He subsequently published the first report of a deceased donor human intestinal transplant in 1967.[3] This transplant was performed without the benefits of modern organ procurement techniques, immunosuppression, critical care management or PN. The patient died within 12 hrs and there was little progress in this field for the subsequent two decades. In the 1980s, intestinal transplantation was again attempted after the establishment of cyclosporine as an effective immunosuppressive agent in 1984.[4,5] In 1987, Dr. Thomas Starzl and colleagues at the University of Pittsburgh performed the first successful multivisceral transplant, in which a portion of the transplant allograft included the entire length of small intestine.[6] Thereafter, intestinal transplants took many forms including isolated intestine, combined intestine and liver, combined stomach, pancreas, and intestine (modified multivisceral), and combined stomach, pancreas, intestine and liver (multivisceral), (see Table 1).

Results from these early transplants were marked by numerous complications and barriers, similar to those experienced with the development of transplantation of other solid organs. In the 1990s, a drug originally known as FK506 was developed, and later became known as tacrolimus (marketed in the United States as Prograf). Routine use of this calcineurin inhibitor coincided with improved outcomes and facilitated modulation of immunosuppression through stable blood levels and a significant decrease in the incidence of rejection.[7,8] Only recently has intestinal transplantation evolved from its status as an experimental intervention, to being the standard of care for select patients meeting specified criteria. Over the last

Table 1. History of intestinal transplantation.

1902	French physician Alexis Carrel implants intestinal grafts into the necks of dogs.
1959–1960	American physician Richard Lillehei describes experimental intestinal transplantation in dogs.
1962	Dr. Richard Lillehei autotransplants cold, preserved small intestine in a dog.
1960s	Eight human intestinal transplants are reported with no survivors. Failure is thought to be related to inadequate immunosuppression.
1967–1968	Parenteral nutrition is developed and is used clinically to provide supplemental nutrition to humans.
1970s	Cyclosporine is developed as an effective immunosuppressive agent by Jean Borel.
Early 1980s	Several centers experiment with clinical human intestinal transplantation with poor success.
1987	First multivisceral transplant at the University of Pittsburgh by Dr. Thomas Starzl.
1988	First international small bowel transplant symposium.
1989	Tacrolimus introduced for immunosuppression with improved outcomes compared to cyclosporine.
2000	Intestinal transplantation qualifies for financial reimbursement in the United States as an approved medical procedure.

decade, intestinal transplantation has grown consistently, but not at a rapid pace. One year graft and patient survival for intestinal transplantation now approaches that for other abdominal solid organ transplants, while long-term results have yet to be determined given the limited number of transplants performed. Recent improvements in clinical outcomes are related to careful donor and recipient selection, improved immunosuppression protocols, refinement in surgical techniques and experienced post-transplant clinical management. Intestinal transplantation remains today as the only definitive curative therapy for patients with intestinal failure who develop serious complications related to long-term use of PN. Expanded use may benefit other patient groups including those with nonresectable tumors, intestinal dismotility syndromes, and portomesenteric thrombosis.

INTESTINAL FAILURE

The primary indication for intestinal transplantation worldwide is intestinal failure. Intestinal failure is a clinical condition characterized by the inability of the gastrointestinal tract to maintain adequate nutrition, fluid and electrolyte balance, or normal growth and development of the body. Acute or chronic loss of the enteric absorptive mass caused by SGS, intestinal dysmotility or enterocyte dysfunction can precipitate intestinal failure. It is critical to recognize that a diagnosis of intestinal failure is independent of intestinal length. Clearly, the shorter the intestinal length, the higher is the risk of intestinal failure. However, short intestinal length is neither necessary, nor adequate, for the diagnosis of intestinal failure. There are many conditions of intestinal dysfunction in which the available enterocyte mass or function is inadequate to provide the body with sufficient nutrition or hydration. It is also essential to recognize that in a number of gastrointestinal diseases, a combination of massive resection and dysmotility of the remnant bowel can be present.[9,10] The most common causes of intestinal failure in children are necrotizing enterocolitis, gastroschisis, intestinal atresia (apple peel syndrome), volvulus, pseudo-obstruction and aganglianosis.[11] In the adult population, ischemia, inflammatory diseases (e.g. Crohn's disease), trauma and tumors (e.g. desmoid) are the most common causes of intestinal failure (Table 2).

Permanent alimentation of patients with enteral access does not constitute intestinal failure, so long as the patient is able to maintain an adequate nutrition and hydration status. The diagnosis of intestinal failure must be entertained when the patient requires long-term PN or intravenous fluids. Since the introduction of PN in 1968 by Dudrick and Wilmore, this therapy experienced dramatic growth and soon became available as

Table 2. Common causes of intestinal failure.

Pediatric	Adult
Gastroschisis	Ischemia
Necrotizing enterocolitis	Inflammatory bowel disease
Intestinal atresia	Volvulus
Midgut volvulus	Tumors
Aganglionosis	Trauma
Pseudo-obstruction	Pseudo-obstruction

the first line treatment for patients with a variety of gastrointestinal diseases.[12] It is estimated that 40,000 people are currently on chronic PN in the United States. As PN became more successful at sustaining life, comorbidities related to the prolonged use of the central venous system became apparent. Hospital readmissions occur in as many as 50% of patients placed on home PN during the years that they are on PN. Catheter-associated infections are responsible for 2/3 of these admissions.

It is very difficult to predict the reversibility of intestinal failure. However, when specific factors and clinical parameters are observed, it is possible to predict the likelihood that chronic PN will be required. For example, it is very likely that pediatric patients with ultra SGS (<20 to 30 cm of small bowel) combined with residual dysmotility, partial loss of the colon and absence of the ileocecal valve will remain on PN in order to achieve adequate growth and development.[9] Half of the children on long term PN will develop varying degrees of cholestatic liver disease. Risk factors associated with the development of liver disease while receiving PN include prematurity, low birth weight, lack of enteral feedings, lipid infusion, and bacterial overgrowth, among others. Clinical findings that may accompany liver disease are hyperbilirubinemia and jaundice, splenomegaly and thrombocytopenia.[13] Gastroesophageal varices and ascites may not be present, even in cirrhotic patients, due to the decrease in venous mesenteric flow that occurs after massive intestinal resections. In adults, intestinal resection resulting in less than 100 cm of jejunoileum and associated with abnormal remnant mucosa, and lack of the ileocecal valve, are predictors of chronic PN dependency. Among those patients with less than 50 cm of jejunoileum, the mortality reaches 40% within 5 yrs.[14,15] The development of cirrhosis associated with chronic PN is a catastrophic situation that leads to death in the majority of patients that are not rescued by transplantation. Unfortunately, once cirrhosis has been established, survival at 1 yr for children is only 20% to 30%.[11] In 2007, policies regarding organ allocation in the United States were amended, giving priority to pediatric patients awaiting combined liver/pancreas/intestinal transplant. Ultimately, early referral remains the best practice for patients at risk of complications related to intestinal failure.[16]

SURGICAL MANAGEMENT OF INTESTINAL FAILURE

Transplantation of the small intestine is indicated for patients who experience life-threatening complications of PN and/or intestinal failure.

The actual indications for intestinal transplantation can be divided into two categories, (1) those related to intestinal failure, and (2) nontraditional indications. In the United States, a governmental agency entitled the Centers for Medicare and Medicaid Services (CMS) administers services related to government supported health care services. The majority of private insurance payers then follow the criteria established by this agency. There are four CMS approved indications for intestinal transplantation, and all are associated with complications related to chronic PN:

(1) Loss of major routes of venous access.
(2) Multiple episodes of catheter associated life threatening sepsis.
(3) Fluid and electrolyte abnormalities in the face of maximal medical therapy.
(4) PN associated cholestatic liver disease.

Nontraditional indications for intestinal transplantation include:

(1) Diffuse mesenteric thrombosis.
(2) Benign/low grade malignant tumors involving the mesenteric root.
(3) Abdominal catastrophes (trauma, radiation, sclerosis, other).

It is estimated that 15% to 20% of patients on chronic PN are potential candidates for intestinal transplantation. The indications for transplantation, and the choice of organs to include in the graft, vary according to the baseline disease, presence and degree of liver disease, number of previous abdominal surgeries and functional quality of other abdominal organs. If biochemical changes related to liver dysfunction are present, a liver biopsy should be part of the work-up for patients awaiting an intestinal transplant. A liver biopsy should be obtained for all patients who have received long-term PN. The presence of cirrhosis or advanced bridging fibrosis is an indication for liver replacement. For patients with moderate liver fibrosis, serial liver biopsies should be performed at regular intervals, and these patients must undergo frequent examination for clinical signs of portal hypertension (Table 3).

Timing of intestinal transplantation, and the components of the evaluation, are patient specific. Patients with ultra SGS (<30 cm of small bowel), or with congenital enteropathies, should be considered early for intestinal transplantation to avoid PN-induced liver injury.[17] Those with functional

Table 3. Minimal indications for listing for isolated intestinal transplantation.

(1) Patient has demonstrated irreversible intestinal failure in the absence of severe liver dysfunction.
(2) The patient meets one of the following criteria:
(i) Thrombosis of two of the six major venous access sites (subclavian, jugular or femoral veins).
(ii) Recurrent catheter related sepsis.
(Two or more episodes of systemic sepsis secondary to line infections within 1 yr).
(iii) A single episode of catheter related fungal infection, septic shock or acute respiratory distress syndrome (ARDS).
(iv) Failure of growth and development in children.
(v) Recurrent dehydration or electrolyte abnormalities resulting in frequent hospital admissions of organ damage.

disease of the intestine may have poor quality of life and are frequently disabled by massive intestinal dilatation, despite the presence of decompressive enterostomies. These patients should also be considered for intestinal transplantation. Doppler ultrasonography of the neck veins and extremities provides a venous map for the anesthesiologist who must place central venous lines for the transplant procedure. It is not uncommon for these patients to have lost one or more of the six major routes of venous access during the course of their illness. Doppler ultrasound of the abdomen can provide an assessment of portal vein patency, which can be an issue in this patient population.

Despite increased general awareness of intestinal transplantation, 60% to 70% of the patients referred for intestinal transplantation have already developed some degree of irreversible liver failure.[18] Mortality on the transplant wait list for intestinal transplant candidates continues to be double that for any other solid organ and reaches 40% to 60%.[19] Early referral of PN patients to specialized centers for intestinal rehabilitation, before irreversible liver function occurs, is crucial to improve outcomes. Furthermore, with the increasing number of patients awaiting liver transplantation, early referral is critical as patients in need of combined liver and intestinal transplantation are competing for the same pool of organs as those awaiting isolated liver transplant. Late referral may result in excessively long transplant wait list times which will impact on survival.

During the waiting time, stable patients should be reevaluated often to assess for deterioration of liver function and for loss of vascular access. Clinical management of PN should be carefully monitored in patients awaiting isolated intestinal transplantation in an attempt to minimize liver damage. As with other solid abdominal organ transplants, absolute contraindications to intestinal transplantation include severe cardio–pulmonary disease, severe systemic infections with multiple organ failure, aggressive malignancy and severe neurologic impairment. HIV infection is now considered a relative contraindication for solid organ transplantation.

Types of transplant grafts (combinations of organs transplanted) can be tailored according to the indication for intestinal transplant and the recipient's liver function. The common element in all variants is transplantation of the small bowel. Inclusion of the colon, spleen, kidney, and abdominal wall is performed as appropriate to the baseline pathology and center preference.[20,21] However, all described modifications are different combinations of the "cluster" concept initially proposed in 1991 by Starzl.[22]

ISOLATED SMALL INTESTINE TRANSPLANT (ISOLATED INTESTINE, ITx)

Isolated transplantation of the small intestine is performed for patients with irreversible intestinal failure in the absence of severe liver dysfunction. In addition, one of the following criteria should be present:

(1) Thrombosis of two of the six major venous access sites (subclavian, jugular or femoral veins).
(2) Recurrent catheter related sepsis (two or more episodes of systemic sepsis secondary to line infections per year (or) one episode of catheter related fungal infection, septic shock or acute respiratory distress syndrome (ARDS).
(3) Failure of growth and development in children.

In certain patients, end stage renal failure can be caused by several years of dehydration and electrolyte imbalances. In these patients, a concomitant renal transplant can be performed. When pancreatic dysfunction in addition to intestinal failure is present (e.g. type I diabetes, cystic fibrosis, chronic pancreatitis), a simultaneous small bowel-pancreas transplant can be performed (see Figure 1).

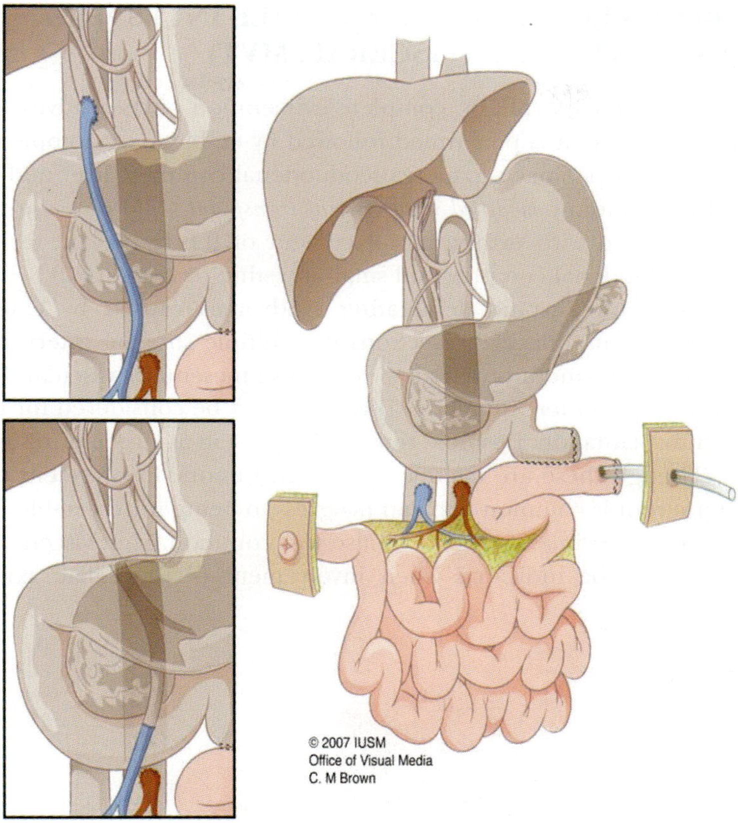

Figure 1. Drawing of isolated intestine.

COMBINED LIVER-SMALL INTESTINE TRANSPLANT

Performed in patients with intestinal failure and irreversible liver disease, transplantation of the liver and intestine is usually performed as a composite graft. In this technique, the native stomach, pancreaticoduodenal complex and spleen are preserved. A portocaval shunt must be performed to provide drainage for the native organs. The donor pancreas is harvested en-block with the intestine and liver. Even though most patients do not have evidence of pancreatic disease, inclusion of the donor pancreaticoduodenal complex avoids hilar dissection by keeping intact the drainage of the common bile duct. Partial graft pancreatectomy keeping only a small portion of the pancreatic head and duodenum has been abandoned in most centers.

COMBINED LIVER-PANCREAS-SMALL INTESTINE TRANSPLANT (MULTIVISCERAL, MVT)

In a *multivisceral graft* (MVT), complete evisceration of the native foregut and remnant midgut is performed followed by en-block orthotopic transplantation of the stomach, pancreaticoduodenal complex, liver and small bowel. In the variant *modified multivisceral transplant* (MMVT), the native liver is preserved with orthotopic placement of the transplant stomach, pancreaticoduodenal complex and small intestine (see Figure 2).

Patients with chronic debilitating syndromes caused by extensive abdominal trauma, massive resections or multiple surgical interventions leading to SGS, dysmotility disorders , extensive mesenteric vascular thrombosis or multiple enterocutaneous fistulas should be considered for multivisceral transplantation. Desmoid tumors can present as large nonresectable lesions. Though these are technically benign tumors, involvement of the mesenteric root is common and can progress to being unresectable. Local recurrence after primary resection is also very common. Multivisceral transplantation may be indicated when involvement of the celiac axis and

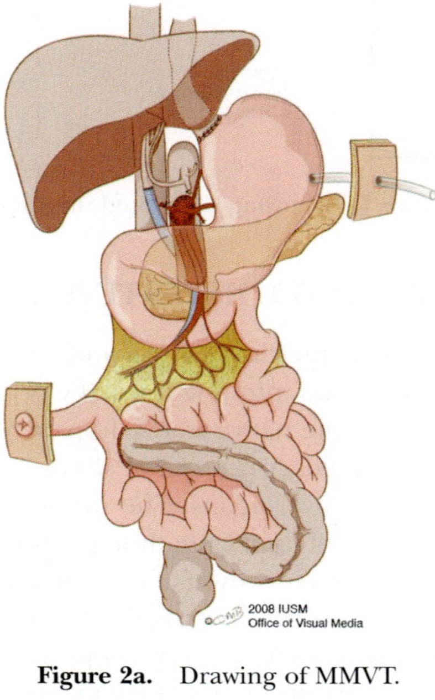

Figure 2a. Drawing of MMVT.

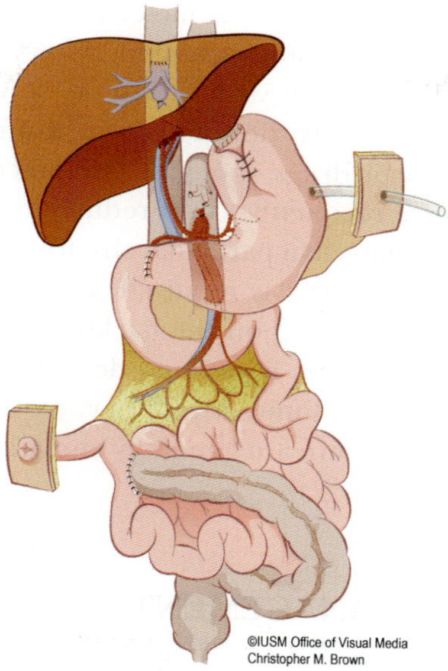

Figure 2b. Drawing of MVT.

mesenteric artery precludes complete resection. In select cases, where the celiac axis is spared, an isolated intestinal transplant or a modified multivisceral transplant can be performed. Intestinal autotransplantation has also been described in select cases in which the native bowel is first resected, then the tumor is resected, and, finally, the native bowel is retransplanted. Multivisceral transplantation may also be indicated in patients with diffuse portomesenteric thrombosis.

Intestinal Donor Selection

In most cases, candidates for intestinal and multivisceral transplants present with a retracted abdominal cavity due to multiple surgeries. For this reason, it is important to consider donors that are 25% to 50% smaller than the recipient. Organs from these smaller donors provide adequate function while requiring less intraabdominal space. Usually young donors, ABO-identical, hemodynamically stable, and with appropriate anatomy are considered. At procurement, selective decontamination of the gut may be performed according to center preference. The use of antilymphocyte antibodies in the donor is utilized by some centers. Unfortunately, there is no evidence that this therapy results in a reduction in rejection episodes or in a decreased incidence of graft vs. host disease (GVHD). Liberal use of cytomegalovirus (CMV) positive donors is now a universal practice with newly available prophylactic drugs, though CMV-infected donors should be avoided in CMV-negative recipients. Graft reduction can be performed as necessary to tailor the organs to a particular size for the recipient, however, more extensive backbench work is required. Reduction in length of the small intestine can be performed on the backbench or after reperfusion. Though living intestinal donors have been described, their use has been very limited. There are a limited number of intestinal transplants performed each year, and there are generally enough intestinal graphs for those on the waitlist.

POSTOPERATIVE MANAGEMENT OF THE INTESTINAL TRANSPLANT RECIPIENT

In the immediate postoperative period, an early concern in the small intestine transplant recipient is the maintenance of the fluid and electrolyte balance. The transplanted small intestine can develop significant edema in the first 24 to 48 hrs after surgery, caused mainly by ischemia-reperfusion injury and fluid sequestration. Edema of the intestinal graft can be deleterious not only for the transplant graft, but also for the surrounding abdominal organs. A significant increase in intraabdominal pressure can lead to abdominal compartment syndrome, resulting in increased ventilation requirements and renal failure. Resuscitation should be carefully balanced between colloid administration and the use of vasopressors to modulate intraabdominal pressures with hemodynamic stability and fluid status. Broad spectrum antibiotics are typically maintained for several days or longer.

Transplant small bowel peristalsis relies entirely on the intrinsic myenteric innervation (Aurbach's plexus and Meissner's plexus), since the extrinsic innervation system is disrupted during organ procurement. Even though the intestine initiates peristaltic movements immediately after reperfusion, peristalsis can be erratic when compared to a normal small bowel. Stoma output is usually present 24 to 48 hrs after transplant and good graft perfusion can be easily assessed at the bedside by inspecting the stoma. A poorly perfused stoma should be evaluated immediately with ileoscopy and abdominal ultrasound with Doppler. This finding could be the result of hyperacute rejection or poor perfusion restricted either to the stoma or to the entire graft.

Though intestinal transplantation offers the opportunity for nutritional autonomy, several steps need to be accomplished during the early stages post-transplant to arrive at that goal. Patients are initially maintained on PN with a slow transition to enteral feedings. Most centers use a low fat, elemental formula for enteral feeds in the first weeks after transplant. Lipids are introduced slowly, 2–4 wks after transplant. Medium-chain triglycerides are directly absorbed by the portal venous system and are used as the main source of lipids in the first few weeks after transplant. Although disruption of the lymphatics occurs during the donor operation, chylous ascites is a rare event after transplant. A more aggressive approach with polymeric formulas has been reported with low incidence of chylous ascites and diarrhea. Gastroparesis can be present in the early postoperative period but usually improves with the use of promotility agents. Enteral formula may be introduced between days 3 and 14. Patients that develop high ostomy output with a normal graft (rejection has been ruled out) can benefit from the addition of fiber combined with loperamide, lomotil, opiates and kaolin-pectin mixture. Once 50% of the caloric requierements are achieved with food and enteral formula, PN is discontinued. The majority of patients receive enteral formula for 4–8 wks after transplant. PN can be stopped in well over 90% of the patients receiving intestinal transplantation. In some pediatric patients, a more complex developmental approach with the learning of eating habits may be required.

REJECTION

Acute cellular rejection remains the most common complication after intestinal transplantation and still occurs with higher frequency when compared with transplantation of other solid abdominal organs. In two recent large center reports, the incidence of acute cellular rejection was as high as 50% in the first 90 days after transplant. The occurrence of rejection in the first 90 days after transplant has a negative impact on long-term graft survival as reported by the latest intestinal transplant registry (ITR) report. The diagnosis of rejection is based on a combination of clinical signs, endoscopic findings and histologic examination. Although high volume stooling is the most common symptom, rejection can also be manifest with fever, vomiting, ileus, cramping, severe abdominal pain and gastrointestinal bleeding. Rejection of the small bowel causes different degrees of mucosal and intramural injuries. Typical histological features of early rejection of the small bowel include an increase in the number of apoptotic bodies, lymphocytic infiltration of the lamina propria, increasing space between the villae, and ulceration. Several biopsies should be taken in the presence of rejection, since the injury can spare segments of the graft. Mucosal injury can lead to damage of the intestinal epithelial barrier, and life threatening episodes of sepsis can occur with bacterial translocation. Augmentation of baseline immunosuppression in response to rejection increases the risk of infectious complications. This cycle, then, leads to high rates of morbidity and mortality in intestinal transplantation.

An ileostomy is generally constructed during the transplant and facilitates endoscopic access to the intestinal graft. Protocols for graft surveillance with serial endoscopy and biopsy differ from center to center. Usually, surveillance ileoscopy is performed once or twice a week for the first 2 to 3 mths, and then monthly for another 6 mths. The ileostomy is closed 3–12 mths post-transplant. Once the normal physiologic transit is reestablished, a colonoscopy is performed every 6–12 mths, or whenever clinically indicated. The use of noninvasive screening for rejection of the intestinal graft is in its infancy. Citrulline, calprotectin , perforin and granzime B have been utilized in monitoring for rejection, however further studies are needed to confirm their applicability. Histological evaluation continues to be the "gold standard" for the diagnosis of rejection. Episodes of mild rejection can usually be treated with a steroid pulse. Progression from mild to moderate or severe rejection may necessitate the use of antilymphocyte preparations (rATG, OKT-3 or Campath). Use of infliximab, an anti-tumor necrosis factor (TNF)-alpha agent, has been reported in a few patients with rejection resistant to steroids and OKT3.

COMPLICATIONS OF INTESTINAL TRANSPLANTATION

As previously discussed, rejection is the primary complication encountered in intestinal transplantation. Unfortunately, this frequently leads to over-immunosuppression and its accompanying complications. In spite of improved surveillance and pharmacologic agents including antibiotics, antivirals and antifungals, sepsis remains the leading cause of death in intestinal transplant patients in both the perioperative and long-term periods. Intestinal recipients experience translocation of bacteria from the compromised bowel pretransplant and experience frequent infections of indwelling catheters. Post-transplant, the increased level of immunosuppression and need for parenteral access continue to result in catheter infections as well as standard postsurgical infections of the urinary system, lungs, and surgical wound. Because of the lengthy and complicated course associated with intestinal disease, patients may be colonized with multidrug resistant bacteria, and infectious processes often have a fungal component. Intraabdominal fluid collections often need drainage, either with reexploration or percutaneous placement of a drainage catheter. Some centers have described post-transplant pancreatitis when the pancreas is included as part of a MVT, but others have not had this experience. Infectious processes can specifically infect the transplanted intestine. The transplant intestine can experience invasive infection with clostridium difficile, CMV, cryptosporidium and other common viruses. These infections generally respond to the same treatments that would be utilized for such infections of the native intestine.

The use of calcineurin inhibitors has dramatically improved outcomes in intestinal transplantation. However, these agents are well-known for their nephrotoxicity. In general, average serum levels for these drugs are maintained at higher levels in intestinal transplant patients when compared to those for recipients of other organs. A decline in renal function has been well described in patients undergoing solid organ transplantation and this decline may be more precipitous in intestinal transplant patients. Kato *et al.* described the incidence of renal insufficiency (glomerular filtration rate <90 mL/min) in children to be 13% at transplant, 48% at 1 yr and 35% at 2 yrs post-transplant.

Post-transplant lymphoproliferative disorder (PTLD) is well defined in intestinal transplantation and remains a persistent problem. Rates of PTLD have remained stable at 6–8% of all recipients in spite of changes in immunosuppression regimens. PTLD has its highest incidence approximately 2 yrs post-transplant. This malignancy is now treatable with antiCD20 antibody (rituximab) and mortality related to PTLD has decreased significantly in recent years. GVHD, relatively rare in kidney, liver and pancreas transplantation is more common in intestinal transplant patients. Transplant intestine contains a disproportionately high concentration of immune-related tissue and has a well defined role in immunologic surveillance. Our center has noted an increased risk of GVHD in patients receiving a greater volume of transplant organs in proportion to their total body mass. Therefore, patients undergoing multivisceral transplant have a higher incidence of GVHD compared to those recipients of either a single solid organ or isolated small intestine.

Surgical complications are not uncommon in intestinal transplantation. Most recipients have had multiple abdominal surgeries prior to reaching intestinal transplantation and have developed dense adhesions. These may result in significant blood loss and hemodynamic instability at the time of transplant. Also, enterotomies are common leading to intestinal spillage and wound contamination. Additionally, there is a loss of abdominal domain resultant from a decrease in organ volume in the peritoneal cavity. This loss of domain can make closure of the abdomen difficult and can result in abdominal compartment syndrome if the abdomen is closed under pressure. Mesh closure of the abdomen is frequently indicated and several centers have utilized abdominal wall transplant or flap closure of the abdomen in conjunction with intestinal transplantation to provide coverage. Additionally, the graft itself can be cut down with a resection of intestine or a portion of the liver to provide the necessary space.

Almost by definition, intestinal transplant patients have a poor nutritional status and this directly impacts wound and anastomotic healing. Wound dehiscence and wound infections are common. Gastrointestinal tract anastomotic leaks are not infrequent. Many multivisceral transplant patients with esophagogastrostomy experience severe reflux symptoms and a gastric "wrap" of the esophagus at the time of transplant has been found to improve symptoms. Intestinal transplant patients have difficulty maintaining their weight and often must have supplemental PN or enteric feeds. Children may experience delays in development and growth (both height and weight), though the majority have normal growth when intestinal function is normal.

TRANSPLANT OUTCOMES

The International Small Bowel Transplant Association (ISBTA) meets biennially to review current research, transplant volume and clinical outcomes in intestinal transplantation. At the meeting, updated results are presented from the ITR and include worldwide data. In the United States, in 2007, 20 centers performed at least one intestinal transplant. Between 2005 and 2007, 28 centers worldwide reporting to the ITR performed 389 intestinal transplants on 377 patients. Types of transplants during this recent period included:

(%)	**Adult** (40%)	(%)	**Pediatric** (60%)
50	Isolated small intestine	36	Isolated small intestine
39	Multivisceral cluster	35	Small intestine / Liver
11	Small intestine/Liver	29	Multivisceral cluster

Leading indications for primary intestinal transplant during this period included:

(%)	**Adult**	(%)	**Pediatric**
24	Ischemia related loss of intestine	20	Gastroschisis
12	Crohn's disease	17	Volvulus
11	Other short gut	13	Necrotizing enterocolitis
10	Intestinal dismotility	9	Aganglionosis/Hirschsprung's
9	Trauma	8	Pseudo-obstruction
7	Volvulus	8	Intestinal atresia
6	Desmoid tumor	6	Microvillous inclusion disease

Transplant outcomes from 2005 to 2007 varied according to the type of transplant performed. For all patients, graft survival at 1 yr was 80% for isolated small intestine and 70% for small intestine/liver and for MVTs. Patient survival at 1 yr was 90% for isolated small intestine, but remained at 70% for small intestine/liver and multivisceral transplant patients. This disparity in graft survival is related to the increased complexity of the multiorgan transplants and the increased severity of illness seen in patients receiving these transplants. Median hospital stay also varies by transplant type and is 30 days for isolated small intestine, 60 days for small intestine/liver and 40 days for multivisceral transplant patients. Of those patients alive at 6 mths post-transplant, 70% are considered to be at full function (modified Karnofsky performance score 90–100%). Of the remainder, 15% of recipients are at partial function and 15% have had their grafts removed.

As with other abdominal and thoracic organs, long-term transplant outcomes for intestinal transplantation were initially poor but have improved with increasing experience. Results from the 1980s included patient survival at 5 yrs of ~40%, with an improvement to 45% in the 1990s. Since 2000, 5-yr patient survival is near 60% for all adult and pediatric recipients. Unfortunately, those with higher risk of death include the very old and very young. Though survival is similar for pediatric and adult patients up to 3 yrs post-transplant, it worsens significantly for pediatric patients when compared to adult patients after 4 yrs. In one report, children less than 1 yr of age faired much worse than those older than 1 yr of age (3-yr survival 12% vs. 52%). According to data from the U.S. Organ Procurement and Transplantation Network (OPTN), 1-yr patient survival for all U.S. intestinal transplants from 2003–2004 improved with increasing age:

	Patient survival	
Age group	1 yr (%)	5 yrs (%)
1 yr and younger	66	46
1–5 yrs	80	58
6–11 yrs	60	46
12–17 yrs	85	77
18 yrs and older	84	65

From the Organ Procurement and Transplant Network (U.S.), 2002–2007.

Quality of Life

Two large intestinal transplant centers have recently published papers assessing the post-transplant quality of life for intestinal recipients. The majority of recipients are able to be weaned from PN within 4 wks of transplantation (median 18 days) and nearly all are free from additional enteral supplementation by 1 yr (median 69 days). There is a significant overall improvement in quality of life as measured by validated "before and after" quality of life questionnaires for intestinal transplant patients compared to those not transplanted (p = 0.01). Subcategory analysis demonstrated improvement in nearly all quality of life areas including anxiety, depression, appearance, stress experience, parenting, optimism, control of impulsiveness, and quality of relationships.

Cost Effectiveness

The cost to maintain a patient on PN ranges from \$75,000–\$150,000 per year, excluding the costs of home nursing, support, equipment and supportive materials. Additionally, PN related complications result in an average of one major hospitalization per year, and catheter related complications are common and costly. Intestinal transplantation has been shown to be a cost effective therapy and is superior to continued PN in appropriately selected patients. Costs for intestinal transplantion, including the initial hospitalization for the transplant range from \$200,000–\$400,000. There are frequent hospital readmissions after transplant, but these admissions decrease markedly after the second year post-transplant. The benefit of transplantation reaches parity with PN after 2–3 yrs post-transplant and is more cost-effective thereafter.

Intestinal transplantation has shown consistent growth over the past 20 yrs with improving outcomes. As with other solid organ transplants, intestinal transplantation has moved out of the experimental realm to now become the standard of care for many patients with intestinal failure. Intestinal transplantation may soon be extended routinely to patients who, while not strictly meeting the criteria for intestinal failure, may benefit from intestinal transplantation such as those with nonresectable indolent tumors or patients with diffuse thrombosis of the porto-mesenteric system. As clinical experience has increased with intestinal transplantation, outcomes have improved. Currently reported 1-yr graft and patient survival is now 80%, which approaches that for other solid abdominal organs. Unfortunately, most of the gains in survival are seen in the first postoperative year, with long-term survival remaining basically unchanged since the early 1990s. Increase in access to intestinal transplantation, and more widespread awareness of this option, will likely result in a consistent increase in the number of yearly transplants for the foreseeable future.

Intestinal transplantation continues to be performed only in situations where all other therapeutic modalities have failed. There are no randomized trials comparing intestinal transplantation to long-term PN to establish guidelines for a timely referral for this treatment option. Late referral remains a crippling problem in the field of intestinal transplantation, with a great number of patients in need of simultaneous liver transplantation at the time of listing for intestinal transplantation. Early referral for isolated intestinal transplant will certainly reduce the need for simultaneous multi-organ transplants, and will, thereby, increase the residual organs available for those in need of (primarily) liver transplantation.

ORGAN PROCUREMENT

The organ procurement operation from a deceased donor is well standardized with little variation among surgeons. The primary goal of the procurement procedure is the safe removal of each individual organ, all of which remain viable for transplantation. Safe preservation of the organs is dependent upon two primary principles: (1) rapid exsanguination and vascular flushing with an appropriate preservation solution, and (2) rapid cooling. The involved organs are carefully dissected and prepared simultaneously. For the abdominal organs, an aortic cannula is placed which is used to flush the arterial system of the abdominal cavity. Some surgeons choose to place a second cannula in the portal vein (through the inferior mesenteric vein) to flush the portomesenteric system. The abdominal aorta is clamped superior to the celiac trunk and near the iliac bifurcation to isolate the abdominal organs. The outflow for the blood and preservation solution is generally through the suprahepatic vena cava at its junction with the right atrium. As the clamps are placed and the preservation solution is infused, iced normal saline is placed throughout the abdominal cavity to topically cool the organs. For living donor kidney and partial liver procurement, the organ/segment resection is performed in the donor with complete dissection performed while vascular inflow and outflow remains intact. Clamps are applied simultaneously and the donor graft is removed, followed by rapid flushing and cooling.

The choice of preservation solution has recently engendered some discussion. In the U.S., there are two primary solutions in use for abdominal organ preservation: University of Wisconsin (UW) and Histidine-tryptophan-ketoglutarate (HTK) solutions. The composition of HTK and UW preservation solutions, and the history behind their development, have been published previously.[23] HTK is a very low viscosity solution that is based upon a buffer system (histidine), with two additional substrates (tryptophan and ketoglutarate). UW is a much more viscous solution which flushes at a slower rate and with a lower total volume. With either solution, preservation of the organs is based upon the primary principle that the osmotic concentration is maintained by metabolically inert substrates with the addition of oxygen radical scavengers. UW is felt to provide organ tolerance to long cold ischemia times in a predictable manner. UW was first compared to HTK in a randomized fashion in liver transplantation over a decade ago and demonstrated clinical equivalence.[24] Subsequent clinical studies have demonstrated essentially equivalent outcomes for these two solutions in deceased donor liver transplantation. The solutions have also been found to be similar in living donor liver transplantation. HTK, with its lower viscosity, may result in better penetration of the microcirculation for a better flush. This may lead to a lower rate of biliary complications and may provide a more thorough flush in livers procured using donation after cardiac death.

Once procured, the organs must be transplanted and reperfused within a strict time limit. Whereas the heart and lung can only tolerate cold ischemia times of 4 and 6 hrs, respectively, the liver can routinely be transplanted with up to 12 hrs of cold ischemia time. The kidney and pancreas can tolerate much longer cold ischemia times ranging from 24 to 48 hrs. Beyond these time constraints, successful transplantation is possible but potential complications arise and there is increased risk of primary nonfunction and graft loss or patient death.

REFERENCES

1. Lillehei RC, Longerbeam JK, Goott B, Goldberg S, Scott WR. (1962) Gastrointestinal transplantation. *Surg Clin N Am* **42**:1191–1217.
2. Lillehei RC, Goldberg S, Goott B, Longerbeam JK. (1963) The present status of intestinal transplantation. *Am J Surg* **105**:58–72.
3. Lillehei RC, Idezuki Y, Feemster JA, Dietzman RH, Kelly WD, Merkel FK, Goetz FC, *et al.* (1967) Transplantation of stomach, intestine, and pancreas: Experimental and clinical observations. *Surgery* **62**:721–741.
4. Calne RY, Rolles K, White DJ, Thiru S, Evans DB, McMaster P, Dunn DC, *et al.* (1979) Cyclosporin A initially as the only immunosuppressant in 34 recipients of cadaveric organs: 32 kidneys, 2 pancreases, and 2 livers. *Lancet* **2**:1033–1036.
5. Borel JF, Feurer C, Gubler HU, Stahelin H. (1976) Biological effects of cyclosporin A: A new antilymphocytic agent. *Agents Actions* **6**:468–475.
6. Starzl TE, Rowe MI, Todo S, Jaffe R, Tzakis A, Hoffman AL, Esquivel C, *et al.* (1989) Transplantation of multiple abdominal viscera. *Jama* **261**:1449–1457.

7. Murase N, Demetris AJ, Matsuzaki T, Yagihashi A, Todo S, Fung J, Starzl TE. (1991) Long survival in rats after multivisceral versus isolated small-bowel allotransplantation under FK 506. *Surgery* **110**:87–98.
8. Iwaki Y, Starzl TE, Yagihashi A, Taniwaki S, Abu-Elmagd K, Tzakis A, Fung J, *et al.* (1991) Replacement of donor lymphoid tissue in small-bowel transplants. *Lancet* **337**:818–819.
9. Fishbein TM, Matsumoto CS. (2006) Intestinal replacement therapy: Timing and indications for referral of patients to an intestinal rehabilitation and transplant program. *Gastroenterology* **130**:S147–S151.
10. DeLegge M, Alsolaiman MM, Barbour E, Bassas S, Siddiqi MF, Moore NM. Short bowel syndrome: Parenteral nutrition versus intestinal transplantation. Where are we today? *Digest Dis Sci* **52**:876–892.
11. Goulet O, Ruemmele F, Lacaille F, Colomb V. (2004) Irreversible intestinal failure. *J Pediatr Gastr Nutr* **38**:250–269.
12. Dudrick SJ, Wilmore DW, Vars HM, Rhoads JE. (1968) Long-term total parenteral nutrition with growth, development, and positive nitrogen balance. *Surgery* **64**:134–142.
13. Suita S, Ikeda K, Nagasaki A, Hayashida Y, Kaneko T, Hamano Y, Nakata M, *et al.* (1982) Follow-up studies of children treated with a long-term intravenous nutrition (IVN) during the neonatal period. *J Pediatr Surg* **17**:37–42.
14. Messing B, Crenn P, Beau P, Boutron-Ruault MC, Rambaud JC, Matuchansky C. (1999) Long-term survival and parenteral nutrition dependence in adult patients with the short bowel syndrome. *Gastroenterology* **117**:1043–1050.
15. Chan S, McCowen KC, Bistrian BR, Thibault A, Keane-Ellison M, Forse RA, Babineau T, *et al.* (1999) Incidence, prognosis, and etiology of end-stage liver disease in patients receiving home total parenteral nutrition. *Surgery* **126**:28–34.
16. Gupte GL, Beath SV, Protheroe S, Murphy MS, Davies P, Sharif K, McKiernan PJ, *et al.* (2007) Improved outcome of referrals for intestinal transplantation in the UK. *Arch Dis Child* **92**:147–152.
17. Kaufman SS, Atkinson JB, Bianchi A, Goulet OJ, Grant D, Langnas AN, McDiarmid SV, *et al.* (2001) Indications for pediatric intestinal transplantation: A position paper of the American Society of Transplantation. *Pediatr Transplant* **5**:80–87.
18. Fryer JP. (2007) Intestinal transplantation: Current status. *Gastroenterol Clin N* **36**:145–159.

19. Freeman RB, Jr, Steffick DE, Guidinger MK, Farmer DG, Berg CL, Merion RM. (2008) Liver and intestine transplantation in the United States, 1997–2006. *Am J Transplant* **8**:958–976.
20. Tzakis AG, Kato T, Levi DM, Defaria W, Selvaggi G, Weppler D, Nishida S, *et al.* (2005) 100 multivisceral transplants at a single center.[see comment]. *Ann Surg* **242**:480–490; discussion 491–483.
21. Levi DM, Tzakis AG, Kato T, Madariaga J, Mittal NK, Nery J, Nishida S, *et al.* (2003) Transplantation of the abdominal wall. *Lancet* **361**:2173–2176.
22. Starzl TE, Todo S, Tzakis A, Alessiani M, Casavilla A, Abu-Elmagd K, Fung JJ. (1991) The many faces of multivisceral transplantation.[erratum appears in Surg Gynecol Obstet 1991 Sep; **173**(3):242]. *Surg Gynecol Obstetr* **172**:335–344.
23. Bretschneider HJ. (1980) Myocardial protection. *Thorac Cardiovasc Surg* **28**:295–302.
24. Erhard J, Lange R, Scherer R, Kox WJ, Bretschneider HJ, Gebhard MM, Eigler FW. (1994) Comparison of histidine-tryptophan-ketoglutarate (HTK) solution versus University of Wisconsin (UW) solution for organ preservation in human liver transplantation. A prospective, randomized study. *Transpl Int* **7**:177–181.

OVERVIEW OF IMMUNOSUPPRESSIVE AGENTS 33

Richard S. Mangus

INTRODUCTION

The majority of current immunosuppressive drugs specifically target T-cell activation, clonal expansion or differentiation in the effector cells. The process of T-cell activation is highly coordinated and involves binding of the T-cell receptor (TCR)-CD3 complex to the combined MHC-antigen expressed on the surface of antigen-presenting cells. Additional cell-bound and secreted co-stimulatory molecules contribute to augmentation of the T-cell activation. As a result of these interactions, multiple signal transduction pathways become operational, leading to induction of cytokine gene expression and stimulation of cellular activation. Interruption of any of the events of T-cell activation by immunosuppressive drugs results in downstream inhibition of cytokine expression and T-cell proliferation. The immunosuppressants cyclosporine (CsA), tacrolimus, and sirolimus suppress the immune response by inhibiting signal transduction pathways within the T-cell. These drugs bind to their intracellular targets, immunophilins, creating composite surfaces that block the activity of unique pathways. For CsA-cyclophilin and tacrolimus-FK-binding protein, the target is calcineurin. Sirolimus and everolimus inhibit the T-cell cycle downstream from the IL-2 receptor. Other available agents include polyclonal and monoclonal antibodies against TCRs, antiinterleukin-2 receptor (IL-2) monoclonal antibodies, and antiproliferative agents such as mycophenolate mofetil and azathioprine.

IMMUNOSUPPRESSION INDUCTION

The use of induction therapy with antilymphocyte monoclonal or polyclonal antibody preparations is now a frequent practice in nearly all transplant centers. The most commonly used induction agents are rabbit antithymocyte globulin (rATG), alemtuzamab, basiliximab and daclizumab. Modifications in the initiation of the immunosuppression regimen, including induction therapy, have more recently translated into decreased episodes of acute cellular rejection in the first 90 days post-transplant. This benefit, then, results in improved short-term patient and graft survival. With the native immune system being depleted and, in essence, reset in the presence of the transplant graft, there was a hope for the development of tolerance with replenishment of immune cells. These induction agents have not produced tolerance to this point, but it is felt by proponents that they may permit a reduction in the required maintenance immunosuppression.

Rabbit Antithymocyte Globulin (rATG, Thymoglobulin)

rATG is prepared by immunizing rabbits with cells derived from fragments of the human thymus gland. Unlike monoclonal preparations directed against specific T-cell antigens, rATG is a polyclonal preparation containing antibodies to a variety of T- and B-cell antigens. Studies have shown that the human thymus, in addition to containing thymocytes that usually express T-cell antigens, also contains 5 to 10% plasma cells.[1] Therefore, the rabbit inoculation results in a preparation that contains antibodies against plasma cell/B-cell antigens, as well as the expected T-cell antigens. In addition to T- and B-cell depletion, studies have shown a possible protective effect against reperfusion injury when thymoglobulin is administered before reperfusion of solid organs.[2] Several mechanisms have been proposed to explain this finding, including a blockade of adhesion molecules, decreased cell surface expression of beta-integrins, as well as endothelial inflammatory cells.

A primary benefit of rATG induction is effective early immunosuppression without renal toxicity. Targeting cell surface antigens using monoclonal and polyclonal antibodies represents an attractive therapy in the prevention of acute rejection after solid organ transplantation, while minimizing initial high doses of tacrolimus (and its side effect of nephrotoxicity). Use of rATG to induce immunosuppression allows a delay in the introduction of calcineurin inhibitors, which may spare renal function in the immediate post-transplant period. An important side effect of rATG is a significant septic-type reaction with administration of the agent which includes hypoxia and pulmonary edema, tachycardia, fever, and shaking chills.

Alemtuzumab (Campath-1H)

Alemtuzumab is a recombinant DNA-derived humanized monoclonal antibody directed against CD52, and has increased in popularity as an induction agent in transplantation over the last decade. Administration of this antibody results in a large depletion of lymphocytes, as well as natural killer cells, monocytes and thymocytes. This broad depletion of immune cells provides an opportunity to "reset" the immune system upon exposure to the transplanted organ.[3] This agent, however, differs from rATG in that it does not appear to deplete plasma cells or memory lymphocytes. Because these cells are not depleted, it appears that there is a lower incidence of post-transplant infectious risk, as these immunocompetent cells remain active. Alemtuzumab has been associated with infusion-related events similar to those seen with rATG, and include instability of blood pressure, rigors, fever, hypoxia, and bronchospasm. Alemtuzumab is also known as Campath.[4]

Daclizimab (Zenapax)

Daclizumab (trade name *Zenapax*) is a humanized monoclonal antibody with high affinity to the T-cell IL-2 receptor. Daclizumab binding is highly specific for an IL-2 receptor subunit which is expressed on activated lymphocytes, but not seen on inactive lymphocytes. Therefore, this agent specifically inhibits IL-2-mediated activation of lymphocytes, a critical pathway in the cellular immune response involved in allograft rejection.

With saturation of the T-cell IL-2 receptors, and prevention of T-cell activation and signaling, B-cell activation may also be impeded. Daclizumab has primarily been studied in kidney transplantation, but is now being employed more across other transplanted organs. Daclizumab is similar to *basiliximab* (Simulect), in that both agents are monoclonal antibodies against the IL-2 receptor of T-cells. Both have been shown to be clinically effective immune suppression medications. Daclizumab has been described as an induction agent and may allow the delayed introduction of calcineurin-inhibitors in the early post-transplant period. Unlike rATG and alemtuzumab, administration related reactions to daclizumab are infrequent and mild, though anaphylactic reaction has been reported.

MAINTENANCE IMMUNOSUPPRESSION

Cyclosporin (CsA, Neoral, Sandimmune)

Initially isolated from a Norwegian soil sample, *Cyclosporin A,* the primary form of CsA, is a cyclic peptide produced by a fungus. CsA binds to the cytosolic protein cyclophilin (immunophilin) of immunocompetent lymphocytes, particularly T-lymphocytes. This complex of CsA and cyclophilin inhibits calcineurin, which is involved in the transcription of IL-2. CsA inhibits lymphokine production and interleukin release and, therefore, leads to a reduced function of effector T-cells. There is a large surface area of interaction of the drug–immunophilin complex. The calcineurin inhibitors, tacrolimus and CsA, have a specificity for their biologic targets that is similar to the interaction between growth factors and their receptors. It is thought that most, if not all, of the therapeutic as well as toxic effects of these drugs, are due to inhibition of calcineurin. Inhibition of the action of calcineurin results in a complete block in the translocation of the cytosolic component of the nuclear factor of activated T cells (NF-AT), resulting in a failure to activate the genes regulated by the NF-AT transcription factor. These genes include those required for B-cell help such as interleukin (IL-4) and CD40 ligand as well as those necessary for T-cell proliferation such as IL-2.

CsA, marketed as Neoral or Sandimmune, remains commonly used throughout the world as it is an inexpensive and effective clinical agent. Side effects are common with long-term therapy and can include renal dysfunction, hirsutism, tremor, hypertension, gum hyperplasia, acne, and headaches.

Tacrolimus (Prograf)

In the 1990s, a drug originally known as FK506 was developed, and later became known as tacrolimus.[5] Routine use of this calcineurin inhibitor coincided with improved clinical outcomes, and facilitated modulation of immunosuppression through stable blood levels and a significant decrease in the incidence of rejection. Although a major component of the immunosuppressive effects of CsA and tacrolimus is accounted for by inhibition of calcineurin, it appears that tacrolimus also inhibits steps distal to calcineurin activation in the T-cell activation cascade. The superiority of tacrolimus over CsA in attenuating rejection episodes in patients with renal, heart-lung, and liver allografts has been documented. This finding is supported by the demonstrated capacity of tacrolimus monotherapy to reverse steroid-resistant allograft rejection episodes.[6,7] This is an important clinical difference between tacrolimus and CsA, as CsA has not been shown to be effective in the treatment of allograft rejection. Though the exact cellular and molecular targets of tacrolimus remain to be fully understood, it has taken its place as the primary maintenance immunosuppressive agent for most organs at most centers. Besides this nephrotoxicity, tacrolimus has also been implicated in the development of post-transplant diabetes, hypertension, hair loss, hyperkalemia and hypertriglyceridemia. There are also neurologic side effects unique to tacrolimus which include a lowered seizure threshold, tremor, peripheral neuropathic-type pain, and mutism.

Sirolimus (Rapamycin, Rapamune)

Sirolimus is the product of the bacterium streptomyces hygroscopicus originally found in a soil sample from Easter Island, also known as "Rapa Nui". Because of this history, and its classification as a macrolide, sirolimus has been marketed as rapamycin and has been found to be an effective immunosuppressant as well as antiproliferative agent. Sirolimus inhibits the response to IL-2 and thereby blocks activation of T- and B-cells. The mode of action of Sirolimus is to bind an intracellular protein, FK-binding protein, in a manner similar to tacrolimus. However, unlike the tacrolimus-bound complex which inhibits calcineurin, the sirolimus-bound complex inhibits the target of rapamycin (TOR) pathway. Inhibition of TOR activation results in the inhibition of T lymphocyte activation and proliferation associated with antigen and cytokine (IL-2, IL-4, and IL-15) stimulation, and the inhibition of antibody production.

Sirolimus has been used in association with tacrolimus in some patients, though the clinical effects of combining these two agents are not well described. The chief advantage sirolimus has over calcineurin inhibitors is that it is less toxic to kidneys. Transplant patients maintained on calcineurin inhibitors long-term tend to develop impaired kidney function or even chronic renal failure. It is possible that this effect can be minimized by using sirolimus instead. Sirolimus can be used alone, in conjunction with calcineurin inhibitors, or with mycophenolate mofetil, so as to provide steroid-free immunosuppression regimes. A well known side effect of sirolimus, impaired wound healing, may limit use of this agent in the immediate postoperative period. The antiproliferative effect of sirolimus has also been used in conjunction with coronary stents to prevent restenosis in coronary arteries following balloon angioplasty. These antiproliferative actions have also led to the study of this drug for its antitumor properties.

Mycophenolate Mofetil (Cellcept)

Mycophenolate mofetil (Cellcept) is frequently given as part of a double or triple drug regimen. It is used interchangeably with azathioprine and has a similar side-effect profile as both are antiproliferative agents. The primary benefit of an antiproliferative agent in conjunction with a CI is an increase in the overall level of immunosuppression. Use of these agents may allow lower dosing of the CI, thus minimizing nephrotoxicity and preserving long-term renal function. The primary side effects of mycophenolate mofetil include gastrointestinal distress that can be manifest as nausea or loose stools and bone marrow suppression resulting in neutropenia and anemia.

Azathioprine (Imuran)

Azathioprine (Imuran) is a DNA synthesis inhibitor through its action as a purine analogue. This drug is one of the oldest known immunosuppressive agents and acts by inhibiting the proliferation of leukocytes (as well as all fast-growing cells). Azathioprine was used in conjunction with steroids as the immunosuppressive regimen first employed in kidney and liver transplantation. This dual therapy was the standard in antirejection therapy until the introduction of calcineurin inhibitors in the late 1970s. Azathioprine is also utilized in patients with certain autoimmune diseases. Its side effect profile is similar to that described for mycophenolate mofetil.

Prednisone

Prednisone is a synthetic corticosteroid that results in a broad suppression of the immune response and is employed in the treatment of a wide variety of disease processes. Prednisone has been an important component of immunosuppression in organ transplantation since its inception. Prednisone taken orally is converted in the liver to prednisolone, an active steroid. This drug suppresses the adrenal glands and results in a variety of side effects including high blood glucose levels, weight gain, poor tissue healing, osteoporosis, glaucoma and Cushing's syndrome.

Additional Medications

Trimethoprim/sulfamethoxazole (Bactrim, Septra) is a combination drug given to immunosuppressed patients for *Pneumocystis carinii* prophylaxis. Patients generally take this for a minimum of 1 yr post-transplant, but may stay on the drug indefinitely. Side effects of this medication include bone marrow suppression and hepatotoxicity. This medication if frequently stopped if the liver function enzymes are elevated in a transplant patient to determine if there is some other etiology of the abnormality.

Ganciclovir (Cytovene) and valganciclovir (Valcyte) are given for cytomegalovirus (CMV) prophylaxis. The choice of antiviral agent, and length of therapy, depends upon the patient's risk category for invasive CMV disease. The lowest risk group is the donor CMV negative and recipient CMV negative, while the highest risk group is the donor CMV positive and recipient CMV negative. These drugs can also result in bone marrow suppression and often must be stopped for severe neutropenia. Fluconazole (Diflucan) is used as antifungal prophylaxis for both topical and systemic disease. It is well known to be hepatotoxic and frequently must be stopped if there is an unexpected elevation in the patient's liver function enzymes. Fluconazole and other antifungals interact with tacrolimus and cyclosporin metabolism so that serum levels of these agents must be closely monitored when antifungals are initiated or stopped. Lamivudine (Epivir) is used for the treatment of chronic hepatitis B and is also employed in the prophylaxis of hepatitis B in patients who receive liver allografts from donors who have been exposed to the hepatitis B virus. Aspirin is given to most transplant patients as an antiplatelet agent to prevent thrombosis of the transplanted graft.

REFERENCES

1. Bonnefoy-Berard N, Flacher M, Revillard JP. (1992) Antiproliferative effect of antilymphocyte globulins on B cells and B-cell lines. *Blood* **79**:2164–2170.
2. Beiras-Fernandez A, Thein E. (2003) Hammer C. Induction of immunosuppression with polyclonal antithymocyte globulins: An overview. *Exp Clin Transplant* **1**:79–84.
3. Magliocca JF, Knechtle SJ. (2006) The evolving role of alemtuzumab (Campath-1H) for immunosuppressive therapy in organ transplantation. *Transpl Int* **19**:705–714.
4. Riechmann L, Clark M, Waldmann H, Winter G. (1988) Reshaping human antibodies for therapy. *Nature* **332**:323–327.
5. Murase N, Kim DG, Todo S, Cramer DV, Fung J, Starzl TE. (1990) FK506 suppression of heart and liver allograft rejection. II: The induction of graft acceptance in rats. *Transplantation* **50**:739–744.
6. (1994) A comparison of tacrolimus (FK 506) and cyclosporine for immunosuppression in liver transplantation. The U.S. Multicenter FK506 Liver Study *Group. N Engl J Med* **331**:1110–1115.
7. Moore R, Lord R. (1994) Tacrolimus (FK506) versus cyclosporin in prevention of liver allograft rejection. *Lancet* **344**:948.

Section 5:
Head/Neck

THYROID 34

Adam C. Alder and Michael A. Skinner

INTRODUCTION

Developments in understanding the thyroid in the late 19th and 20th centuries have made surgical treatment of thyroid disorders relatively common and morbidity free. Thyroid disease is uncommon in children. Thyroid cancer is rare in general while thyroid nodules and lesions become more common with age. In children, thyroid lesions more commonly represent neoplastic processes. The impact of thyroid dysfunction on maturation and growth, while mostly medically managed, can be dramatic. In this chapter, the background of development and normal physiology of the thyroid gland are discussed, followed by pathologic conditions. The chapter concludes with operative techniques and tips along with appropriate preoperative workup and postoperative care guidelines.

EMBRYOLOGY

The thyroid gland is derived from a bud that forms from the base of the tongue and migrates to the low midline of the neck. This budding structure forms the thyroglossal duct which moves inferiorly and develops into a bilobed structure. By 6 wks of age, the thyroglossal duct is usually reabsorbed completely. If this structure persists, it may present as a midline neck mass — the thyroglossal duct cyst. This cystic structure may present acutely as an abscess or mass or, chronically, as an abscess or an infected, draining fistula. Treatment includes antibiotics followed by removal of the thyroglossal duct cyst in its entirety. Abscesses should be drained and the thyroglosssal duct should be removed after resolution of inflammation. Resection involves removal of the thyroglossal duct from its origin at the base of the tongue, through the middle of the hyoid bone by resecting this central portion of the bone, and the cyst itself (the Sistrunk procedure) (see Chapter 39 — Neck Cysts).

Ectopic thyroid may also present as a midline neck mass. Ultrasound of the thyroid gland is routinely obtained in the workup of a midline neck mass to ensure the presence of normal thyroid tissue. If the midline mass is the only thyroid tissue, controversy exists regarding resection of the midline tissue. This functional thyroid tissue may prevent replacement hormone treatment, although hormone supplementation is often required for hypothyroidism or control of the size of the mass. Some advocate complete resection as neoplasms may arise within the tissue and there is no guarantee that hormone replacement will be prevented. We advocate resection and hormone replacement.

C-cell migration from the fourth pharyngeal pouch occurs during the descent of the thyroid early in the development of the embryo. These cells produce calcitonin and are the cells of origin for medullary thyroid carcinoma, which can occur sporadically, familially or as part of MEN 2A or 2B.

PHYSIOLOGY

The blood supply is from the superior and inferior thyroid arteries. The superior thyroid artery arises as the first branch of the external carotid artery. It courses with the external branch of the superior laryngeal nerve which innervates the cricothyroid muscle. Injury to this nerve results in a loss of voice quality and strength.

The inferior thyroid artery arises from the thyrocervical trunk. The recurrent laryngeal nerve runs along the same course as the inferior thyroid artery and the nerve should be identified prior to ligation of the branches of the artery during thyroid resection. This artery also supplies both the inferior and superior parathyroid glands.

The thyroid gland contains two main cell types: follicular cells and the parafollicular cells or c-cells. Follicular cells produce thyroxine (T_4) and triiodothyronine (T_3). Production of these hormones requires iodine. This process is controlled by thyroid stimulating hormone (TSH) from the pituitary gland. If iodine is not present, the individual may develop cretinism, which is characterized by mental and growth retardation, hypothyroidism, nodular goiter and follicular thyroid carcinoma.

Production of T_4 and T_3 is completed by the enzyme thyroid peroxidase. Regulation of T_3 and T_4 release is by the hypothalamic-pituitary-thyroid axis. TSH acts as a the major regulator of thyroid hormone release. There are negative feedback loops of TSH and circulating levels of T_3 and T_4.

Evaluation of thyroid function centers around three blood tests: TSH, T_3 and T_4 levels. The relationship between these three blood levels determines whether the individual is hypo-, eu- or hyperthyroid. Evaluation of clinical symptoms is also important. Dosing of thyroid replacement is also managed by the level of TSH in a treated patient. Routine use of thyroglobulin and calcitonin levels is common after resection of the thyroid gland. Post-thyroidectomy elevation of thyroglobulin or calcitonin may represent recurrence of tumor.

NON-NEOPLASTIC THYROID CONDITIONS

Hypothyroidism

Disorders of hypothyroidism are rarely treated surgically. These disorders are generally related to defects in the hypothalamic-pituitary-thyroid axis. Rarely, there is a pathologic condition related to failure to respond to normal stimuli, such as a defect in the thyroid receptor gene.

In neonates, the most common cause of hypothyroidism is thyroid gland dysgenesis, which accounts for 90% of cases. This abnormality is usually identified by screening programs. Because of transplacental passage of maternal thyroid hormones, neonates are asymptomatic even in the presence of no active thyroid tissue.

Goiter and Thyroiditis

A goiter is found in about 3% of the population when children are specifically surveyed for abnormalities of the thyroid. Goiter refers to an enlargement of the thyroid and may be the result of nodules or diffuse hypertrophy. There may be either euthyroid or hyperthyroid conditions. The etiology of the goiter may be related to any of the diagnoses listed in Table 1.

Most thyroid goiter in areas where iodine supplementation is common is simple colloid goiter also known as adolescent or nontoxic goiter. Diagnosis

Table 1. Differential diagnosis of goiter in children.

Autoimmune Mediated	Chronic lymphocytic (Hashimoto's) thyroiditis
	Graves' disease
	Simple colloid goiter
Compensatory	Iodine deficiency
	Medications
	Goitrogens
	Hormones or receptor defect
Inflammatory Conditions	Acute suppurative thyroiditis
	Subacute thyroiditis

is made by documenting normal thyroid function levels and the diffuse nature of the thyroid enlargement is revealed by thyroid imaging by scintigraphy or by ultrasound. The majority of thyroid glands in patients with nontoxic goiter become normal in adulthood. This regression occurs as frequently with, as without, treatment with thyroid hormone and therefore does not require treatment with thyroid hormone replacement unless there is evidence of hypothyroidism.

Thyroiditis

Thyroiditis is classified in three types: chronic (Hashimoto's), subacute (de Quervain's) and acute. Chronic lymphocytic thyroiditis, also called Hashimoto's thyroiditis, is a common cause of diffuse thyroid enlargement in children. Adolescent females are most commonly affected as a part of a spectrum of autoimmune thyroid disorders. Associated conditions include juvenile rheumatoid arthritis, Addison's disease, and type I diabetes mellitus. Typically patients are euthyroid and progressively become hypothyroid. About 10% present with symptoms of hyperthyroidism and may develop thyrotoxicosis, sometimes referred to as hashitoxicosis. There are typically high titers of circulating antithyroglobulin and antimicrosomal antibodies and histologic evaluation reveals infiltration by B-cell lymphocytes.

Children most often present with thyroid gland enlargement which prompts an evaluation. On palpation, the thyroid gland is granular or pebbly or may be mildly tender. Laboratory evaluation should include TSH initially. An assessment of serum thyroid antibodies can confirm the diagnosis in patients suspected to have the condition. An ultrasound of the thyroid will reveal a diffuse hypoechogenicity and scintigraphy reveals patchy uptake. Rarely, fine needle aspiration may be required if no antibodies are identified.

Treatment of euthyroid patients with Hashimoto's thyroiditis is typically expectant. Initiation of thyroid hormone replacement in euthyroid patients does not change the typically benign course of this disease. Thyroid function should be monitored every 6 mths to assess for development of hypothyroidism, which should prompt thyroid replacement. Most patients' symptoms will resolve along with thyroid enlargement and detectable serum antibodies.

Subacute thyroiditis (de Quervain's thyroiditis) is caused by a virus and is rare in children. The thyroid gland is typically tender and swollen. Usually TSH is slightly suppressed because of leak of thyroid hormone from the inflamed thyroid follicles. Scintigraphy reveals low levels of thyroid uptake which differentiates this process from Graves' disease. Microscopic examination typically reveals granulomas and epithelioid cells. The mainstay of treatment is control of symptoms with nonsteroidal anti-inflammatory agents and corticosteroids with duration of symptoms being approximately 2–9 mths followed by complete resolution of the condition.

Acute suppurative thyroiditis is the result of a bacterial infection of the thyroid gland. Patients may appear ill with evidence of sepsis and an acutely inflamed thyroid gland. Most are euthyroid. Identified organisms are typically staphylococci or mixed aerobic and anaerobic flora. This infection is sometimes related to a congenital pharyngeal sinus which predisposes patients to the condition. Antibiotics alone are required in the absence of an abscess, which may require incision and drainage. Aspiration of the abscess under ultrasound guidance has been reported although it may require repeated treatment.

Hyperthyroidism

With rare exceptions, hyperthyroidism in children is caused by diffuse toxic goiter, or Graves' disease. This condition is an autoimmune syndrome

Table 2. Causes of hyperthyroidism in children.

Graves' Disease (toxic diffuse goiter)
Toxic nodular goiter
Subacute thyroiditis
Neonatal thyroiditis
Thyroid-secreting hormone-secreting pituitary tumor
McCune–Albright syndrome
Thyrotropin receptor mutation

in which antibodies are made against the TSH receptors on the follicular cells of the thyroid gland. Most often the onset of the condition is delayed 2–3 wks after delivery. The ratio of males to females affected is 1:5 with the peak incidence of onset in adolescence. Symptoms develop gradually over time with initial reported symptoms including nervousness, emotional lability, and declining performance at school. Later symptoms include weight loss and increased sweating, palpitations, heat intolerance, and malaise. True exophthalmos is unusual in children, but a conspicuous stare is common. A smooth goiter is commonly identified on physical exam which may be associated with a bruit when auscultated. Laboratory evaluation reveals typical findings associated with elevated thyroid hormone production, i.e. elevated free T_4 levels and suppressed TSH. Occasionally, there is an isolated elevation of T_3, referred to as T_3 toxicosis. Identification of TSH-stimulation immunoglobulins confirms the diagnosis of Graves' disease.

The management of Graves' disease involves medical management with antithyroid medications or ablation of the thyroid gland with radioactive ^{131}I. Surgical resection is required for patients with symptoms refractory to medical treatment. Treatment often begins with initiation of anti-thyroid medications. The most commonly used medications are propylthiourocil (PTU) and methimazole. Both medications reduce circulating thyroid hormone levels by inhibiting organification of iodide by the follicle cells and coupling of iodotyrosines. Methimazole is preferred because of its less frequent dosing and higher potency. TSH must be monitored for elevated levels which indicate over treatment and should prompt a reduction in dose. Once free T_4 and T_3 levels are normal, the dose of methimazole should be reduced to 10 mg and maintained to keep thyroid hormone levels normal. Methimazole and PTU have a serious side-effect of idiosyncratic agranulocytosis. Initial symptoms of a sore throat and fever should prompt a neutrophil count. If low, these medications should be stopped which will allow the granulocyte count to recover in 2–3 wks. Parenteral antibiotics are recommended during the intervening period. Other side effects include nausea, minor skin reactions, urticaria, arthralgias, arthritis, and fevers.

Remission of Graves' disease has been reported in 25% in treated patients if medication is discontinued after 2 yrs and another 25% every 2 yrs. Persistent circulating TSH receptor antibodies are associated with lower rates of remission. Failure to respond to antithyroid medications or a severe reaction to the medications used for treatment should prompt definitive ablation of the thyroid. This involves either radioactive ablation with ^{131}I or surgical resection. Both treatment options have benefits and risks. Radiologic ablation is effective, but doesn't prevent future hypothyroidism. Ablation may also require additional larger doses of radiation to render the gland completely hypofunctional. There does not appear to be teratogenic or carcinogenic effects related to the use of ^{131}I.

Surgical resection for treatment for Graves' disease is recommended for disease refractory to medical treatment. Subtotal thyroidectomy is the procedure of choice and is appropriate for those who fail medical management or who refuse radioactive ablation. Details of the procedure are discussed later. In Graves' disease, the thyroid gland is enlarged and engorged with blood. There may be compressive symptoms related to the enlarged gland. Prior to any surgical treatment, patients should be rendered euthyroid with antithyroid medications. Symptoms of hyperthyroidism can be controlled with β-adrenergic-blocking agents like propranolol. Lugol's solution, an aqueous solution of elemental iodine and potassium iodide, should be administered 4 to 7 days before surgery to reduce the glands engorgement and vascularity. Frequently, patients will need postoperative thyroid hormone replacement because of hypothyroidism. There is a risk of recurrence of hyperthyroidism affecting as many as 5% in 1 yr and up to 50% in 25 yrs. Postoperative monitoring of thyroid function and assessment of symptoms of hyperthyroidism should be repeated regularly.

NEOPLASTIC THYROID CONDITIONS

Thyroid Nodules

Thyroid nodules may be the initial finding of thyroid cancer, although this risk is reported to be about 20% of the total number of nodules identified. Often patients are referred to the clinic after an initial evaluation of a thyroid mass. Initial evaluation in the surgical clinic should include a careful history to assess for clinical evidence of thyroid function. Past medical conditions especially those that might have predisposed to exposure to radiation assist in predicting the risk of thyroid malignancy. Assessment of the family history for thyroid cancer or thyroid conditions is imperative as well. A careful exam of the neck including the thyroid and lateral nodal chains should be completed. Evidence of adenopathy is suspicious of an advanced malignancy. A TSH level is obtained to confirm the level of

Table 3. Differential diagnosis of solitary thyroid nodules in children.

Adenoma
Carcinoma
Thyroid cyst
Ectopic thyroid gland
Lymphovascular malformation
Thyroglossal duct remnant
Germ cell tumor

thyroid function. Imaging provides additional information that assist in differentiating a solitary nodule from a multinodular or diffuse goiter. Ultrasound evaluation, when performed by experienced radiologists or surgeons, readily identifies the nodule although it cannot differentiate between a malignant or benign lesion. It may also identify enlarged lymph nodes. The next step in the evaluation of a thyroid nodule is the decision of whether to obtain a fine needle aspiration biopsy (FNA). The FNA is a highly sensitive and specific test in adults and is commonly used. In children, the test often requires sedation and its utility may not be as great given the higher likelihood of malignancy. In adolescents, FNA can be very useful. The result of the FNA is typically one of four — it may confirm malignancy, identify benign cells, be indeterminate or be inadequate for diagnosis.

Thyroid nodules in prepubertal children should be removed in all cases because of the difficulty in establishing the benign nature of the lesion and the unknown natural history of thyroid nodules in such children. In older patients, if FNA confirms a benign lesion, it may be observed with serial ultrasound examinations. If there is demonstrated growth of a benign lesion, the FNA cannot confirm a benign nodule, or in patients with established malignancy, the nodule should be removed. Occasionally, preoperative scintigraphy may provide assistance in determining the anatomy of the thyroid and aberrant nodules.

Extent of resection in the case of an indeterminate nodule should be limited to lobectomy. This limits the risk to the recurrent laryngeal nerve and parathyroid glands. Sometimes total or subtotal thyroidectomy may be indicated because of a high likelihood of malignancy; for example, in a patient with radiation exposure, enlarging nodule or family history of thyroid disease.

Thyroid Carcinoma

Thyroid malignancies in children are unusual with a reported incidence of one to two cases per million individuals under 20 yrs of age. The peak incidence is between 10 and 18 yrs of age and is twice as common in girls as boys. There has been a decline in the number of thyroid malignancies probably owing to the less common use of external beam radiation for the treatment of benign diseases. Radiation is a significant predisposing factor whose importance in the development of thyroid cancer has been confirmed by reports from areas affected by nuclear catastrophes. There is typically a 4–6 yr latency from exposure to development of thyroid cancer with a reported increase in thyroid tumor incidence of more than 60-fold.

Childhood malignancies also predispose a child to the development of thyroid malignancy. Hodgkin's lymphoma is the most common first malignancy associated with the development of thyroid cancer which is related to both the radiation as well as the alkylating agents used in its treatment. There is a median lag time of about 12 yrs to the recognition of thyroid disease.

Both sporadic and familial thyroid cancers are related to genetic events including the RET proto-oncogene resulting in constitutive activation of the tyrosine kinase molecule. This gene event has been associated with papillary cancers as well as other types of thyroid malignancies.

Thyroid malignancies usually present clinically as a nodule or mass that may be associated with cervical adenopathy in a euthyroid patient. After obtaining a careful history and a complete physical exam, TSH levels are assessed to confirm normal thyroid function. Ultrasound examination provides details about size, location and associated nonpalpable nodules and enlarged lymph nodes. The ultrasound may also provide evidence of invasion of adjacent structures. FNA; if obtained, may identify malignant cells or be indeterminate.

Much debate remains about the recommended treatment of thyroid malignancies in terms of the extent of resection. Clear guidelines include removal of all abnormal tissue which may involve subtotal or total thyroidectomy along with central or modified lymph node dissection. The advantages of total surgical extirpation of the thyroid include more effective postresection radioactive iodine treatment and easier surveillance for recurrence using serum thyroglobulin and scintigraphy. However, the extent of surgical resection determines the risk of injury to the recurrent

Table 4. Thyroid cancer staging.

Papillary thyroid cancer	
Stage I	Cancer is found only in the thyroid
Stage II	For <45 yrs: Cancer beyond thryoid For>45 yrs: Cancer limited to thyroid, but>1 cm
Stage III	Age>45 yrs and Spread outside thyroid, but not beyond neck or lymph nodes
Stage IV	Age>45 yrs and Tumor has spread to other parts of the body – Lungs – Bones
Follicular thyroid cancer	
Stage I	Cancer is found only in the thyroid
Stage II	For <45 yrs: Cancer beyond thryoid For> 45 yrs: Cancer limited to thyroid, but> 1 cm
Stage III	Age> 45 yrs and Spread outside thyroid, but not beyond neck or lymph nodes
Stage IV	Age> 45 yrs and Tumor has spread to other parts of the body – Lungs – Bones
Medullary thyroid cancer	
Stage I	Lesion <1 cm
Stage II	Lesion ≥ 1 cm and>4 cm
Stage III	Positive lymph nodes
Stage IV	Spread beyond the thyroid.

laryngeal nerve and parathyroid glands. Complications related to these structures occur more frequently in younger children than in older patients. Proponents of less aggressive resection argue that most thyroid cancers in children are well differentiated and have an indolent course and, therefore, survival is not improved by more extensive resection. After resection, patients with confirmed malignancy may undergo radioactive ablation of any residual thyroid tissue.

Surveillance for recurrence should include evaluation with serum thyroglobulin level and antithyroglobulin antibody titers. Elevation of the thyroglobulin after near total removal of the thyroid indicates possible recurrence and should prompt scintigraphy. Exam of the neck should also be completed regularly as well as screening or directed ultrasound. Recurrence of thyroid cancer is most common in the lungs and the neck. The risk of recurrence is reported to be 30% after 20 yrs and, therefore, surveillance should be long term. Most episodes of recurrence can be effectively treated with radioiodine ablation. Long-term survival is determined by extent of residual disease after resection and age at time of diagnosis. Relapse-free survival at 20 yrs has been reported to be 10% for those age 10 yrs or younger and 48% for those older than age 10.

Multiple Endocrine Neoplasia

About 5% of thyroid malignancies are medullary thyroid cancers (MTC) which arise from the parafollicular cells. These neural crest cells migrate to the thyroid from the fourth pharyngeal pouch and release calcitonin. While sporadic cases of MTC occur, this malignancy is also part of the multiple endocrine neoplasia (MEN) 2 syndrome. The MEN 2 syndrome has two subtypes. MEN 2A, which is associated with pheochromocytoma and parathyroid adenomas, is less virulent than MEN 2B, which is associated with pheochromocytoma, neurofibromatous disease and Marfanoid habitus. A third type of familial syndrome, familial medullary thyroid carcinoma syndrome (FMTC), has also been described. In each case, medullary thyroid cancer is almost certain to occur, and may occur very early in life. These syndromes are related to a mutation in the RET proto-oncogene that predisposes to the syndrome. Prophylactic total thyroidectomy and surveillance with calcitonin levels is recommended in those at risk. Patients who develop MTC should have total thyroidectomy and central lymph node (level VI) dissection. These tumors are not radioiodine sensitive. Those at risk who are known to have MEN 2A should undergo thyroid resection by age five. As MEN 2B is more virulent, their glands should be removed in infancy. There is genetic testing available to identify those at risk in relatives of an individual known to have MTC.

OPERATIVE TECHNIQUE

After induction, a roll is placed under the shoulders and the neck is extended. The patient is placed in a semi-fowler position with the knees bent over pillows. The arms should be tucked and appropriately padded. The neck from the lower chin to the upper chest should be prepped with an antiseptic solution.

Every step of the operation should be completed in as bloodless a manner as possible. It is the preference of the authors to use sterile water as irrigation to clean-up the field, if bleeding should occur, once hemostasis is obtained. Bipolar cautery and tissue sealing devices (Ligasure) are used routinely by the authors.

A collar incision is made 2–3 cm superior to the suprasternal notch from sternocleidomastoid to sternocleidomastoid. The incision is made following the Langer lines and symmetry should be the goal. After the skin is incised sharply, the subcutaneous tissue is divided exposing the platysma, which is divided along the length of the incision. After obtaining hemostasis, inferior and superior flaps are made from the thyroid notch superiorly to the suprasternal notch inferiorly by elevating the platysma with Allis or Lahey clamps and dividing the thin areolar tissue. Self-retaining retractors may be used to retract the skin flaps. The strap muscles are divided longitudinally in the midline along the avascular plane.

The operation is then continued toward the lobe with the thyroid pathology. The strap muscles are dissected away from the underlying gland by retracting the strap muscles with a small retractor or Allis clamps. Dissecting close to the muscles keeps bleeding to a minimum. The middle thyroid vein is encountered and should be tied in continuity and divided. This allows the thyroid lobe to be retracted up and medially. Often, a figure-of-eight suture in the substance of the lobe or a noncrushing clamp aids in medial retraction. Dissection is continued inferiorly along the capsule of the thyroid until the inferior pole is encountered. The lateral dissection of the thyroid lobe is completed by moving superiorly, staying within the capsule of the gland. A blunt curved hemostat placed across the superior pole aids in lateral and medial displacement of the vascular bundle. A window is created between the upper medial border of the thyroid gland and the cricothyroid muscle. Dissection of the fibrous tissue allows for identification of the external branch of the superior laryngeal nerve in this window. Once the nerve is identified, the superior pole can be divided close to the thyroid capsule. The remnant vascular pedicle should be suture ligated as it may retract up into the neck. Alternatively, the vascular pedicle is taken with bipolar cautery.

An inspection for the parathyroid glands and the recurrent laryngeal nerve can be made now that the thyroid lobe is mobilized and retracted medially. Parathyroid glands are pink to tan colored and are usually associated with a lobule of fat. The superior gland is typically located on the posterior surface of the upper portion of the lobe of the thyroid. The inferior gland is typically located inferior to the inferior thyroid artery and may be as far inferior as the inferior thymic ligament or in the thymus itself. Searching for a difficult to identify parathyroid gland should include inspection along the tracheo-esophageal groove, inside the carotid sheath, and in the thymus. If the parathyroid is inside the substance of the thyroid lobe, it will not be possible to identify or preserve. Care must be taken to avoid injury to the blood supply to the parathyroid. This can be accomplished by ensuring dissection along the capsule of the thyroid gland and avoiding cautery away from the substance of the thyroid. If any concern exists regarding the viability of an identified parathyroid gland, it should be preserved and reimplanted in a muscle belly in the neck or forearm.

After completing mobilization of the thyroid and strap muscles laterally to the carotid sheath, the inferior thyroid artery is identified coursing medially toward the junction of the middle to lower third of the thyroid lobe. Care should be taken to identify the recurrent laryngeal nerve as it courses along the tracheoesophageal groove. The nerve can be palpated as a cord within the connective tissues lateral to the trachea. Gentle dissection with a fine tipped instrument, being careful not to induce bleeding, facilitates identification of the white longitudinal fibers of the nerve. It should be identified along its course so that the branches of the artery can be safely ligated adjacent to the capsule of the gland. Caution should be exercised to ensure bloodless dissection with the capsule of the gland. Any tissue that is not "see-through" should be clamped and tied or divided with bipolar cautery. After division of the branches of the inferior thyroid artery, the remaining attachment is limited to fibrous soft tissue anterior to the trachea. This is divided with cautery. Attention is then turn to the opposite side for total thyroidectomy or the resection is concluded by including the isthmus in the specimen by dividing and ligating at the border of the remaining thyroid lobe.

After ensuring hemostasis, the wound is closed in layers reapproximating the strap muscles in the midline with absorbable suture followed by the platysma and then skin. It is our preference to use a 5-0 prolene suture in a subcuticular technique followed by steri-strips. The prolene suture is left with tails that allow for removal on POD #1.

POSTOPERATIVE ORDERS

Patients are generally extubated and placed on the floor after recovery. Clears are generally begun the night of the procedure then advanced to a regular diet the following morning. An overnight stay is generally all that is needed for postoperative observation. Clinical signs of hypocalcemia and bleeding are the indications for observation. For lobectomy patients, serum testing of calcium levels is generally not required. For total thyroidectomy patients, initiation of calcium and vitamin D (ergocalciferol) replacement can be pursued by means of several strategies.

Some advocate immediate postprocedure assessment of parathyroid hormone levels. Because of the short half life of this hormone, a normal value (> 20 pm/dL) in the recovery area confirms functional parathyroid tissue and no further testing is necessary. If the level is intermediate, (10–20 pm/dL) a morning assessment of the calcium level is justified with initiation of calcium replacement if symptoms of hypocalcemia ensue. For low levels (< 10 pm/dL), calcium replacement is begun before symptoms ensue and calcium levels checked to ensure adequate replacement.

Another approach to postoperative calcium levels includes the routine assessment of ionized or total serum calcium the morning after surgery. Initiation of calcium replacement for symptoms or low levels is initiated. For very low levels, activated vitamin D (ergocalciferol) is given in addition to calcium replacement.

Initiation of thyroid hormone replacement can be a difficult decision in the immediate postoperative period. Synthetic thyroid hormone is given early on when the indication for thyroidectomy is benign disease. When the indication is thyroid malignancy, initiation of thyroid hormone replacement may be delayed until after treatment with radioactive iodine (^{131}I). After treatment is completed, thyroid hormone replacement is initiated to both replace lost hormone as well as suppress production of TSH levels.

COMPLICATIONS

Hypocalcemia

Historically, the major complication of thyroid surgery was hypocalcemia. The cause of this problem was poorly understood until the identification of the parathyroid glands and their function was identified. Now that the function of parathyroid hormone and the parathyroid glands is understood, the identification and protection of the parathyroid tissue is a routine part of thyroidectomy. When parathyroid glands are identified, their blood supply should be meticulously preserved. If the tissue appears ischemic, then a biopsy should be performed to confirm the histology. The remainder of the gland should be preserved in an iced saline solution and, when convenient during the procedure, minced and implanted in either the forearm musculature or the sternocleidomastoid.

When symptoms of hypocalcemia are identified during the postoperative period, treatment should be initiated urgently. Patients and their families should be warned about the signs related to hypocalcemia and what to do when identified. If taking P.O, then oral calcium citrate should be given and repeated each hour until the symptoms subside. Activated vitamin D aids in the absorption of the supplemental calcium. If not taking PO or if symptoms are severe, intravenous administration of calcium gluconate should be administered until symptoms subside. If symptoms persist, then administration via continuous drip may at times be required. Transition to scheduled medication or oral medications can be completed once symptoms resolve. Lifelong calcium and vitamin D supplementation may be required for the minority of those who have hypocalcemia. It is much more likely that a temporary drop in calcium levels will recover.

Nerve Injury

The recurrent laryngeal nerve and external branch of the superior laryngeal nerve are at risk during thyroidectomy. The external branch of the superior laryngeal nerve innervates the cricothyroid muscle which is important for tone and strength of voice. Injury to this nerve results in voice weakness which can be troublesome for professional opera singers and public speakers.

More concerning for the general population is injury to the recurrent laryngeal nerve. This branch of the vagus nerve has critical functions related to voice and movement of the vocal cords. Vocal cord dysfunction may be related to stretching, contusion or division of the nerve. In the first two cases, the nerve recovers function along with resolution of the voice changes. When divided, the nerve may be repaired by grafting or repairing the nerve. As well, medialization thyroplasty or injection of the vocal cord is possible to move the affected vocal cord to the midline to provide improved apposition to the functional side. Unilateral nerve injuries are managed expectantly, especially when symptoms are limited to changes in voice. Assessment for cord function should be a routine part of preparation for reoperation in the neck. This is most frequently done using flexible laryngoscopy in the clinic setting.

Bilateral nerve injuries can be life-threatening because of the midline position of the paralyzed vocal cord. This acts as a laryngeal obstruction and requires immediate reintubation or emergent tracheostomy or cricothyroidotomy. As before, function may return if the nerves are only stretched or contused. If divided, surgical options include chronic tracheostomy and nerve repair or grafting.

Tracheoesophageal Injury

Injury to the trachea or esophagus is uncommon in thyroid surgery. These structures are in the surgical field and are at risk especially when confronted by invasive or bulky lesions. Tracheal injury can be repaired when recognized during the operation by debridement of devitalized tissue and primary repair with monofilament, absorbable sutures placed around the tracheal rings in an interrupted fashion. Prompt extubation aids with prevention of fistulas by returning the patient to the natural negative pressure respiratory physiology. Extensive involvement of the trachea with a malignant lesion, such as with anaplastic thyroid cancers, may require tracheostomy for safe management.

Esophageal injuries are also repaired at the time of injury by debridement and primary repair with interrupted absorbable suture. Use of a muscle flap over the repair can be used to aid with healing. In the rare case of a missed injury, control of oral and gastric secretions and placement of a gastrostomy tube may be required.

REFERENCES

1. Skinner MA. (2006) Surgical diseases of the thyroid and parathyroid glands. In: JL Grosfeld, JA O'Neill, AG Coran, EW Fonkalsrud (eds.), *Pediatric Surgery*, 6th edition, pp. 850–860. Mosby, Philadelphia.

2. Kapila K, *et al.* (2010) Fine needle aspiration cytology of the thyroid in children and adolescents: Experience with 792 aspirates. *Acta Cytol* **54**(4):569–574.
3. Scholz S, *et al.* (2011) Thyroid surgery at Children's Hospital Boston: A 35-year single-institution experience. *J Pediatr Surg* **46**(3):437–442.
4. Pawelczak M, *et al.* (2010) Outcomes of children and adolescents with well-differentiated thyroid carcinoma and pulmonary metastases following ^{131}I treatment: A systematic review. *Thyroid* **20**(10):1095–1101.

PARATHYROID 35

Adam C. Alder and Michael A. Skinner

INTRODUCTION

The parathyroid gland is the major determinant of serum calcium in the pediatric patient. These glands arise from the branchial pouches and descend into the neck in a relatively predictable pattern. Abnormalities in secretion of parathyroid hormone (PTH) are rare in children.

Hypoparathyroidism is a condition treated most often with calcium and vitamin supplementation along with novel methods for hormone delivery. It may be the result of iatrogenic injury or an acquired absence of the glands.

Hypersecretion of PTH or hyperparathyroidism (HPT) can be categorized into three types: primary, secondary and tertiary HPT. Surgical techniques including new minimally invasive and directed parathyroidectomy have been developed to minimize the risks of surgery in the neck, namely recurrent laryngeal nerve injury, hypoparathyroidism and recurrence of HPT.

In this chapter, we describe the embryology of the parathyroid glands and major pathologic conditions related to the gland, and then provide a description of the technical aspects of parathyroidectomy including preoperative work-up and postoperative care. We conclude by describing the common complications of the parathyroidectomy.

PATHOPHYSIOLOGY

Embryology

As the thyroid bud descends from the foramen lacerum, nests of tissue arising from the third and fourth branchial pouches descend and come to rest posterior to the lobes of the thyroid gland. Interestingly, the inferior parathyroid gland arises from the third branchial pouch and descends along with the thymic tissues. The superior gland arises from the fourth branchial pouch. Histologically, the normal parathyroid gland is relatively fatty while a paucity of adipose tissue and sheets of parafollicular cells is typical of adenoma and hyperplastic glands.

Physiology

PTH is the primary regulator of serum calcium with actions on osteoclasts and osteoblasts as well as the gut in the absorption of calcium. Vitamin D activity is also closely tied to the activity of PTH. In the presence of intact PTH, osteoclasts take up elemental calcium from bone and mobilize it into the serum; gut absorption of calcium increases and activation of vitamin D to 10, 25-dihydroxycalciferol is promoted. The level of PTH released is typically controlled by a negative feedback loop utilizing a calcium receptor on the parathyroid tissue. Failure of this feedback loop leads to the pathologic conditions related to hypersecretion of PTH. Chronic hypocalcemia also results from an overall pathologic state related to elevated levels of PTH which is most common in individuals with chronic kidney disease.

HYPERPARATHYROIDISM

Primary

Primary HPT is characterized by normal to elevated serum calcium and inappropriately elevated serum PTH. When the negative feedback regulation of serum calcium and PTH secretion is functional, elevations in serum calcium are associated with inhibition of release of PTH. When calcium levels decline, PTH secretion is stimulated to counteract the change. Often the identification of elevated serum calcium is an incidental finding, leading some to suggest screening for the abnormality, as the disease will be found in 1/500 to 1/1000 patients. In the setting of hypercalcemia, several etiologies must be ruled out. An intact PTH level should be obtained. A history of cancer treatment, familial hypercalcemia hypocalciuria, or active supplementation with large doses of dietary calcium could be causes of hypercalcemia unrelated to unregulated PTH release. If the calcium level is elevated and a PTH level is in the upper range or above normal, localization should be sought as the most common cause of primary HPT is parathyroid adenoma. An adenoma loses its sensitivity to the negative feedback regulation and becomes autonomous. Often subtle symptoms of hypercalcemia are identified by thorough investigation for bone pain, kidney stones, sluggish mentation, depression and abdominal crampy pains.

Localization of the parathyroid glands can be accomplished using ultrasound and nuclear scintigraphy — Sestamibi scan. When concordant, the identification of a single abnormal gland is highly suggestive of parathyroid adenoma, which is present in 70–80% of cases of primary HPT, and allows for directed resection of the specific parathyroid gland when used in conjunction with rapid intraoperative hormone level assay.

If there is no specific gland identified to be abnormal or the localizing studies are discordant, then the elevated levels of hormone may be related to hyperplasia of the parathyroid glands. Often this is associated with the multiple endocrine neoplasia (MEN) syndrome or another familial HPT syndrome. A detailed family history as well as review of systems including screening for additional endocrinopathies (gastrinoma, insulinoma, pheochromocytoma, medullary thyroid carcinoma) should be completed expeditiously. Genetic testing and screening tests may also be indicated.

Secondary

When elevated PTH levels are found in the presence of chronically low calcium levels, the pathologic state is referred to as secondary HPT. In this type of HPT, the feedback mechanism for control is intact, albeit blunted by down regulation of the PTH receptors. It has also been suggested that the accumulation of N- and C-terminus particles of PTH act to blunt the response of the body to the hormone. While the prolonged presence of elevated PTH can have significant consequences, the underlying cause of low calcium must be identified and managed. Commonly the hypocalcemia is the result of chronic kidney failure. Other etiologies include lack of dietary sources of calcium and vitamin D deficiency. Treatment of the underlying causative problem assists greatly in the management of secondary HPT and should be done early to facilitate return to a normal physiologic state. If low calcium and elevated PTH levels persist, complications of growth, skeletal development, kidney function, or cardiac dysrhythmias can arise.

The treatment of secondary HPT is mainly medical involving calcium supplementation, phosphate binders, dietary changes and treatment of metabolic acidosis. The use of calcitriol is helpful in restoring the low calcium levels. Indications for surgery include: failure of medical management and development of complications from HPT such as calciphylaxis. Surgical therapy should include complete resection of all parathyroid tissue and reimplantation of a portion of one gland, preferably in the forearm. Some advocate preservation of additional tissue for future use should the implanted graft fail.

Tertiary

Unlike in secondary HPT where the normal function of the feedback loop controlling the level of PTH release remains intact and stimulated by chronically low levels of calcium, tertiary HPT occurs when the feedback loop fails to correct HPT despite correction of the calcium level and is characterized by chronically elevated PTH levels and hypercalcemia. These patients are at high risk for complications related to elevated calcium and PTH. Dietary restrictions, medications (Calcinet) and prevention of secondary parathyroid disease are the mainstay of medical therapy. Surgical indications include failure of medical management and complications attributable to the HPT.

Surgical management includes complete resection of parathyroid tissue and reimplantation of a portion of a gland, preferably in the forearm. Some advocate preservation of additional parathyroid tissue in case of graft failure.

PARATHYROID CARCINOMA

Parathyroid carcinoma represents an exceedingly rare condition in children. It is characterized by severely elevated PTH levels and associated severe hypercalcemia. Patients typically suffer from complications of the severe hypercalcemia notably bone pain, peptic ulcer disease and altered mental status. Sometimes a palpable mass is noted on physical exam.

Surgical management is indicated in all instances after correction of the severe electrolyte disturbances. Severe hypercalcemia is treated by giving normal saline boluses along with bisphosphonates and furosemide to help lower the calcium level. Surgical management is by completing four gland exploration and excision of abnormal glands *en bloc* with any involved and attached tissue, be it thyroid, strap muscle, etc. Any abnormal lymph nodes should be removed as well. Pathology will confirm an invasive component of the tumor.

MEN

Patients with HPT who have a family history of thyroid abnormalities, HPT, gastric ulcers or episodes of hypertension need to be evaluated for MEN 1 and MEN 2A. Appropriate blood tests can screen for the syndromes. Positive tests should be confirmed with genetic testing and followed up with appropriate treatment. Those identified as afflicted with an MEN syndrome are unlikely to have an adenoma, but rather suffer from parathyroid hyperplasia and require four gland exploration with reimplantation of half a gland in the forearm musculature. Long-term follow-up for sequelae of MEN is necessary.

MANAGEMENT

Operative Technique

The patient is positioned as for thyroid surgery with the patient in a semi-fowler position and the neck extended. The shoulders are placed on a roll. Review of preoperative imaging for concordance and the anticipated location of the adenoma is useful. Some surgeons perform an intraoperative ultrasound for incision planning and confirmation of the site of the involved gland. This is not critical when a four gland exploration is planned.

When performing directed parathyroidectomy, it is the authors' preference to use a midline low collar incision that is limited in length initially. A lateral approach at the anterior border of the sternocleidomastoid muscle at the level of the located gland has been advocated by some when localizing studies are concordant and the intraoperative ultrasound identifies a likely lesion. Dissection follows sharp skin separation through the platysma and flaps are created superiorly and inferiorly as for thyroidectomy. The strap muscles are split in the midline and the dissection exposes the thyroid lobe laterally. Unless four gland exploration is intended, the contralateral planes should not be violated in case of future need for neck operations. The inferior gland resides typically posterior to the lower pole, but may be in the same area as the inferior thyroid artery. Care must be taken to protect the recurrent laryngeal nerve (RLN) when dissecting around the branching inferior thyroid artery. The location of the inferior gland may be variable, but will be anterior and inferior to the RLN.

The superior gland is commonly located posterior to the superior lobe of the thyroid. The gland will be located posterior and superior to the course of the RLN. Exploration for "missing" glands must include an evaluation of the carotid sheath. If no abnormal gland is identified in any of the indicated locations, then resection may be indicated to remove an intraldoar gland.

To facilitate limited exploration for an abnormal parathyroid gland, intraoperative PTH assay is routinely included. Assessment of the baseline level should be completed prior to skin incision to prevent inadvertent elevation of the baseline as the result of manipulation of the glands. After identification of the suspected gland a 5-, 10- and 20-min PTH level should be obtained. In order to be confident that the correct gland has been removed, the level should fall by greater than one half *and* into the normal range. Failure to achieve both of these criteria results in a higher than acceptable risk of leaving abnormal parathyroid tissue and mandates further search for abnormal parathyroid tissue.

Closure of the operative field should be completed after ensuring hemostasis. It is the authors' preference to use sterile water for irrigation which facilitates identification of any areas of hemorrhage. The strap muscles are closed with interrupted figure-of-eight sutures composed of absorbable suture material. The platysma is approximated with simple interrupted absorbable suture. Our preference is to close the skin with a fine polypropylene suture using a subcuticular technique and dressed with steri-strips. The tails of the skin suture are left out for removal on postoperative day one. Alternately, an absorbable monofilament suture may be used on the skin and steri-strips or liquid adhesive used for a dressing.

When a four gland exploration is needed, a larger collar incision is required. Care should be made to identify all parathyroid tissue. Supernumerary glands occur in 3.7% of patients. Routine biopsy of suspected glands confirms their identity. The authors do not routinely use a drain. Preservation of the harvested tissue in iced saline allows for reimplantation. The authors do not recommend implantation into the muscle belly of the sternocleidomastoid as occasionally implants become hyperplastic and cause recurrent symptoms. This mandates resection and would result in reoperative neck surgery with its attendant risks. To implant into a muscle belly of the forearm, an incision is made over the muscle and portions of the finely minced section of gland are placed in multiple locations in the muscle belly which are then closed and marked with colored polypropylene suture. The skin incision closed in routine fashion.

Postoperative Orders

Patients are generally sent to recovery and, if directed parathyroid gland resection is completed, may be discharged home with appropriate supervision and pain medications. For some, observation overnight with a clear liquid diet and pain medication is indicated, especially if bilateral evaluation of the glands has been completed.

Routine PTH level assay makes postoperative surveillance and treatment reliably predictable. If postresection levels stabilize in the normal range, then no further measurement or treatment is necessary. A postresection "bone hunger" has been reported and may require calcium supplementation during the immediate postoperative period.

If PTH levels are low, calcium supplementation is required and should be maintained till postoperative follow-up confirms normal levels of PTH. Signs and symptoms of hypocalcemia are watched for in the postoperative period. The Tchvostek sign is elicited by tapping the side of the cheek over the masseter muscle. A positive sign is found when the corner of the mouth retracts. A Trousseau's sign is described as tetany of the forearm musculature when a blood pressure cuff is used to occlude blood flow to the forearm. Symptoms of periorbital and fingertip paresthesia are the result of hypocalcemia. Education for signs and symptoms of hypocalcemia should be completed and routine surveillance until stabilization should be obtained in patients too young to report symptoms.

Follow-up of calcium and PTH measurement confirms recovery of calcium turnover. The wound is monitored for healing during routine clinic visits. Calcium supplementation may be weaned after stabilization of the PTH and calcium levels. For those who have undergone three and a half gland resection, this may take some weeks.

Minimally invasive techniques for exploration and removal of the parathyroid glands has been described and is favored in highly specialized centers. We do not have experience with this technique and refer interested readers to the papers describing the novel technique.

COMPLICATIONS

The major complications of parathyroid resection are incomplete removal of abnormal glandular tissue, nerve injury and hypocalcemia. With routine intraoperative PTH assay, the risk of leaving abnormal tissue when the level falls by half and into the normal range is very low. When this does not occur, exploration of the remaining parathyroid glands is mandated. In cases of recurrent or persistent disease, preoperative directed venous sampling can be effective in identification of a possible location of a candidate lesion. Typical aberrant locations of parathyroid glands are well described. Ectopic glands occur in up to 20% of individuals and may be located in the carotid sheath, the retro-esophageal space, the thymus or within the substance of the thyroid gland itself. Inability to locate a gland or persistent or recurrent disease should prompt a systematic and complete assessment of the possible aberrant locales up to and including thymectomy and thyroid lobectomy in the appropriate patient. Intraoperative ultrasound is another useful adjunct.

Recurrent laryngeal nerve injury during parathyroidectomy is rare. Injury is more frequent in the setting of a four gland exploration. Care must be taken to look for nonrecurrent variants of the laryngeal nerve when exploring for the superior glands which occur more frequently on the right than the left. This configuration is present in less than 1% of the general population, but is more frequent when there exists congenital vascular anomalies. Recurrent laryngeal nerves in the typical course are at more risk during identification of an inferior gland. Careful attention to use of electrocautery is important and it is the authors' preference to use bipolar cautery to minimize spread of electrical diathermy.

Hypocalcemia is rare in the setting of directed parathyroidectomy which makes this technique attractive when preoperative imaging is concordant and the intraoperative hormone assay is confirmatory of complete resection of abnormal glands. Calcium supplementation is likely to be required in the immediate postoperative period as a result of upregulated calcium metabolism. Simply, serum calcium is depleted in the setting of persistently high PTH levels and upon correction of the PTH level may fail to recover because of chronically depleted tissue stores. This may result in transient hypocalcemia despite normal PTH levels and requires replacement of calcium to prevent symptoms. Typical supplementation involves calcium carbonate 300 mg PO twice daily. The amount of calcium supplementation may be increased up to 1200 mg PO daily if there is concern for hungry bone syndrome or low levels of PTH are measured at the time of operation. Bisphosphonates have been used to attenuate the degree of hungry bone syndrome in adults with primary HPT. Experience with its use in children is limited. Active vitamin D (calcitriol) is added when severe hypocalcemia is anticipated or measured and when symptoms are present. This is given at 0.25 μg/dose by mouth.

When symptoms occur they must be rapidly treated. For inpatients with venous access, calcium gluconate may be given intravenously. For patients at home or taking a diet, they should take calcium carbonate 300 mg by mouth every hour until symptoms resolve. The supplementation should be continued at 300 mg PO four times daily. Admission for treatment is required with persistent symptoms or intolerance of oral replacement. PTH levels can recover and reassessment of the need for calcium supplementation should be planned. Synthetic PTH is being investigated as a novel therapy that is intended to be more physiologic and provide better control of calcium levels.

CONCLUSION

HPT is a rare finding in pediatric patients. Primary HPT is treated surgically and has a favorable prognosis. Secondary and tertiary HPTs are medically managed with surgical treatments reserved for failed medical management and complications. Surgical resection has a favorable risk profile and, when meticulously performed, has few sequelae. Main complications include residual abnormal glandular tissue, nerve injury, and hypocalcemia. New techniques for resection include directed parathyroidectomy and minimally invasive endoscopic resection.

REFERENCES

1. Skinner MA. (2006) Surgical diseases of the thyroid and parathyroid glands. In: Grosfeld JL, JA O'Neill, AG Coran, EW Fonkalsrud (eds.), *Pediatric Surgery*, 6th edition, pp. 850–860. Mosby, Philadelphia.
2. Bae JO, Skinner MA. (2010) Endocrine disorders and tumors. In: GW Holcomb III, JP Murphy (eds.), *Aschcraft's Pediatric Surgery*, 5th edition, pp. 1037–1054. Saunders, Philadelphia.
3. Sanchez CP. (2003) Secondary hyperparthyroidism in children with chronic renal failure. *Pediatr Drugs* **5**:763–776.
4. Sosa JA, Tuggle CT, Wang TS, *et al.* (2008) Clinical and economic outcomes of thyroid and parathyroid surgery in children. *J Clin Endocrinol Metab* **93**:3058–3065.
5. Iqbal CW, Wahoff DC. (2009) Diagnosis and management of pediatric endocrine neoplasms. *Curr Opin Pediatr* **21**:379–385.
6. Wang TS, Roman SA, Sosa JA. (2008) Predictors of outcomes following pediatric thyroid and parathyroid surgery. *Curr Opin Oncol* **21**:23–28.
7. Fiedler AG, Rossi C, Gingealewski CA. (2009) Parathyroid carcinoma in a child: An unusual case of an ectopically located malignant parathyroid gland with tumor invading the thymus. *J Ped Surg* **44**:1649–1652.
8. Kollars J, Zarroug AE, van Heerden J, *et al.* (2005) Primary hyperparathyroidism in pediatric patients. *Pediatrics* **115**:974–980.

LARYNGEAL AND TRACHEAL DISORDERS 36

Charles M. Leys

CLINICAL PRESENTATION

Tracheal and laryngeal lesions can cause acute life-threatening airway obstruction, requiring immediate diagnosis and management. The most common sign of upper airway obstruction is stridor, which may be associated with labored respirations, tachypnea, use of accessory muscles of respiration, sternal and intercostal retractions, hypoxia, cyanosis, and mental status changes. Chronic airway obstruction may present with similar signs and symptoms, but may also produce failure to thrive, poor weight gain, pulmonary hypertension, and pectus excavatum. Airway obstruction may also present with dysphagia, sore throat, cough, and changes in vocal character (hoarseness, weak cry). A muffled cry suggests obstruction at the level of the pharynx. A barking cough is associated with laryngeal inflammation and edema. Characteristics of the stridor can indicate the level of obstruction. A high-pitched inspiratory stridor suggests a lesion above the glottis, such as laryngomalacia or vocal cord paralysis. Biphasic stridor, with high pitch on inspiration and low pitch on expiration, typically indicates a fixed obstruction in the subglottis or trachea. Expiratory stridor indicates an intra-thoracic obstruction, such as tracheomalacia.

DIAGNOSIS AND WORK-UP

The differential diagnosis for respiratory distress or cyanosis in infancy (Table 1) includes congenital heart disease and central nervous system

Table 1. Conditions causing cyanosis or respiratory distress.

Congenital heart disease
CNS disorders
Maternal anesthesia
Birth Trauma (subdural hematoma)
CNS malformations
Gastrointestinal disorders
Tracheoesophageal fistula
Gastroesophageal reflux
Airway malformations and obstructions
Choanal atresia
Pierre–Robin syndrome (micrognathia)
Nasopharyngeal mass (teratoma, encephalocele)
Hypertrophy of tonsils, adenoids
Craniofacial abnormalities
Subglottic stenosis
Laryngomalacia, tracheomalacia, bronchomalacia
Vocal cord paralysis
Laryngeal neoplasms (hemangioma, lymphangioma)
Laryngeal web, atresia
Laryngeal papillomatosis
Infectious (croup, epiglottitis)
Laryngeal clefts
Laryngeal cysts and laryngocele
Tracheal stenosis, web
Vascular rings
Mediastinal masses
Foreign body
Trauma

(CNS) etiologies, such as maternal anesthesia, birth trauma, and CNS malformations. If the cyanotic infant makes a vigorous effort to breathe, cardiac and CNS disorders typically can be ruled out. The approach to evaluating a patient with suspected airway obstruction will differ between newborns and older children.

A newborn with respiratory distress should have immediate suctioning and have the tongue pulled forward to assess for patency above the larynx. If distress continues, a chest radiograph should be obtained to evaluate for etiologies other than airway obstruction, such as pneumothorax, diaphragmatic hernia, hyaline membrane disease, lobar emphysema, or agenesis of a lung. If airway obstruction is severe and persists, direct laryngoscopy should be performed to visualize the base of tongue, epiglottis, and larynx. If the larynx is patent, an endotracheal tube should be placed. If the obstruction is less severe, the infant is monitored and a systematic evaluation can be completed. A careful head and neck physical exam will detect micrognathia (Pierre–Robin syndrome), cleft lip and palate, or a compressing mass in the neck, tongue, or nasopharynx. Compressing mass lesions may also be visualized on lateral soft tissue radiographs of the head and neck and standard chest radiographs. Small catheters can be passed through each nare to assess for posterior choanal atresia. Passing a small catheter into the stomach will document esophageal patency. If the distress is mild, a barium contrast study can be obtained, which may find esophageal stenosis, trachea–esophageal fistula (TEF), vascular ring compressing the trachea or esophagus, swallowing dysfunction with aspiration, or gastroesophageal reflux.

Evaluation of an older child begins with assessment of the child's overall appearance, which will often dictate how quickly further evaluation and intervention should proceed. Presence of anxiety, restlessness, and diaphoresis are ominous signs of impending airway compromise. Level of consciousness should be determined, as immediate airway management will be required in the unconscious or obtunded child. Bradycardia is a late indicator of severe hypoxia. The best initial study is plain radiographs of the neck, with both lateral and antero–posterior views. A chest radiograph is also important to evaluate for foreign bodies, mediastinal mass, or pulmonary conditions that may account for the respiratory compromise. If time permits and initial radiographs are not diagnostic, airway fluoroscopy can provide additional dynamic information, and a contrast esophagram may show a vascular ring or gastroesophageal reflux.

A complete evaluation of an infant or child with stridor will often include awake flexible nasopharyngoscopy and laryngoscopy with topical anesthetics. This allows visualization of the dynamics of supraglottic tone, vocal cord mobility, and the impact of some fixed lesions, though the scope should not be advanced through the glottis. Flexible endoscopy should not be performed in a child with supraglottitis (formerly called epiglottitis), as this may precipitate complete obstruction. For suspected pathology distal to the glottis, endoscopy should be performed in the operating room.

MANAGEMENT

Nonsurgical initial interventions for the child with acute airway obstruction may include simply observation in a closely monitored setting. Humidified oxygen will improve oxygenation and clearance of secretions. Nebulized racemic epinephrine will reduce mucosal edema and can be helpful in inflammatory conditions. Additional adjuvant therapies include corticosteroids, antibiotics, and inhaled helium/oxygen mixture (heliox). Antibiotics can prevent bacterial superinfection, which is common in cases of virally mediated inflammation. Heliox improves oxygen delivery by reducing airway turbulence and gas resistance. Nasal airways can be easily inserted in most children and are helpful for pharyngeal obstruction. Oral airways can be used briefly, but are not tolerated by most children. Endotracheal intubation remains the mainstay of airway intervention for severe airway obstruction. Tube size can be estimated by the formula: size = (age in years + 16) ÷ 4. If airway visualization is difficult due to trauma or unstable cervical spine, emergent transtracheal oxygenation may be achieved with a 16-gauge needle inserted through the cricothyroid membrane.

Surgical management of acute airway obstruction will begin with endoscopy. Under anesthesia, the larynx can be visualized initially with direct laryngoscopy followed by rigid pediatric laryngoscopes for a more detailed exam. The subglottic airway is evaluated and secured with a rigid ventilating bronchoscope, which can also be utilized for various interventions. If the airway cannot be controlled by the translaryngeal approach, tracheostomy remains the preferred airway. However, emergent tracheostomy should be avoided due to higher complications such as bleeding, pneumothorax, pneumomediastinum, and injury to surrounding structures. In rare cases, cricothyroidotomy may be required, utilizing a small endotracheal tube or tracheostomy tube.

LARYNGEAL AND SUBGLOTTIC LESIONS

Laryngotracheal Stenosis

Laryngeotracheal stenosis may be congential or acquired, and most commonly involves the subglottis, though it may also involve the supraglottis, glottis, or upper trachea. Congenital stenosis is rare and results from failure or incomplete recannalization of the larygneal lumen by the 10th week of gestation. Most cases of congential stenosis improve with laryngeal growth and may not require surgical management. The diagnosis may be suggested by lateral neck radiographs and confirmed by endoscopy. Acquired subglottic stenosis is typically caused by prolonged endotracheal intubation and is much more difficult to manage. Severe airway obstruction may necessitate initial tracheostomy, followed by subsequent laryngotracheplasty. grade I lesions (0 to 50% obstruction) and many grade II lesions (51% to 70%) can be managed with endoscopic laser techniques. Grade III (71% to 99%) and grade IV (no visible lumen) lesions will require open surgical reconstruction, such as anterior cricoid split with cartilage graft or partial cricotracheal resection.

Laryngomalacia

Laryngeomalacia is the most common laryngeal anomaly and cause of stridor in infancy. The clinical sign is inspiratory stridor that worsens with feeding or agitation and improves when positioned prone with the neck extended. The symptoms result from collapse of supraglottic laryngeal structures during inspiration. The diagnosis is confirmed by awake flexible laryngoscopy, which will demonstrate the cyclic collapse of supraglottic tissue and often an omega shaped epiglottis. Symptoms are typically present at birth, peak at 6–8 months, and resolve by 18–24 months, so most patients will not require surgical intervention. Many of these patients have gastrointestinal reflux disease and benefit from anti-reflux therapies. Surgical intervention may be indicated for severe laryngomalacia with life-threatening obstruction or complications of hypoxia. Supraglottoplasty involves microsurgical removal of the redundant prolapsing tissue and release of the aryepiglottic folds. This procedure is highly successful, but some patients will require revision or tracheostomy until it resolves spontaneously.

Laryngeal Webs and Atresia

Congenital laryngeal webs and atresia are rare anomalies that result from prenatal failure of recanalization of the larynx. Most are located at the glottic level, though they can be supraglottic or subglottic. They manifest as airway obstruction and weak or absent cry at birth, and the diagnosis can be easily confirmed with a laryngoscope. A thin web may be ruptured by intubation or may be lysed by endoscopic electrocautery or laser. Thick webs and atresia require urgent tracheostomy and subsequent reconstruction. If atresia is suspected on prenatal ultrasound, an ex utero intrapartum treatment (EXIT) procedure may be life-saving.

Laryngeal and Laryngotracheal Clefts

Laryngeal and laryngotracheal clefts are rare congenital defects that result from incomplete midline separation of the developing trachea and esophagus. Most clefts involve only the supraglottic larynx but the cleft length can vary and extend down to the carina or main stem bronchi. Associated anomalies are common, including TEF in 20–27%. Of all patients with TEF, 6% will have an associated laryngeal cleft, often discovered after TEF repair when the child has persistent aspiration. Clinical symptoms of a cleft include congenital inspiratory stridor, cyanosis with feedings, aspiration, and recurrent pulmonary infections. Symptom severity increases with length of cleft. Diagnosis is made by endoscopic exam. Clefts limited to the supraglottic larynx do not require surgical repair, and treatment includes swallowing therapy and gastroesophageal reflux therapy. Clefts extending below the vocal cords will require surgical repair and either tracheostomy or short-term stenting via endotracheal intubation.

Laryngocele

A laryngocele is a fluid or air filled saccular dilatation of the laryngeal ventricle. It produces severe airway obstruction and stridor in neonates, requiring emergent intubation and needle aspiration of the cyst. The cyst can refill, so management includes laryngoscopy with unroofing of the cyst.

Vocal Cord Paralysis

Vocal cord paralysis may be congenital or acquired and unilateral or bilateral. Causative factors include ligation of patent ductus arteriosus, conditions with elevated intracranial pressure, birth trauma with stretch injury, or an inflammatory insult. In most infant cases, a cause cannot be identified, and it often resolves in 4–6 weeks. Unilateral palsy produces stridor with mild symptoms and does not require specific therapy. Bilateral palsy may resolve with treatment of an intracranial condition or with observation for cases of injury related to stretch or inflammation.

If it does not resolve, or is not expected to recover, tracheostomy is often required. The posterior glottis can be opened to relieve the airway obstruction using a variety of surgical procedures, including arytenoidectomy and lateral fixation of the cord.

Laryngeal Hemangioma

Laryngeal hemangiomas are typically located just below the glottis, but can be in the trachea. Patients are usually asymptomatic at birth, but often develop stridor by age 3 months. Approximately 50% are associated with cutaneous hemangiomas. The classic finding on lateral neck radiograph is asymmetric subglottic narrowing, and the diagnosis is confirmed by endoscopy *without* biopsy. As with cutaneous hemangiomas, these lesions have a rapid growth phase, which slows by age 12 months, followed by spontaneous involution over months to years. Therefore, lesions without symptoms may not require specific therapy. Options for the management of symptomatic lesions include tracheostomy, partial resection with laser or cryotherapy, open surgical resection, systemic or intralesional corticosteroids, and systemic interferon α-2a.

Recurrent Respiratory Papillomatosis

Recurrent respiratory papillomatosis is caused by human papillomavirus and produces stridor, hoarseness, wheezing, and upper airway obstruction. It is the most common laryngeal tumor in children, most commonly in children 18 months to 5 yrs old. Diagnosis is made by endoscopy. Some lesions regress spontaneously in adolescence, but most require surgical ablation using laser or cryotherapy techniques. Complications of surgical therapy include scarring, stenosis, and laryngeal web formation.

TRACHEAL LESIONS

Tracheal Stenosis

Tracheal stenosis is most commonly acquired and caused by endotracheal intubation in older children and adolescents. Infants more commonly develop stenosis in the subglottic region after intubation. Congenital tracheal stenosis is rare, usually resulting from complete cartilaginous tracheal rings, which is often associated with other anomalies. Symptoms include biphasic stridor and respiratory distress. Radiographs should be obtained, but the diagnosis is confirmed by endoscopy. Congenital stenosis is most often treated with either segmental resection and anastomosis or slide tracheoplasty. Acquired stenosis often can be treated with endoscopic techniques, which may include dilation, stenting, laser, or cryotherapy.

Tracheomalacia

Tracheomalacia produces expiratory stridor with increased respiratory effort or coughing, resulting from dynamic collapse of soft and pliable tracheal cartilage. This differs from larygnomalacia, which produces inspiratory stridor, though the two can coexist. Other symptoms include a "barking" cough, recurrent pneumonia, and acute life-threatenting apnea spells. Spells may occur during meals and can progress to cyanosis, bradycardia, and arrest. Primary or isolated tracheomalacia resolves by 18 months of age. Secondary tracheomalacia results from an associated condition, such as vascular ring, TEF, or long-term ventilation with a cuffed endotracheal tube or tracheostomy. The diagnosis may be suggested by airway fluoroscopy, but is easily established by bronchoscopy with spontaneous ventilation. Mild to moderate cases do not require surgical intervention, as the condition improves with time. Infants with severe tracheomalacia may benefit from aortopexy, in which the ascending aorta and aortic arch are sutured to the posterior table of the sternum. This utilizes the native attachments between the aorta and trachea to pull the anterior tracheal wall forward and expand the lumen. This can be performed via left thoracotomy or thoracoscopic approach. Tracheostomy remains an option if aortopexy fails to resolve the symptoms.

Vascular Compression Anomalies

Congenital anomalies of the great vessels can result in vascular rings that compress the esophagus and trachea, causing dysphagia and stridor. Symptoms can be subtle, so a high index of suspicion is needed to make the diagnosis. Significant compression will cause stridor, chronic cough, recurrent bronchitis or pneumonia, feeding difficulties with failure to thrive, and reflex apnea (apnea during feeding or vagal stimulation). The most symptomatic type of vascular ring is a double aortic arch, which forms a tight complete ring around both the trachea and esophagus. This occurs when the embryonic dorsal fourth right arch fails to regress and crosses behind the esophagus to the left side of the chest, often remaining the dominant arch. Diagnosis is suggested by a contrast esophagram showing posterior indentation of the esophagus on lateral view. Further imaging with magnetic resonance or computed tomographic angiography can further define the nature of the anomaly. Treatment consists of dividing the minor arch and lysis of residual adhesions to the trachea and esophagus, most often performed via left thoracotomy. A complete ring may also be formed by a right aortic arch with a left ligamentum arteriosum, which is treated the same as a double arch. Other anomalies of the great vessels may produce a symptomatic but incomplete vascular ring. Innominate artery compression occurs when the innominate artery origin is displaced to the left of midline and causes anterior tracheal compression as it courses from left to right. The esophagram will be normal, but bronchoscopy will find flattened distal tracheal rings, and the compression may appear pulsatile. Mild symptoms will resolve with growth, but severe cases may require aortopexy. The most common mediastinal vascular anomaly is an aberrant right subclavian artery arising from the descending aorta and coursing posterior to the esophagus. This can cause dysphagia but will not produce airway obstruction. A pulmonary artery sling, the least common vascular ring anomaly, occurs when the left pulmonary artery arises as a branch off the right pulmonary artery and passes between the trachea and esophagus as it courses to the left lung. This usually produces severe airway obstructive symptoms and is frequently associated with complete tracheal cartilaginous rings. Repair requires cardiopulmonary bypass to permit division and reimplantation of the left pulmonary artery, with translocation anterior to the trachea. Tracheal reconstruction is performed concurrently if complete rings are present.

REFERENCES

1. Thompson DM, Cotton RT. (2006) Lesions of the larynx, trachea, and upper airway. In: JL Grosfeld, JA O'Neill Jr, EW Fonkalsrud, *et al.* (eds.), *Pediatric Surgery*, 6th edition, pp. 983–1000. Mosby Elsevier, Philadelphia, PA.
2. Potsic WP, Wetmore RF. (2006) Otolaryngologic disorders. In: JL Grosfeld, JA O'Neill Jr, EW Fonkalsrud, *et al.* (eds.), *Pediatric Surgery*, 6th edition, pp. 813–834. Mosby Elsevier, Philadelphia.
3. Grosfeld JL. (2003) Disorders of the upper airway. In: JA O'Neill Jr, JL Grosfeld, EW Fonkalsrud, *et al.* (eds.), *Principles of Pediatric Surgery*, 2nd edition, pp. 325–338. Mosby, St. Louis.

LYMPHADENOPATHY 37

Nicholas F. Fiore

CLINICAL PRESENTATION

Neck lymphadenopathy typically presents as an enlarged neck mass noted by a family member or pediatrician. Palpable lymphadenopathy is present in many or even most preschool and primary school children and may generate significant anxiety for families. Often the presentation is acute and may be accompanied by tenderness, fever, and erythema. Nodes due to infectious or inflammatory conditions follow an upper respiratory infection, an oropharyngeal infection, or an allergic response. Those associated with malignancy may be asymptomatic or may present with systemic or constitutional symptoms such as malaise, weight loss, night sweats, pruritis, chronic cough, orthopnea, or new onset dyspnea. Although the diagnosis may seem relatively simple on the surface, the management of neck lymphadenopathy requires finesse and involves a judgment by the clinician with input from the family and pediatrician.

When evaluating adenopathy it is important to note the duration of the presence of mass, changes in the mass, recent illness, history of trauma, fevers, weight loss, fatigue, travels, as well as a family history of blood dyscrasias or lymphoma. A history of constitutional or systemic symptoms, pet exposures, exposure to tuberculosis or human immunodeficiency virus (HIV) may further direct the workup and treatment.

PATHOPHYSIOLGY/INCIDENCE

The anterior cervical chain drains the oropharynx, and any oropharyngeal infection has the potential to cause lymphadenopathy. Because lymphadenopathy is so prevalent, the challenge to the clinician lies in distinguishing inflammatory and/or infectious causes from malignant ones such as lymphoma. In general, nodes due to inflammatory conditions enlarge acutely, are tender, often cause overlying erythema, and follow an infection. Those nodes which are firm, fixed, nontender, and often larger than 2 cm, as well as those in the posterior triangle or supra clavicular fossa, raise a higher index of suspicion for malignancy. History is very important in directing the workup for neck adenopathy. Complete blood count (CBC) with differential, chest X-ray, purified protein derivative (PPD), HIV assay, and monospot or EBV titers are obtained as suggested by history. The differential diagnosis includes viral lymph node hyperplasia, cat-scratch disease, bacterial infection, fungal infection, mumps, mono or EBV, lymphoma or other malignancy, HIV-related adenopathy, or actinomycosis.

CLASSIFICATION

Acute Suppurative Lymphadenitis

The patient with acute suppurative lymphadenitis is most likely a preschooler older than 1 yr of age who presents with a unilateral, rapidly-enlarging, mass associated with tenderness and erythema and possibly a fever. This is most commonly incited by a tonsillitis or pharyngitis. Penicillin-resistant staphylococci, group A streptococci or both are the classic causative organisms, but more recently methicillin-resistant *Staphylococcus aureus* (MRSA) enters the differential. If the node is indurated and the patient not toxic, an observational period is often warranted during which a 5–10 day course of treatment with a broad-spectrum cephalosporin or ampicillin with a beta-lactamase inhibitor is initiated. Clindamycin or Bactrim are reasonable choices if MRSA is suspected or prevalent in a certain area. One can expect a clinical response within 72 hrs.

The common bacterial-associated lymphadenitis is managed in an outpatient setting without further diagnostic tests and often resolves without requiring further workup or treatment. If the patient displays signs of toxemia, has poor oral intake, or peristent fevers (especially in an infant), a more aggressive approach may be pursued, including inpatient admission and intravenous antibiotics. Imaging studies are often confusing and not helpful because distinguishing induration from purulence may be difficult. An ultrasound may indicate whether a mass is solid or cystic, and a Computed Tomography (CT) with intravenous contrast will evaluate the neck for signs of occult pathology such as a peritonsillar abscess. Clinical evaluation supersedes imaging modalities as these studies often prompt premature attempts at drainage. A CBC is probably the only lab test required in this clinical setting.

Antibiotics are utilized until the node abscesses at which time drainage is needed. Incision and drainage in the operating room results in prompt resolution of the abscess and symptoms, and culture and sensitivity-directed antibiotic therapy treats any residual cellulitis. A small incision is made over the point of maximal fluctuance and the loculations are bluntly divided. Once cultures are obtained, the wound is irrigated with normal saline. Loose packing with iodoform gauze keeps the wound from closing prematurely and is removed on postoperative day one or two. Recently, we have had good luck making a small incision over the point of maximal fluctuance, breaking up loculations, irrigating the cavity and placing a vessel loop exiting through a small, separate stab incision (See Chapter 88, Skin Abscesses). The vessel loop is tied to itself and a dry dressing applied. The vessel loop is removed sometime within the next week. The patient is discharged the day of or following the procedure as signs of systemic infection rapidly regress. Needle drainage is generally not recommended as it may need to be repeated and is challenging in the absence of sedation.

Viral-associated

Viral infection is the most common cause of acute lymph node enlargement. It presents as acute onset, bilateral, often tender adenopathy with clusters of small nodes. As spontaneous resolution occurs within several weeks, reassurance of the family is the primary therapy.

Mycobacterial Lymphadenitis

Atypical mycobacterial lymphadenitis most commonly presents with unilateral lymph node enlargement with minimal systemic symptoms, since the infection is a localized process. This is in contrast to *Mycobacterium tuberculosis* infections which are a systemic process. Most atypical mycobacterial infections result from a pharyngeal or tonsilar portal of entry. They present as high cervical, submandibular, preauricular, and even parotid adenopathy. On exam, the nodes are tender, firm, and even rubbery. Inciting bacteria include *M. avium intracellulare, M. scrofulaceum, M. fortuitum,* and *M. chelonei.* Workup usually demonstrates a normal chest radiograph and a negative or equivocal PPD. The definitive diagnosis is made from postexcision cultures, although specific skin antigen tests may be helpful. Persistent adenopathy more than 3 mths prompts excision as atypical mycobacterial infections are not responsive to anti-tuberculous medications.

The adenopathy from *M. tuberculosis* is an extension of a primary pulmonary process resulting from exposure to *Mycobacterium tuberculosis* and does not occur in the absence of pulmonary inoculation. It often presents as asymptomatic supraclavicular adenopathy and is suspected with a positive PPD. A negative PPD excludes the diagnosis of *M. tuberculosis* (TB). Chest films are a necessary part of the workup but are most often normal. Adenopathy secondary to TB infection is treated with anti-tuberculosis medications for 6–24 mths and resolves in several months. In certain instances the nodes develop caseous necrosis and chronic drainage. This instance necessitates complete excision because an incisional biopsy may result in a chronic draining sinus.

Cat-scratch

Infection from *Bartonella henselae* results in nonbacterial chronic lymphadenopathy. As a result of a cat scratch, a papule forms at the inoculation site. Over the next several weeks, tender regional lymphadenopathy develops. The patient may develop mild systemic symptoms including malaise, headache, vomiting, and low grade fever. The diagnosis is suggested by a history of exposure and the identification of a papule; it is confirmed by polymerase chain reaction assay from the pus. Management is expectant, unless the node becomes necrotic at which time excision is indicated.

OPERATIVE MANAGEMENT

The decision regarding whether or not to recommend biopsy of cervical adenopathy is challenging because the patient and family often arrive in the office expecting the surgeon to give them a definitive diagnosis. Many expect biopsies of nodes which seem clinically benign. In general, biopsy is justified in cases where nodes are greater than 1 cm and persist more than several months. Those patients with nodes greater than 2 cm, firm, fixed and asymptomatic should proceed directly to biopsy. A complete blood cell count and chest radiograph to look for mediastinal involvement is indicated as preoperative workup. Although most nodes are benign histologically, concern over delaying a diagnosis of a malignancy is in the back of a surgeon's mind. An honest discussion with the family and a phone call to the referring pediatrician are reassuring to the family.

Once the decision is made to proceed with biopsy, informed consent is obtained. The general risks include bleeding, infection, recurrence, peripheral nerve injury, or need for further procedures. The family should understand that the goal of the operation is to obtain a representative sample of the mass, and not necessarily complete excision of the involved area. The surgeon should review the local anatomy preoperatively to consider the location of the spinal accessory, greater auricular, transverse cervical and lesser occipital nerves. The area in question is marked preoperatively, and may include marking the proposed incision in the natural neck skin folds. Otherwise the folds may be distorted or absent once the patient is positioned in the operating room. Local anesthesia is infiltrated without limiting the ability to palpate the node preoperatively. An incision approximating the size of the nodal packet is made in or parallel to the skin lines and can be carried sharply through the platysma. Thereafter, the dissection proceeds bluntly working directly on top of the node. Once it is freed circumferentially, the node pedicle can be cauterized close to the capsule. Additional nodes may be taken as safely possible, but the goal is histologic diagnosis and not a complete excision. Once hemostasis is assured, the platysma is reapproximated with interrupted braided dissolvable suture and the skin closed with subcuticular monofilament suture.

It is extremely important to insure the nodes are processed correctly or the chance for diagnosis may be lost completely. The node is sent fresh for "lymph node protocol" which includes culture for aerobic, anaerobic, fungal, acid fast bacilli, and fungus. Touch preps or frozen sections may be helpful but are often not conclusive.

COMPLICATIONS/FOLLOW-UP

The patient is seen in follow-up in 1–2 wks. Definitive pathology results return within several days and a phone call to the family with the often "good news" is welcomed. Occasionally the wound becomes infected and is allowed to heal by secondary intention. A wound which continues to drain raises the possibility of a mycobacterial or cat-scratch infection which requires complete excision of the affected area to treat effectively.

Managing neck lymphadenopathy may be considered mundane pediatric surgery. Nevertheless, that which seems simple to the surgeon is often a frightening event for the family members who are paralyzed with the possibility of malignancy. The surgeon must exercise judgment in determining whether gentle reassurance, antibiotics, drainage, or biopsy is indicated. Ultimately, the surgeon is rewarded with an extremely appreciative family.

REFERENCES

1. Grosfeld Jay L. (2004) Cervical cysts, sinuses, and other neck lesions. In: JA O'Neil, JL Grosfeld, EW Fonkalsrud, *et al.* (eds.), *Principles of Pediatric Surgery*, 2nd edition, pp. 302–303. Mosby, St. Louis.
2. Newman KD, Hayes-Jordan AA. (2006) Lymph node disorders. In: JL Grosfeld, JA O'Neil, EW Fonkalsrud, *et al.* (eds.), *Pediatric Surgery*, 6th edition, pp. 844–848. Mosby Elsevier, St. Louis.
3. Mattei P. (2003) Benign skin lesions. In: P Mattei (ed.), *Surgical Directives: Pediatric Surgery*, pp. 674–675. Lippincott Williams and Wilkins, Philadelphia.

NECK CYSTS AND SINUSES 38

Nicholas F. Fiore

CLINICAL PRESENTATION

Most neck cysts and sinuses present as an asymptomatic subcutaneous mass or visible pit in the skin. The differential diagnosis for those presenting in the midline include thyroglossal duct cysts, dermoid cysts, and lymph nodes. They are subcutaneous, mobile, and firm and nontender if they are not infected. Thyroglossal duct cysts present in school age children within the first 2 to 10 yrs of life, often enlarging if associated with a viral illness. Dermoid cysts and lymph nodes may be noted at anytime. Branchial remnants present as pits, masses, or cartilaginous remnants in the lateral neck area and are usually at the medial border of the sternocleidomastoid muscle. Pits often drain mucoid material. Cysts and sinuses are at risk for infection. When infected, they are more challenging to remove, and the risk for recurrence increases.

THYROGLOSSAL DUCT CYSTS

Embryology

The thyroid diverticulum develops from the foramen cecum at the base of the tongue, and during the forth to seventh week descends to its pretracheal position. The duct itself, which may pass in front of, behind, or through the hyoid bone, obliterates often leaving the pyramidal lobe of the thyroid as its only remnant. Failure of migration leads to a lingual thyroid seated in the tongue or near the foramen cecum. This thyroid tissue, the sole source of the thyroid hormone production, may function normally, but is more often dysgenetic and renders the patient hypothyroid. Descent may be arrested anywhere in this pathway leaving a sublingual or ectopic thyroid. Persistent elements of the duct result in a thyroid duct cyst and may contain thyroid tissue 25% of the time, even the face of a normally-descending thyroid. Histologically, the duct is lined with stratified squamous or ciliated, pseudostratified columnar epithelium with mucous-secreting glands. Seventy five percent of thyroglossal cysts present as smooth, midline neck masses measuring 1–3 cm. Classically they are described as moving with swallowing or tongue protrusion due to tethering to the foramen cecum. Most thyroglossal duct cysts are located in the midline or just off the midline below the hyoid bone; 25% are submental, 3% are lingual, and 7% suprasternal in location. They often enlarge associated with a viral syndrome or pharyngitis, and may become infected with oral flora.

Work-up

The diagnosis is suspected when a midline neck mass is noted. Additionally, a dermoid, lymph node, branchial remnant, lipoma, hemangioma, and cystic hygroma are potential causes. Although the work-up is controversial, an ultrasound of the neck and thyroid often suffices. The mass is typically cystic and contains echogenic material which potentially distinguishes it from a lymph node or dermoid. If the thyroid gland cannot be readily palpated on physical exam, an ultrasound demonstrating a normal thyroid gland is reassuring that excision of the palpable mass will not result in the unexpected removal of the sole thyroid tissue. A thyroid scan is indicated in the face of hypothyroidism or nonpalpable thyroid. A Computed Tomography (CT) may be indicated if the presentation is unusual; in this circumstance it becomes necessary to demonstrate the relationship of the mass to other structures. In addition a CT may be obtained if there is concern that the mass is a malignancy or a metastatic node. Thyroid function tests are obtained when the mass is identified as solid ectopic thyroid or when the cyst is found to contain thyroid tissue following excision.

Treatment

Once the diagnosis is made, the patient is scheduled for elective excision as an outpatient. To prevent recurrence, the cyst, its tract, and the central portion of the hyoid bone is removed in a procedure described by Sistrunk. Once anesthesia is induced, a roll is placed under the shoulders to extend the neck. A horizontal incision is made in the skin lines over the mass (or an ellipse-shaped incision if there is skin involvement) and subplatysmal flaps are developed in a cephalad and caudad direction. The dissection is carried cephalad to the hyoid bone and then inferior and superior to it, often including a portion of the sternohyoid muscle. The central portion of the hyoid bone is skeletonized and divided, removing the centrum. A small core of tongue musculature is excised at the level of the foramen cecum and the defect closed with absorbable suture. Hemostasis is achieved and the wound is irrigated and approximated by bringing together the strap muscles, platysma, and the skin. No attempt is made to bring the hyoid bone together and a drain is usually not necessary. As long as the patient has adequate pain control and is able to drink well, the patient is released from the recovery room.

Infected or inflamed masses are treated with antibiotics, and those that do not resolve with antibiotics are treated with incision and drainage. Excision is undertaken 4–6 wks later, once the acute inflammation has resolved. Incision and drainage of an infected cyst is avoided if possible since a draining sinus has an increased risk for recurrence. Care should be taken to remove the entire central portion of the hyoid bone in conjunction with the cyst, without separating the duct or leaving the posterior aspect the bone. Incomplete excision of the central hyoid bone or cyst rupture increases the chance for recurrence.

Complications and Follow-up

The recurrence rate is approximately 3%, and usually occurs within the first month following surgery. Seroma, hematoma, and wound infection are other complications. Injury to the hypoglossal nerve is avoided by keeping the dissection medial to the cornua of the hyoid bone. Injury to the trachea or thyroid cartilage is avoided by careful identification of the landmarks. Recurrences are managed by reexcision, removing the scar tissue with a small margin of tissue around it; reexcision is delayed until the primary inflammation resolves in 4–6 wks. Follow-up is scheduled in 2 wks and then again in several months. Careful preoperative evaluation avoids hypothyroidism. There may be an increased risk of developing papillary thyroid carcinoma in the ectopic thyroid, especially in the patient older than 50 yrs of age.

DERMOID CYSTS

Like thyroglossal duct cysts, dermoids (or dermoid cysts) present as midline neck masses along the lines of embryonic fusion in the suprasternal notch or upper neck in the pretracheal *fascia*. They consist of an ectodermal wall with epidermis and epidermal appendages within the cyst wall. Because they are at risk for infection and have a theoretical risk for developing malignancy, dermoids are excised electively. It may be difficult to distinguish dermoids from thyroglossal duct cysts preoperatively or even intraoperatively, although dermoids are filled with keratinaceous material and thyroglossal duct cysts with mucoid material. If the etiology of the mass is uncertain, a Sistrunk procedure is recommended.

MIDLINE CERVICAL CLEFTS

Midline cervical clefts present as a 1–2 cm long and 4–6 mm wide vertically-oriented, thinly epithelialized patch in the low anterior midline neck. They occur secondary to inadequate fusion of paired arch tissue and may have an associated skin tag, sinus tract, or cartilaginous remnant. Treatment is excision with z-plasty closure.

BRANCHIAL CLEFT ANOMALIES

Embryology

There are six paired branchial arches on either side of the neck in the primitive embryo. The arches, consisting of ectoderm, endoderm, and mesoderm are made of depressions externally, and clefts and pouches internally. The arches, pouches and clefts either obliterate or persist to form the structures of the neck and jaw. The dorsal portion of the first cleft forms the external auditory canal. The first pouch forms the eustachian tube, middle ear cavity, and mastoid air cells. A remnant of the second pouch forms the palatine tonsil and supratonsillar fossa. The inferior parathyroids evolve from the third pouch, and the superior parathyroid glands and thymus evolve from the fourth pouch. Branchial anomalies result from the incomplete involution of these structures. The migration of these developing structures predicts and defines the pathway, location, and relationship of a particular anomaly to other structures.

Branchial anomalies are equally common in males and females, with 75–90% being second branchial and 8–20% being first branchial remnants. The spectrum consists of cysts which present later in childhood or adulthood as painful masses, sinuses, fistulas, skin tags, or cartilages — which usually present in infancy or within the first decade of life. Ten to fifteen percent are bilateral. These anomalies are located medial to the anterior border of the sternocleidomastoid muscle as a pit or skin dimple draining mucoid material. A cyst is located on the anterior border of the sternocleidomastoid below the hyoid and lateral to the carotid artery. Typically, they are diagnosed later in life, often when enlarged or infected.

Treatment

A noninfected second branchial anomaly is excised in an elective fashion, often in infants between 3–6 mths of age. The fistula tract runs through the platysma and turns medial above the level of the hyoid bone, over the hypoglossal and glossopharyngeal nerves between the carotid bifurcation, and enters the pharynx at the tonsillar fossa. The tract is lined with squamous, columnar, or ciliated epithelium and may be a complete fistula or may end blindly as a sinus. An infected remnant is treated with antibiotics and possibly needle drainage. Incision and drainage is avoided as it may distort the anatomy and increases the risk of recurrence. During excision, a lacrimal duct probe or large monofilament suture helps to define the tract. The fistula tract is excised in its entirety up to tonsillar fossa, where it is suture-ligated. A second stepladder incision may be required in the older patient. Cartilaginous remnants may involve the skin, subcutaneous tissue or muscle and usually are not associated with a sinus tract.

Third branchial cysts and sinuses arise in the same area as the second but travel between the hypoglossal and glossopharyngeal nerves posterior to the carotid and penetrate the thyrohyoid membrane and enter the piriform sinus. During resection, endoscopy is used to identify the pyriform sinus and the end of the tract. The rarer fourth branchial remnant presents as a recurring left neck abscess, often involving the thyroid and entering the piriform sinus. Excision may require left hemithyroidectomy.

First branchial remnants are challenging to diagnose and treat. Type I remnants are a duplication of the external auditory canal and consists of squamous lining. They parallel the external auditory canal and present just in front or behind the ear. Type II remnants present with drainage below the angle of the mandible and subsequent infection, nonpurulent ear drainage, or as a cystic tympanic membrane lesion of middle ear lesion with a sinus or abscess above the hyoid bone. A careful otoscopic exam is necessary in the evaluation and CT is helpful to track its course in relationship to the facial nerve and middle ear. Excision is hazardous secondary to risk of facial nerve injury and requires exposure of the trunk and peripheral nerve branches. A superficial or deep parotidectomy may be required and excision of the cartilaginous and squamous lining of the external auditory canal. Facial nerve monitoring is typically used intraoperatively.

CONCLUSION

Often the etiology of neck cysts and sinuses is discernible with a careful history and examination. A clear understanding of the embryology and judicious use of ancillary studies guide the surgeon and help to plan the operative course. Excision is definitive treatment, and recurrences are uncommon. Infected cysts require antibiotic therapy and attempts are made to avoid operative drainage because this increases the risk of recurrence. Nearly all neck cysts and sinuses are histologically benign, but if left in situ can develop into a malignancy.

REFERENCES

1. Cook SP. (2003) Thyroglossal duct cysts and related disorders. In: P Mattei (ed.), *Surgical Directives: Pediatric Surgery*, pp. 175–178. Lippincott Williams and Wilkins, Philadelphia.
2. Smith CD. (2006) Cysts and sinuses of the neck. In: JL Grosfeld, JA O'Neil, EA Fonkalsrud, *et al.* (eds.), *Pediatric Surgery*, 6th edition, pp. 861–873. Mosby Elsevier, St. Louis.
3. Grosfeld JL. (2003) Cervical cysts, sinuses, and other neck lesions. In: JA O'Neil, JL Grosfeld, EW Fonkalsrud, *et al.* (eds.), *Principles of Pediatric Surgery*, pp. 295–304. Mosby, St. Louis.

Section 6: Thorax

Newborn Thoracic Masses

CONGENITAL LUNG MALFORMATIONS

39

Alan P. Ladd

INTRODUCTION

Malformations of the congenital lung are historically divided into congenital cystic adenomatoid malformations (CCAM), bronchopulmonary sequestration (BPS) and congenital lobar emphysema (CLE). These lesions are felt to be congenital lesions of the developing lung and not acquired, developmental lesions, largely based on their availability for prenatal diagnosis. Each represents a particular variant in the developmental process, but lesions have been described with a hybrid-type presence of multiple pathologic lesions.

CLINICAL PRESENTATION

The presentation of these congenital lung lesions remains highly variable and includes either their incidental detection during prenatal screening sonography, postnatal development of cardiopulmonary insufficiency from either mass effect or internal shunting of blood flow, or by their recognition as part of an infectious pulmonary process with concurrent identification of a pulmonary parenchymal lesion.

The antenatal detection of malformations of the lung by prenatal surveillance approached only 17% among retrospective analysis of intrathoracic malformations that have gone onto resection.[1] Thus, the true incidence for these lesions is difficult to quantitate. When encountered prenatally, the congenital masses of the lung may present as either an echogenic mass with an absence of intraparenchymal cystic structures or a heterogenic mass with cysts 5 mm or more in diameter.[2] Though the latter lesions may be easily identified as CCAM lesions, the former lesions may not be discernible between CCAM and BPS, unless a systemic arterial supply allows for the clear diagnosis of BPS. The antenatal progression of these masses also is quite variable. Both CCAM and BPS lesions may enlarge or regress with no clear factors evident to predict their natural history. Periods of CCAM growth often occur between the 20th and 26th weeks of gestation with regressions often demonstrated in the third trimester.[3] Approximately 15% of CCAM lesions and nearly 70% of BPS lesions will show regression before birth. The developments of polyhydramnios, pleural effusion, or hydrops convey the greatest risk to the developing fetus. The presence of hydrops in the fetus with CCAM is often a sign of impending demise and often initiates consideration for fetal intervention.[2,4]

The postnatal discovery of congenital lesions of the lung often correspond with the development of pulmonary symptoms related to mass effect or infection complicating those elements of the malformation with communication to the distal airways. The possible spectrum of presenting signs and symptoms for these malformations spans from either the immediate pulmonary collapse from extrinsic compression of the normal airway and developing lung to its incidental discovery on computed tomography. Cases of expansive compression on the antenatal airway and parenchyma may result in pulmonary hypoplasia and corresponding pulmonary vascular hypertension leading to hypoxemia and need for extracorporeal oxygenation in attempts to stabilize the infant prior to surgical intervention. Infants may experience cardiovascular collapse from preferential left-to-right shunting within a BPS lesion with systemic arterial supply. Overinflation of communicating elements of the malformation to the distal bronchiolar airspaces may additionally provide compression of an otherwise normal airway leading to respiratory failure. These progressively expansive lesions, as in CLE, may then require immediate surgical resection in order to eliminate the mass effect on the airway and/or circulatory systems. Delayed identification of heterogeneic cystic and/or solid lesions of the lung during the evaluation of infectious pulmonary problems eventually lend to the identification of intrapulmonary lesions with bronchiolar connections. Such lesions may not be fully recognized from findings of infectious pulmonary infiltrates by standard roentgentograms, until the evaluation by computed tomography identifying an intrinsic mass with associated airspace disease.

PATHOPHYSIOLOGY

No true data exists as to the relative incidence of congenital lung malformations in the general population or prevalence within annual rates of birth. The largest single-institution series reported individually or through cumulative reviews grossly depicts an annual series of 5–10 such patients presenting per year to tertiary-care, pediatric hospitals.[5]

Congenital Cystic Adenomatoid Malformation

CCAM is characterized by the hyperplastic, adenomatoid overgrowth of terminal respiratory bronchioles that form cysts of varying sizes. These intraparenchymal masses tend to be discrete entities within the developing lung with connections to the tracheobronchial tree, though rarely contain cartilage and are not true cysts.

Historically, CCAM has been classified by early descriptive terms put forth by Stocker in 1977.[6] This classification delineated CCAM merely by the presence and nature of the associated cystic formations. Type I denoted lesions with large, often multiloculated cysts greater than 2 cm in diameter; where as type II lesions contained smaller cysts of less than 2 cm. Type III designations included those processes without cystic formation on gross inspection. Unfortunately, this classic categorization does not appropriately identify the overlapping described among hybrid types or the characterization of atypical forms. This "adenomatoid" formation may be more accurately described as a pulmonary hyperplastic process that is analogous to a pathologic growth from large airway obstruction, a possibility that may portend a physiologic etiology for these lesions.[1]

Large cyst type CCAM lesions often present early in infancy related to their relative expansion from air trapping. These enlarging lesions compress the adjacent lung leading to pulmonary function compromise and the possibility of cardiovascular collapse from mediastinal shift. Lesions that convey a significant mass effect may result in the development of pulmonary hypoplasia from its impact on normal parenchymal growth, and the possibility of resultant pulmonary vascular hypertension similar to that described for congenital diaphragmatic hernias. Thus patient morbidity will be impacted by the remaining degree of pulmonary hypoplasia evident, even following complete CCAM resection. Lesions are mostly confined to a single lobe and consist of cystic processes often greater than 2 cm in size, that may be multiple or multi-loculated. Up to

25% of these lesions may have an associated systemic arterial supply.[1] Other large cystic processes of the lung that may be mistaken for CCAM include low-grade cystic pleuropulmonary blastoma, cystic intraparenchymal lymphangioma and pneumatocele. Small cyst type CCAM demonstrate a pattern of maldevelopment that closely resembles pathology from airway obstruction during development and this pattern of maldevelopment may represent a malformation sequence of pathology. These small cyst type lesions show regional replacement of the associated lung parenchyma with variable amounts of associated alveolar parenchyma. Reports of sarcomas arising from these adenomatoid malformations may represent low-grade cystic pleuropulmonary blastoma development. Bronchioloalveolar carcinoma and rhabdomyosarcoma have been seen in older patients in association to large cyst type of CCAM.[3] This relationship to neoplastic change is often the touted rational for recommendations of surgical resection.

Bronchopulmonary Sequestration

BPS is a cystic mass of lung parenchyma without communication to the tracheobronchial tree. This nonfunctional tissue is characterized by its anomalous systemic blood supply, and thus often classified as a vascular anomaly. While the lesions typically acquire inflow from vessels arising from the aorta and other arterial supplies, their venous drainage is also variable and includes systemic, bronchial, or azygous venous drainage.[5] The occurrence of bronchial cartilage portends a possible communication with the foregut in these rare occurrences. Lesions of BPS develop as either intralobar or extralobar lesions. Intralobar lesions account for the majority of sequestrations with common investing pleura as the normal lung. They are characteristically found within the basilar segments of the lower lobes of the lung. Extralobar lesions are commonly found within the lower hemithoracies, as well as possible locations in the mediastinum, pericardium and within the diaphragm.

Though identified to a lesser extent in contemporary series, associated conditions to BPS have been reported to occur in up to 65% of patients and include congenital diaphragmatic hernia, diaphragmatic eventration, esophageal duplications and tracheoesophageal fistula.[5] Rarely, extralobar variants may communicate with the digestive tract, with connection to the esophagus most likely in these cases.[1]

Congenital Lobar Emphysema

Congenital lobar overinflation, often termed CLE, is an additional cause of cystic airspace anomalies. The etiology for this disorder is felt to be secondary to either intrinsic anomalies of the lung leading to partial obstruction of the airway, as in the case of bronchomalacia or lobar bronchus stenosis, or from extrinsic compression of the airways from a mass, such as bronchial cysts or vascular malformations.[5] In either form, it is felt to cause an air-trapping physiology that results in airspace enlargement without other alveolar anomalies. The process of partial airway compression leads to enlargement of the lobes and compression of adjacent parenchyma and a thoracic mass effect.

CLE lesions may be identified as a prenatal lesion if able to exclude microcystic CCAM lesions with an increased echogenicity or lack of systemic arterial blood supply evident in BPS. Regression of these lesions has also been described antenatally, but their clinical course may be more symptomatic during the postnatal course as prominent air trapping may occur, especially with utilization of positive pressure modalities for ventilation. These lesions commonly affect the upper lobes of the lung, with a higher rate of occurrence within the left upper lobe. Requirements for resection often are dependent upon the degree of mass effect on the mediastinum from the profound air-trapping that can occur postnatally. In these cases, a formal lobectomy is required.

Bronchogenic Cyst

Bronchogenic cysts (BC) commonly occur in a mediastinal location, often above the level of the tracheal bifurcation. BC are felt to arise from abnormal budding from the developing foregut or tracheobronchial anlage. These solitary unilocular cysts are filled with fluid or mucous and lined with pseudostatified ciliated columnar respiratory epithelium with notable goblet cells and smooth muscle. Diagnosis is confirmed by the presence of hyaline cartilage plates within the wall of the lesion. Though seen to attach to either the trachea or bronchus, they show no airway communication with these structures. Additional rare locations of presentation include locations from the suprasternal region to below the diaphragm. They may also present as intraparenchymal lesions or within the hilum of the lung, again without parenchymal communication. Nonspecific changes of airway parenchyma may be seen as these lesions may cause compression of nearby tissue.[1,5]

Lesions can gradually enlarge with the accumulation of fluid or mucous production. BC may become symptomatic with their compression of adjacent airways. The cysts may become infected or present as a cause for hemoptysis in the pediatric patient.

Prenatal detection of BC has been reported with the potential for development of a thoracic mass effect leading to mediastinal shift or extrinsic distal airway compression and lobar overinflation.

DIAGNOSIS/WORK-UP

With the increased use of sonographic prenatal screening and defined characterization of lung malformations of the developing fetus, the identification of these prenatal lesions is improving. The current ability for prenatal identification of these lesions, however, is approximately 17% of lesions undergoing eventual resection.[1]

With the identification of these lesions by screening ultrasonography, follow-up assessment with high-resolution sonography should be performed to further characterize the lesions with attempts to determine their etiology, especially with the search for systemic arterial supplies. Ultrafast MRI analysis will also allow for the identification of systemic feeding vasculature, as well as potential communicative processes to either the tracheobronchial tree or the foregut. Lesions with significant components of mass effect, pleural effusion, polyhydramnios, or hydrops fetalis should be referred to a fetal intervention center for possible fetal or early postnatal intervention.[2,5]

Each of the above noted lesions are recognized to have aspects of enlargement and growth during the antenatal course. Regression has also been described for each of these lesions, with an as yet unidentifiable stimulus for decompression during the latter stages of antenatal development. Cystic lesions with associated mass effect and mediastinal shift may be amenable to fetal interventions of thoracentesis, thoracoamniotic shunting, or rare ex-utero intrapartum, fetal lesion resections. With these lesions, the development of hydrops portends a lethal outcome, necessitating early fetal evaluation for the potential of intervention. Prospective predictors of risk for hydrops has only been elucidated in CCAM lesions by the determination of a CCAM volume ratio (length × height × width × 0.52) divided by head circumference. A ratio of greater than 1.6 has been found to be predictive for increased risk of hydrops in over 80% of these fetuses and may be useful in defining close ultrasound observation and early fetal assessment for intervention.[2,6]

MANAGEMENT

With the identification of isolated cystic lesions as in BC or extrapulmonary BPS, the recommended management is surgical resection by either open or thoracoscopic techniques. Though no data is available as to the natural history of lesions found incidentally or prenatally, the potential risks for malignant degeneration of CCAM, and the potential risk of a secondary infection within CCAM, BPS, and BC lesions has been provided as rationale for the resection of these lesions. Thoracic computed tomography is often required for definitive description and localization of these lesions in the postnatal period, especially if not clearly recognized on standard chest radiographs. Operative timing for elective resection is felt to be optimal between 3 and 6 months of corrected postnatal age to minimize associated anesthetic risks. Though the systemic nature of the arterial supply to extrapulmonary BPS avoids pulmonary hilar dissections, the nature of these elastic vessels to retract into the mediastinum or subdiaphragmatic origins of their feeding vessels offers additional consideration during their resection.[5]

Earlier intervention for lesions with associated thoracic mass effect and cardiopulmonary insufficiency may be required in these emergent conditions. Cardiovascular and pulmonary support in symptomatic lesions presenting shortly after birth or in the early newborn period require immediate resection and occasional adjunctive support with extracorporeal oxygenation to support any underlying pulmonary hypoplasia and associated pulmonary vascular hypertension. Lesions with associated overinflation, as in cases of intralobar CCAM and CLE, require lobectomy for complete and definitive resection. Reports have described the option for segmental lobectomy for lesions such as intrapulmonary BPS, but such interventions risk incomplete resection and morbidity of parenchymal air leakage.

Pneumonias that develop within the lesions associated with connections to the tracheobronchial tree (CLE, CCAM) are felt to be caused either by retained secretions or secondary bacterial seeding of the mucous contents. Parenteral antibiotics will allow for eradication of the majority of the infectious organisms, but complete clearance is often not feasible in these disordered parenchymal lesions. Thus, identification of concurrent malformations of the lung with pulmonary infections requires early clearance of the infection. Prophylactic antibiotic coverage of the remaining contents within the malformation is continued until clinical evidence for resolution of the inflammatory aspects is achieved prior to operative resection being considered.

POSTOPERATIVE CONSIDERATIONS

Children reaching operative intervention for these congenital malformations of the lung achieve a nearly 100% survival following resection. Morbidity is conveyed to the postoperative care of children with resultant pulmonary hypoplasia and associated pulmonary hypertension as a result of compression during lung development. Associated conditions, largely consisting of cardiac anomalies and congenital diaphragmatic hernias, may impact overall survival of these children.

Given the potential for malignant degeneration of lesions such as CCAM, incomplete resections could convey an increased risk of morbidity within the patient's lifetime. In most reported series, single lobectomy was the technique most utilized, but with the advent of better visualization technology in the employment of thoracoscopic surgery, thoracoscopic lobectomy should offer the benefits of complete resection and that of less postoperative pain and less impact on growth considerations of the developing chest wall.

REFERENCES

1. Langston C. (2003) New concepts in the pathology of congenital lung malformations. *Semin Pediatr Surg* **21**(1):17–37.
2. Kitano Y, Flake AW, Crombleholme TM, *et al.* (1999) Open fetal surgery of life-threatening fetal malformations. *Semin Perinat* **23**:448–461.
3. Johnson, AM and Hubbard AM. (2004) Congenital anomalies of the fetal/neonatal chest. *Semin Roentgen* **39**:197–214.
4. Adzick NS, Harrison MR, Crombleholme TM, *et al.* (1998) Fetal lung lesions: management and outcome. *Am J Obstet Gynecol* **179**:884–889.
5. Shanti CM and Klein MD. (2008) Cystic lung disease. *Semin Pediatr Surg* **17**(1):2–8.
6. Adzick NS and Kitano Y. (2003) Fetal surgery for lung lesions, congenital diaphragmatic hernia, and sacrococcygeal teratoma. *Semin Pediatr Surg* **12**(3):154–167.

CONGENITAL DIAPHRAGMATIC HERNIA AND INDICATIONS FOR ECMO

40

Troy Perry and Bryan J. Dicken

INTRODUCTION

Congenital Diaphragmatic Hernia (CDH) was first described in 1754 with further reports through the 1800's. Modern surgical repair found its beginnings in 1940 when Ladd and Gross reported a survival rate of >50% with diaphragmatic repair in the postnatal period. CDH is now a well-defined clinical entity with an incidence of 1.7 to 5.7/10,000 live births. This number is a conservative estimate as approximately one third of infants with CDH are stillborn.

CDH defects occur on the left side in 85 to 90% of cases, but can occur on the right or bilaterally. The commonest defect, known as a Bochdalek hernia, involves the posterolateral region of the diaphragm. Anterior regions, known as Morgagni hernias, can also be affected.

Etiology

CDH occurs when the developing diaphragm fails to fully close the pleuroperitoneal canals during embryologic development. During the normal sequence of events, the pleuroperitoneal canals close by 8 wks gestation followed by a return of the midgut into the abdomen at weeks 9 and 10. Lung development largely occurs after this period. Clinical sequelae are seen as a result of herniation of abdominal viscera through the diaphragmatic defect, into the thorax, thereby acting as a physical barrier for normal lung development by occupying the pleural space. This results in pulmonary hypoplasia and pulmonary hypertension characteristic of CDH.

PATHOPHYSIOLOGY

Embryology

Development of the diaphragm begins at 4wks gestation with in-folding of the body wall anteriorly and posterolateral to form the septum transversum and pleuroperitoneal membranes, respectively. Complete formation ends at 8 wks with fusion of all investing tissues to close the pleuroperitoneal canals, first on the right followed by the left. The fully developed diaphragm consists of four components: (1) The septum transversum, which forms the floor of the pericardium and central tendon of the diaphragm; (2) The pleuroperitoneal membranes, which form the dorsolateral portions bilaterally; (3) Esophageal mesentery, which forms the crura; and (4) The muscular components. Classically, the pleuroperitoneal membrane was thought to extend from its dorsolateral location towards the septum transversum anteriorly, and esophageal mesentery medially resulting in closure of the pleuroperitoneal canals. More recent studies have suggested that closure of the canals results from expansion of the posthepatic mesenchymal plate (PHMP). The PHMP is closely associated with the serosa of the underlying abdominal organs. This provides an explanation for the early closure of the right canal as the large right lobe of the liver provides a superior scaffold on which the PHMP may expand.

Fetal lung development occurs in four stages: (1) Embryonic (3–6 wks): Begins with a diverticulum off of the laryngotracheal groove and ends with the development of lung buds, (2) Pseudoglandular (7–16 wks): Defined by the development of bronchial airways, (3) Canalicular (17–24 wks): In this phase, primitive alveolar air sacs develop. Early potential for gas exchange is the major feature, and (4) Saccular (25 wks to term): Alveolar airspaces continue to develop during this phase and type II pneumocytes mature to provide surfactant synthesis.

Associated Anomalies

Associated anomalies are found in 40–50% of all cases of CDH. Below is a list of common abnormalities seen with CDH.

Chromosomal abnormalities are identified in up to 30% of CDH infants, and are associated with worse outcomes. Abnormalities include trisomy 18, 13, and 21; as well as various deletions and translocations. Multiple syndromes are associated with CDH, including Fryns Syndrome, Simpson–Golabi–Behmel syndrome, pentalogy of Cantrell and several others.

Cardiac anomalies occur in 24–36 % of infants. The most common defects found are ventricular septal defects, atrial septal defects and coarctation of the aorta. Others include transposition of the great vessels, tetralogy of Fallot, double outlet right ventricle, and hypoplasia of the left ventricle with or without aortic hypoplasia.

Gastrointestinal (GI) malformations (11%) commonly include Meckel's diverticulum and anal atresia.

Skeletal anomalies are found in 32% of infants with CDH and include limb reduction and costovertebral defects.

Bronchopulmonary malformations occur in 7–18% of cases. Tracheal malformations and pulmonary sequestration are the most common anomalies seen.

Neural tube defects are commonly seen in stillborn infants with CDH.

Midline anomalies include omphalocele, cleft palate, and esophageal atresia.

PRESENTATION AND DIAGNOSIS OF CDH

Routine ultrasound identifies >70% of CDH cases in the antenatal period. Findings on ultrasound depend on the side of the defect, but polyhydramnios is present in up to 80% of all cases. Findings with left-sided defects include intrathoracic stomach, visible peristalsis, and mediastinal shift. Right sided defects are more difficult to diagnose, as herniated liver appears similar to lung tissue, however identification of the intrathoracic gallbladder or hepatic vessels with Doppler is diagnostic. Once suspected on ultrasound a Magnetic Resonance Imaging (MRI) may be performed to confirm the diagnosis.

Clinical diagnosis after birth is generally made in the first 24 hrs with the onset of respiratory distress. Earlier onset occurs with increasing severity of pulmonary hypoplasia and persistent pulmonary hypertension (PPHN). This may be anticipated based on antenatal imaging. Physical findings include a scaphoid abdomen and barrel chest; the latter of which may be larger on the side of the defect, and expands asymmetrically with distention of herniated GI contents. Infants may have absent breath sounds on the side of the defect and heart sounds in the right hemithorax due to mediastinal shift with left sided defects. Diagnosis is confirmed with chest radiography demonstrating herniated abdominal contents in the chest that replace aerated lung, mediastinal shift, and paucity of air in the intraabdominal bowel.

Prognostic Factors

Anatomic considerations may be used to predict outcomes. Relative to the left, right sided lesions carry a worse prognosis with a higher proportion of infants requiring extracorporeal membrane oxygenation (ECMO), (40% vs. 15%) and a lower overall survival (50% vs. 75%). Coexisting anomalies and liver herniation are also associated with poor outcomes.

Parameters based on antenatal imaging are frequently used to predict outcomes by estimating the degree of pulmonary hypoplasia. These include:

(1) Lung-to-head ratio: Fetal ultrasound has utility beyond diagnosis as it may be used to predict prognosis. Lung-head ratio (LHR) is calculated using ultrasound to estimate contralateral lung size and divided by head circumference. The ratio must be calculated between 23 to 26 wks gestation. An LHR less than one is generally associated with poor survival and increased morbidity.

(2) Fetal MRI and total lung volume: Recently MRI has been used to predict prognosis by estimating total lung volume. The study is performed between 32 to 34 wks gestation and measures the total lung volume by combining the areas of the left and right lungs. A normal fetus at 32 wks will have a lung volume of 72 mL. Measurements of <20 mL in infants with CDH is associated with poor survival (35%) and increased

need for ECMO (86%), conversely measurements of >40 mL predict a survival of 90% and only a 10% need for ECMO.[1]

(3) Echocardiography and pulmonary artery (PA) measurements: PA diameters are measured using echocardiography in the third trimester and after birth. PA diameter serves as a surrogate marker of pulmonary hypoplasia. PA growth through the third trimester as measured with serial echocardiography is associated with improved survival. The absolute size of both the left and right PA conferring increased survival is >2 mm at birth.[2]

Measures of Pulmonary Function

Pre and Postductal Oxygen Saturation: The degree of shunting may be estimated by obtaining pre and postductal oxygen saturations most commonly from the right and left arms respectively. A drop in oxygen saturation in the postductal distribution suggests a significant right to left shunt.

Preductal measurements on blood gas or oximetry represent the capacity of the lungs to ventilate and oxygenate. Preductal measurements are frequently used to determine eligibility for ECMO; either alone, or as part of the indices below. Many centers will not offer ECMO to infants with peak preductal saturations <85% in the first 24 hrs as this suggests overwhelming pulmonary hypoplasia.

Modified Ventilatory Index (MVI): MVI is used to predict prognosis, and may be combined with other parameters to identify a need for ECMO. Values >40 suggest a poor prognosis with conventional ventilation. Like $AaDO_2$, MVI is now infrequently used. (respiratory rate (RR); peak inspiratory pressure (PIP)).

$$MVI = (RR \times PIP \times PaCO_2)/1000.$$

Oxygenation Index (OI): OI is most frequently used in algorithms to guide the initiation of ECMO. Values >40 indicate a need for immediate action (mean airway pressure (MAP)).

$$OI = (MAP \times FiO_2 \times 100)/PaO_2).$$

TREATMENT STRATEGIES AND FAILURE: INDICATIONS FOR ECMO

As treatment for CDH evolved, it was recognized that mortality was associated with pulmonary hypoplasia and PPHN, and not inherent to the defect alone. Interventions directed at managing these conditions preoperatively have led to improved survival.

Ventilation management: Protecting lung tissue from further insult is essential in initial resuscitation efforts. This begins with immediate intubation after delivery and nasogastric tube decompression to maximize lung expansion. "Gentle ventilation" strategies to avoid lung barotrauma have been developed in high volume centers. When on conventional mechanical ventilation, suggested values for PIPs range from 20 to 25 cm H_2O and MAPs from 12 to 18 cm H_2O. Permissive hypercapnia is inherent to gentle ventilation strategies and $PaCO_2$ levels <64 torr are generally acceptable.[3]

The use of surfactant to improve pulmonary function in CDH is not recommended as it is linked with increased mortality.

Inability to maintain oxygenation at the above airway pressure limits is often an indication for high frequency oscillatory ventilation (HFV) or ECMO.[4] The following are ventilation parameters indicating a need for ECMO:

(1) PIPs >30
(2) MAPs >18
(3) OI >40 or sustained OI >25 for 4 hrs
(4) Unable to sustain preductal SaO_2 >85%
(5) Failure of HFV

Pulmonary Hypertension and Cardiovascular Management

PPHN in infants with CDH is caused by decreased cross-sectional area of the pulmonary vascular bed leading to varying degrees right to left shunting through the ductus arteriosus. This manifests as poor postductal tissue perfusion. Clinical endpoints such as capillary refill, urine output and lactate levels are utilized to assess adequate tissue oxygenation.[3] Systemic vascular resistance should be increased to a mean arterial pressure of 40 to 50 torr using inotropes and fluids. This reduces the degree of right to left shunt and improves tissue perfusion. ECMO should be considered in cases where repeat fluid boluses are required with high dose inotropes to overcome PA pressures.

Inhaled nitric oxide (iNO) is used to treat PPHN caused by CDH, but evidence is lacking to recommend its routine use. It has been used however as both a rescue and bridging therapy to delay the need for ECMO. Its effectiveness is unclear and some centers have found an increased mortality with iNO. The variable results suggest that the type or duration of iNO delivery plays a role in efficacy. Some institutions report high survival rates without ECMO, utilizing iNO for several weeks as a definitive therapy.[5]

Failure to overcome significant PPHN resulting in tissue hypoxia is an indication for ECMO.[4] The following are cardiovascular parameters indicating a need for ECMO:

(1) Failure to maintain a mean arterial pressure > 50 with inotropic support and adequate volume resuscitation
(2) Persistent metabolic acidosis with lactate > 45 mg/dL
(3) Mixed venous O_2 saturation < 60%

Pre-ECMO Investigations

Once the decision has been made to start an infant on ECMO certain investigations are required to confirm eligibility and facilitate treatment.

Imaging: Cranial ultrasound is performed to identify intraventricular hemorrhage, which is a contraindication for ECMO. Echocardiography is required to assess the degree of cardiac dysfunction, right to left shunting, and identify cardiac anomalies that may be incompatible with life or confound ECMO support, e.g. coarctation. Significant right ventricular dysfunction on echo may indicate a need for venoarterial (VA) ECMO.

Bloodwork: laboratory investigations include Complete Blood Count (CBC), crossmatch, PT/INR, PTT, fibrinogen, urea, creatinine, calcium, magnesium, glucose, lipase, ALT, AST, and total bilirubin. These are required in anticipation of potential bleeding complications, and to assess for end-organ dysfunction.

Consent: A thorough discussion with parents outlining the potential outcomes and expected prognosis after ECMO including both immediate outcomes and future quality of life.

Contraindications to ECMO

(1) Prematurity defined as gestational age < 30 wks or weight <1.5 kg. These patients carry a high risk of intracranial hemorrhage.
(2) Preexisting intracranial hemorrhage > grade II.
(3) Active bleeding or underlying coagulopathy.
(4) Inability to achieve a best SaO_2 > 85% or $PaCO_2$ < 50 torr*
(5) Mechanical ventilation > 14 days. These patients have severe bronchopulmonary dysplasi (BPD).
(6) Multiple congenital anomalies or severe neurologic impairment
(7) Overwhelming sepsis
(8) Parental refusal

VV and VA ECMO

The choice between VA and venovenous (VV) ECMO typically depends on the need for cardiac support (VA), or mere respiratory support of hypoxia (VV). The choice for CDH infants is not clear as these patients often have a need for both. VA provides the most comprehensive support, but also comes with added risks. Table 1 outlines the major features of both VA and VV ECMO.

Outcomes with ECMO

Overall survival with ECMO varies greatly by institution between 44 to 86%. This range likely reflects variations in pre-ECMO care and patient selection for ECMO. A number of variables have been studied to identify prognostic factors for infants starting on ECMO, in order to facilitate better patient selection.[7] Pre-ECMO factors predictive of worse outcomes include birth weight <3000 g, gestational age <38 wks, antenatal diagnosis, and 5-min Apgar score <7. Post-ECMO factors include duration of ECMO> 14 days and development of renal complications.

Table 1. Comparison of features for VA and VV ECMO. (Adapted from Fortenberry J[6])

	VA ECMO	VV ECMO
Cannulation site(s)	Internal jugular vein, right atrium or femoral vein plus right common carotid, axillary or femoral artery, or aorta.	Internal jugular vein only, jugular–femoral, femoral–femoral, sapheno–saphenous, or right atrium.
Usual PaO_2 achieved	60–150 torr	45–80 torr
Indicators of sufficient oxygenation	Mixed venous saturation or PaO_2 and calculated oxygen consumption.	Cerebral venous saturation; O_2 difference across the membrane; PaO_2, pre-membrane saturation trend.
Cardiac effects	Decreased preload, increased afterload; CVP varies, pulse pressure low; coronary oxygenation provided by left ventricular blood; "cardiac stun".	Minimal effects; CVP and pulse pressure unaffected; may improve coronary oxygenation and reduce right ventricular afterload.
Oxygen delivery capacity	High	Moderate, improves with additional drainage sites.
Circulatory support	Partial to complete	Improved delivery of oxygen to coronary and pulmonary circulation can improve cardiac output.
Effect on pulmonary circulation	Moderately to markedly decreased.	Unchanged or improved with oxygenated blood.
Presence of right to left shunt	Decreased hemoglobin saturation of blood in aorta.	Increase hemoglobin saturation of blood in aorta.
Presence of left to right shunt	Potential pulmonary congestion and systemic hypoperfusion.	Potential pulmonary congestion and systemic hypoperfusion.
Recirculation	None	Major impact on oxygen delivery.

Despite its wide spread use, the utility of ECMO for CDH has yet to be proven. Reports of outcomes are highly variable with some non-ECMO centers producing similar survival rates to centers using routine ECMO.[5]

SURGICAL MANAGEMENT

Timing of Repair

Improved recognition of postnatal physiology in CDH infants led to a marked shift in the timing of repair, with emergent repairs making way for a strategy of delayed repair. Physiologic changes that accompany the CDH infant involve the postdelivery "honeymoon" period of relative respiratory and cardiovascular stability, followed by a progressive deterioration in respiratory status. The resulting hypoxemia initiates a vicious cycle of worsening PPHN, and ultimately respiratory failure. Delaying surgical repair allows for a period of medical stabilization, which may or may not include ECMO support. The preoperative period may extend from several days to several weeks.

In the non-ECMO infant, delaying definitive repair until the child has been successfully weaned from vasoactive agents and maintained on low ventilator settings is reasonable. Some centers have further suggested serial echocardiography to guide timing of repair based upon improvement or stabilization of the PPHN. Additional factors to consider include total body fluid status, spontaneous diuresis, and the infant's spontaneous ventilatory effort. Currently, however, there are no recommendations to guide optimal timing of surgery.

Operative Repair

Most surgeons approach the repair of CDH through a subcostal incision. The incision should be approximately one fingerbreadth below the costal margin, to allow sufficient abdominal *fascia* and muscle on the cephalic aspect of the wound to allow for a tension-free closure of the diaphragmatic defect.

The next step is to reduce the contents of the hernia from the chest. Gentle upward traction on the costal margin to "break the seal" and downward traction on the herniated viscera usually reduces the contents into the abdominal cavity. It is helpful to have a nasogastric tube in place at the time of surgery to facilitate decompression of the GI tract. Once reduced, the bowel can be packed inferiorly and medially out of the operative field to completely demonstrate the extent of the defect. Beginning medially, the posterior aspect of the diaphragm rim can usually be "unrolled" from the retroperitoneum. The anterior rim should be similarly identified. A hernia sac, present in approximately 20% of cases, is excised to minimize recurrence. If sufficient diaphragm is present, a primary closure using interrupted nonabsorbable sutures is completed, often with pledgets. Care should be taken to avoid excessive tension on the repair so as to avoid recurrences. If the hernia defect is large, or is under excessive tension, a prosthetic patch repair is preferable. A chest tube is not usually necessary in uncomplicated CDH repairs. A chest tube may be required in patients repaired while on ECMO, where anticoagulation is necessary, or in patients with a persistent air leak. The chest tube should be left to water seal only, as negative pressure may add barotrauma and perpetuate pulmonary hypertension.

Once the hernia has been repaired, the abdominal packs are removed, and the abdomen closed in layers. Occasionally abdominal closure is not possible due to a loss of abdominal domain, or due to unacceptably high abdominal pressures. Under these conditions, temporary closure may be accomplished with an abdominal silo, followed by definitive closure later.

Operative Repair while on ECMO

Surgical repair of CDH while on ECMO follows the same general principles outlined above; however, the required anticoagulation necessitates a greater emphasis on meticulous hemostasis. Prior to initiating surgery, optimization of activated clotting times (ACT) to 160–200 secs, and the use of Aminocaproic acid (Amicar) or Transexamic acid may reduce bleeding. In addition, platelet levels should be maintained greater than 100,000 mm^3 and fibrinogen levels greater than 1 g/L for 24 hrs postoperatively. Finally, liberal use of fibrin glue along raw surfaces, particularly the retroperitoneal diaphragm edge, may be useful. Careful application of these principles has resulted in some centers reporting bleeding complications as low as 12.5% compared to 26% in the Extracorporeal Life Support Organization (ELSO) registry. Recent data has suggested an improved survival for infants repair after ECMO compared to those repaired while on ECMO, even while controlling for factors associated with severity of CDH.

POSTOPERATIVE MANAGEMENT

CDH infants should have regular assessments using a systems based approach to guide management and identify complications. There are special considerations in addition to the standard postoperative complications of infection and bleeding.

Neurologic complications are common with nearly half of CDH infants developing some degree of intracranial hemorrhage during hospitalization. If suspected, MRI will provide a definitive diagnosis.

Postoperative PPHN is a significant cause of mortality, and close cardiovascular monitoring should be continued postoperative using the same principles outlined above to manage blood pressure and shunting, with special attention to volume status. Peri-operative echocardiography is a useful adjunct to predict, and assess postoperative PPHN. A preoperative PA pressure to systemic pressure ratio (PSR) > 0.9 measured on echocardiography is a strong predictor of postoperative mortality. In infants with significant PPHN, and right-to-left shunt despite optimization of contributing factors, sildenafil is often considered as a rescue therapy. Sildenafil has been shown to improve pulmonary hypertension and cardiac output, however little data is available to support its use.

Postoperative pulmonary management follows closely to preoperative goals. Gentle ventilation strategies should be continued, allowing for modest hypercapnia ($PCO_2 < 64$) and oxygenation ($SaO_2 > 90\%$). Early respiratory complications after repair include pneumonia, pneumothorax, and chylothorax. Chylothorax occurs in 10–30% of infants after CDH repair, and is associated with significant morbidity. Diagnosis is confirmed with pleural fluid analysis. Initial management includes tube thoracostomy and total parenteral nutrition; octreotide infusion may be considered, but is of unproven benefit. Patients failing conservative management based on persistently high chest tube outputs require surgery to ligate the thoracic duct.

Enteral feeding should be initiated shortly after repair, and is safe in infants still on ECMO. The nasojejunal route of enteral feeding is generally preferred because of the high incidence of gastroesophageal reflux (GER). Introduction of oral feeds can begin as tolerated when the infant no longer requires mechanical ventilation. Anti-reflux procedures at the time of CDH repair may improve GER in the first 6 mths of life, but have failed to demonstrate long-term benefit.

Acute kidney injury (AKI) is common amongst infants with CDH. The cause is multifactorial owing to the critically ill state, but it is an independent risk factor for mortality. Because neonates often develop nonoliguric renal failure, low urine output does not necessarily preclude the end sequelae of AKI. Serial measurements of serum creatinine can identify infants at risk, and prompt early intervention.

Table 2. Long-term complications and suggested follow-up for infants with CDH.

	Complications	Suggested follow-up
Neurodevelopment	Developmental delay, and behavioral disorders.	Neurodevelopment evaluations at discharge, then annually.
Hearing	Sensorineural hearing loss.	Auditory brainstem evoked response or otoacoustic. emissions screen with all health checks*.
Cardiac	Cardiac anomalies, and PPHN.	Echocardiography at discharge, then as recommended by cardiology.
Respiratory	Bronchospasm, aspiration, pneumonia, pulmonary hypoplasia, chronic lung disease.	Pulmonary function tests as indicated at 6 and 18 mths; RSV prophylaxis during first 2 yrs.
Gastrointestinal	GER foregut dysmotility, bowel obstruction and volvulus.	Upper GI study, pH probe and/or gastric scintiscan at discharge and 1 yr as indicated.
Musculoskeletal	Pectus deformities, chest wall asymmetry, and scoliosis.	Physical exam, chest radiograph and/or computed tomography.
Diaphragmatic hernia	Recurrent hernia, and prosthetic patch infection.	Chest radiograph at discharge, and with all health checks* if patched repair.

*Routine health checks should be completed as recommended for all children at 1–3, 4–6, 9–12, and 15–18 mths of age, then annually up to the age of 16 yrs.

Sepsis is a devastating complication in CDH infants, and should always be considered if clinical status declines. Common sources include pneumonia, arterial and venous catheters, and infected prosthetic patch. Strict infection control protocols have been shown to improve survival.

LONG-TERM FOLLOW-UP AND LATE COMPLICATIONS

Many infants with CDH that survive beyond the neonatal period will have significant morbidities affecting multiple organ systems. Because of their complex needs, they require close follow-up by a multidisciplinary team. Table 2 outlines common abnormalities and suggested follow-up in addition to routine health checks.

REFERENCES

1. Lee TC, Lim FY, Keswani SG, *et al.* (2011) Late gestation fetal magnetic resonance imaging — derived total lung volume predicts postnatal survival and need for extracorporeal membrane oxygenation support in isolated congenital diaphragmatic hernia. *J Pediatr Surg* **46**(6):1165–1171.
2. Okazaki T, Nakazawa N, Ogasawara Y, *et al.* (2011) Increase in fetal pulmonary artery diameters during late gestation is a predictor of outcome in congenital diaphragmatic hernia with liver herniation. *J Pediatr Surg* **46**(12):2254–2259.
3. Logan JW, Rice HE, Goldberg RN, Cotten CM. (2007) Congenital diaphragmatic hernia: A systematic review and summary of best-evidence practice strategies. *J Perinatol* **27**(9):535–549.
4. Antonoff MB, Hustead VA, Groth SS, Schmeling DJ. (2011) Protocolized management of infants with congenital diaphragmatic hernia: effect on survival. *J Pediatr Surg* **46**(1):39–46.
5. Tam YS, Cheung HM, Tam YH, *et al.* (2012) Clinical outcomes of congenital diaphragmatic hernia without extracorporeal membrane oxygenation. *Early Hum Dev* **88**(9):739–741.
6. Fortenberry J. (2005) In K Van Meurs (ed.), *ECMO Extracorporeal Cardiopulmonary Support in Critical Care*, 3rd edition, p. 88. Extracorporeal Life Support Organization, Michigan.
7. Seetharamaiah R, Younger JG, Bartlett RH, Hirschl RB. (2009) Group OBOTCDHS. Factors associated with survival in infants with congenital diaphragmatic hernia requiring extracorporeal membrane oxygenation: A report from the Congenital Diaphragmatic Hernia Study Group. *J Pediatr Surg* **44**(7):1315–1321.

ESOPHAGEAL ATRESIA AND TRACHEOESOPHAGEAL MALFORMATIONS 41

Frederick J. Rescorla

INTRODUCTION

Esophageal and tracheoesophageal fistulas are relatively common neonatal surgical conditions affecting between 1–3,000 to 4,000 live births. The first description was in 1670 however it was not until 1939 that the first staged repair occurred followed by the first primary repair in 1941. Although there have been many refinements in the clinical management with advanced neonatal care, pediatric anesthesia and improved care of low birth infants, this still remains a challenging problems in some children particularly those with long gap esophageal or those born prematurely with respiratory distress.

PATHOPHYSIOLOGY

Embryology

Although esophageal atresia and tracheoesophageal fistula are relatively common foregut anomalies, the embryologic events are not completely understood. The trachea and esophagus both develop from the embryologic foregut as a median diverticulum. At 22 days gestation the endoderm differentiates into a ventral respiratory portion and a dorsal esophageal segment. The separation of these two is thought to occur by the formation of lateral longitudinal tracheoesophageal folds that subsequently fuse in the midline and create the tracheoesophageal septum. At 6 to 7 wks of gestation, the separation between the two is complete. One theory is that incomplete fusion of the folds results in a defective tracheoesophageal septum allowing an abnormal connection between the trachea and esophagus. Another theory is that there is imbalance in the growth of the cranial and caudal folds leading to esophageal atresia and the presence of a fistula.

Esophageal atresia and TEF is usually a sporadic occurrence. There is a slightly increased incidence among twins and various environmental teratogens including oral contraceptives and methimazole have been implicated. Chromosomal abnormalities are found in 6–10% of children with Trisomy 18 being more common than Trisomy 21. Various genes have been identified with an association with esophageal atresia and tracheoesophageal fistula.

Classification

Several classifications have been reported, however the most common is that of the Gross classification of types A through E based on the presence or absence, as well as location of the fistula (Figure 1). Type A, pure esophageal atresia occurs in 5–13% of cases. Both ends of the esophagus end blindly, and as noted in the figure, the major problem is the lack of distal esophageal length. Type B, esophageal atresia with proximal fistula occurs in 1% of cases. This also has a major problem with the lack of distal esophageal length and can be difficult to differentiate from type A on initial clinical evaluation. Type C, esophageal atresia with distal tracheoesophageal fistula is the most common subtype accounting for 78–86% of cases. Type D, esophageal atresia consists of both proximal and distal fistulas and accounts for <1% of cases. Type E or H-type TEF without esophageal atresia appears in approximately 2–6% of cases. Although this is discussed with neonatal esophageal atresia, in view of the lack of esophageal obstruction, the clinical presentation is often later in life.

Associated Anomalies

Associated congenital anomalies are very common and occurred in 65% of 227 children treated at out institution. Congenital heart disease is the most common defect occurring in 13–38% of cases. Vertebral defects occur

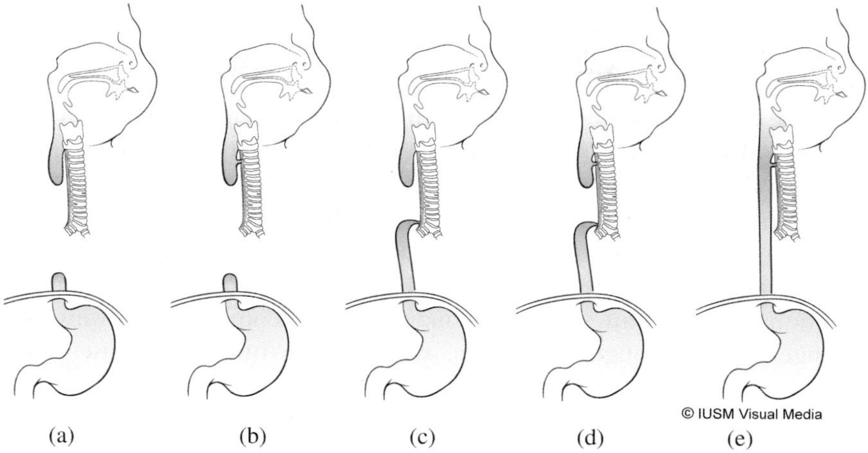

Figure 1. Classification system for esophageal atresia and tracheoesophageal fistula.

in 6–21% of cases. Other gastrointestinal abnormalities include duodenal atresia, malrotation and imperforate anus in 13%, renal anomalies in 5–15% and vertebral defects in 6–21%. The vertebral anomalies are usually located in the thoracic region. The VACTERL association represents a constellation of potential abnormalities in the vertebral, anorectal, cardiac, tracheoesophageal, renal, and limb areas. The VACTERL association was initially listed as VATER representing vertebral, anal, tracheoesophageal and radial dysplasia. This was later changed to include cardiac and limb anomalies. In a series of over 400 patients, 23% had at least two of the VACTERL defects. TEF has also been associated with CHARGE syndrome consisting of coloboma, heart defects, choanal atresia, developmental retardation, genital hypoplasia, and ear abnormalities. In view of these potential associations, all children with esophageal atresia and TEF undergo evaluation with spine films, echocardiogram, renal ultrasound and a careful examination of the extremities and anorectal region.

CLINICAL PRESENTATION

Prenatal diagnosis of esophageal atresia and tracheoesophageal fistula is difficult. It is occasionally suspected based on a third trimester ultrasound demonstrating polyhydramnios with or without fluid in the stomach. Some reports have noted an upper neck pouch thus suspecting a blind ending esophagus. The most common presentation after birth is excessive salivation due to blockage of secretions in the proximal esophageal pouch, respiratory distress and symptoms related to aspiration of secretions. Abdominal distention can occasionally occur as air passes through the fistula into the gastrointestinal tract. In children born prematurely who develop severe respiratory distress and require ventilatory support, the development of significant abdominal distention can be severe and in addition the gastrointestinal tract may be more compliant allowing the passage of air through the fistula, thus making inflation of the lungs difficult.

DIAGNOSIS

The diagnosis of esophageal atresia and TEF is usually confirmed by attempting to pass an orogastric tube into the stomach. The tube usually stops at 8–12 cm from the lips. A chest X-ray is then obtained along with a portion of the abdomen to evaluate the location of the tube, as well as to check for the presence of air in the gastrointestinal tract. As noted in Figure 1, patients with type A or B will not have air in the gastrointestinal tract below the diaphragm. It is reasonable to allow at least 4 hrs of life prior to definitively assuming that there is no distal fistula as there have been some reports showing absence of gas initially. The presence of air in the stomach usually confirms the presence of a distal fistula, thus making the diagnosis a type C or D. Contrast studies are not indicated and are associated with the risk of aspiration into the tracheobronchial tree due to the potential presence of a fistula.

Risk Stratification

Timing of operative repair must be individualized to the clinical state of the child accounting for associated conditions, respiratory status and physiologic status including he potential presence of pneumonia related to aspiration. Waterston in 1962 reported a classification system in which group A, the best clinical status, were those with birth weight over 2.5 kg and in good condition. Group B were birth weights between 1.8 and 2.5 kg and in good condition, or with the presence of moderate pneumonia or moderate anomalies, although there were no strict criteria concerning the status of the anomalies. Group C, which were considered the highest risk, were birth weight <1.8 kg or any other weight with severe pneumonia or severe associated anomalies. This did allow stratification based on risk, although others over the years have questioned the validity as intensive care management of small babies has advanced. The Montreal classification, reported by Poenaru in 1993, eliminated the weight and considered group I those with no ventilator dependence and minor or major anomalies, and those with ventilator dependence and minor anomalies. Group II included ventilator dependence and major anomalies or those with life threatening anomalies regardless of pulmonary status. Spitz in 1993 reported a classification system in which group I were birth weight >1500 g without major cardiac disease, group II, birth weight <1500 g or major cardiac disease, and group III birth weight <1500 g and major cardiac disease. Subsequent retrospective reviews have suggested the Spitz classification system the most reliable at predicting prognosis thus pointing out the serious morbidity and mortality related to cardiac defects, as well as indicative of the improved survival related to advanced respiratory support.

MANAGEMENT

Basic management of all children consists of oral esophageal suction catheter, intravenous fluid support and antibiotics. Based on the above classification system, infants with distal tracheoesophageal fistula and stable respiratory and cardiac status can undergo operative repair within the first 24 hrs of life. Small infants above 1000 g can undergo operative repair if they are stable.

Operative Management Type C or D

These defects include esophageal atresia with distal TEF, with or without proximal TEF. The first successful repair of esophageal atresia and tracheoesophageal fistula was performed by Cameron Haight in Ann Arbor, Michigan in 1941. Prior to that, in 1939 there were reports of a staged repair using initial gastrostomy with subsequent ligation of the fistula and esophageal replacement through an antethoracic skin tube. The classic approach is through a right thoracotomy with division of the fistula and primary end-to-end anastomosis. The presence of a right aortic arch occasionally can make the operative approach from the right difficult and some have recommended going through the left chest in the presence of a right aortic arch. Although we usually try to discern the location of the arch based on the echocardiogram, this is not always possible. An echocardiogram should also carefully evaluate for the presence of a vascular ring.

The operative preparation by the anesthesiologist is critical to the management of these children. An awake intubation is usually performed to allow spontaneous breathing during the initial phase of the procedure. An attempt is made to position the endotracheal tube bevel to occlude the fistula. Intraoperative flexible bronchoscopy through the tip of the endotracheal tube often aids in diagnosing the presence of the distal esophageal fistula as well as allowing positioning of the endotracheal tube. In addition, if desired, catheter occlusion of the tracheoesophageal fistula can be performed using a small Fogarty catheter and others have reported utilization of a bifurcated tracheal tube although this is rather difficult. One lung ventilation with left main stem intubation is another possibility. We generally attempt to position the endotracheal tube to occlude the fistula and use spontaneous breathing until the fistula is controlled. In addition, bronchoscopy usually allows the evaluation of a proximal pouch fistula although this needs to be evaluated intraoperatively during the dissection of the proximal pouch.

The patient is positioned for a right posterolateral thoracotomy with proper support. A small 10 Fr replogle tube or 10 or 12 Fr red rubber catheter is placed in the proximal esophageal pouch to allow the anesthesiologist to gently put pressure on this to aid the surgeon in identifying the proximal pouch. The latissimus dorsi muscle and serratus anterior muscle can be spared during the operative approach with a thoracotomy. By sparing the serratus anterior one can avoid the winged scapula. The fourth intercostal space is identified and the intercostal muscle divided. An extrapleural dissection is performed after dividing the intercostal muscles. A moistened cotton tipped applicator is useful for separating the pleura from the undersurface of the ribs. A small infant rib spreader and the intact pleura is dissected superiorly and posteriorly. The azygos vein is identified and usually marks the site of the fistula. After division of the azygos vein the fistula can usually be identified and encircled with a vessel loop. Care must be taken to avoid extensive dissection of the esophagus as small feeding vessels are important as the blood supply to the distal esophagus. Sutures are placed on the tracheal side and the fistula is divided and closed with interrupted or running 5/0 PDS (Ethicon Johnson & Johnson, Somerville, NJ). The suture line is placed under saline and the anesthesiologist provides gentle ventilation to check the closure. Mediastinal pleura should be placed over the tracheal suture line to reduce the risk of recurrence of a tracheoesophageal fistula.

Gentle pressure is placed on the proximal pouch by the anesthesiologist who advances the esophageal tube. A traction suture of 3/0 silk can be placed through the esophagus and tube and then with manipulation of the suture there is no excessive tension on the esophagus. The proximal esophagus must be mobilized to the thoracic inlet separating it very carefully from the trachea. Care should be taken to stay on the esophageal side during this division to avoid an injury of the trachea. Very rarely a type D variant with a proximal fistula will be encountered at this time. If there is an adequate length to the two esophageal segments, a primary anastomosis can be performed at this time. Occasionally the distal esophagus must be mobilized slightly however, care should be taken to preserve the blood supply to this segment of the esophagus.

If the distance between the two segments is 2 cm or greater and it is not felt that a safe anastomosis can be performed, the surgeon has the option of performing a circular myotomy as described by Livaditis. This is generally performed approximately 2 cm above the blind end of the proximal tip and can be made with a Beaver blade to divide the longitudinal circular smooth muscle allowing the esophagus to stretch on the submucosa and mucosa. A second myotomy may be required, but this is very difficult to do on the proximal esophagus and may need to be performed on the distal esophagus, again taking care to avoid injury to the blood supply.

Although the original description by Haight was a two layer anastomosis, most currently use a single layer anastomosis with 4/0 or 5/0 suture material. Silk suture may be used but has been associated with increased leak and stricture rate in some reports. Most surgeons use monofilament absorbable 4/0 PDS or Maxon sutures. Most centers utilize an end to end anastomosis but there have been reports of end-to-side with ligation but not division of the tracheoesophageal fistula. This has been noted with a lower leak and stricture rate but does have a higher recurrent TEF rate. A 12 Fr chest tube or flat drain can be placed in the posterior mediastinal space to provide drainage should a leak occur. Some have abandoned use of extrapleural drainage tubes, however we generally place a tube or a drain.

The thoracosopic technique has been popularized by Lobe and Rothenberg and the primary advantage is to avoid any sequelae of a thoracotomy in a young child. The thoracoscopic technique follows the same principles as that of the open procedure although knot tying has been more difficult. The fistula in these cases is divided with either suture ligature or a clip.

Timing of surgery

The common clinical scenarios which result in the discussion about the timing of surgery are that of the presence of associated cardiac anomalies or severe respiratory distress. In children with cardiac anomalies, discussions with the pediatric cardiologist and pediatric cardiac surgeons determine the order of procedures. If the cardiac procedure must be performed immediately over the first few days of life, an occluding catheter such as a Fogarty placed through the fistula can occlude the fistula and allow a time period for performing the cardiac procedure. It using a Fogarty catheter, contrast in the balloon allows visualization on X-ray and the effectiveness of this can be determined by films demonstrating minimal intestinal gas. Care of this tube is essential as dislodgement could possibly lead to complete tracheal occlusion. We therefore generally leave this catheter at least 1 cm below the carina and secure the catheter to the endotracheal tube. We also believe that it is important to not over distend the catheter and therefore try to simply have the amount of fluid in the balloon to just occlude the fistula. In some of these cases we have placed a gastrostomy tube and with this in place it is rather simple to determine by the leak through the G-tube whether the fistula is effectively being occluded and it is also possible to determine the lowest volume possible in the catheter balloon to stop the leak from the gastrostomy tube.

In children with severe respiratory distress requiring significant ventilatory support, occlusion of the fistula by some manner as mentioned above is usually necessary. If the child is less than 1000 g we will usually try to ligate or divide the fistula relatively early on and then defer the anastomosis until the child is older and in a stable condition. If the child is over 1000 g and it is anticipated that the child will stabilize, we may wait and divide the fistula and perform a primary anastomosis at the initial procedure.

Esophageal Atresia and Distal TEF with Severe Respiratory Distress

The management of a child with a distal fistula and severe respiratory distress is complicated when positive pressure ventilation is required. The fistula may be the path of least resistance allowing air to preferentially enter the gastrointestinal tract. Various maneuvers can be utilized to manage this. The endotracheal tube can be positioned with a bevel occluding the fistula, a maneuver which usually requires flexible bronchoscopy. A gastrostomy tube will relieve the abdominal and gastric distention but will allow air to continue to pass out through the tube. The gastrostomy tube can be placed under water in order to add PEEP to the system, but air can still pass distally. Another option at the time of gastrostomy placement is to encircle the distal esophagus with a vessel loop and occlude the distal esophagus thus effectively closing the fistula.

Another option is to place a Fogerty catheter alongside the endotracheal tube and either with bronchoscopic guidance or fluoroscopy passes the catheter into the fistula. The catheter should be placed down to confirm that it is actually in the fistula and the balloon then inflated and positioned below the carina and left in place to occlude the fistula. We have left this in up to 2 wks to occlude the fistula while a child underwent life threatening cardiac surgery prior to TEF repair. This cannot be left in at a high pressure for a long time as it can lead to ischemia of the fistula. Another option is to perform an urgent thoracotomy with either ligation or a division of the tracheoesophageal fistula followed by a delayed esophageal repair when the child is stable.

Esophageal Atresia without a Distal Fistula

Patients with Gross type A or B have the difficult problem of having a short distal esophagus. In the past, these children often underwent a cervical esophagostomy with an esophageal replacement at approximately 1 yr of age. In the late 80's and early 90's the utilization of delayed repair was popularized and this is currently utilized at most centers. With this strategy an initial gastrostomy is placed and it is often useful to perform bronchoscopy at this time to evaluate for the possibility of a proximal fistula which may not be readily apparent from initial evaluation. The stomach is often very small in these infants and even placing the gastrostomy and trying to bring it up to the abdominal wall can be difficult. The feeds are advanced slowly but eventually brought to a high volume. After the gastrostomy is placed, feedings are advanced and often taken to a high volume in order to increase the stomach size and also promote reflux into the distal esophageal pouch.

If a proximal fistula is present (type B), it is reasonable to try to defer division until the time of definitive reconstruction unless respiratory problems occur due to aspiration from the proximal pouch into the trachea and then it may need to be closed at an earlier time. The gap between the two segments is measured utilizing contrast injected into the stomach in order to reflux the distal esophagus and a bougie placed orally into the proximal esophagus to measure the distance. The gap is usually described in terms of the number of vertebral bodies which takes into account the child's size. Exploration is usually performed at around 3 mths of life. We generally perform a standard extrapleural approach with mobilization of both ends and primary repair, often with one or two circular myotomies. If a long gap (>2 cm) remains and the surgeon does not feel a primary repair is possible, thoracoscopy can be utilized to directly visualize the two ends and mobilize them in order to assess feasibility of primary repair. In addition a thoracoscopic Foker procedure can be performed in which sutures are placed into the proximal and distal segments and external traction applied in an attempt to decrease the gap.

Foker reported a technique in which at the initial procedure, either as a thoracotomy or by thoracoscopy, an assessment is made after dissecting out the two ends of the esophagus as to whether a primary anastomosis is possible. If it is not possible, tension pledgetted traction sutures are placed using horizontal mattress sutures into the two ends of the esophagus. Internal or external traction is then applied. The sutures are brought out of the back above and below the incision and tied with a silastic buttons. The sutures are shortened between one and three times per day to maintain tension until the two ends of the esophagus are observed to be 1 cm apart on radiologic evaluation at which time operative repair is performed. Internal traction sutures are placed to the vertebral *fascia* and utilized for smaller gaps where they are left in place for 3 to 4 days. This has been reported to be successful managing between long gaps however, a high percentage of these patients do subsequently require an anti-reflux procedure. At the time of primary repair, one or two circular myotomies are often required to gain adequate length for the anastomosis.

At the time of definitive repair, the surgeon should be prepared for alternative methods should the gap not be able to be bridged with the native esophagus. The various options include a gastric pull-up, reverse gastric tube and colonic interposition.

An alternative method reported by Kimura utilized a cervical esophagostomy with advancement of this down the anterior chest wall combined with a spiral myotomy to gradually increase the length of the esophagus in an extrathoracic location. We have utilized this technique with one child referred to our center with a cervical esophagostomy and successfully completed a delayed primary repair of the esophagus.

POSTOPERATIVE MANAGEMENT

It is very common to leave the endotracheal tube in place until a time when the child is clearly prepared for extubation. Should reintubation be required, it is very important to have skilled personnel to directly visualize the cords and reduce risk of injury to the esophageal anastomosis. A nasogastric tube is usually placed during the initial procedure and this can be used for early feeds on postoperative day two or three. Most centers utilize drip feeds in order to minimize reflux. Gastrostomy tubes are not routinely utilized in children with esophageal atresia and distal tracheoesophageal fistula. A contrast study is performed on postoperative day seven as long as a leak is not noted with the presence of saliva in the drain or chest tube. If the child is stable and a small leak is present with a small amount of fluid coming from the anastomosis, one can simply wait another 5 to 7 days before performing the esophagram. Most small leaks will seal unless there is a complete disruption of the anastomosis. Over 95% of these resolve spontaneously.

Postoperative strictures are fairly common and are more common if a leak has been present with a rate of approximately 50%. Reports of the incidence of strictures are between 17–40%. This is difficult to tell from some series as routine dilatation has been part of the management of some centers. It should be noted that the distal esophagus is smaller than the proximal esophagus and there will be a caliber change at the anastomosis due to the long standing *in utero* obstruction of the proximal esophagus. If dilatation is needed a balloon dilator or a wire guided system is useful for dilatation. The rate of leak is high in type A primary repair as is subsequent gastroesophageal reflux requiring antireflux procedure.

Recurrent Tracheoesophageal Fistula

Recurrence of a tracheoesophageal fistula has been reported between 3–15% with many noting it around 9%. It is usually located at the site of the original fistula and it is also thought that a previous leak or excessive tension can increase the incidence of recurrent TEF. Children usually present with cough, choking or cyanosis with feeds or recurrent pneumonia. Endoscopic treatments with cauterization or fibrin glue or the placement of Surgisis (Cook Inc., Bloomington, Indiana) plugs have been reported although many of these have a fairly high recurrence rate. There have also been reports of placing Surgisis prophylactically between the trachea and esophagus at the time of initial TEF repair. Although the endoscopic maneuvers can be utilized, if the fistula persists, division and interposition of pericardium or intercostal muscle flap should be performed.

Tracheomalacia

This is defined as generalized or localized weakness of the trachea that allows the anterior and posterior walls of the trachea to come together during expiration. This generally occurs in 8–15% of patients with TEF and often requires long term ventilatory support. Aortopexy has been reported to have good success with managing this and can be performed through a left or right anterior thoracotomy, through a sternotomy or also thoracoscopically. Some children with severe tracheomalacia do require tracheostomy.

Gastroesophageal Reflux

Gastroesophageal reflux is extremely common in this population occurring in 35–60% of patient and is likely due to an intrinsic motor dysfunction of the esophagus. Reflux can lead to esophageal strictures and if a stricture fails to improve with dilatation and reflux is noted, an antireflux procedure is indicated. Most patients with type A undergoing primary repair require an antireflux procedure.

H-TYPE TRACHEOESOPHAGEAL FISTULA

Tracheoesophageal fistula without esophageal atresia usually occurs at the cervical level or at least above the second thoracic vertebral body. The diagnosis is usually delayed past infancy with symptoms consisting of coughing or choking during feeds with liquids usually causing more symptoms than solids. The diagnosis is usually made during the first 3 yrs of life, but we have seen children as old as 9 yrs of age present with this diagnosis. A high index of suspicion is needed in a child affected with these symptoms. Contrast studies of the esophagus may demonstrate the fistula however, if there is a high index of suspicion, a balloon or double balloon technique to inject contrast under pressure may be successful in demonstrating the fistula. If there is a high index of suspicion, rigid bronchoscopy if useful and is a very accurate method of detecting the site of the fistula. At bronchoscopy the fistula is located in the posterior membranous wall and a small flexible catheter such as a 3 or 4 Fr Fogarty or ureteral catheter can be passed through the fistula into the esophagus and with the use of contrast and fluoroscopy the diagnosis can be confirmed.

Operative management for an H-type fistula can usually be performed through a right cervical incision. It is useful to place a catheter through the fistula to allow identification once the esophagus is identified. If a Fogarty is used with a balloon this can be pulled back and with gentle traction placed on the catheter by the anesthesiologist the fistula can usually be identified. Care must be taken to avoid injury to the vagus nerve and recurrent laryngeal nerve during this dissection. The fistula is encircled and divided and each side closed with 4/0 sutures of PDS, Maxon or vicryl. One of the strap muscles should be mobilized and placed in between the two suture lines and tacked in place with fine sutures to prevent a recurrent fistula. We generally leave a drain in these pending an esophagram on postoperative day number six or seven, and usually place a nasogastric tube to allow feeds during this time.

OUTCOME

A review from our institution demonstrated a significant incidence of dysphagia, respiratory infections, gastroesophageal reflux disease and choking, which occurred most frequently during the first 5 yrs of life. This tends to improve as the children grow older. As the children start to eat more solid food and swallow larger pieces of meat such as hotdogs without properly chewing them, these sometimes become stuck at the anastomosis and require esophagoscopy for removal. Our institution demonstrated that approximately 50% of the children weighed less than the 25th percentile during the first 5 yrs of life and this decreased to 30% at 10 yrs of age.

The overall survival for infants with esophageal atresia and tracheoesophageal fistula is >90% with most deaths due to a complex cardiac or chromosomal abnormalities which are incompatible with life. Long term follow-up by pediatric surgeons is important to monitor for motility disorders, gastroesophageal reflux, as well as the potential development of esophagitis and Barrett's esophagus.

In Waterston's original report in 1962, the survival was 95% for group A, 68% for group B and 6% for group C. Utilizing the Spitz classification with 357 patients treated at Great Ormond Street Hospital in London between 1980 and 1992 the survival was 97% for group I, 59% for group II and 22% for group III.

SELECTED REFERENCES

1. Engum SA, Grosfeld JL, West KW, *et al.* (1995) Analysis of morbidity and mortality in 227 cases of esophageal atresia (EA) and/or tracheoesophageal fistula (TEF) over two decades. *Arch Surg* **130**(5):502.
2. Poenaru D, Laberge JM, Neilson IR, *et al.* (1993) A new prognostic classification for esophageal atresia. *Surgery* **113**(4):426.
3. Rothenberg SS. (2002) Thoracoscopic repair of tracheoesophageal fistula in newborns. *J Pediatr Surg* **37**(6):869–872.
4. Spitz L, Kiely E, Brereton RJ, Drake D. (1993) Management of esophageal atresia. *World J Surg* **17**(3):296.
5. Waterston BJ, Bonham-Carter RE, Aberdeen E. (1962) Esophageal atresia with tracheoesophageal fistula: a study of survival in 218 infants. *Lancet* **1**:819–822.
6. Foker JE, Linden BC, Boyle EM, Jr, *et al.* (1997) Development of a true primary repair for the full spectrum of esophageal atresia. *Ann Surg* **226**:533, discussion 541.

PECTUS EXCAVATUM 42

Scott A. Engum

CLINICAL PRESENTATION

Pectus excavatum (PE) is a posterior intrusion of the chest wall into the thoracic cavity. Although frequently noted at birth, antenatal diagnosis is rare. The majority of patients will remain asymptomatic in the childhood years. It is not uncommon for patients to not notice the depression until a pubertal growth spurt and 80% of patients are male.[1] It is not uncommon to see scoliosis in 15–20% of patients. PE can be a component of several rare syndromes and include King–Denborough syndrome and spinal muscular atrophy.[2,3]

Concern about the appearance of the chest prompt many patients to seek evaluation with our without other symptoms. A large percentage of patients with PE are self-conscious about their body image and this creates interpersonal difficulties. During adolescence, body image is of great importance. This is the time when the person is establishing an independent identity, choosing a trade, and beginning involvement with the opposite sex, and those patients afflicted with a PE deformity may have reduced capacity to carry out these actions. Many have tried to push this off as "only cosmetic", however Lawson and others have developed and validated tests for body image effects specific to PE.[4]

Many patients perceived exercise intolerance and efforts to dissect the cause have led to pulmonary function studies. Both spirometry and plethysmography show that lung volumes are modestly decreased. Kelly and colleagues found FVC to be 77% of predicted, FEV1 was below average in 83%, and the FEF25–75% was below average in 73% of patients.[5]

In a follow-up study the FVC was 90% predicted, FEV1 was 89% and FEF25–75% was measured at 85% predicted.[2] The only rational physiologic explanation for the decreased spirometry values is the chest wall deformity since pulmonary parenchyma and airways of the lung are unaffected.

PATHOPHYSIOLOGY

Incidence

In a 1975 Collaborative Perinatal Project Chung noted a varied incidence of PE from 38/10,000 births among white infants to 7/10,000 births among black infants to 20/10,000 infants categorized as other.[6] A Nigerian survey of 2195 autopsied patients by Odelowo showed no patients with PE indicating the infrequent occurrence in the African region.[7] In the United States, PE constitutes 90% of all chest wall defects.

Classification

Classically, the PE deformity has been described as a "cup", which is a focal defect, or "saucer", which presents as a broad deformity. With the increased use of Computed Tomography (CT) scans and further studying of preoperative photography, additional types of patients have been noted and include the long trench/furrow (not uncommonly asymmetrical), and the mixed carinatum/excavatum deformities. The frequency of occurrence is unclear; however, the "cup" deformity is most common.[8] Daunt and coworkers examined normal children to obtain values for the pectus index and found this value to be 2–2.3.[9]

Pathology

In the embryo, the normal sternum appears during the 6th week of embryology as a pair of parallel mesenchymal bands of condensed mesenchyme. Cells migrate from two lateral plates on either side of the anterior chest wall to fuse in the midline by the 10th week of gestation in a ventrolateral and craniocaudal fashion. The plates begin to chondrify almost at once. At about the same time, a median cranial rudiment called the presternum appears and is associated with the developing shoulder girdle. The lateral bands then fuse with the presternum cranially and with the tips of the ribs laterally. During the 7th week, the sternal bands join at their cephalic ends and gradually fuse in the midline. This fusion progresses with the decreasing rapidity and ceases during the 10th week. The most caudal portion — the xiphoid process — however, often remains bifid. At about the 6th month, the paired suprasternal cartilages appear cranially and laterally to the presternum. These usually fuse with the presternum to form part of the manubrial articulation with the clavicle. From 8 months to 4 yrs after birth, the ossification centers are established.[10]

Most frequently, PE involves the lower sternum near the xiphoid and affects the adjacent cartilages. There are a number of attachments that exert forces on the sternum and include the articulation with the clavicles and the upper costal cartilages, the xiphoid process to the linea alba and the most medial fibers of the rectus abdominis, in addition to the posterior fibers to the diaphragm.

Unfortunately, the etiology for PE remains unknown. Mechanical forces may play a role in development and acquired forms of the condition are noted in patients with congenital diaphragmatic hernia. Patients with connective tissue disorders such as Marfan's syndrome, Ehlers–Danlos syndrome, or Sprengle's deformity suggest an instrinsic cartilage abnormality.[1] Evaluation of cartilage removed in a surgical case have shown mechanical property concerns as relates to stress and strain deformation, abnormal cartilage content, and electron microscopy. Histological evaluation has been unremarkable.[11,12]

In a large series of North American patients evaluated by Nuss, 43% of patients gave a family history of PE, and 4% a family history of pectus carinatum. A number of inheritance patterns have been documented and include autosomal dominant, autosomal recessive, X-linked, and multifactorial in different families. There is a tendency in some families to have similar morphology over generations.[1]

DIAGNOSIS

Preoperative imaging is important and an inexpensive, readily available chest radiograph is sufficient for some experienced surgeons to complete severity indices measurements. Most believe that a CT scan of the chest is advantages to show the three dimensional (3D) skeleton and degree of cardiac compression/displacement. In addition, the cephalocaudad extent of the depression is more easily visualized, as well as cartilage deformity, and calcifications. Utilizing a CT scan, the pectus radiographic index can be determined by measuring the internal thoracic diameter from left to right divided by the distance from the back of the sternum to the front of the vertebral body. Magnetic Resonance Imaging (MRI) can be utilized, but it is less convenient and time consuming with little benefit other than radiation exposure.

Cardiac evaluation may have right atrial/ventricular compression or mitral valve prolapse which can be present in approximately 18% of patients. Mitral valve prolapse is secondary to compression on the heart and one may note resolution of this finding in half of surgically treated patients and dysrhythmias have been noted in 16% of patients. The hemodynamic effects of PE continue to strike controversy. Bevegard in 1962 showed on right heart catheterization that patients with a 20% or greater decrease in physical work capacity from the supine to sitting position had a shorter distance from the sternum to the vertebrae. In addition, the increase in stroke volume from rest to exercise was 18.5%, compared to 51% in normal subjects.[13] Others have shown that the stroke volume was 31% lower and cardiac output was 28% lower in upright vs. supine exercise.[14] In some patients, despite the severe PE noted, there may be no compression of the heart as noted on a CT scan and continued controversy exists due to the lack of objectively measured PE severity correlated to the amount of cardiac compression. Future studies will need to clarify this position, however, summarization shows a compression of the right heart that causes a decreased stroke volume, and when combined with a decrease in movement of air within the lungs (restrictive pulmonary condition) there is a diminished cardiopulmonary capacity in severe cases of PE.

Deformity of the chest wall led many investigators to attribute the symptomatic improvement after surgery to an improvement in pulmonary function. Some investigators have shown decreased values for FVC, FEV1, maximal voluntary ventilation, and diffusing capacity of the lung compared to normal patients and with exercise testing that the maximal oxygen uptake and oxygen tension were significantly lower than normal controls, but this was related to cardiovascular rather than a pulmonary cause.

SURGICAL MANAGEMENT

Prior to any operation, it is important to note any asymmetry, costal flaring, sternal torsion/rotation, cephalad extent of the depression, and the presence/absence of narrowed anterior/posterior diameter of the chest.

The clinical utility of careful preoperative appraisal lies in the guiding expectations of the family and to determine which procedure will give the patient the best outcome. Review of the CT scan with the patient and family preoperatively aids in communicating the extent of the deformity and to offer realistic expectations and outcome. It is not uncommon to obtain preoperative photographs to allow for comparison to postoperative results.

Surgical correction of primary PE has been shown to carry low operative risk across centers in North America. Thus, the surgical treatment for a severe case should not be withheld due to a primary care physician's lack of knowledge or importance of the deformity to the child or parents. Operative repair is readily accomplished in teenagers, close to the age of skeletal maturity.

The indications for surgery include a pectus radiographic index of 3.25 or greater along with cardiac and/or pulmonary compression, restrictive and/or obstructive pulmonary lung disease, previously failed repair, or formal cardiology evaluation illustrating mitral valve prolapse, murmur, or conduction abnormality.[15]

The modern open surgical repair is often attributed to the modifications made by Ravitch and Welch. Ravitch initially recommended excising all deformed cartilages with the perichondrium and isolating the sternum, except at its attachments to the manubrium. Welch preserved the perichondrium to allow costochrondral regeneration. To this day, principles of open repair include resection of deformed cartilage with preservation of the perichondrial sheaths, sternal osteotomy (transverse posterior or wedge anterior), remodeling of the sternum, and fixation of the sternum in its new position. Addition of a stabilizing bar in 1961 by Adkins represents a major turning point in the treatment of PE by reducing perioperative pain and hospital duration, as well as recurrence of the chest deformity. The stabilizing bar bridges the sternum and ribs, avoids a flail chest and the paradoxical breathing that can occur along with resultant pulmonary complications. One disadvantage of the bar is that they require a second surgery for removal.[5]

The push for minimally invasive surgery also brought about further modifications to the traditional open procedure. Fonkalsrud recently described an open repair of PE with minimal cartilage resection. In this technique, a chevron inframammary incision with midline extension is performed. Myocutaneous skin flaps are raised to expose the deformed costal cartilages, but unlike the traditional Ravitch repair, only a short segment of cartilage is resected medially (3–8 mm) and a second in proximity to the costochondral junction laterally, using these as small hinges at either end. Care is taken to preserve the perichrondrium. The xiphoid process is removed, and the retrosternal space is mobilized up to the level of posterior angulations. A transverse wedge osteotomy is made across the anterior sternal table, and the lower sternum is elevated gently, fracturing the posterior table. For patients with an asymmetric deformity, in addition to raising the sternum, it is twisted to correct one-sided angulation. A steel strut can then be positioned to stabilize the repair for 6 months. The xiphoid sternum and costal cartilages are sutured back to sternum before closing to increase chest wall stability. Reattaching the sternum provides additional stabilization and fills a void in the lower chest. Minced cartilage or bone chips from the previous resections can be placed in any spaces where the costal cartilage does not make contact with the newly positioned sternum or ribs to promote cartilage regeneration. Finally, the pectoralis and abdominal muscles are reapproximated.[16]

A revolution across the entire surgical community occurred during the 1990s with the dissemination and uptake of "key hole surgery". Nuss and colleagues shifted the paradigm in PE surgery with publication of their results using minimally invasive techniques. The Nuss procedure involves lateral transverse chest incisions and the placement of one or two temporary retrosternal steel bars fitted to the individual patient and bent like a "U". The sternum is elevated by using the patients own chest wall for support without cartilage resection. In response to a number of concerning complications, including pericarditis, ventricular injury, and thoracic outlet syndrome, techniques have been modified to improve patient safety.[5] Thoracoscopy is now routinely performed to directly visualize dissection, and steel struts may be stabilized laterally by a number of techniques. A severe asymmetrical or mixed deformity with sternal protrusion does not respond as well to the Nuss operation and may be better treated by the open Ravitch procedure. Park has reported excellent results in asymmetrical PE using an asymmetrically bent bar and the Nuss procedure.[17]

The use of prostheses to fill the pectus deformity in carefully selected patients may also provide excellent early cosmetic results; however, implants do not address the underlying physiologic burden, may migrate away from the midline resulting in worse cosmesis, and tend to be very expensive.

POSTOPERATIVE MANAGEMENT

The patient undergoes a thoracic epidural in the operating room at the time of the surgical case and this provides adequate postoperative pain control along with supplemental oral medications and intravenous narcotics. Stool softeners are initiated as this time as well. The patient is admitted to a ward bed, restricted to bed rest on the first day along with no side lying or rolling. The patient is up in a chair on postoperative day one and consultation with respiratory therapy for incentive spirometry and physical therapy for postoperative activity guideline education is initiated.

COMPLICATIONS/FOLLOW-UP

Many patients with PE have perceived exercise intolerance; however, investigations have yielded mixed results. A meta-analysis in 2006 showed the average cardiovascular function increased by greater than one half standard deviations following the surgical repair of PE. Unfortunately, many papers in the study had flaws in study design and a conclusive answer continues to elude the surgical community.

Concern about the appearance of the chest prompt many patients to seek evaluation with our without other symptoms. A large percentage of patients with PE are self-conscious about their body image and this creates interpersonal difficulties. Many have tried to push this off as "only cosmetic", however Lawson[4] and others have developed and validated tests for body image effects specific to PE. Marked improvement in psychosocial functioning was noted after repair; however the severity of the PE depression on CT scan did not correlate with the patients' or parents' perception of body image concerns.

Postoperatively, three patients that had studies performed showed the cardiac index increased by 38% and was attributed by an increased stroke volume. In more recent studies, a diminished stroke volume has been demonstrated by cardiac catheterization, oxygen saturation studies, CT scan and echocardiogram with improvement following surgery.

Pulmonary function test have failed to document consistent improvement resulting from surgical repair. Some studies have shown a decrease in functional test due to chest wall rigidity following surgery. Workload studies have shown improvement in exercise tolerance following surgical repair. Although patients reported a subjective improvement in their exercise tolerance, pulmonary function after a minimally invasive chest wall repair was shown by Sigalet to be reduced at 3 mths and maximal oxygen uptake was reduced while cardiac function was enhanced with an increase in stroke volume.

REFERENCES

1. Nuss D, Kelly RE, Croitoru DP, *et al.* (1998) A 10-year review of a minimally invasive technique for the correction of pectus excavatum. *J Pediatr Surg* **33**:545–552.
2. Kelly RE, Shamberger RC, Mellins R, *et al.* (2007) Prospective multicenter study of surgical correction of pectus excavatum; design, perioperative complications, pain, and baseline pulmonary function facilitated by internet-based data collection. *J Am Coll Surg* **205**(2):205–216.
3. Bach JR, Bianchi C. (2003) Prevention of pectus excavatum for children with spinal muscular atrophy type 1. *Am J Phys Med Rehabil* **82**(10):815–819.
4. Lawson M, Cash T, Akers R, *et al.* (2003) A pilot study of the impact of surgical repair on disease-specific quality of life among patients with pectus excavatum. *J Pediatr Surg* **38**(6):916–918.
5. Kelly RE. (2008) Pectus excavatum: Historical background, clinical picture, preoperative evaluation and criteria for operation. *Semin Pediatr Surg* **17**:181–193.
6. Chung CS, Myrianthopoulos NC. (1975) Factors affecting risks of congenital malformations. I. Analysis of epidemiologic factors in congenital malformations. Report from the Collaborative Perinatal Project. *Birth Defects Orig Artic Ser* **11**(10):1–22.
7. Odelowo EO. (1989) Congenital chest wall malformations in Nigerians. *Afr J Med Sci* **18**(4):263–268.
8. Cartoski M, Kelly RE, Nuss D, *et al.* (2006) Classification of the dysmophology of pectus excavatum. *J Pediatr Surg* **41**:1573–581.
9. Daunt SW, Cohen JH, Miller SF. (2004) Age-related normal ranges for the Haller index in children. *Pediatr Radiol* **34**(4):326–330.
10. Engum SA. (2008) Embryology, sternal clefts, ectopia cordis, and Cantrell's pentalogy. *Semin Pediatr Surg* **17**:154–160.
11. Kelly RE, Jr, Lawson ML, Paidas CN, *et al.* (2005) Pectus excavatum in a 112-year autopsy series: Anatomic findings and the effect on survival. *J Pediatr Surg* **40**:1275–1278.
12. Feng J, Hu T, Liu W, *et al.* (2001) The biomechanical, morphologic and histochemical properties of the costal cartilages in children with pectus excavatum. *J Pediatr Surg* **26**(12):1770–1776.

13. Bevegard S. (1962) Postural circulatory changes at rest and during exercise in patients with funnel chest, with special reference to factors affecting the stroke volume. *Acta Med Scand* **171**:695.
14. Beseir GD, Epstein SE, Stampfer M, *et al.* (1972) Impairment of cardiac function in patients with pectus excavatum, with improvement after operative correction. *N Engl J Med* **287**:267.
15. Nuss D, Kuhn MA. (2007) Our approach: MIS repair of pectus excavatum. *Contemp Surg* **63**(9):444–451.
16. Fonkalsrud EW. (2009) 912 Open pectus excavatum repairs: Changing trends, lessons learned: One surgeon's experience. *World J Surg* **33**:180–190.
17. Park HJ, Jeong JY, Jo WM, *et al.* (2010) Minimally invasive repair of pectus excavatum: A novel morphology-tailored, patient-specific approach. *J Thor Cardio Surg* **139**(2):379–386.

Chest Wall Anomalies

PECTUS CARINATUM 43

Scott A. Engum

CLINICAL PRESENTATION

Pectus carinatum (pigeon breast) is more frequent in boys with the typical disease process recognized during the early adolescent years and becomes progressively more severe until full skeletal maturity has been achieved, after which, little change occurs throughout adulthood. One typically notes a symmetrical protrusion of the body of the sternum and costal cartilage. Some patients can have an associated lateral depression of the ribs. Fewer patients can present with an asymmetrical protrusion or a mixed deformity with components of protrusion and depression. Patients may indicate some component of tachypnea with physical exertion or reduced endurance and this is felt to be related to reduced respiratory excursion of the thorax and a fixed increase in anterior to posterior diameter of the chest. Some patients may complain of pain in the area of the deformed cartilages. Symptoms commonly became more severe during the adolescent years of rapid skeletal growth, causing progressive limitations in exercise tolerance. Up to a third of patients may experience exertional wheezing or worsening asthmatic symptoms.

PATHOPHYSIOLOGY

Incidence

Pectus carinatum occurs less frequently than excavatum at a ratio of 1:5. It occurs four times more frequently in boys and an overall prevalence of 0.6%.[1]

Classification

The most frequent form is a symmetrical protrusion of the body of the sternum (gladiolus) and costal cartilages, termed chondrogladiolar. Protrusion can also be asymmetrical with the deformity limited to one side of the sternum, and the costal cartilages producing a keel-like protrusion. A mixed deformity where the patient has both protrusion and a depression component occurs. In this variety, the sternum is often rotated posteriorly toward the depressed side and can be seen in conjunction with Poland's syndrome. The least frequent presentation is chondromanubrial, where the protrusion is primarily the manubrium and the superior costal cartilages with a relative depression of the body of the sternum. This is frequently associated with premature fusion of the sternal sutures and a broad comma-shaped or Z-shaped sternum and there is an increased incidence of congenital heart disease in these patients.[2]

Pathology

The origin is poorly understood and most believe it is associated with an excessive growth of the ribs and/or costal cartilage. There appears to be a genetic predisposition with a positive family history noted in more than 25% and some component of connective tissue abnormality such as scoliosis is noted in up to 15% of patients.

DIAGNOSIS

Children can present with a wide spectrum of protrusion deformities from mild to severe and the diagnosis is typically made on physical exam during a clinic. When these individuals are observed during physical exertion, patients frequently will compensate with tachypnea and wider diaphragmatic excursions. Controversy remains, however, regarding the association of pectus carinatum and respiratory dysfunction because reported physiologic studies on these patients are sparse.

In younger patients presenting with a pectus carinatum, a chest radiograph may be warranted to rule out any associated mediastinal process (tumor). In the typical adolescent patient, further work-up is not necessary. If any evaluation is performed, it is typically a chest radiograph or computerized tomographic scan and will show an increased anterior to posterior diameter, a somewhat narrow width, and a narrow cardiac silhouette in most patients. A pectus radiographic index may range from 1.2 to 2.1 with a normal individual at approximately 2.5. Some third party payers are mandating a pectus radiographic index of less than 2.0 prior to any authorization for surgical correction.

SURGICAL MANAGEMENT

Nonoperative treatment with compressive orthotics has been reported to gain similar outcomes by exploiting the moldable nature of growing bone and cartilage with selective application of external force on the chest wall. Haje and colleagues designed the first brace in Brazil in the 1990s.[3] At present, one can use a custom-fitted thoracic brace or a low profile brace with compression plates and aluminum struts. Some protocols will have the patient were the brace for 23 hrs a day for 3 to 6 mths or until the defect has flattened. At that point, 16 hrs daily wear was continued for 3 to 6 mths allowing the patient to participate in school activities without the brace. Patients are allowed to remove the brace for sporting events throughout all stages of treatment protocol. The maintenance phase requires nightly bracing after complete subjective improvement is noted and continues until linear growth ceases, to prevent recurrence.[4] It is not uncommon to reevaluate patients on an every 3-month basis to ensure proper fit of the device. The biggest challenge to successful treatment lies in the fact that this process is most often noted in young adolescent boys who pose significant compliance issues. Patients with some component of significant asymmetry, excavatum or a sternal angulation of more than 20° may be better served with an open Ravitch repair.

A typical open Ravitch repair can be performed with a transverse incision identical to that performed with a pectus excavatum. All deformed cartilage is removed and an osteotomy is performed that allows the posterior plate of the sternum to fracture which returns the sternum to a normal position. If a mixed deformity is encountered, a wedge-shaped osteotomy is often required and closure of the osteotomy will elevate and rotate the sternum into the correct position. In the chondromanubrial form, it is not uncommon to need to take a wedge of the anterior plate of the sternum at the point of maximal protrusion and at times create a second osteotomy at the site of the second angle of the Z-shaped sternum. Others have been able to accomplish the procedure with a single osteotomy if the sternum is more comma-shaped and truncated. A support bar is typically not necessary in routine cases, however, in the mixed deformity, it may be required.

Fonkalsrud has advocated a progressively less extensive open repair compared to the classic Ravitch with small segments of cartilage (12 mm length) resected adjacent to the sternum and laterally at the level where the chest wall was at the desired level. In this case, only the lower two or three perichondrial sheaths were detached from the sternum. After the transverse anterior sternal osteotomy with lowering and straightening of the lower sternum, the lower perichondrial sheaths were reattached to the sternum. An Adkins strut was used for most of these patients and autologous cartilage chips were placed in the perichondrial sheaths at both ends to promote healing.[5]

Similar to the Nuss procedure where pressure is exerted beneath the sternum, Hock describes a minimal access treatment utilizing a two lateral transverse incision at the mid-axillary line where a bar is inserted into the chest at the lateral intercostal space and subsequently exits at the sternocostal interspace lateral to the carinatum and then back into the chest at the opposite lateral sternal intercostal space. The bar will then exert anterior pressure on the sternum, pushing it posteriorly and supported by the patient's own thorax.[6] Others have utilized a similar anterior pressure, but left the support bar external to the chest and secured laterally with fixation plates attached to the ribs for support.

Kim and associate describe a thorascopic approach where an asymmetrical (unilateral) pectus carinatum was treated with excision of the abnormal cartilage from within the thorax using electrocautery and angled bone rongeur. Two spaced out segments measuring 5 mm each were removed from each deformed rib to optimally affect the depression of the chest wall. A chest binder is then worn postoperatively for up to 1 yr.[7]

POSTOPERATIVE MANAGEMENT

The patient undergoes a thoracic epidural in the operating room at the time of the surgical case and this provides adequate postoperative pain control along with supplemental oral and intravenous medication. Stool softeners are initiated early. The patient is admitted to a routine ward bed, restricted to bed rest on the first day along with no lying on their side or rolling. The patient is up in a chair on postoperative day 1 and consultation with respiratory therapy for incentive spirometry and physical therapy for postoperative activity guideline education is initiated. The typical length of a hospital stay is 4 days.

COMPLICATIONS/FOLLOW-UP

Complications are infrequent but include infection, bleeding, pneumothorax, pneumonia, wound related concerns. Blood transfusion is rare. Results are overwhelmingly successful and recurrence is rare. If reoperation is necessary, it is typically related to a repair of the deformity occurring at an early age prior to complete development.

REFERENCES

1. Shamberger RC, Welch KJ. (1987) Surgical correction of pectus carinatum. *J Pediatr Surg* **22**:48–53.
2. Shamberger RC. (2006) Congenital chest wall deformities. In: JL Grosfeld, JA O'Neill, EW Fonkalsrud, AG Coran (eds.), *Pediatric Surgery*, 6th edition, pp. 894–930. Mosby-Elsevier, Philadelphia.
3. Haje SA, Bowen JR. (1992) Preliminary results of orthotics treatment of pectus deformities in children and adolescents. *J Pediatr Orthop* **12**(6):795–800.
4. Kravarusic D, Dicken BJ, Dewar R, *et al.* (2006) The calgary protocol for bracing of pectus carinatum: A preliminary report. *J Pediatr Surg* **41**:923–926.
5. Fonkalsrud EW. (2009) 912 open pectus excavatum repairs: Changing trends, lessons learned: One surgeon's experience. *World J Surg* **33**:180–190.
6. Hock A. (2009) Minimal access treatment of pectus carinatum: A preliminary report. *Pediatr Surg Int* **25**:337–342.
7. Kim S, Idowu O. (2009) Minimally invasive thoracoscopic repair of unilateral pectus carinatum. *J Pediatr Surg* **44**:471–474.

Chest Wall Anomalies

POLAND SYNDROME 44

Scott A. Engum

CLINICAL PRESENTATION

The anterior chest wall functions to protect the intrathoracic viscera and upper abdominal organs. In addition, the semi rigid chest wall maintains a relative negative pressure for inspiration and positive pressure for expiration. Lastly, the chest wall provides a base for upper limb movement. A variant of the pectus abnormalities, there is a combination of the absence of pectoralis major and minor muscles, ipsilateral breast hypoplasia, and absence of the segments of two to four ribs (generally some combination of the second to fifth, the second being least frequently involved). This is a diverse disease process that can include ipsilateral hand (webbing of the fingers), and arm abnormalities (shortening — brachysymphalangism) in many cases.[1]

Prenatal ultrasound diagnosis is possible by identification of severe hypomelia, ipsilateral chest wall asymmetry, and thoracic hemivertebra. Due to its variability in presentation, Poland's syndrome may remain undiagnosed at birth.[2]

Clinical presentation depends on the extent of tissue involvement and the number of associated conditions. Many children may be found to have minimal bone/cartilage deformity requiring no surgical intervention, while the rare patient will show diffuse hypoplasia of the chest wall that may not have a surgical option. Most patients fall between these extremes and are noted to have localized excavatum deformities (commonly on the right), with or without a contralateral carinatum and buckling of the parasternal cartilages. The costosternal pectoralis major is always absent with the pectoralis minor missing or hypoplastic in 75%.[1] It is common to have thinner soft tissue coverage over the affected area in addition to a hypoplastic nipple that may be situated higher on the chest wall. There can be associated alopecia of the anterior chest wall or axilla and infrequently, regional muscular involvement noted in either hypoplastic or absent serratus (Sprengel's deformity — winging of the scapula from deficiency), latissimus dorsi, or trapezius muscles.[3,4]

Breast development typically lags behind the contralateral chest wall and commonly is smaller and higher than the normal side. Cardiopulmonary compromise is infrequent and dextroposition without other intracardiac lesions predominates. Lung herniation can occur in up to 8% of patients and may warrant early intervention, however, endothoracic *fascia* is described as a tough and resilient layer capable of restraining the lung and providing enough support for later surgery.[5,6]

Limb anomalies are present in most cases and involve ipsilateral syndactyly involving the middle 3 fingers. There is no correlation between the severity of chest wall and hand anomalies.[1]

Other deformities can include craniofacial abnormalities, thoracic tumors, scoliosis, hypoplasia of the rib cage and lungs, upper extremity hypoplasia, breast and nipple hypoplasia, and deficiencies of the skin, subcutaneous tissues, sweat glands, hair of affected areas and involvement of adjacent muscles such as the serratus, latissimus dorsi, and the external oblique. The most commonly associated syndromes are Mobius (bilateral or unilateral facial nerve palsy combined with ocular abductor palsy) and Klippel–Feil (cervical vertebral and brain stem abnormalities). Malignancies are also noted and particularly leukemia or lymphoma. Other disorders include renal agenesis, ureteral reflux, Adams–Oliver syndrome, Parry–Romberg syndrome, and congenital hemangioma.[7–11]

PATHOPHYSIOLOGY

Incidence

An accurate incidence of the disease is unknown; however, data suggest that Poland's syndrome occurs in approximately one in every 30,000 to 100,000 live births.[1] Men are affected three times as often as women, with right-sided deformities twice as common. Unfortunately, there are likely an increased number of males with unequal chest growth typically not seeking evaluation and treatment. Patients with milder disease process may go undetected until late in adolescence and into puberty when chest wall or breast growth asymmetry is noticed, especially by the female patient.

Pathology

Lallemand in 1826 is credited as the first to describe an absence of the pectoralis muscle alone and in 1835, Bell was the first to record the condition. Froriep in 1839 described a woman with the paired absence of the pectoralis and ipsilateral syndactyly and this was substantiated with a description of the same condition by Poland in 1841. The most accurate understanding of the clinical manifestation occurred with Thomson's work in 1895.[12] Furst in 1900 thoroughly described a cadaver dissection and proposed that the two groups of malformations of the chest and hand are so often present together, that they must be a syndrome. Bing in 1902 presented 14 cases of a 102 patients he had collected with pectoral absence. Brown and McDowell documented the first review of the syndrome in 1940, followed by Clarkson proposing the name "Poland's syndactyly" for the syndrome in 1962.[13] The use of eponyms in medicine has been questioned to classify diseases as it is not uncommon to credit one person for the achievements of many as described in Poland's syndrome. However, the eponym may serve as a value in grouping together a number of related symptoms and signs under one common name.[14]

The etiology of Poland's syndrome remains unknown. There are three mechanisms of pathogenesis that have been described. One theory relates to genetic inheritance, and there has been sporadic and familial occurrence, however, twin studies have shown no strong genetic corollary and no abnormalities in any chromosome. The phenotypic mosaicism results from a postulated lethal mutation of an upper limb bud cell line and the extent of the deformity in such a mosaic depends ton the timing of cell death. Early mutations could explain a severe chest wall and limb anomaly, whereas a late mutation may produce more localized defects.[15]

The second source relates to teratogenic effects of environmental factors. Limited studies have shown a two-fold risk of developing Poland's syndrome in children whose mothers smoked during pregnancy; however, there is little follow-up work. Prenatal administration of misoprostol and cocaine abuse has also been implicated.[16]

A more common theory focuses on vascular compromise during embryogenesis. It is thought that a mesodermal change (growth of ribs drive the subclavian artery into a defective configuration resulting in the artery becoming hypoplastic) resulting in injury, thrombosis, or embolus to the subclavian artery during the sixth or seventh week of development and results in a cascade of developmental alterations and is referred to as subclavian artery supply disruption sequence. Any early fetal low flow state could alter development of the limb bud and explain the anomalies. The malformation that ensues is dependent on the degree of arterial occlusion/low flow and location of involvement (more proximal the occlusion, the more severe).[16,17]

DIAGNOSIS

Physical examination is the hallmark for initial diagnosis of this disorder. Documenting a full examination of the affected extremity as well as the implications of a muscle transfer is important. In addition, a Computed Tomography (CT) scan of the chest wall has proven helpful in assessing the configuration for reconstruction. Preoperative identification of clinically important vascular supply to proposed muscle flaps whether by CT or Magnetic Resonance Imaging (MRI) three dimensional (3D reconstruction) are critical for surgical planning because a myocutaneous flap that is being considered may have some component of hypoplasia and could contribute to postoperative graft failure.

SURGICAL MANAGEMENT

Surgical correction began in the mid-20th century and was dominated by Mark Ravitch's experience and reviews.[5] He was the first to report successful correction of the chest wall component in 1952.

The ideal procedure is done as a single stage with an individualized approach, which combines thoracic and plastic surgical expertise after the patients growth spurt. Early intervention in the young are discouraged as this may lead to similar reductions in anterior chest wall growth as noted in the classic Ravitch procedure unless significant skeletal involvement compromises pulmonary or cardiac function. Early repair for protection of mediastinal structures is occasionally needed with the surgical technique concentrating on improving the chest wall support while leaving the soft tissue reconstruction for a second stage later. In these cases, a 2-stage approach is appropriate.

Delayed surgery allows for detailed tissue assessment, contralateral matching, and prevention of recurrence. Surgical reconstruction is indicated for patients with significant deformities of the chest wall and the overlying soft tissue, inadequate protection of the mediatstinum, paradoxical movement of the chest wall, aplasia/hypoplasia of the breast in females, and a cosmetic defect. In most cases, the chest wall defect will not affect ventilation and single lung ventilation of the contralateral side can be contemplated to reduce the risk of lung injury during chest wall defect repair.

In shallow defects, an implant or muscle flap can be placed directly over the defect. This can be done through small incisions or an endoscopic approach. In some cases, customized tissue implants for localized defects can be developed and placed in the patient with the understanding that the implant may need adjustment in the future.

The goal of the deep defect is to provide a stable base to place an autologous tissue transfer (rib graft, or pedicle/free musculocutaneous muscle flap) or a form of implant. Severe chest wall hypoplasia or agenesis is repaired with synthetic mesh, rib grafting, sternal osteotomy, or contralateral cartilage resection when a carinatum deformity is present.[1,6] Prosthetic mesh overlay with or without rib and cartilage transfer is recommended as this reduces the risk of recurrence while still providing a stable base for any implants. Gore-Tex, Prolene, or Marlex meshes are used most often. The prosthetic material is sutured to the edges of the defect and to the sternum. The mesh is put under tension to provide a firm base layer for the implant or muscle. Sternal depression or torsion can be corrected with an osteotomy. When necessary, subperichondrial cartilage resection can be performed. The defect can be bridged by contralateral rib harvest for split rib grafts or splitting the cartilage from the normal upper and lower borders of the defect and rotating the pieces over the ends of the adjacent hypoplastic rib ends. Implants or muscle are placed directly over the defect. The latissimus dorsi is most commonly used as a muscle or musculocutaneous flap. The ipsilateral latissimus dorsi muscle is normal in most cases and provides a reliable source of soft-tissue augmentation of the anterior chest.[18–20]

Reconstruction of the female breast deformity remains controversial. Some advocate delaying reconstruction until the breasts are fully mature and then reconstructing with autologous tissue, such as a transverse rectus abdominis muscle flap. Others have advocated insertion of a tissue expander in early adolescence with periodic expansion of the breast throughout puberty allowing for adjustment of breast size to match to opposite breast until sexual maturity. At this time the expander can be removed and replaced with a permanent breast implant.

With the evolution of regenerative medicine, tissue engineering may play a role in the future repair of Poland's syndrome.

POSTOPERATIVE MANAGEMENT/FOLLOW-UP

This is a diverse disorder that affects a small subset of children with chest wall deformities. Diffuse hypoplasia without a correctable depression is problematic. Excellent results may be obtained by localized repair without the need for large scale rib or sternal reconstruction, but understanding the correctable components of the chest wall deformity are critical to allow the patient, family, and surgeon to arrive at appropriate postoperative expectations. Children with extensive disease will require a team approach and complications such as bleeding, infection, and seroma are not uncommon. Recurrence of the defect can occur and are noted more frequently when the disorder was repaired at an earlier age. Reoperation can occur for implant failure or migration, rib graft migration, or muscle flap atrophy. Reports have shown the value of covering an implant with muscle for best results. The concavity below the clavicle created by the hypoplastic muscle can be problematic for females and these self image issues should be considered.

REFERENCES

1. Shamberger RC, Welch KJ, Upton J III. (1989) Surgical treatment of thoracic deformity in Poland's syndrome. *J Pediatr Surg* **24**:760–765.
2. Paladini D, D'Armiento MR, Martinelli P. (2004) Prenatal ultrasound diagnosis of Poland syndrome. *Obstet Gynecol* **104**:1156–1159.
3. Alexander A, Fokin MD, Robicsek F. (2002) Poland's syndrome revisited. *Ann Thorac Surg* **74**:2218–2225.
4. Moir CR, Johnson CH. (2008) Poland's syndrome. *Semin Pediatr Surg* **17**:161–166.
5. Ravitch MM. (1977) Poland's syndrome. In: MM Ravitch (ed.), *Congenital Deformities of the Chest Wall and their Operative Correction*, pp. 233–271. WB Saunders, Philadelphia, PA.

6. Haller JA, Jr, Colombani PM, Miller D, *et al.* (1984) Early reconstruction of Poland's syndrome using autologous rib grafts combined with latissimus muscle flap. *J Pediatr Surg* **19**:423–429.
7. Kuklik M. (2000) Poland–Mobius syndrome and disruption spectrum affecting the face and extremities: A review paper and presentation of five cases. *Acta Chir Plast* **42**:95–103.
8. Erol M, Caksen H, Tan O, *et al.* (2004) Report of a girl with Klippel–Feil syndrome and Pland anomaly. *Genet Couns* **15**(4):469–472.
9. Ahn MI, Park SH, Park YH. (2004) Poland's syndrome with lung cancer. *Acta Radiol* **41**(5):32–34.
10. Francken GA, Monette RJ, Czarnecki DJ, *et al.* (1992) Localized large benign fibroma of the pleura in Poland's syndrome. *AJR Am J Roentgenol* **159**(2): 428–429.
11. Athale UH, Warrier R. (1998) Poland's syndrome and Wilms tumor; an unusual association. *Med Pediatr Oncol* **30**(1):67–68.
12. Thomson J. (1895) On a form of congenital thoracic deformity. *Teratologia* **2**:1–12.
13. Clarkson P. (1962) Poland's syndactyly. *Guy's Hosp Rep* **111**:335–346.
14. Ram AN, Chung KC. (2009) Poland's syndrome: Current thoughts in the setting of a controversy. *Plastic Reconstr Surg* **123**(3):949–953.
15. Farina D, Gatto G, Leonessa L, *et al.* (1999) Poland syndrome: A case with a combination of syndromes. *Paminerva Med* **41**:259–260.
16. Martinez-Frias ML, Czeizel AE, Rodriguez-Pinilla E, *et al.* (1999) Smoking during pregnancy and Poland sequence: Results of a population-based registry and a case-conrol registry. *Teratology* **59**:35–38.
17. Poland's syndrome. National Institutes of Health-National Human Genome Research Insitute. Available at http://www.genome.gov/14514230.
18. Marks MM, Argenta LC, Izenberg PH, *et al.* (1991) Management of the chest-wall deformity in male patients with Poland's syndrome. *Plast Reconstr Surg* **87**(4):674–678.
19. Seyfer AE, Icochea R, Greaber GM. (1988) Poland's anomaly: Natural history and long-term results of chest wall reconstruction in 33 patients. *Ann Surg* **208**(6):776–782.
20. Urschel HC, Jr. (2000) Poland's syndrome. *Chest Surg Clin North Am* **10**(2): 393–403.

JEUNE'S SYNDROME 45

Scott A. Engum

CLINICAL PRESENTATION

Newborns present with a small, narrow, bell-shaped chest and some degree of respiratory distress varying from negligible to rapidly fatal. The most common and prominent clinical presentation is alveolar hypoventilation caused by impaired chest expansion as a result of short horizontally placed ribs and the resultant lung hypoplasia. Associated skeletal abnormalities that occur include short, stubby extremities with short and wide bones. The clavicles can be in a fixed and elevated position. The pelvis may be small and hypoplastic. Initial cases reported resulted in neonatal deaths, however, today, there are a number of articles illustrating patient survival. Efforts have shown the ability to diagnose and follow fetuses affected by this condition. This does allow for prenatal consultation to occur with pediatric surgical specialists that will be involved in the postnatal care of the infant.[1]

In older children, symptoms can range from minor to severe and occur after an uneventful open pectus excavatum repair at an early age. Most patients continue in the postoperative period asymptomatic and are able to participate in all vigorous physical activities. As they get older they begin to experience shortness of breath with activities, which can progress to "asthma" type symptoms, obstructive sleep apnea, increasing shortness of breath at rest, orthopnea, complete intolerance of exercise, and recurrent pneumonias. In their teenage years, they can become bedridden, may be placed on continuous oxygen and unable to participate in school. In spite of vigorous medical management, most patients' clinical status and pulmonary function studies deteriorate. Pulmonary function testing typically reveals forced vital capacity (FVC) of only 30% to 50% and forced expiratory volume in 1 second (FEV1) to be 30% to 60% of predicted values.[2]

PATHOPHYSIOLOGY

Incidence

Otherwise known as asphyxiating thoracic dystrophy, the frequency of this condition is approximately 1 per 100,000 to 130,000 live births for the congenital variety and there is no data reported for the acquired conditions.[3]

Classification

This form of osteochondrodystrophy can be classified as congenital, occurring at birth or an acquired condition following an open (Ravitch) pectus excavatum repair at an early age.

Pathology

Jeune's syndrome in the neonate was described in 1954 and is inherited in an autosomal recessive pattern and is not associated with chromosomal abnormalities.[4,5] This syndrome has variable expression and extent of pulmonary impairment. The chest is narrow in the transverse and sagittal axes which create horizontal ribs that are short and wide with splayed costochondral junctions and little respiratory motion. Microscopic evaluation of the cartilage reveals disordered and poorly progressing endochondral ossification that leads to shortened rib length. Pathologic assessment show normal bronchial development with fewer alveolar divisions.

In 1996, Haller described a group of children who had previously undergone repair of pectus excavatum chest wall deformities utilizing the traditional "open" Ravitch-type approach with subperichondrial resection of deformed cartilages and a transverse sternal osteotomy. The development of restrictive lung disease is unusual after pectus excavatum repair, however in some patients there is a disruption of the normal growth centers of the affected ribs when too aggressive a resection has been performed at too early an age (typically 4 yrs or younger).[2] Unfortunately, an early aggressive approach to pectus excavatum (surgical repair prior to 7 yrs of age) was advocated in the 1970s and 1980s.[6] The mechanical cause of the restrictive pulmonary process is poor growth of the bony thorax combined with increased rigidity of the chest wall limiting air flow characteristics with subsequent decrease in vital capacity.

DIAGNOSIS

Initial physical exam will illustrate the clinical findings previously discussed and an anteroposterior chest radiograph will illustrate the short horizontal ribs and narrow chest. A lateral radiography demonstrates the short rib ends at the midaxillary line and abnormal flaring at the costochondral junction. A Computed Tomography (CT) scan of the thorax, with three-dimensional (3D) reconstruction can better characterize the patient and allow for improved preoperative planning. This study not only shows the severe narrowing of the bony thorax, but the marked reduction in the volume of the lungs. Pulmonary function studies can be completed and will demonstrate a severe restrictive pulmonary disorder.

SURGICAL MANAGEMENT

A number of techniques have been described with the basic goal to expand the thoracic volume and allow for improved lung expansion which then increases the efficiency of the work of breathing and allows the generation of a higher negative intrathoracic pressure. Most approaches involve a median sternotomy with graft interposition (synthetic or autologous) to keep the two sternal halves apart. This in turn increases the chest wall circumference and subsequent lung expansion. Staged procedures may be required with progressive chest wall expansion to match the growth of the child.[3]

Davis utilized a lateral thoracic expansion technique where ribs and underlying tissue is divided in a staggered fashion, and then placed the ribs in fixation with titanium plates, to allow for gradual chest enlargement. This author has documented rib healing and periosteal new bone formation as early as 3 wks postoperatively.[7,8]

Campbell describes a vertical expandable titanium rib (VEPTR) procedure. Vertically oriented titanium struts are attached to ribs and/or transverse processes of the spine and progressively lengthened with a series of procedures to allow progressive expansion of the chest cavity.[9]

Treatment of acquired asphyxiating thoracic dystrophy following a pectus repair remains controversial. Minor abnormalities in pulmonary function probably do not need to be treated unless progression to more severe or debilitating symptoms occurs. Some surgeons perform a redo "open" type of procedure. This redo procedure is modified as Haller described with the placement of an anteriorly angled modified Rehbein splint to maintain sternal elevation and rib distraction.[2] Others have performed a sternal elevation procedure with mild improvement in pulmonary function and higher level of technical difficulties.

Weber and colleague utilized a modified median sternotomy approach with interposition of multiple rib grafts, lateral osteotomy of the ribs (2–6 bilaterally), opening of the pleura, and wedging of the sternum in a permanently opened position (4–8 cm).[10]

POSTOPERATIVE MANAGEMENT/FOLLOW-UP

Many surgeons will never have the opportunity to care for a congenital variety of Jeune's syndrome. It is not uncommon to remain intubated postoperatively for several days and standard methods of care are instituted as described with anterior chest wall deformity therapy. Three-dimensional imaging studies can be performed postoperatively to document increases in chest volume. Despite improvements in perioperative and postnatal care, many of these infants will eventually die of their disease.

In the acquired variety, close monitoring of the postoperative pectus excavatum patient may show more individuals affected by this process than is reported. Following surgery, one would hope that there would be improvement in oxygen use and subsequent weaning with the patient having the ability to return to school and begin an exercise program. Long-term follow-up of functional outcome of most patients remains unreported. This condition has not been described as a complication of the Nuss procedure (minimally invasive repair of pectus excavatum), even when the Nuss repair was performed on younger children.

REFERENCES

1. Chen CP, Lin SP, Liu FF, *et al.* (1996) Prenatal diagnosis of asphixiating thoracic dysplasia (Jeune syndrome). *Am J Perinatol* **13**(8):495–498.

2. Haller JA, Colombani PM, Humphries CT, *et al.* (1996) Chest wall constriction after too extensive and too early operations for pectus excavatum. *Ann Thorac Surg* **61**:1618–1625.
3. Phillips JD, van Aalst JA. (2008) Jeune's syndrome (asphyxiating thoracic dystrophy): Congenital and acquired. *Semin Pediatr Surg* **17**:167–172.
4. Jeune M, Beraud C, Carron R. (1955) Asphyxiating thoracic dystrophy with familial characteristics. *Arch Fr Pediatr* **12**(8):886–891.
5. Morgan NV, Bacchelli C, Gissen P, *et al.* (2003) A locus for asphyxiating thoracic dystrophy, ATD, maps to chromosome 15q13. *J Med Genet* **40**(6):431–435.
6. Haller JA, Jr, Scherer LR, Turner CS, *et al.* (1989) Evolving managment of pectus excavatum based on a single institutional experience of 664 patients. *Ann Surg* **209**(5):578–583.
7. Davis JT, Ruberg RL, Leppink DM, *et al.* (1995) Lateral thoracic expansion for Jeune's asphyxiating dystrophy: A new approach. *Ann Thorac Surg* **60**(3):694–696.
8. Davis JT, Long FR, Adler BH, *et al.* (2004) Lateral thoracic expansion for Jeune syndrome: Evidence of rib healing and new bone formation. *Ann Thorac Surg* **77**(2):445–448.
9. Campbell RM, Jr, Smith MD, Mayes TC, *et al.* (2004) The effect of opening wedge thoracostomy on thoracic insufficiency syndrome associated with fused ribs and congenital scoliosis. *J Bone Joint Surg* **86**-A(8):1659–1674.
10. Weber TR, Kurkchubasche AG. (1998) Operative management of asphyxiating thoracic dystrophy after pectus repair. *J Pediatr Surg* **33**:262–265.

Section 7:
Abdomen

PRENATAL CONSIDERATIONS — ABDOMINAL WALL DEFECTS

46

Cynthia Gingalewski

INTRODUCTION

Abdominal wall defects in newborns are common. With advances in prenatal screening, the majority of abdominal wall defects are identified prior to birth, such that appropriate parental prenatal counseling about perinatal expectations can be performed. Omphalocele and gastroschisis comprise the spectrum of congenital body wall defects and occur in 4–5 per 10,000 live births. Although in the same category of defects, their pathophysiology and outcomes are very different. The etiologic factors contributing to the development of gastroschisis and omphalocele are unknown; however, environmental factors and a young maternal age are thought to play a large role in the development of gastroschisis, while advance maternal age and genetic factors have more of a role in the development of an omphalocele.[1,2]

OMPHALOCELE

Etiology

The body wall defect of omphalocele consists of a midline defect that allows for the herniation of abdominal viscera into the umbilical cord, resulting in a membrane covered defect. It is thought to occur at 3–4 wks gestation when the cranial, caudal and two lateral embryonic folds normally meet to form the abdominal wall. If the cranial fold is primarily involved then the defect is associated with defects of the lower sternum, diaphragm, and pericardium and is associated with cardiac defects, collectively known as the Pentology of Cantrell. If the defect is primarily with the caudal fold then the omphalocele is associated with a bladder extrophy or cloacal extrophy.

Associated Anomalies

Other anomalies are commonly associated with the omphalocele (30%) and a thorough assessment for other anomalies should be undertaken, that should include a fetal Magnetic Resonance Imaging (MRI). In addition a fetal karyotype should be obtained to evaluate for chromosomal abnormalities. Fetuses with omphalocele are at increased risk for cardiac defects (50%) and should undergo a fetal echocardiogram. The overall survival of infants with omphalocele is largely dependent upon associated anomalies (Table 1). Families need to be counseled extensively about the risk of associated anomalies and their impact on the survival of the fetus. In some circumstances, counseling families about termination of pregnancy is appropriate.

Mode of Delivery

In all circumstances families should be aware that early fetal delivery is not warranted unless there is evidence of fetal distress (abnormal biophysical

Table 1. Associated anomalies with omphalocele. Omphaloceles have a high risk of both chromosomal anomalies (30%) as well as cardiac defects (50%).

Beckwith–Wiedemann syndrome
Trisomies 13, 18, 21
Lethal omphalocele-cleft palate syndrome
Marshall–Smith syndrome
Meckel–Gruber syndrome
Cardiac defects
Cloacal extrophy

profile, intrauterine growth retardation). Maximization of lung development and fetal growth is extremely important.

A distinction needs to be made between an Omphalocele and a giant Omphalocele (>5 cm, containing fetal liver). This not only has an impact upon fetal and infant survival but also on the mode of delivery and the surgeons' ability to close the abdominal wall defect. All giant omphalocele should be delivered by cesarian section.[3] This avoids birth dystocia, sac rupture and liver injury. In smaller omphaloceles, there has not been a prospective randomized controlled clinical trial of vaginal delivery vs. elective cesarian section, thus the mode of delivery is dependent upon the comfort level of the maternal–fetal medicine specialist. Deliveries should be planned and require communication between the maternal–fetal medicine specialists, neonatologists and pediatric surgeons.

Perinatal Plan of Care

Informing families of realistic expectations for the perinatal care of babies with omphaloceles relieves anxieties and allows families to plan for extended care of other children at home. Again, the outcomes and length of stay is very much dependent upon associated anomalies, the presence of a giant omphalocele and the degree of pulmonary insufficiency. Families need to be prepared for long hospitalizations and multiple surgeries. Outcomes for giant omphaloceles can be separated into immediate/short term outcomes and long term outcomes. In a large series of patients from Children's Hospital of Philadelphia, all giant omphaloceles that survived pregnancy required intubation at birth.[4] Two thirds of these infants had respiratory insufficiency requiring prolonged intubation with the average length of time on the ventilator was longer than 2 months. Evaluation of the infants chest at birth for a long, narrow thorax (the so called "dog chest") is a strong indicator of pulmonary hypoplasia (Figure 1). Parents should be counseled for the possibility of prolonged ventilator requirements, and the possibility of a tracheostomy and home ventilation.

Most families are most anxious about the closure of the abdominal wall. Primary closure should be attempted for small omphaloceles (< 3 cm). This facilitates earlier enteral feeding and decreases the risk for sepsis, liver dysfunction and cholestasis. For larger defects and for those patients with multiple anomalies, a delayed closure should be undertaken. The omphalocele sac should be covered (xeroform, sulfasalazine, or Aquacele). Aquacele has

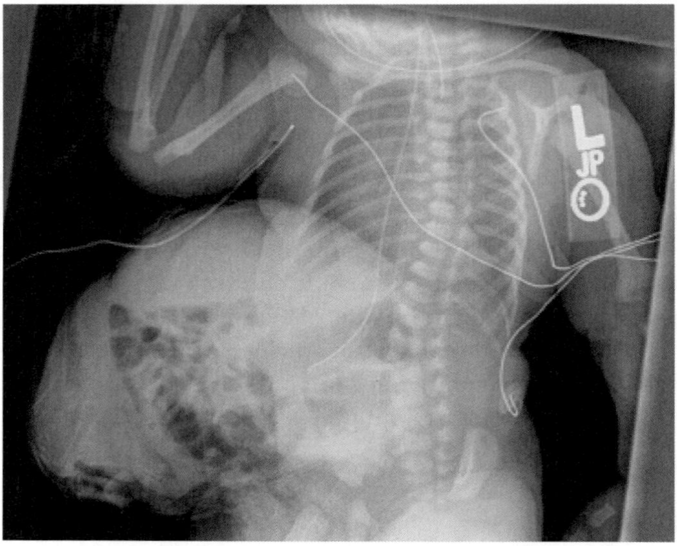

Figure 1. Chest X-ray of infant with giant omphalocele. Classic appearance of the elongated "dog chest" that is indicative of pulmonary hypoplasia with giant omphaloceles.

become standard at our institution because it is easy to apply, absorbs fluids and once adherent does not need to be changed, so it simplifies treatment for the nursing staff and eventually the parents. The amnion sac eventually becomes epithelialized (several weeks to months depending upon the size). Then typically between 1–2 yrs of age a definitive repair is performed.

Long term outcomes from isolated small omphaloceles are good in general. With giant omphaloceles, both gastrointestinal and pulmonary complications are common. These include gastroesophageal reflux disease, oral aversion and failure to thrive. Prenatal counseling should include talking about the possible need for a surgical gastrostomy tube and possible surgical procedures for gastroesophageal reflux disease.[4] Also common occurrences are asthma, recurrent pulmonary infections, and chronic lung disease.

Parents should also be aware of the fact that infants with omphaloceles have malrotation with the risk of midgut volvulus (although rare). In addition, postclosure there is the risk for adhesive small bowel obstructions (13%), the highest risk being within the first year of life.[5]

GASTROSCHISIS

Etiology

Ultrasound diagnosis of gastroschisis can be made after 11 wks of gestation when the intestinal contents have returned into the peritoneal cavity. Gastroschisis can be differentiated sonographically from omphalocele by the lack of a membranous covering. The etiology of the abdominal wall defect which is consistently to the right of the umbilical cord has many theories, but all are speculative. Fetuses with gastroschisis have few associated anomalies (10%), and in contrast to the omphalocele, it is rare to have chromosomal abnormalities. Young maternal age is the only consistent risk factor, in combination to an environmental event. This has included cigarette smoking, cocaine use, water toxins, etc.[6] There have been multiple reports that the incidence of gastroschisis in increasing in both the United States and Europe.

Mode of Delivery

As with omphaloceles, there is no benefit to the fetus with gastroschisis to deliver preterm. Vaginal delivery can safely be performed in most circumstances and delivery at a center with pediatric surgery facilities decreases the risk of morbidity.[7] In a randomized, controlled, clinical trial of elective preterm delivery at 36 wks gestation, there was no differences in length of stay, time on total parenteral nutrition (TPN), incidence of necrotizing enterocolitis (NEC) or sepsis when compared to those infants who delivered when onset of labor occurred.[8,9] It should be stressed to parents that the overall outcomes for infants born with gastroschisis in children's hospitals in the United States is excellent with survival >95%.[10] If delivery by the maternal–fetal medicine specialist is to be at a hospital without pediatric surgical services immediately available, the infant should be warmed, the intestine covered and the infant hydrated while a transfer to a nearby children's hospital is arranged.

Perinatal Plan of Care

The majority of infants with gastroschisis can be considered "simple",[11] that is isolated gastroschisis without evidence of other associated anomalies including intestinal atresia. The remaining 10–15% of newborns have complex gastroschisis and as such can be anticipated to have a significantly longer length of stay and time to full enteral feeds. They are also at higher risk to develop NEC, and short bowel syndrome. The difference in the hospitalizations should be stressed to parents prenatally, especially those with radiographic indicators of intestinal atresia (early dilated intraabdominal intestinal loops).[12,13] But it should also be understood that the presence of dilated bowel loops is not associated with increased risks of adverse perinatal outcomes.[14–17]

Parents should be informed of the various methods of intestinal coverage and abdominal wall closure. Primary closure in the operating room, primary sutureless closure at the bedside, and silo placement should all be discussed and the indications for their use. In general the type of closure has no impact on infant outcome.[18] Multiple clinical reports comparing various techniques have failed to show significant differences in outcomes as measured by length of stay, TPN use, time to enteral feeds, incidence of sepsis, or NEC. However there does tend to be a shorter length of ventilatory support for those infants with a primary sutureless closure and for those who have a temporary silastic silo placed.[19,20]

The average time to full enteral feeds for infants with gastroschisis is 3 wks, but parents should know this is just an average time. This time can be prolonged by the occurrence of line sepsis, NEC, and bowel ischemia. Complex gastroschisis stays are typically longer.

Parents should also be aware of the fact that similar to infants with omphaloceles, all infants with gastroschisis have malrotation and carry a risk of midgut volvulus (although rare). In addition, postclosure there is a greater risk for adhesive small bowel obstructions (25%) the highest risk being within the first year of life.[5]

In general the overall survival is >90% and developmental data suggests normal outcomes.[7]

SUMMARY

Omphalocele and gastroschisis comprise the spectrum of abdominal wall defects. And although they are placed in the same congenital anomaly category, they behave very differently and carry significantly different prognoses. Prenatal counseling of families carrying fetuses with these diagnoses will allow them to make informed decisions about continuing the pregnancy as well as what to realistically expect in the perinatal period and beyond.

REFERENCES

1. Frolov P, Alali J, Klein MD. (2010). Clinical risk factors for gastroschisis and omphalocele in humans: A review of the literature. *Pediatr Surg Int* **26**(12):1135–1148.
2. Mann S, Blinman TA, Wilson D. (2008). Prenatal and postnatal management of Omphalocele. *Prenatal Diag* **28**(7):626–632.
3. Lurie S, Sherman D, Bukovsky L. (1999). Omphalocele delivery enigma: The best mode of delivery still remains dubious. *Eur J Obstet Gyn R B* **82**(1):19–22.
4. Biard JM, Wilson RD, Johnson MP, *et al.* (2004). Prenatally diagnosed giant omphaloceles: short and long-term outcomes. *Prenatal Diag* **24**(6):434–439.
5. VanEijck FC, Wijnen RM, VanGoor H. (2008). The incidence and morbidity of adhesions after treatment of neonates with gastroschisis and omphalocele: A 30 year review. *J Pediatr Surg* **43**(3):479–483.
6. Feldkamp ML, Carey JC, Sadler TW. (2007). Development of gastroschisis: Review of hypotheses, a novel hypothesis, and implications for research. *Am J Med Genet A* **143**:639–652.
7. Holland AJ, Walker K, Badawi N. (2010). Gastroschisis: An update. *Pediatr Surg Int* **26**(9):871–878.
8. Logghe HL, Mason GC, Thornton J, *et al.* (2005). A randomized controlled trial of elective preterm delivery of fetuses with Gastroschisis. *J Pediatr Surg* **40**(11): 1726–1731.
9. Reigstad I, Reigstad H, Kiserud T, *et al.* (2011). Preterm elective caesarean section and early enteral feeding in gastroschisis. *Acta Paediatrica.* **100**(1):71–74.
10. Lao OB, Larison C, Garrison MM, *et al.* (2010). Outcomes in neonates with gastroschisis in US Children's Hospitals. *Am J Perinatology* **27**(1):97–101.
11. Molik KA, Gingalewski CA, West KW, Rescorla FJ, Engum SA, Scherer LR, Grosfeld JL. (2001) Gastroschisis: A Plea for Risk Categorization. *J Pediatr Surg* **36**(1):51–55.
12. Nick AM, Bruner JP, Moses R, *et al.* (2006). Second trimester intra-abdominal bowel dilatation in fetuses with Gastroschisis predicts neonatal bowel atresia. *Ultrasound in Obstetrics and Gynecology* **28**(6):821–825.
13. Huh NG, Hirose S, Goldstein RB. (2010). Prenatal intraabdominal bowel dilatation is associated with postnatal gastrointestinal complications in fetuses with gastroschisis. *Am J Obstetrics and Gynecology* **202**(4):396.e1–396.e6.
14. Tower C, Ong SS, Ewer AK, *et al.* (2009). Prognosis in isolated Gastroschisis with bowel dilation: A systematic review. *Arch of Disease in Childhood Fetal and Neonatal Edition* **94**(4):F268–F274.
15. Mears AL, Sadiq JM, Impey L. (2010). Antenatal bowel dilatation in Gastroschisis: A bad sign? *Pediatr Surg Int* **26**(6):581–588.

16. Alfaraj MA, Ryan G, Langer JC, *et al.* (2011). Does gastric dilation predict adverse perinatal or surgical outcome in fetuses with gastroschisis? *Ultrasound in Obstetrics & Gynecology* **37**(2):202–206.
17. Garcia L, Brizot M, Liao A, *et al.* (2010). Bowel dilation as a predictor of adverse outcome in isolated fetal gastroschisis. *Prenatal Diag* **30**(10):964–969.
18. Machidu M, Takamizawa S, Yoshizawa K. (2008). Umbilical cord inverting technique: a simple method to utilize the umbilical cord as a biologic dressing for sutureless gastroschisis closure. *Pediatr Surg Int* **27**(1):95–97.
19. Pastor AC, Phillips JD, Fenton SJ. (2008). Routine use of a SILASTIC spring loaded silo for infants with Gastroschisis: a multicenter randomized controlled trial. *J Pediatr Surg* **43**(10):1807–1812.
20. Riboh J, Abrajano CT, Garber H. (2009). Outcomes of sutureless gastroschisis closure. *J Pediatr Surg* **44**(10):1947–1951.

Abdominal Wall

GASTROSCHISIS 47

Kim Molik

HISTORY/INTRODUCTION

Once considered lethal, abdominal wall defects now have an excellent survival. Initially thought to be variants of the same process, we now recognize two major types of abdominal wall defects.

Omphalocele is a defect which arises from the umbilicus itself and is contained by a layer of amnion protecting the viscera from *in utero* insult. Gastroschisis is a defect which arises to the right of an otherwise normal umbilicus. The intestines are not enclosed in any membrane and have been exposed to amniotic fluid *in utero,* resulting in a chemical peritonitis. The two defects are easily distinguishable at birth by physical examination as well as by prenatal ultrasound. It is important to make this distinction as the operative management and postoperative care is somewhat different for each of these maladies.

PATHOPHYSIOLOGY

Embryology

Several theories attempting to explain the etiology of gastroschisis have been proposed. None have been proven.

(1) A vascular insult to the abdominal wall resulting in local ischemia and perforation of the abdominal wall.
(2) Premature involution of the right umbilical vein resulting in local abdominal wall weakness and eventual herniation.
(3) Environmental insults including cocaine, smoking, and other vasoactive substances.
(4) Abnormal development of the abdominal wall.

Incidence and Epidemiology

Gastroschisis occurs in 2.5:10,000 births. However, many studies are now documenting an increase in the incidence of gastroschisis throughout the United States. Many recent retrospective studies have linked young maternal age with gastroschisis and many consider maternal age a risk factor. Women less than 20 yrs of age have a 16x greater risk of delivering an infant with gastroschisis than those 30 yrs of age. The average maternal age of those with gastroschisis in this country is 19 yrs old. Some studies also link young paternal age as well. Gastroschisis mainly affects nonhispanic whites while African American and Asian populations less commonly. Other potential risks include primigravida and maternal smoking, but these have not been proven.

Antenatal Care

Two-thirds of infants with gastroschisis are diagnosed *in utero* by ultrasound. The remaining 1/3 most likely did not have prenatal care or routine ultrasound examinations. The second trimester alpha-feto protein may be elevated as well. There is no "treatment" prenatally for gastroschisis. Fetal closure is experimental and although some have recommended amniotic fluid exchanges to prevent bowel inflammation, this has not been proven and is not routinely performed in the United States. Infants with gastroschisis may be delivered by routine vaginal delivery with cesarean section reserved for maternal indications only. Although 19% of infants suffer from intrauterine growth retardation, 80% are born greater than 32 wks gestation. Gastroschisis is usually an isolated defect and other serious congenital anomalies are rare. Commonly infants with gastroschisis may have an associated inguinal hernia or undescended testes.

MANAGEMENT

Postnatal Care

There are several aspects to the care of an infant with gastroschisis:

(1) Airway assessment. Most infants with gastroschisis are born near term and have mature stable airways. However, some premature infants may require endotracheal intubation. Continuous positive airway pressure (CPAP) is not recommended as it may worsen intestinal distension.
(2) Fluid resuscitation. Infants with gastroschisis rapidly lose fluids from the exposed intestine. They require immediate intravenous access and fluid resuscitation to prevent hemodynamic collapse. A foley catheter, although not routine, may be necessary.
(3) Thermal stability. As with fluid loss, infants with gastroschisis also rapidly lose heat from the exposed intestine. They require overhead radiant warmers as well as warmed linens and minimization of unnecessary exposure.
(4) Care of the intestine. After examining the intestine to confirm viability and assessing for other defects, the intestine must be covered (Figure 1). If an immediate repair is planned, simple coverage with

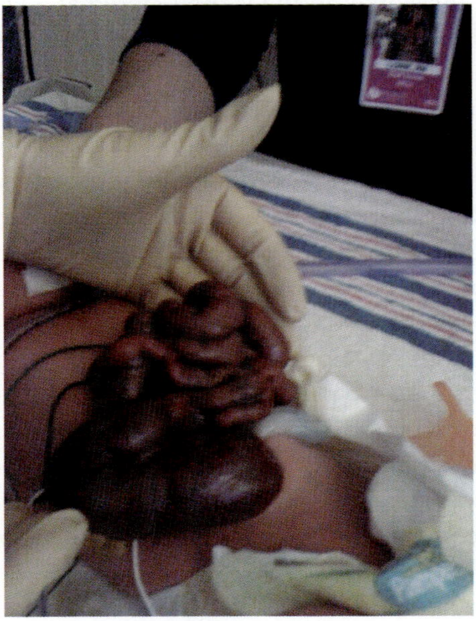

Figure 1. Gastroschisis defect.

warm saline soaked gauze and plastic covers will be sufficient. If a silo is planned, that can usually be performed at the bedside. A nasogastric tube is essential to allow bowel decompression and facilitate closure of the defect.

(5) Infants with gastroschisis must still receive all the usual postnatal treatments including vitamin K and routine eye treatment.

Operative Treatment

There are several options to closing the defect in gastroschisis:

(1) Immediate repair. Several years ago, this was the treatment of choice. It has fallen away in favor of immediate bedside silo placement. After intubation, the infant is taken to the operating room where the bowel is again inspected for additional anomalies, the defect is usually enlarged and the swollen and irritated bowel is placed into the abdominal cavity. The fascial defect may be closed using a variety of techniques. During the fascial closure, the mean airway pressure is monitored to assure no respiratory or ventilatory compromise will result from closing the defect. Occasionally, the *fascia* is unable to be closed and only the skin is reapproximated using permanent suture. The resulting incisional hernia is then closed at a later time.

(2) Silo placement with delayed fascial closure. This is the more popular approach used today. Essentially a silo, either preformed or manually sewn, is placed around the fascial defect. A preformed silo can usually be placed at the bedside without anesthesia (Figure 2). A manually sewn silo usually requires the use of general anesthesia and the operating room. Regardless, once the silo is placed, the contents of the silo are gradually reduced into the abdominal cavity over the course of 3–5 days. Once all the intestines are fully reduced, the infant is taken to the operating room for definitive fascial closure.

(3) Surgical treatment of Complicated Gastroschisis. Approximately 10% of infants with gastroschisis will have a segment of intestine that is either stenotic, ischemic or atretic. This increases the complexity of the repair chosen. There are three options. First is to perform a primary repair. This may be hazardous depending on the condition of the intestine. The second option is to perform a ileostomy with delayed takedown. Of course locating a spot for the ostomy may be difficult and the electrolyte and nutritional complications may make this option

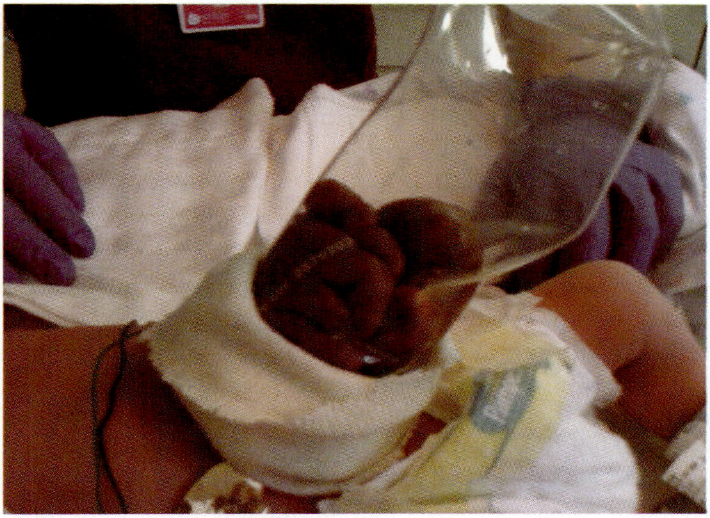

Figure 2. Silo coverage of gastroschisis defect.

unattractive. The last option is to "clip and drop" the segments and plan for delayed anastomosis. During this period however, the child will be completely TPN dependent and require a nasogastric tube for decompression. Not surprisingly, these additional intestinal anomalies add 2–4 wks of hospital stay and may increase the number the number of operative procedures required. These infants who are labeled as "Congenital gastroschisic" account for the majority of the morbidity and mortality associated with gastroschisis.

POSTOPERATIVE CONSIDERATIONS

Postoperative Care

The postoperative care of infants with gastroschisis focuses on the management of bowel function and providing adequate nutrition for healing and growth.

(1) Adynamic ileus. All infants with gastroschisis have a period of adynamic ileus. Many believe the extent of the ileus is related to the amount of intestinal inflammation present at birth. This has never been scientifically proven however. The average time to initiate feeds is 14 days and

the average time to achieve goal feeds is approximately 4 wks. Similar to all bowel surgery, feeds are started when the nasogastric drainage clears and bowel movements begin. Intestinal transit is usually slower than the normal infant and results in the delay to achieving goal feeds. Frequently, feedings are interrupted because of abdominal distension and emesis. Prokinetics and rectal suppositories are frequently used and may be temporarily helpful. Once feedings are initiated, breast milk may be used if available. Otherwise, "standard" formulas are tried. Occasionally, an infant may require a soy formula. However, elemental formulas are not usually necessary.

(2) Parenteral Nutrition. Parental nutrition is essential to the care of an infant with gastroschisis. Because the period of adynamic ileus may extend up to 6 wks in complicated cases, adequate calorie intake cannot be overemphasized. Hyperalimentation may be administered by either a surgically placed central catheter or by a percutaneous peripherally inserted central line. Peripheral intravenous lines do not allow for the high amount of dextrose and triglycerides required. However, central line infections do occur and can add to the hospital stay and occasionally the morbidity. They must be treated aggressively and may require removal or replacement of the catheter.

Long Term Outcomes

Overall survival is 91%. Those infants that do not survive usually succumb to infectious complications of long term parenteral nutrition. Short bowel syndrome does occur in infants with gastroschisis and requires long term follow up. For those seriously affected, an intestinal or multivisceral transplant may be considered. Necrotizing enterocolitis can occur but not commonly. The risk of adhesive bowel obstruction is similar to those who undergo laparotomy for other conditions. Infants with gastroschisis do have anatomical nonrotation of the intestine; however, midgut volvulus is uncommon. Parents may be counseled that the appendix is not in the usual location and that appendicitis may need to be diagnosed with Computed Tomography (CT) imaging. Otherwise, longterm developmental, cognitive, and nutritional outcomes are excellent.

REFERENCES

1. Klein MD. (2006) Congenital defects of the abdominal wall. In: JL Grosfeld, JA O'Neill, EW Fonkalsrud, AG Coran (eds.), *Pediatric Surgery*, 6th edition. Mosby Elsevier, Philadelphia, PA.
2. Vu LT, Nobuhara KK, Laurent C, *et al.* (2008) Increasing prevalence of gastroschisis: population-based study in California. *J Ped* **152**(6):807–811.
3. Henrich K, Huemmer HP, Reingruber B, *et al.* (2008) Gastroschisis and omphalocele: Treatments and long-term outcomes. *Ped Surg Int* **24**(2):167–173.
4. Skandalakis J, Gray SQW, Ricketts R. (1972) The anterior abdominal wall. In: J Skandalakis (ed.), *Embryology for Surgeons*, 2nd edition, pp. 540–593. Williams & Wilkins, Baltimore.
5. Feldkamp ML, Carey JC, Sadler TW. (2007) Development of gastroschisis: Review of hypotheses, a novel hypothesis, and implications for research. *Am J Med Genet A* **143**(7):639–652.

OMPHALOCELE 48

David J. Hobbs and Marc G. Schlatter

INTRODUCTION

Omphaloceles are congenital abdominal wall defects containing variable abounts of herniated abdominal viscera. The clinical presentation of infants born with this condition depends greatly upon the size of the defect and the presence of other congenital anomalies which can pose significant challenges to those caring for them. This chapter highlights the presentation, management, and outcomes of infants born with omphaloceles.

CLINICAL PRESENTATION

The midline abdominal wall omphalocele defect is characterized by a translucent membranous sac composed of amnion and peritoneum separated by Wharton's jelly (Figure 1). The umbilical cord inserts into this membranous sac. The defect can be centered in the upper, mid, or lower abdomen and ranges in size from 4 cm up to very large to defects that extend to the costalchondral margins. The abdominal wall muscles are essentially intact but displaced laterally. Infants with large omphaloceles often have concomitant pulmonary hypoplasia and may experience respiratory distress shortly after birth or following attempts at visceral reduction. The size and location of the defect as well as the presence of respiratory failure have important implications for management.

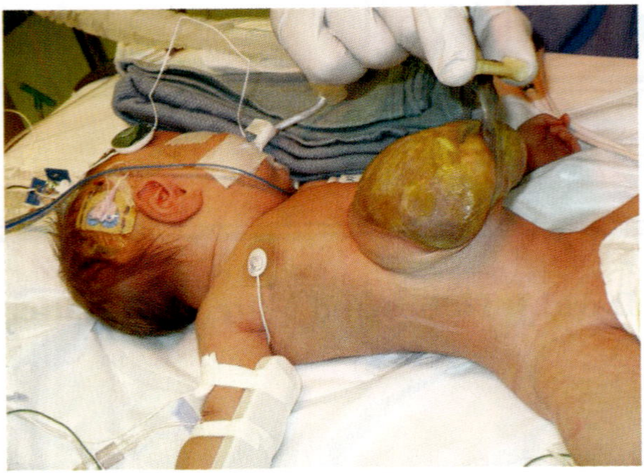

Figure 1. Newborn infant with omphalocele.

PATHOPHYSIOLOGY

Incidence

Omphalocele is among the most common congenital abdominal wall defects. The incidence of omphalocele is approximately 2/10,000 live births with a slight male predominance. The true incidence may even be higher due to underreporting of stillbirths and voluntary terminations of pregnancy with sonographic evidence of abdominal wall defects.

Classification

Central abdominal wall fascial defects larger than 4 cm are considered omphaloceles and typically contain multiple loops of intestine, variable amounts of liver or spleen, and possibly the gonads. Large defects that extend to the costalchondral margins are known as *giant omphaloceles* (Figure 2). Smaller defects (less than 4 cm) are often referred to as *umbilical cord hernias.*

Embryology

Although no specific etiology has been identified for omphaloceles in humans, there are two prevailing embryologic explanations to support the

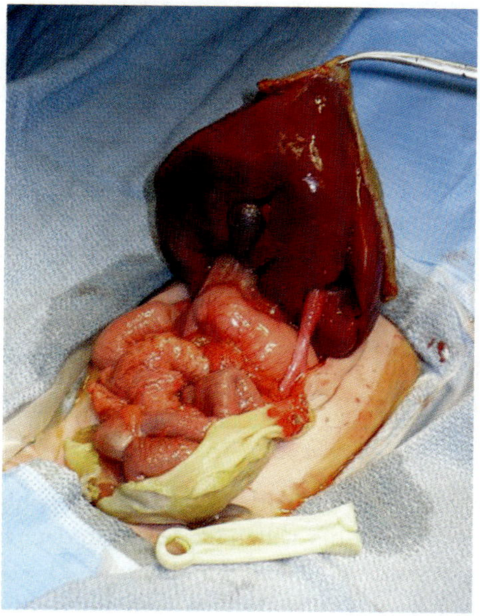

Figure 2. Giant omphalocele with extensive multivisceral herniation.

formation of this congenital anomaly. The first explanation suggests that the developing midgut undergoes rapid cellular proliferation around the 4th to 5th weeks of gestation at a faster pace than the growth of the abdominal wall leading to a physiologic herniation of the viscera into the umbilical cord. Failure of the viscera to retract back into the abdominal cavity by 12 wks of gestation is thought to result in an omphalocele. The second explanation suggests that failure of lateral mesoderm ingrowth around 4 to 7 wks of gestation may give rise to omphalocele.

Associated Conditions

Omphalocele can be associated with a number of chromosomal abnormalities and conditions in 50% to 70% of cases.

As many as 45% of patients with omphalocele will have concomitant congenital heart disease (ventricular and atrial septal defects, ectopia

Table 1. Conditions associated with omphalocele.

(1)	Cardiac disease: ventricular and atrial septal defects, ectopia cordis
(2)	Chromosomal abnormality
(3)	Beckwith–Wiedemann syndrome: macroglossia, organomegaly, hypoglycemia
(4)	Down's syndrome
(5)	Musculoskeletal
(6)	Neural tube defects
(7)	Pentalogy of Cantrell: omphalocele, diaphragmatic hernia, sternal cleft, ectopia cordis, cardiac defect
(8)	OEIS: omphalocele, exstrophy, imperforate anus, spinal defects
(9)	Gastroesophageal reflux
(10)	Cryptorchidism

cordis, coarcation of the aorta) with progression to pulmonary hypertension,[1] and 10–40% of patients will have associated chromosomal abnormalities including trisomies 12, 13, 15, 18, and 21 (Down syndrome).[1] Musculoskeletal and neural tube defects, and Beckwith–Wiedemann syndrome (macroglossia, organomegaly, hypoglycemia) have also been associated with omphalocele.[1,2] Small omphalocele size may correlate with fewer cardiac anomalies but an increased prevalence of gastrointestinal anomalies.[3]

DIAGNOSIS

Prenatal Ultrasound

The diagnosis of omphalocele cannot be conclusively determined in the first trimester, since the resolution of the physiologic herniation occurs at or around 12 wks gestation. If an abdominal wall defect is detected antenatally, a follow-up examination should be performed to identify which viscera are present in the sac, the relationship between the umbilical cord and the defect, and the presence of growth retardation. In a report from 19 European antenatal registries,[4] the sensitivity of antenatal ultrasound examination in detecting omphalocele was 75% with a mean gestational age at first detection of 18 +/– 6 wks gestation.

Diagnostic Tests

Prenatal screening by maternal serum alpha fetoprotein (AFP) testing in combination with ultrasound in the second trimester will identify the majority of omphaloceles. Serum AFP may be significantly elevated (more than four times greater than normal) in the second-trimester.[5] Elevated amniotic fluid AFP and Acetylcholinesterase (AchE) was found in 20% and 27% of those with omphalocele, respectively.[6]

MANAGEMENT

Preoperative

The prenatal management of omphalocele has been facilitated by advancements in prenatal diagnoses and the provision of centralized perinatal care composed of a multidisciplinary team of maternal/fetal obstetrical specialists, pediatric surgeons, and neonatologists. Prenatal discussions with families provide them the opportunity to anticipate the potential challenges of postnatal care.

Although variable opinions exist regarding the optimal mode of delivery for infants with omphalocele, available data doesn't provide significant evidence to favor cesarean section over a vaginal approach.[7] The actual mode of delivery is often based upon other obstetric indications and maternal wishes.

Regardless of the mode of delivery, care should be exercised to avoid damage or rupture of the omphalocele sac, which increases the risk of infection, intestinal and/or hepatic injury. Infants with omphaloceles may demonstrate fluid and heat loss, which is offset by the administration of maintenance intravenous fluids via peripheral venous access, preferably in an upper extremity and avoiding the use of the umbilical vessels. The omphalocele sac is best wrapped with a loose, nonadherent covering followed by mildly compressive gauze that wraps around the infant as well in order to provide some stability for the viscera within the sac. Overly moist dressings may accentuate heat losses and also adhere to the sac as they dry out and therefore are best avoided. A nasogastric tube should be placed to keep the intestines decompressed. There is little urgency to the closure of omphalocele. A judicious delay to closure will allow for appropriate preliminary management, clinical stabilization, and thoughtful planning,

Table 2. Initial management and evaluation.

(1) Assess respiratory status; intubate if necessary
(2) Obtain peripheral venous access (avoid umbilical vessels)
(3) Assess size and content of omphalocele sac
(4) Place nasogastric tube (NG) tube to low intermittent suction
(5) Gently wrap with nonadherent gauze followed by supportive gauze
(6) Echocardiography

taking into account several considerations including the size and severity of the defect, as well as the presence of associated pulmonary, cardiac, and/or suspected chromosomal abnormalities (Table 2).

Cardiac defects are common and echocardiography with cardiology consultation is indicated, especially prior to surgery. Those with larger defects often have some degree of pulmonary hypoplasia with a predisposition to right-to-left shunting due to hyperactivity of smooth muscle cells within the pulmonary vasculature.[8] Early respiratory compromise may necessitate immediate intubation with conventional and/or high frequency ventilation. Further compromise of the infant's respiratory status may require the administration of nitric oxide to reduce pulmonary pressures, and possibly extracorporeal membrane oxygenation support (ECMO).

Infants with omphalocele and Beckwith–Wiedemann syndrome may require additional attention to careful glucose management as a result of a relative hyperinsulinemic state from their organomegaly. Incidentally, infants with Beckwith–Wiedemann syndrome have a higher incidence of developing malignancies (i.e. Wilms' tumor and hepatoblastoma) within the first 2 yrs of life and will require follow-up screening following the initial successful management of the omphalocele.

Surgical Considerations

The goal of surgical management is two fold; to return the viscera to the abdominal cavity and to close the fascial and skin defect if possible. A diminished abdominal domain resulting from herniated viscera during development predisposes these patients to an abdominal compartment syndrome, especially with reduction of the viscera that is too forceful or vigorous. In this condition, high intraabdominal pressures cause further respiratory compromise (high peak pressures, elevated CO_2), diminished blood flow to viscera and kidneys (oliguria, acidosis), and reduced venous return (hypotension). This process can be self-perpetuating and may worsen until release of the abdominal pressure. This complication may be averted by the decision to carry out the goals of surgical management (reduction of viscera and fascial closure) in stages at different settings.

At the time of operative closure (whether primary, staged, or delayed), the omphalocele sac and abdomen are first prepared with an antiseptic. Excess umbilical cord should be ligated near the omphalocele sac and removed distally. The skin is incised circumferentially around the defect and generous skin flaps are elevated from the fascial layer. The membranous sac is excised and the umbilical vessels and urachus are ligated. Omphalocele sac that is adherent to the liver should remain *in situ* to avoid bleeding. It may be helpful to manually stretch the abdominal wall prior to reduction of the intestines followed by the liver. Primary closure may not be possible and monitoring of either the infant's ventilatory pressures (peak inspiratory pressure less than 25 mm Hg) or intraabdominal pressures (gastric via NG tube or bladder via urinary drainage catheter) may be required especially as fascial sutures are placed and approximated in order to determine whether primary closure is safe. In the event of a tight fascial closure causing high intraabdominal pressures, options to consider may include the placement of abdominal patch (i.e. Gore-tex) sutured to the fascial edges to increase the abdominal domain or placement of the viscera within a prosthetic silo that will allow slow reduction of the abdominal viscera over a period of days to 1-wk. Another option may involve the temporary closure of the skin only, with an anticipated return to the operating room at a much later date to repair the resultant abdominal wall hernia. This later option has been largely replaced by staged reduction and closure with a preformed silo (Figure 3). If primary fascial closure is possible, pediatric surgeons have traditionally approximated both the *fascia* and skin transversely, resulting in a horizontal "bunching" of the abdominal wall. Another alternative has been a transverse fascial closure accompanying a "purse-string" approximation of the skin edges in order to approach a more "normal" appearance of an umbilicus. One of the authors has implemented and successfully utilized a "triangular" variation of fascial closure that is applicable for both primary closure of omphaloceles and gastroschisis defects for the past 15 yrs with excellent results (Figures 4 and 5). The "triangular" fascial closure facilitates a more normal contour of the abdominal wall and appearance of the "neo-umbilicus".

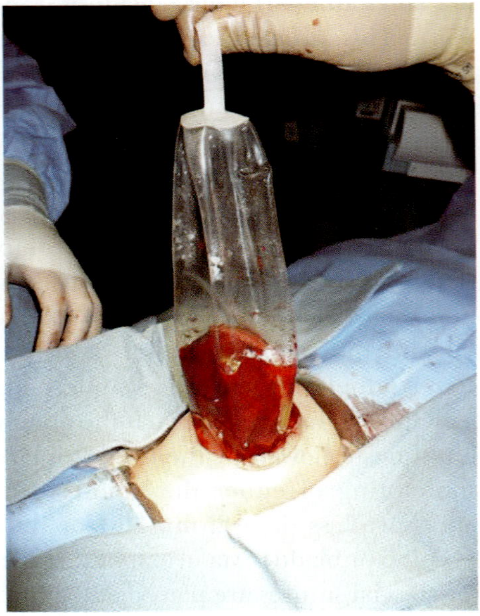

Figure 3. Staged reduction of large omphalocele using preformed silo.

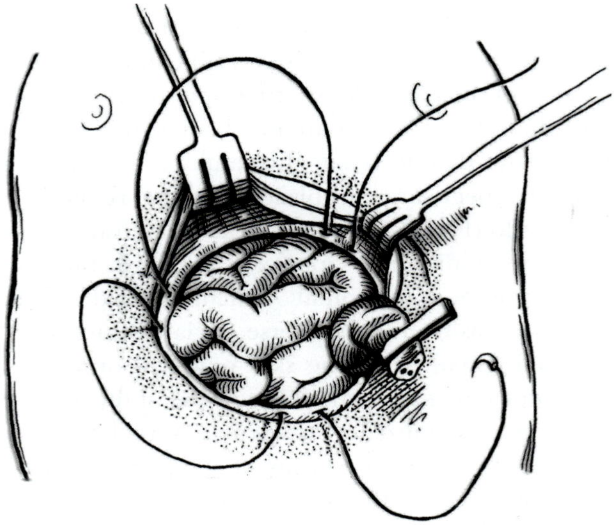

Figure 4. Triangular fascial closure — step 1.

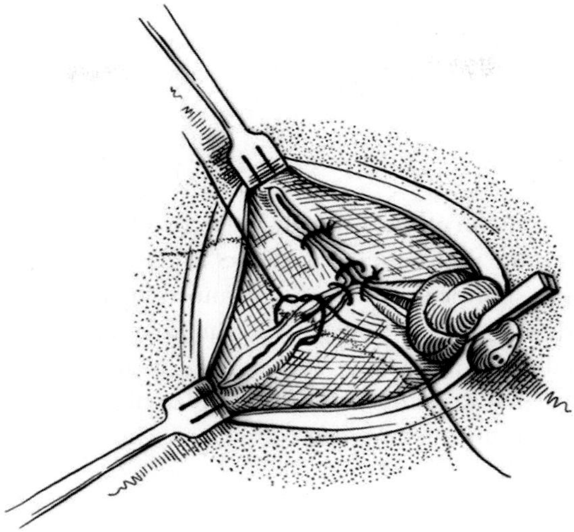

Figure 5. Triangular fascial closure — step 2.

In the event that the patients with large omphaloceles are too clinically unstable for surgical intervention due to significant cardiac, pulmonary, chromosomal co-morbidities, or very large size, the omphalocele sac may be left alone or "painted" with various antimicrobial agents, with either method resulting in the eventual epithelialization of the omphalocele membrane. These infants can then be considered for delayed repair at the 1–2 yrs of life if their other conditions stabilize.

Postoperative Considerations

Immediate postoperative concerns include the development of further respiratory insufficiency and/or abdominal compartment syndrome, especially when primary fascial closure has been accomplished. Besides the pressure related complications that can occur with primary fascial closure, the incidental "kinking" of the hepatic veins from reduction of the liver may contribute to impaired venous return and subsequent metabolic acidosis.

In addition, the abdominal wall should be carefully assessed for the development of ischemia or cellulitis. If unsafe high abdominal pressures are avoided, the patient with primary closure will demonstrate eventual accommodation of the viscera and more normal pressures. Since many patients with omphalocele will have a significant delay in gastrointestinal function, parenteral nutritional support is important.

OUTCOMES

Outcomes of omphalocele are mostly reflective of the associated conditions present, not the abdominal wall defect itself or its repair, although the latter may lead to significant morbidity or mortality if attention is not paid to the risk of developing an abdominal compartment syndrome. Survival rates for omphalocele range from 70% to 95%. Mortality is often related to the associated cardiac and chromosomal abnormalities. Antenatal exteriorized liver and respiratory complications at birth are predictors of adverse outcome with omphalocele.[1,9]

Patients may require late reoperation for repair of an abdominal wall hernia, intestinal atresia, or undescended testicles. Bowel obstruction and recurrent nonspecific or functional abdominal complaints are not uncommon. In the absence of significant co-morbidities, the vast majority of patients may experience good health, and the quality of their educational and social life is comparable to that of the general population.[10,11]

REFERENCES

1. Nicholas SS, Stamilio DM, Dicke JM, Gray DL, Macones GA, Odibo AO. (2009) Predicting adverse neonatal outcomes in fetuses with abdominal wall defects using prenatal risk factors. *Am J Obstet Gynecol* **201**:383.e1–6.
2. Mann S, Blinman TA, Wilson RD. (2008) Prenatal and postnatal management of omphalocele. *Prenat Diag* **28**:626–632.
3. Kumar HR, Jester AL, Ladd AP. (2008) Impact of omphalocele size on associated conditions. *J Pediatr Surg* **43**(12):2216–2219.
4. Vachharajani AJ, Rao R, Keswani S, Mathur AM. (2009) Outcomes of exomphalos: An institutional experience. *Pediatr Surg Int* **25**(2):139–144.
5. Barisic I, Clementi M, Häusler M, Gjergja R, Kern J, Stoll C. (2001) Euroscan Study Group. Evaluation of prenatal ultrasound diagnosis of fetal abdominal wall defects by 19 European registries. *Ultrasound Obstet Gynecol* **18**(4):309–316.
6. Saller DN Jr, Canick JA, Palomaki GE, Knight GJ, Haddow JE. (1994) Second-trimester maternal serum alpha-fetoprotein, unconjugated estriol, and hCG levels in pregnancies with ventral wall defects. *Obstet Gynecol* **84**(5):852–855.

7. Tucker JM, Brumfield CG, Davis RO, Winkler CL, Boots LR, Krassikoff NE, Hauth JC. (1992) Prenatal differentiation of ventral abdominal wall defects. Are amniotic fluid markers useful adjuncts? *J Reprod Med* **37**(5):445–448.
8. Segel SY, Marder SJ, Parry S, Macones GA. (2001) Fetal abdominal wall defects and mode of delivery: A systematic review. *Obstet Gynecol* **98**:867–873.
9. Kamata S, Usui N, Sawai T, Nose K, Fukuzawa M. (2008) Prenatal detection of pulmonary hypoplasia in giant omphalocele. *Pediatr Surg Int* **24**(1):107–111.
10. Biard JM, Wilson RD, Johnson MP, Hedrick HL, Schwarz U, Flake AW, Crombleholme TM, Adzick NS. (2004) Prenatally diagnosed giant omphaloceles: Short- and long-term outcomes. *Prenat Diagn* **24**(6):434–439.
11. Koivusalo A, Lindahl H, Rintala RJ. (2002) Morbidity and quality of life in adult patients with a congenital abdominal wall defect: A questionnaire survey. *J Pediatr Surg* **37**(11):1594–1601.

UMBILICAL HERNIA, URACHAL AND OMPHALOMESENTERIC REMNANTS

49

Nicole Sharp and Danny Little

CLINICAL PRESENTATION

Umbilical anomalies present with a wide array of signs and symptoms generally depending on pathophysiology. Pediatric surgeons and their house officers are often the first to be consulted when there is an unusual umbilicus. Umbilical hernias are usually noted early in life. When prompted, many parents will admit that another family member had an umbilical hernia. Although up to 80% will close spontaneously by 5 yrs of age, many children are still referred for early evaluation. Of note, there are some infants and toddlers who will demonstrate a giant proboscoid hernia during the first 2 yrs of life. These unique cases often prompt early surgical intervention. Children with urachal or omphalomesenteric remnants commonly present with a mass at the umbilicus, drainage, or infection. They may be diagnosed as newborns but late presentation in the childhood years is not uncommon.

EMBRYOLOGY OF THE UMBILICUS

The normal umbilicus is in a midline ventral position at the level of the iliac crests overlying the third and fourth lumbar vertebrae. It is characterized as a depression consisting of the mammelon (umbilical cord remnants) and the cicatrix (intra and extraembryonic coelom). These areas are surrounded by a slightly raised region referred to as the cushion.

Development of the anterior abdominal wall is dependent on differential growth of embryonic tissue. The embryo consists of a dorsally located amnion and a ventrally located yolk sac. The yolk sac is divided into two portions: intracoelomic and extracoelomic. The primitive gut is formed by the intracoelomic portion which communicates with the extracoelomic cavity through the vitelline duct (omphalomesenteric duct). The vitelline duct typically involutes during the seventh or eighth week of gestation. The embryo is attached to the chorion, the precursor to the placenta, by a connecting stalk composed of extraembryonic mesoderm from which the umbilical vessels develop. During the third week of gestation, the allantois develops as a diverticulum off of the yolk sac. While the allantois has no known role in humans, it serves as a reservoir for the developing renal system in lower vertebrates. The distal hindgut (cloaca) and the urogenital sinus separate into the urogenital sinus ventrally and the anorectal canal dorsally. The developing bladder remains connected to the allantois via the urachus. In normal development, apoptosis occurs leading to obliteration of both the vitelline duct and urachus. Failure of apoptosis, results in omphalomesenteric remnants and urachal remnants, respectively. The obliterated embryonic urachus becomes the median umbilical ligament. After birth, the umbilical arteries become the medial umbilical ligaments, while the umbilical vein becomes the ligamentum teres (round ligament of the liver).

During the fourth gestational week, the disk-shaped trilaminar embryo begins to form the umbilical ring through folding of the lateral wall (somatopleure) and ventral flexion. The umbilical ring is the transition from epidermis to amnion and surrounds the umbilical cord. The umbilical cord consists of the yolk stalk which contains the vitelline (omphalomesenteric) duct, the umbilical arteries, the umbilical vein, the allantois and Wharton's jelly. The 6th through 10th gestation weeks are marked by rapid intestinal growth causing the developing midgut to herniate through the umbilical ring. As the body wall continues to grow, the intestines are incorporated back into the coelomic cavity after rotation and fixation. The umbilical ring contracts and is typically closed by birth.

PATHOPHYSIOLOGY AND TREATMENT OF CONGENITAL UMBILICAL DISORDERS

Umbilical Dysmorphology

A single umbilical artery is the most common irregularity of the umbilical cord, occurring in up to 1% of births. This condition may be detected during a routine second trimester ultrasound. It is difficult to say if a single artery poses a problem for the baby, given that many of these newborns are completely healthy. However, one-third of these babies will have congenital chromosomal anomalies (including Trisomy 18), renal, neurologic or cardiac anomalies.

Umbilical dysmorphology is also associated with other syndromes including Robinow's, Reiger's, and Aarskog's syndromes (Table 1).

Delayed Separation of the Umbilical Cord

Typically the umbilical cord will separate from the umbilicus within the first month postnatally. Frequently, the house officer will be asked to evaluate an infant who has delayed separation of the umbilical cord. Families will often admit to the use of various topical treatments including antimicrobials, iodine, and/or isopropyl alcohol. Delayed separation may signify an underlying immune disorder.

Umbilical Hernia

Hernias of the umbilicus are a common condition presenting as a visible protrusion during periods of increased intraabdominal pressure such as crying, coughing or straining. The umbilical ring closure is incomplete. Incidence is difficult to accurately portray but has been estimated around 10–25%. There is no sex predilection. Risk factors include prematurity, low birth weight, and African American race. Most umbilical hernias are isolated anomalies. However association with Trisomy 21, hypothyroidism, mucopolysaccharidoses, and Beckwith–Wiedemann syndrome does exist. Umbilical hernias commonly contain omentum or segments of small bowel, but most are easily reducible through the umbilical ring. The defect size is variable.

Most umbilical hernias, even large hernias, resolve spontaneously. Diameter and sharpness of the fascial defect is often thought to be a

Table 1. Syndromes associated with umbilical dysmorphology.

Robinow's syndrome
Flat, poorly epithelialized umbilicus
Flat facial profile
Mesomelic shortening
Genital hypoplasia
Rieger's syndrome
Broad umbilicus with prominent stalk
Redundant umbilical skin
Goniodysgenesis
Hypodontia
Aarskog's syndrome
Prominent umbilicus
Short stature
Facial dysplasia
Syndactyly
Genital anomalies

predictor of spontaneous regression. Hernias with diameters greater than 2 cm or those with thin fascial edges are less likely to close spontaneously. Initial management is usually observation. A parent may be taught to routinely check the fascial defect, while the child is sleeping. This evidence may help the pediatric surgeon determine if spontaneous closure is occurring. Children with umbilical hernias will often point to their hernia during times of abdominal discomfort. Thus, a prudent house officer should educate the parents on the nature of visceral pain and reinforce the concept that the umbilical hernia is unlikely to be the source of any discomfort. Although very uncommon, when the house officer is asked to reduce an incarcerated umbilical hernia, we suggest milking the air out of the intestine by applying steady pressure on the incarcerated mass. Persistent incarceration or strangulation requires urgent surgical exploration.

Relative indications for surgery include the uncommon "symptomatic" hernia, increasing size of hernia with regards to the fascial opening, or hernia persistence past the age of 3 to 5 yrs. Some surgeons may consider repair concurrent with other surgical procedures. If surgical intervention is pursued, a curvilinear infraumbilical incision is made. The cicatrix is raised by incising the underlying subcutaneous fat with care to avoid injury to the overlying skin. The tissue around the fascial defect and hernia sac is cleared. Management of the hernia sac is variable. Some surgeons prefer to open the hernia sac, reduce the hernia contents, and trim the sac back to the *fascia*. Others advocate dissecting the hernia sac free and returning it back to the abdomen unopened. As described by Gross, transverse closure is recommend followed by preservation of the umbilical appearance. The use of interrupted fascial sutures with knots "buried" is recommended. Skin is closed with fine subcuticular sutures. The final repair is reinforced with Tegaderm™ pressure dressing left in place for 5 days to prevent hematomas or seromas. There are numerous methods to manage troubling redundant skin including V-Y advancement flap, purse-string techniques and umbilicoplasty.

Omphalomesenteric Remnants (Vitelline Duct Remnants)

Patent vitelline ducts are among the most common congenital malformations with an incidence of 2%. Among these, Meckel's diverticulum is most prominent. Other types of remnants include fistulas, sinuses, cysts, mucosal remnants or even congenital bands. The type of lesion is determined by the stage at which the obliteration of the vitelline duct was arrested during development. Signs of feces draining from the umbilicus indicate the vitelline duct is uniformly patent from umbilicus to terminal ileum. Other symptoms may include prolapse of the proximal and distal ileum through the patent duct. Some patients may present with a mechanical intestinal obstruction due to the remnant attachments to the abdominal wall serving as a fulcrum for the intestines to wrap around, as an isolated midgut volvulus. Subtle symptoms may be recognized with small duct remnants necessitating fistulography to delineate the anomaly. Treatment involves prompt surgical intervention. An infraumbilical incision is recommended, allowing for a full exploration of the umbilical structures. Any bands attached to the umbilicus should be ligated. The vitelline duct is then traced back to the ileum and divided with care to ensure hemostasis of omphalomesenteric vessels. Fistulae should be treated with wedge excision and transverse repair of the ileum. Periodically a Meckel's diverticulum may be found attached to a vitelline band. Formal excision is required. On rare occasions, the vitelline duct may originate from the appendix. Umbilicoplasty should be performed at the conclusion of the case. Cystic remnants may be a source of infection or abscess. Initial treatment is surgical drainage followed by delayed excision of the remnant. Of note, there have been rare descriptions of spontaneous regression of vitelline duct remnants.

Uracal Remnant

A patent urachus is a result from failure of closure of the allantoic duct. The incidence of a patent urachus is 1/1000 live births. A patent urachus should be suspected if there is drainage of clear fluid or urine from the umbilicus. Other signs and symptoms may include peri-umbilical granulation tissue, umbilical rash, pain, purulent drainage, retraction of umbilicus during micturition, swelling or erythema. These symptoms may result from an associated granuloma, fistula, sinus or cyst. Similar to omphalomesenteric remnants, the type of urachal lesion that forms is determined by the stage at which obliteration of the allantois was arrested during development. If a granuloma is noted, initial treatment is application of silver nitrate. If the lesion persists after serial treatments, further evaluation may be needed. Ultrasound is preferred, although CT may be useful as well. A probe can be used to see if a sinus or fistula is present. Further investigation of any of these lesions (fistula, sinus, cysts or granulomas) can be obtained with use of fistulography. Historically, injection of indigo carmine directly into the tract was recommended with observation of the color of the draining fluid or urine. The relationship between a patent urachus (serving as a "pop-off") and major urethral obstruction is unclear. A voiding cystourethrogram may be considered. Urachal remnants may become infected. There is a rare risk of rupture into the peritoneal cavity. In addition, benign and malignant neoplasms have been found in association with these anomalies. Due to these risks, surgical therapy is recommended. Typically an infraumbilical incision is used to explore and identify all umbilical structures. Sinuses and cysts should be excised in an infraumbilical approach. The patent urachus is often ligated and transected at the level of the bladder. Broad-based connections with the bladder are closed with absorbable sutures in a two-layer fashion. Some advocate excision of a ventral bladder cuff due to the risk of recurrence or urachal carcinoma with ligation alone.

Umbilical Polyp

This is a rare anomaly resulting from persistence of all or part of the omphalomesenteric duct or urachus. Tissue is firm, red and often has a mucoid secretion. The polyp may communicate directly with the ileum or bladder leading to drainage of fecal material or urine, respectively. Silver nitrate will not be effective. Therefore, treatment is surgical excision of the entire remnant as discussed above for vitelline duct and urachal remnants.

PATHOPHYSIOLOGY AND TREATMENT OF ACQUIRED UMBILICAL DISORDERS

Umbilical Granulomas

Umbilical granulomas are common and present as a small mass of granulation tissue following cord separation. Granulomas range from 1 mm to 1 cm in size and consist of true granulation tissue with fibroblasts and capillaries. The tissue is often soft and vascular, red in color, and pedunculated in appearance. Treatment consists of single or multiple applications of silver nitrate. The house officer should warn the family that this procedure will be uncomfortable for the child. Additionally, the silver nitrate can stain the child's clothing and a gauze can be placed over it after treatment. Alternative diagnoses, like umbilical polyps or sinuses, should be suspected if there is a lack of response to treatment.

Umbilical Infections

Necrotic tissue of the umbilical cord is an excellent medium for infection. Fortunately, aseptic delivery and cord care techniques have dramatically decreased the risk of umbilical infections. Omphalitis refers to a localized umbilical infection characterized by purulent umbilical discharge and periumbilical cellulitis. The house officer should be aware that progression to necrotizing fasciitis and umbilical gangrene can occur. Frequent exams (documented in the chart) are necessary as intravenous antimicrobial therapy is initiated. Umbilical remnants may also be a source of umbilical infection, as discussed above. Risk factors include delivery at home, low birth weight, use of umbilical catheters and septic delivery. The umbilicus is susceptible to bacterial, fungal, viral and parasitic infections. Common microbial isolates include *Staphylococcus aureus, Streptococcus pyogenes,* and *Escherichia coli.* Tetanus infection is extremely rare. Surgical intervention in the form of debridement may be needed in cases of severe, rapid infection or associated abscess formation.

OTHER CONGENITIAL AND ACQUIRED CONDITIONS OF THE UMBILICUS

Albeit rare, other congenital or acquired conditions may affect the umbilicus. Any dermatoses including seborrheic dermatitis, contact dermatitis, pilonidal disease or psoriasis could be implicated. Starch, talc, or other chemicals may cause a foreign body reaction. Concretions of keratinous and sebaceous material may form omphaliths. Pancreatic or endometrial tissue may be found at the umbilicus.

Tumors of the umbilicus include pyogenic granulomas, hamartomas, hemangiomas, dermatofibromas, neurofibromas, granular cell tumors, teratomas, desmoid tumors, lipomas, melanoma, urachal adenocarcinoma, squamous cell carcinoma, basal cell carcinoma and sarcomas. Inclusion cysts, keloids, nevi and other skin lesions may also be associated with the umbilicus. Metastatic tumors of the stomach, pancreas, endometrium, ovary, cervix, colon, small intestine, gall bladder, lung, prostate, and breast may affect the umbilicus. Suprapubic dermoid sinuses have been reported and may represent a variant of a dorsal urethral duplication. Bladder or cloacal exstrophy may be associated in an unusually low set umbilicus or may be incorporated into the open bladder plate. An appendico-omphalic anomaly occurs when a fistula or extension of the appendiceal artery connects the appendix to the umbilicus. Enteric fistulas may also occur with Crohn's disease, perforated appendicitis, colonic perforations or gallbladder perforations. As one can clearly see, a broad differential is required when caring for these children.

REFERENCES

1. Skandalakis J, Gray SQW, Ricketts R. (1994) The anterior abdominal wall. In: J Skandalakis (ed.), *Embryology for Surgeons,* 2nd edition, pp. 540–593. Williams & Wilkins, Baltimore.
2. Zinner MJ, Ashley SW. (2007) Hernias. In: Maingot (ed.), *Maingot's Abdominal Operations,* pp. 122–123. Appleton & Lange, Norwalk, Conn.

3. Kokoska ER and Weber TR. (2003) Umbilical and supraumbilical disease. In: M Ziegler, R Azizkhan & T Weber (eds.), *Operative Pediatric Surgery*, pp. 537–542. McGraw-Hill Companies, New York.
4. Cilley RE. (2006) Disorders of the umbilicus. In: JL Grosfeld, JA O'Neill, AG Coran & E Fonkalsrud (eds.), *Pediatric Surgery*, 6th edition, pp. 1143–1154. Mosby Elsevier, Philadelphia, PA.

INGUINAL HERNIAS AND HYDROCELES

50

Frederick J. Rescorla

INTRODUCTION

Inguinal hernias represent one of the most common surgical conditions treated by pediatric surgeons. Inguinal hernias in infants and children are generally indirect inguinal hernias but may rarely be femoral hernias or direct inguinal hernias.

PATHOPHYSIOLOGY

Embryology and Anatomy

The processus vaginalis is first noted at approximately 3 mths of fetal life as a peritoneal diverticulum extending through the internal inguinal ring. The gonads form on the nephrogenic ridges in the retroperitoneum during the 5th week of gestation. The testis is attached to the scrotum by the gubernaculum and the ovary to the labia via the round ligament. Testicular descent starts around the 3rd month of gestation and the testis reaches the internal inguinal ring by about 7 mths. It then further descends down the canal and is preceded in its descent by the processus vaginalis. As the testis descends through the abdominal wall, the layers of the abdominal wall become part of the cord with the internal spermatic *fascia* a continuation of the transversalis *fascia,* the cremasteric muscle fibers from the internal oblique and the external oblique contributing to the external spermatic *fascia*. The processus vaginalis is located anteromedial to the cord structures and the scrotal portion of it forms the tunica vaginalis. The female anlage of the processus is the canal of Nuck which leads to the labia majora. The canal of Nuck also closes around the 7th month of fetal life and ovarian descent is completed into the pelvis.

Several studies have noted the incidence of a patent processus vaginalis at birth to be as high as 40–60% whereas in adults at autopsy, 5% have a patent processus. A patent processus can close after birth, but the rate of closure decreases with advancing age. Patency of the processus vaginalis can result in an indirect inguinal hernia. Indirect inguinal hernias are more common on the right, thought to be related to the later descent of the right gonad. Abnormalities related to failure of obliteration of the processus vaginalis lead to several common anatomic possibilities (Figure 1). Normal anatomy is defined as the lower processus vaginalis forming the tunica vaginalis with the processus vaginalis being obliterated from the tunica vaginalis up to the internal inguinal ring. A hydrocele results from fluid coming from the peritoneal cavity, down a narrow processes vaginalis resulting in a fluid collection within the tunica vaginalis. In many children the size may change gradually with time, although on physical examination pressure on the hydrocele sac often results in no change due to the fact that the connection is very small. This small communication from the hydrocele sac to the peritoneal cavity allows fluid to pass back and forth to the hydrocele, however the opening is not large enough to allow the intestine to enter the internal ring. Hydroceles may be limited to the scrotum

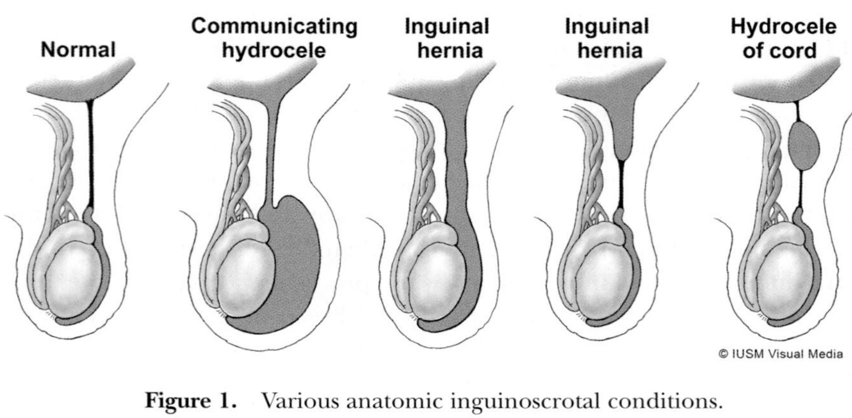

Figure 1. Various anatomic inguinoscrotal conditions.

or involve the inguinoscrotal region. A hydrocele of the cord occurs when a segment of the processus contains fluid without communication to the scrotum or internal ring. An inguinal hernia results when the processus vaginalis is patent from the internal ring down a variable distance towards the scrotum. A complete inguinal hernia is generally defined as one in which the tunica vaginalis communicates freely from the internal ring allowing intestinal contents to go back and forth into the scrotum.

Incidence and Associated Defects

Approximately 0.8–5% of all children will develop an inguinal hernia. Right sided hernias are twice as common as that on the left and the male to female ratio ranges from 5:1 to 10:1. The incidence of inguinal hernia is higher in premature infants with the rates between 10 and 30%, with term newborns generally having a rate between 3–5%. Approximately 10% of infants with hernias have bilateral hernias at initial presentation.

Children with increased intraabdominal pressure have a higher incidence of inguinal hernias. This includes children with ventriculo-peritoneal shunts or peritoneal dialysis catheters as well as the presence of abdominal wall defects. As mentioned above premature children have a higher incidence as do children with connective tissue disorders. Children with Cystic Fibrosis have a hernia incidence as high as 15% and this may be related to higher intraabdominal pressure associated with this chronic pulmonary condition. Hernias are also commonly seen in association with undescended testis.

CLINICAL PRESENTATION

Most children with inguinal hernias are noted with an asymptomatic inguinal or inguinoscrotal mass. If this is visible on initial presentation to the physician an attempt should be made at reduction. Transillumination allows the differentiation of a hydrocele or communicating hydrocele as well as the rather rare occurrence of a hydrocele of the cord in which a fluid filled sac is separated from the tunica vaginalis as well as from the internal inguinal ring. Usually physical examination allows identification of a normal cord proximal to the hydrocele thus differentiating hydroceles from hernias.

Not infrequently a child is referred to a surgeon with the history of either a parent or primary care physician identifying a hernia which is not apparent on initial exam with the surgeon. Various maneuvers can be utilized to increase the abdominal pressure in an attempt to reproduce the hernia, however some will not be observed during the clinic visit. If the child can cooperate, the physician can ask them to push their abdominal wall out or they can put their thumb in their mouth and "blow" on their thumb to increase their intraabdominal pressure. Particular care should be taken if the child has an associated retractile testis as this can sometimes be mistaken for an inguinal hernia. If the hernia cannot be reproduced during the visit and if the history is excellent or if a physician has seen the hernia most pediatric surgeons will proceed with operative repair.

INITIAL MANAGEMENT

It is important at the initial presentation to ensure that the hernia is not incarcerated. This can generally be performed by simply reducing the abdominal contents back into the abdominal cavity. If the hernia is not readily reducible, the surgeon's fingers can be made to create an inverted "V" at the level of the external ring and the other hand utilized to reduce the contents deep to the external oblique and into the peritoneal cavity. Transillumination should be performed first as some children sent in with a reported incarcerated hernia actually have a simple hydrocele. If the hernia cannot be reduced, sedation may be utilized in an attempt to reduce the incarcerated hernia and if this is unsuccessful, emergent operative repair should be undertaken.

Young girls not infrequently present with an asymptomatic incarcerated ovary and an attempt should be made to reduce the ovary. If it is not reducible, we generally proceed with operative repair either that day or in the next day or two, cautioning the family to be very observant and contact us immediately should pain or tenderness or increased swelling occur in this area.

Children with hydroceles, with or without communication, can generally be observed until approximately 1 yr of age as spontaneous closure will occur in many of these cases. Children with a history of incarceration which can be reduced easily, are generally scheduled for operative repair within the next few days. At our institution if the surgeon or emergency room physician is needed to reduce the hernia, the child is admitted and the hernia repaired in the next 24 hrs.

Premature infants who are hospitalized due to their prematurity are often noted with inguinal hernias and the timing for operative repair often raises considerable discussion. At our institution we generally repair the hernias prior to discharge however this occasionally is surgeon dependant and may sometimes be delayed in the presence of other co-morbidities or in children who may require another major operative intervention at a later time.

OPERATIVE TECHNIQUE

Indirect inguinal hernias are repaired through an open or a laparoscopic technique. In the open technique, an inguinal crease incision is utilized to enter the groin. Scarpa's *fascia* is divided and the external oblique identified and traced down to the inguinal ligament. This is then traced inferiorly until the external ring is identified. The external oblique is opened in the direction of it's fibers with care taken to avoid injury to the ilioinguinal nerve which is identified and carefully preserved. The hernia sac is identified by gently spreading the cremasteric fibers. The hernia sac is then elevated and the cremasteric fibers further taken off of the hernia sac. The vessels are identified on the lateral aspect of the hernia sac. These are gently taken down in a lateral direction, pushing them away from the hernia sac. The vas is usually the last cord structure identified and must be clearly identified and separated from the hernia sac.

After the vas and vessels are definitely separated, the hernia sac is doubly clamped and divided. The proximal portion is traced to the level of the internal ring with separation of the vas and the vessels carefully away from it. This can be aided by gentle traction on the distal cord structures. High ligation should be accomplished at the level of the internal ring with absorbable or nonabsorbable sutures. It is not necessary to remove all of the distal sac. If there is an associated hydrocele, we generally excise the distal sac to the level of the testes and then excise the anterior portion of the tunica vaginalis. Distal dissection of the sac should be very carefully performed to avoid injury to the cord structures.

The operation for a hydrocele is identical and care should be taken to properly ligate the processus vaginalis at the level of the internal ring. The distal sac of the hydrocele should be opened widely and either excised down to its junction with the testis and epididymis or else everted behind the cord structures and sutured in a marsupialization type fashion (Bottle procedure).

Various laparoscopic techniques have been utilized to enable suture ligation of the processus vaginalis at the level of the internal ring, leaving the entire distal sac in place. Most reports have noted a higher recurrence rate which has decreased over time with the surgeon's experience, however many reports still have higher recurrence rate (0.4–4.1%) than noted in large open repair series (0.2–0.5%).

Contralateral Patent Processus Vaginalis

The management of the contralateral side in patients with unilateral hernias has been a topic of debate and controversy for many years. Early data in the pediatric surgical literature demonstrated a high incidence of contralateral patent processus vaginalis (CPPV) in young children at the time of unilateral hernia repair with some demonstrating an incidence as high as 57% in children younger than 2 yrs of age. A series by McGregor followed a large number of children undergoing unilateral inguinal hernia repair over a 32-yr period and identified a contralateral hernia rate of 28%. More recent reports following for a contralateral hernia after unilateral repair have found lower rates with these generally between 5–14%, however the follow-up in many of these papers is less than 2 yrs. The basic question is whether or not it is worthwhile assessing for a CPPV and then repairing it to prevent the development of a hernia at a later date. Some pediatric surgeons only repair the symptomatic side and do not assess for a CPPV.

Patients presenting with a left sided inguinal hernia have an associated increase risk of CPPV and reports in girls have demonstrated a higher rate of CPPV. Prior to the advent of laparoscopy surgeons had several options. Some would perform routine contralateral exploration in children who were premature or perhaps less than 1 or 2 yrs of age with some extending this to a higher age in girls. In addition, other maneuvers to assess for a CPPV were available to surgeons including palpation for the "silk glove sign", however this technique has not been proven to be reliable. Ultrasound has been utilized and this has been shown to be reliable in some studies. Other techniques have included performing a herniogram with injection of dye into the peritoneal cavity and radiologic evaluation of the contralateral side. Pneumoperitoneum has also been utilized however this has not been a reliable study. Intraoperative probing using a Bakes dilator from the symptomatic side and probing the contralateral internal ring has also been utilized however this also has not been proven reliable.

The introduction of laparoscopy allowed surgeons to evaluate the contralateral side either by passing a laparoscope through the symptomatic hernia sac or through the umbilicus or a higher abdominal stab incision. At our institution this is performed through the hernia sac thus avoiding an additional abdominal wall puncture (Figure 2). Low pressure insufflation (8 mm Hg) is utilized with a rigid 70° telescope. A recent evaluation of data from our institution (1508 children over 4 ½ yrs) demonstrated a 32% CPPV rate for right hernias and a 42% rate for left hernias. The CPPV rate was highest in premature neonates (46%) and in infants less than 6 mths of age (45%). After 6 mths of age the CPPV rate was 19–24%. This data also demonstrated a higher incidence of CPPV in girls over 2 yrs compared to boys over two. At our institution contralateral evaluation is generally offered to boys less than 2 yrs of age and girls up to 8–10 yrs of age; however this is somewhat surgeon dependent.

Incarceration

The incidence of incarceration is higher in premature neonates and the younger infant group. In addition, injury to the bowel with incarceration is more common in the premature and younger infants. These children

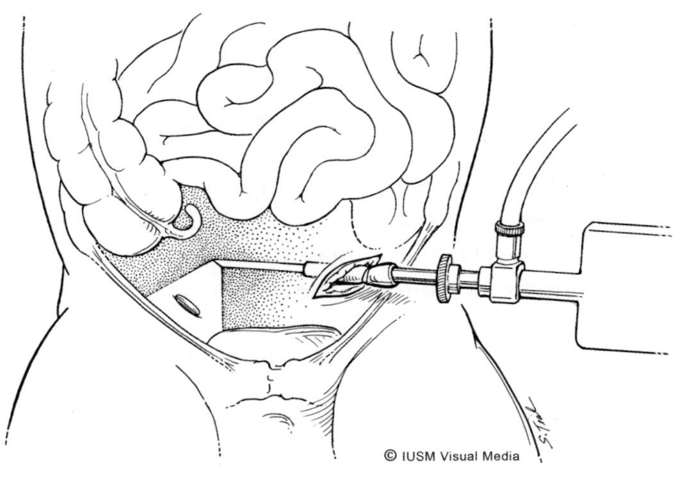

Figure 2. Laparoscopic evaluation of a CPPV, use of a reusable trocar and a 70° telescope.

generally present with a tender irreducible inguinal mass with or without a scrotal mass. Occasionally it may be difficult to differentiate an incarcerated inguinal hernia from a large tense hydrocele which extends up to the level of the internal ring. For most hydroceles the surgeon can palpate cord structures proximally towards the level of the internal ring allowing differentiation of incarceration from hydrocele. Other maneuvers include a rectal examination with palpation of the internal ring. Ultrasound may be useful in these select cases to differentiate fluid from intestinal contents.

For reduction, one hand is used to make an inverted "V" which is placed at the level of the external inguinal ring and reduction is then attempted from the distal portion of the incarceration attempting to reduce the contents below the level of the external oblique *fascia,* through the inguinal canal and into the peritoneal cavity. Over 90% of incarcerated hernias can be reduced with a small percentage requiring emergency operation. Sedation is occasionally helpful however this is rarely utilized at our institution and if the pediatric surgeon cannot reduce the hernia, the child is generally taken for operative exploration.

If the hernia can be reduced, the child is generally admitted to the hospital and taken to the operating room in the next 24 hrs for operative repair. This allows some of the edema to resolve, however these hernias are often still difficult to repair. If the hernia cannot be reduced the child is taken for operative immediate reduction and exploration. If the hernia reduces spontaneously with induction of anesthesia the hernia sac should still be opened. Cloudy contents or bloody fluid would generally require evaluation of the peritoneal cavity to make sure that the bowel is not injured. This can be accomplished by delivering the bowel out through the hernia sac with another option to place a laparoscope through the hernia sac to visualize the peritoneal cavity. Bowel injury is quite rare occurring in perhaps 1–2% of incarcerated hernias. If the bowel is compromised, a resection can be performed through the hernia sac or a separate abdominal incision with the bowel delivered out to accomplish the resection and anastomosis. The testis should be inspected on the affected side as it can sometimes be compromised from a vascular standpoint. Most surgeons leave the testis in place even if it is discolored. Occasionally an ovary may be incarcerated and compromised and unless the ovary is definitely necrotic, we generally reduce this into the peritoneal cavity and repair the hernia.

Sliding Hernias

Sliding hernias are relatively uncommon however are more frequent in young girls with the fallopian tube and ovary part of the sliding defect. The management options include distal ligation with inversion of the sac and closure of the internal ring, sometimes with a purse string suture of the peritoneum. Occasionally the round ligament and fallopian tube can be separated from the hernia sac and placed back in the abdominal cavity allowing a standard high ligation however care must be taken to avoid injury to the fallopian tube. Another option is to make an incision in the peritoneum on each side of the sliding structure, fold it into the abdomen and then carefully close the peritoneum.

COMPLICATIONS AND OUTCOMES

The recurrence rate in some laparascopic series has been as high as 4.1% however this has generally dropped down to 1% and 2% in most series with increased experience. A recent report from our institution of over 1500 open hernia repairs identified a recurrence rate of 0.2% with a 2.9 +/− 1.6 yr follow-up. The recurrence rate has been noted to be higher in children with increased abdominal pressure such as those with ventriculo-peritoneal shunts or ascites and is known to be higher in the presence of connective tissue disorders. Damage to the vas or vessels is a rare complication. We generally quote an incidence of less than 0.5% for recurrence, infection and injury to the vas deferens.

The most common cause of an early recurrent hernia is a missed hernia sac and in these repeat exploration should be performed by an experienced surgeon. Another cause of recurrence is a direct or femoral hernia which was missed at the initial exploration, or acquired direct hernia as a result of injury to the floor during the initial procedure. Some very large chronic indirect inguinal hernias can lead to dilatation of the internal ring and partial closure of the ring is necessary at the initial procedure.

Anesthesia and Risk of Postoperative Apnea and Bradycardia

Children with prematurity have an increased risk of postoperative apnea and bradycardia and overnight monitoring of these children is necessary until they achieve an adequate level of maturity. This is usually defined by the postconceptual age which is gestational age plus chronologic age in weeks and is utilized to determine which children require overnight observation. Reports in the literature recommend observation for premature children with postconceptual ages less than 51 to 60 wks. At our institution we generally keep infants less than 54 wks postconception for overnight observation. Term infants over 1 mth of age do not require overnight observation.

REFERENCES

1. Bhatia AM, Gow KW, Heiss KF, *et al.* (2004) Is the use of laparoscopy to determine presence of contralateral patent processus vaginalis justified in children greater than 2 years of age? *J Pediatr Surg* **39**:778–781.
2. Rescorla FJ, West KW, Engum SA, *et al.* (1997) The "other side" of pediatric hernias: The role of laparoscopy. *Am Surg* **63**:690–693.
3. Schier F, Montupet P, Esposito C. (2002) Laparoscopic inguinal herniorrhaphy in children; a three-center experience with 933 repairs. *J Pediatr Surg* **37**:395–397.

PYLORIC STENOSIS 51

Mustafa Kabeer

CLINICAL PRESENTATION

Infantile hypertrophic pyloric stenosis causing gastric outlet obstruction in the newborn period is a common problem encountered in pediatric surgery. The classic presentation of pyloric stenosis occurs in the 2–6 wk old infant, usually male, with progressively worsening symptoms of nonbilious emesis mostly described as projectile. Approximately 10% of patients have blood tinged emesis related to the gastric irritation from prolonged vomiting. The child may have a prolonged period of these episodes and may present with significant dehydration manifesting in the history as less frequent wet diapers. This disorder can occur at any point from birth to 3 mths of age and may affect premature babies as well. Occasionally babies can become emaciated if this has continued for long periods of time. Due to decreased enteric flow from the pyloric obstruction, many of these infants exhibit an indirect hyperbilirubinemia which resolves within a week after pyloromyotomy.

PATHOPHYSIOLOGY

Pyloric stenosis was first described in an autopsy report in London in 1717 by Mr. Patrick Blair. Since then, Dr. Harald Hirschsprung described further case reports in 1887. It was successfully treated by several individuals in the early 1900's by performing extramucosal pyloroplasty but finally culminated into the definitive operation of pyloromyotomy by Dr. Ramstedt in 1912.

The etiology of pyloric stenosis is still not well understood but seems to suggest a decrease in neuronal nitric oxide synthase. The plasma nitrite concentration is high in babies with pyloric stenosis and low in normal controls but is normalized after pyloromyotomy.[1] This may be due to the decreased expression of neuronal nitric oxide synthase.[1] This may also be manifest as lower plasma arginine levels related to decreased nitric oxide synthesis.[2] The process causes the pylorus to undergo concentric hypertrophy to the point of symptomatic luminal obstruction.

The incidence of pyloric stenosis is between 2–4/1000 live births predominantly occurring in males (4:1 male:female). It is noted more frequently in Caucasian than in African American or Asian babies. The majority (90%) occur sporadically but there are familial cases (7%) suggesting some genetic linkage. There is a suggested link to chromosome 16q24 although there may be variable expression due to locus heterozygosity.[3] There is a much higher likelihood of developing pyloric stenosis if the mother had pyloric stenosis than if the father had it. Transmission rate to boys is 19% and 7% to girls if the mother has pyloric stenosis and 5% to boys and 2.5% to girls if the father had pyloric stenosis.[4] There have also been reports of increased risk of pyloric stenosis with blood types B and O. There may even be some link with an increased risk of pyloric stenosis as a result of formula feeding versus strict breast feeding.[5]

DIAGNOSIS/WORK-UP

A physical exam will often reveal a palpable mid-epigastric mass which is the hypertrophied pylorus referred to as the palpable "olive". It is usually located in the right upper quadrant just lateral to the midline and near the liver border. Some infants may have either a distended stomach or may be crying from hunger thus making it difficult to palpate. Ultrasound has become a routine form of imaging to diagnose the problem and provide dimensions relating to its hypertrophy. The commonly used criteria based on ultrasound measurements are a pyloric muscle thickness of 4mm (Figure 1) and a pyloric channel length of at least 1.6 cm (Figure 2). It should be mentioned that premature babies or babies only a few weeks old, especially those that may be either small for gestational age (SGA) or have intrauterine growth retardation (IUGR) may still have pyloric stenosis without meeting the measurement criteria. Babies less than 21 days old with pyloric stenosis have ultrasound dimensions for muscle wall thickness at

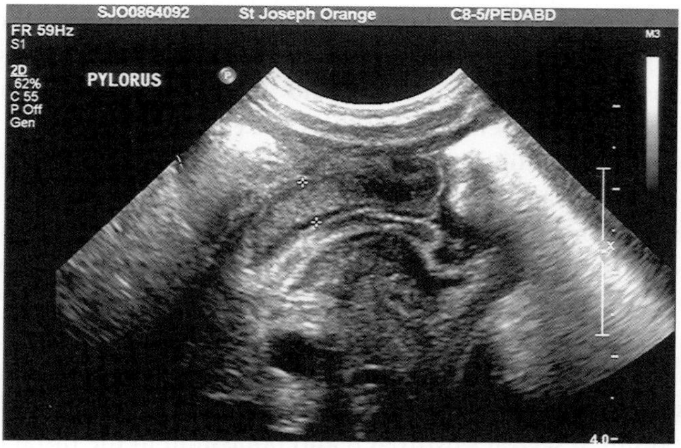

Figure 1. Ultrasound: pyloric muscle thickness.

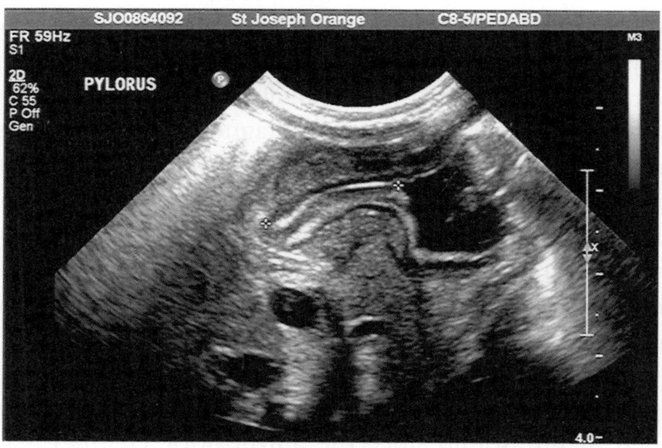

Figure 2. Ultrasound: pyloric channel length.

3.5 mm.[6] Serial ultrasound can be used in patients that present early in their course and have a history consistent with pyloric stenosis but do not meet radiographic criteria. One study documented the rate of pyloric hypertrophy to vary from 0.17 mm/day up to 0.5 mm/day.[7] In these instances, it will help to assess the clinical history and also to evaluate for emptying of gastric contents on imaging studies. This may be seen as fluid or air bubbles traversing the pyloric channel during upper gastrointestinal (UGI) series or ultrasound, respectively. An UGI series to evaluate for pyloric stenosis may be especially useful in cases where the diagnosis may involve classic symptoms and history but a normal ultrasound. There may also be other causes of persistent nonbilious emesis that this could help elucidate.

Laboratory evaluation is a critical component in evaluating and treating these infants. Many babies with pyloric stenosis lose gastric acid due to ongoing emesis and acquire metabolic alkalosis. This alkalosis is manifested in the electrolyte panel as hypokalemia, hypochloremia and hyponatremia in association with an increase in serum bicarbonate. Serum potassium levels may be within normal parameters but the total body potassium is usually low and as such needs to be replaced. With increasing dehydration, the body makes more aldosterone to conserve sodium and water. In order to save the sodium, it secretes hydrogen and potassium in the distal tubules of the kidney. This leads to a paradoxical aciduria even though the body is alkalotic. Because the serum chloride is also low, the renal tubules absorb bicarbonate along with the sodium and this exacerbates the alkalosis.

The differential diagnosis includes gastroesophageal reflux, antral hypertrophy, foveolar cell hyperplasia, pylorospasm, duodenal or pyloric web or even due to increased intracranial pressure from an intracranial process. Many of these may be correctly diagnosed with an UGI series but any reason for suspecting intracranial pathology should be evaluated with a head Computed Tomography (CT)/Magnetic Resonance Imaging (MRI) and an appropriate neurosurgical consultation. Focal foveolar hyperplasia is considered a rare cause of gastric outlet obstruction and can mimic pyloric stenosis. However, one study suggests that this incidence may be higher, up to 12%, and may lead to increased incidence of ongoing postoperative emesis.[8] An extended myotomy helped alleviate this problem. Antral hypertrophy also mimics symptoms of pyloric stenosis but may be distinguished by ultrasound since the antropyloric channel may be long but the pylorus is not thickened. This may be seen in infants with congenital heart disease who have been on prostaglandin E_1 infusion (PGE_1).[9]

MANAGEMENT

Fluid and Electrolyte Correction

Correction of electrolytes is mandatory preparation for operative correction. Fluid resuscitation is initiated with normal saline boluses to correct hypovolemia and hypochloremia. Potassium is supplemented once urine output is adequate. Maintenance intravenous fluid should contain potassium. Minor correction can be accomplished with potassium at 20 meQ/L of fluid but severe hypokalemia must be corrected with 40 meQ/L of potassium and even additional potassium riders. Repeat monitoring of electrolytes is helpful to monitor progress. A normal potassium level after correction of alkalosis, as evidenced by serum bicarbonate less than 30 mMol/L, and a serum chloride greater than 100 mMol/L is evidence of adequate preparation. The use of intravenous cimetidine or Prilosec® has been shown to correct severe alkalosis within the same day of admission.[10] This could allow these infants to avoid a prolonged stay in the hospital with ongoing metabolic derangement and at the same time, allow for quicker surgical intervention.

Lack of adequate resuscitation and electrolyte correction prior to surgery leaves babies at risk of apnea, prolonged intubation or death. All babies should be monitored with either apnea monitors or pulse oximetry after the operation. There is no role for narcotics either during the operation or for postoperative pain since the risk of apnea and hypoxia increase substantially with its use. The risk for apnea is magnified further by any uncorrected alkalosis since the infant compensates with hypoventilation and respiratory acidosis. Close attention should also be paid during induction of anesthesia since there is a high risk of aspiration from increased gastric residual. The gastric residual may be substantial if the baby also had undergone a contrast study such as an UGI. It is unnecessary to delay the operation due to NPO status since all babies with pyloric stenosis should be treated as if they have a full stomach. All infants with pyloric stenosis should undergo gastric tube decompression prior to induction of anesthesia.

Operative Technique (Open)

A pyloromyotomy is effective treatment for pyloric stenosis. The operative approach can be either open or laparoscopic. The open technique can be performed via a right upper quadrant transverse incision (Figure 3), a supraumbilical or infraumbilical incision. The supraumbilical incision has been noted to have a much higher incidence of infection if antibiotics are not given.[11] The right upper quadrant incision can be carried down transversely through all of the tissues from skin, through anterior and posterior rectus sheath and muscle or the anterior rectus sheath can be divided longitudinally after creating a subcutaneous space and then spreading the rectus muscle and then dividing the posterior rectus sheath transversely.

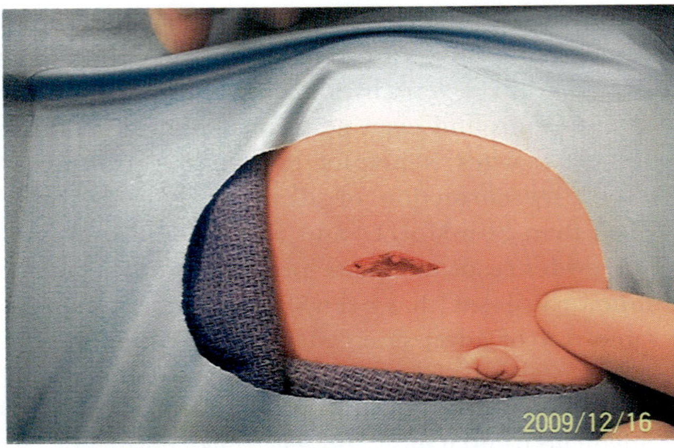

Figure 3. Open pyloromyotomy. Right upper quadrant incision.

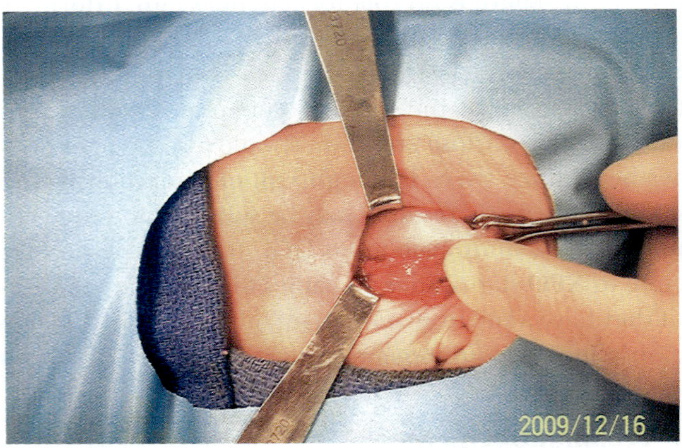

Figure 4. Open pyloromyotomy. Delivering the pylorus.

This avoids dividing rectus muscle and allows for closure of the rectus sheath in two perpendicular directions thus significantly reducing the risk of wound herniation. The pylorus is ultimately brought out of the cavity (Figures 4 and 5) via these incisions and then divided (Figures 6 and 7) and separated (Figures 8 and 9) taking great care to avoid perforation of the inner lining. A technique where the pylorus remains in the abdominal cavity and the muscle is separated using skin hooks to provide the tension needed to separate the muscle has been described.[12]

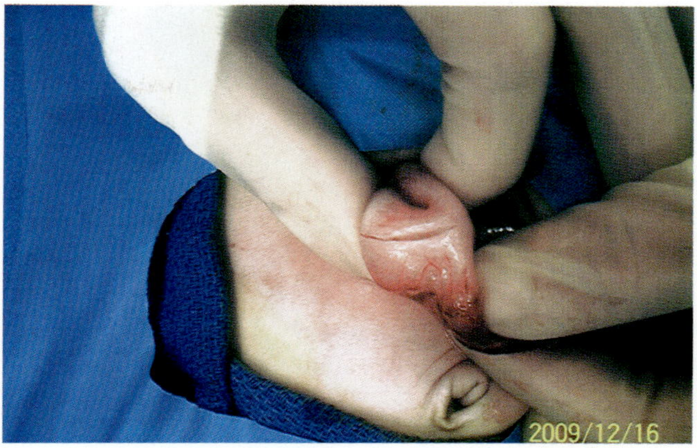

Figure 5. Open pyloromyotomy. Hypertrophied pylorus.

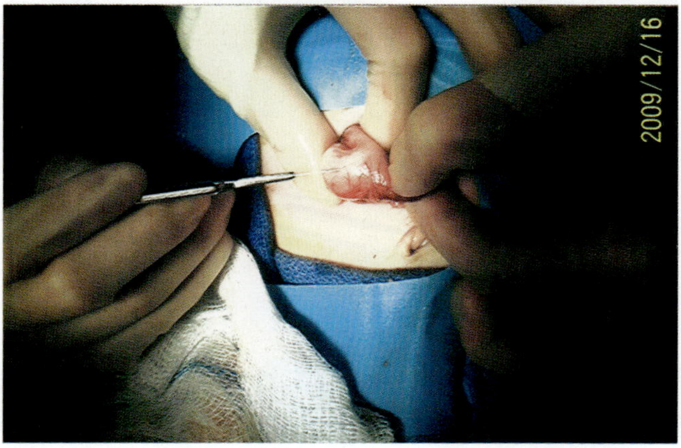

Figure 6. Open pyloromyotomy. Incising the pylorus.

Laparoscopic Technique

A very nice alternative is to perform it laparoscopically. The initial incision is placed below the umbilicus with insertion of a Veress needle and a sheath into the peritoneal cavity (Figures 10 and 11). Subsequently, the abdomen is insufflated to a pressure of 8 mm Hg and then a 3 or 5 mm trocar is inserted through this radially expanding sheath. A stab incision is made in the right upper quadrant and in the left upper quadrant under direct

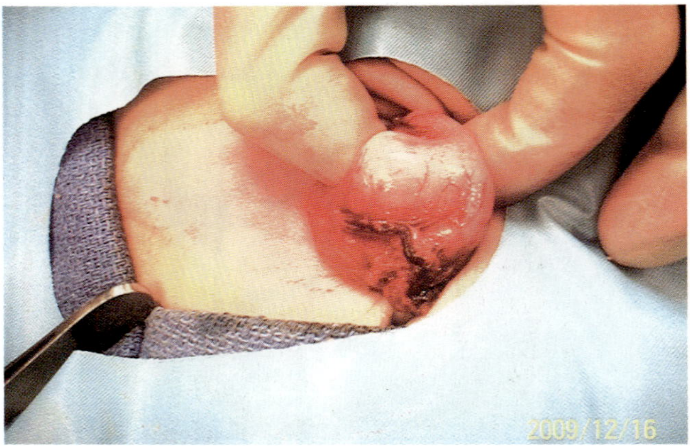

Figure 7. Open pyloromyotomy. Incision on the pylorus.

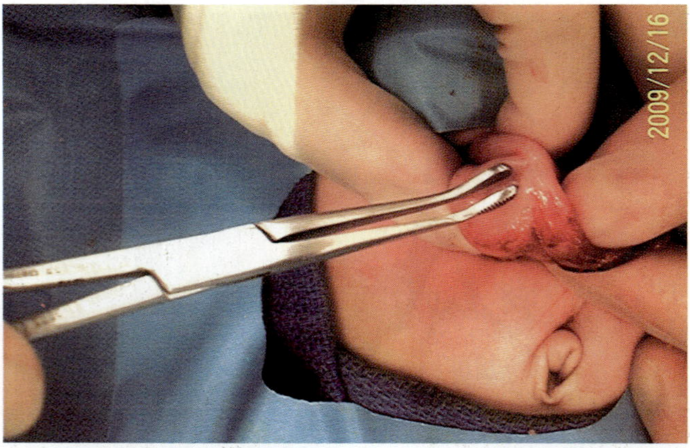

Figure 8. Open pyloromyotomy. Muscle separation.

visualization. A 3 or 5 mm box grasper is passed through the right upper quadrant incision and is utilized to grasp the pylorus from the duodenal end and stabilize it (Figure 12). A cutting instrument is passed from the left upper quadrant incision to cut the pylorus (Figure 13) and subsequently the pyloric spreader is passed through this incision (Figures 14 and 15). The proper instruments are essential to this operation (Figure 16). The

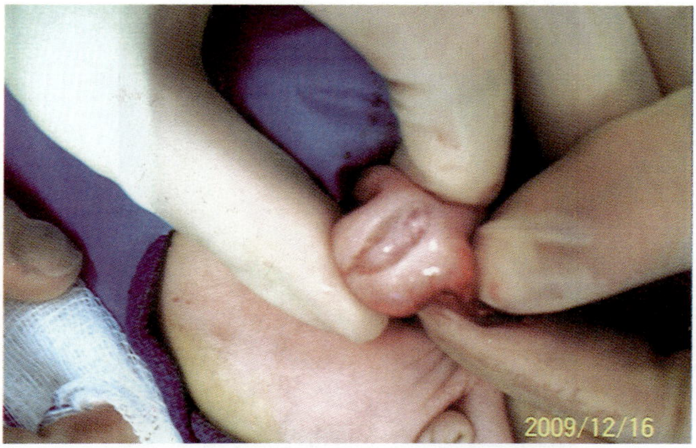

Figure 9. Open pyloromyotomy. Complete pyloromyotomy.

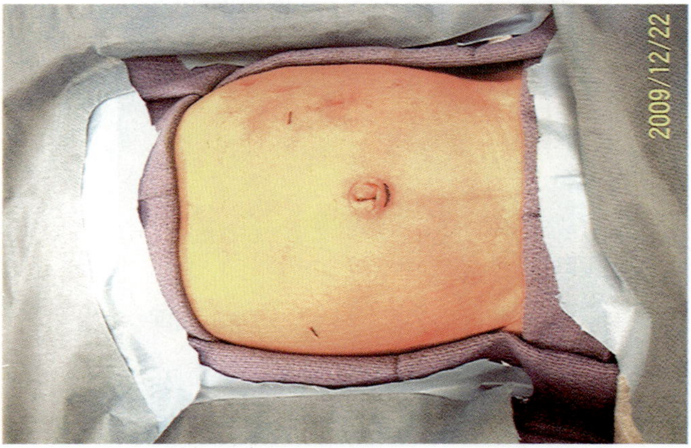

Figure 10. Laparoscopy pyloromyotomy. Incision sites.

grasper should be a box grasper and not a serrated or toothed grasper as it may injure the duodenum. The ideal cutting instrument was the "Banana" blade which is a sheathed arthroscopy blade. Unfortunately, this is no longer being manufactured. Others have tried the introduction of a nonsheathed beaver blade on its handle either directly or through a 5 mm trochar. A bovie cautery with an extended insulated blade tip can also be introduced directly into the peritoneal cavity through the left upper

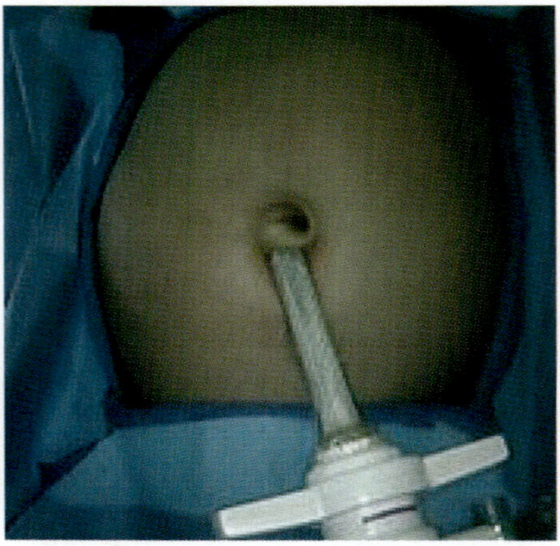

Figure 11. Laparoscopy pyloromyotomy. Single trochar insertion.

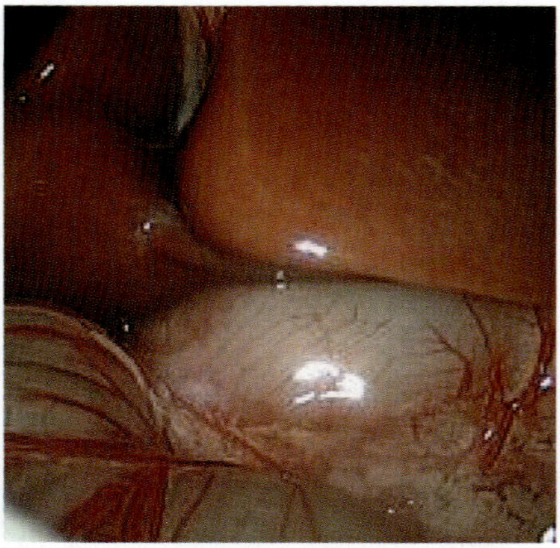

Figure 12. Laparoscopy pyloromyotomy. Box grasper to stabilize pylorus.

quadrant incision and may be used for incising the hypertrophied pylorus. This can also provide hemostasis at the same time.

Studies have varied in their analysis of laparoscopic versus open approaches. It becomes clear that there is a learning curve to a laparoscopic approach and the complications become less frequent over time. Most of these complications are perforations or incomplete myotomy.[13,14]

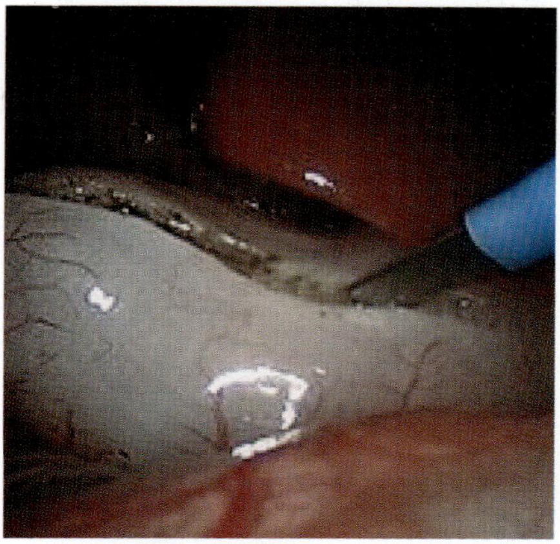

Figure 13. Laparoscopy pyloromyotomy. Incising the pylorus.

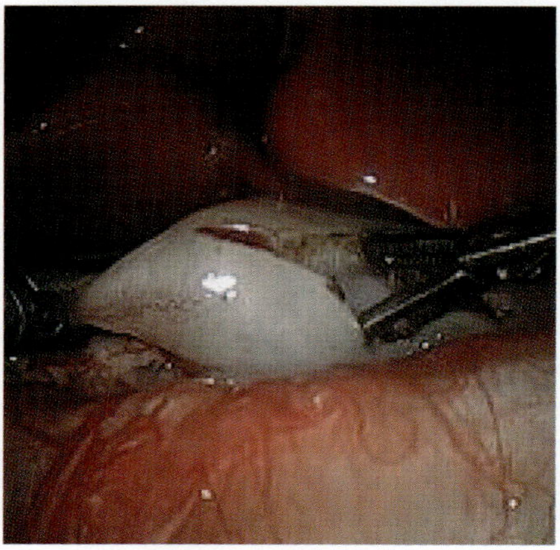

Figure 14. Laparoscopy pyloromyotomy. Pyloric spreader.

Many studies suggest there is a shorter time to full feedings and a shorter length of stay with a laparoscopic approach.[13,15] Others show no difference in length of stay and yet others show an increased length of stay due to the increased complication rate.[14,16] Some studies have shown a similar complication rate to the open procedure and yet others have shown an overall decreased complication rate if wound infections are included.[13,15]

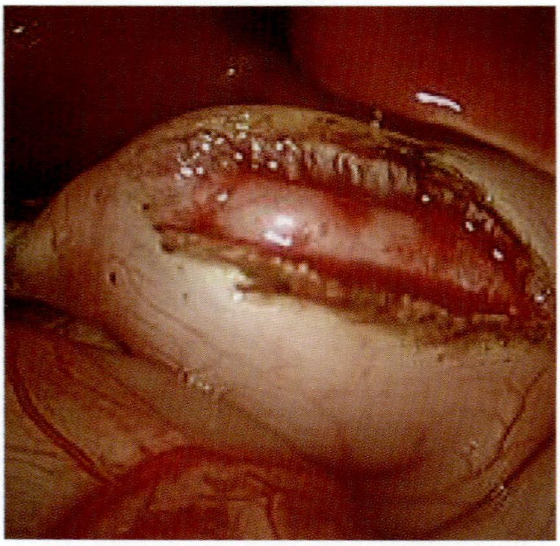

Figure 15. Laparoscopy pyloromyotomy. Completed myotomy.

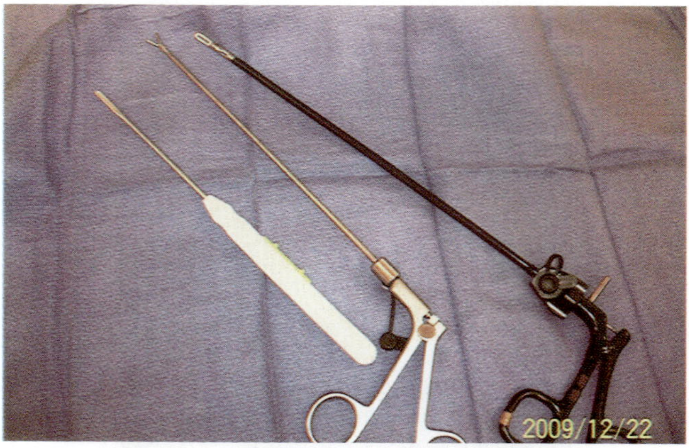

Figure 16. Laparoscopy pyloromyotomy. Laparoscopic instruments.

The laparoscopic approach does seem to have the same or lower risk of postoperative emesis.[15,17] Emesis correlated inversely with weight on admission and with chloride and potassium levels and correlated directly with anion gap.[18] Incidence of postoperative emesis may correlate with increased preoperative dehydration and electrolyte imbalance.

POSTOPERATIVE CONSIDERATIONS

Feedings may be started 2–6 hrs after an uncomplicated pyloromyotomy. Various feeding regimen are utilized. Pedialyte is given as the first two feeds at 15 cc q 3 hrs and then converted to ½ strength formula and then full strength formula. Volumes are increased by 15 cc every other feed until goal feeding is achieved. The baby is then discharged on ad lib feedings. Another option is to advance feeds to 100 mL/kg/day and then release the infant and allow the family to continue the advancement at home.

There are many sources of morbidity in postsurgical patients with pyloric stenosis. Infants are at risk of wound infection since many still have an umbilicus which has not epithelialized. Most wound infections occur near the umbilical incision. Preoperative antibiotic prophylaxis is advised for laparoscopic or open procedures where an incision is placed in proximity to the umbilicus. Apnea may occur in alkalotic patients or those treated with narcotics for pain control where the drive for ventilation is suppressed. Perforation usually occurs due to overly aggressive attempts at myotomy on the duodenal side of the pylorus, whereas incomplete pyloromyotomy usually occurs due to inadequate myotomy on the gastric side of the pylorus. The suspicion of perforation is alleviated by having the anesthesiologist instill 30–45 cc of air via the nasogastric tube (NG) tube after the operation. If air is seen leaking from the myotomy site as bubbles, the patient should be explored. A perforation may be very small and therefore easily missed. Usually, it is seen as a tiny puckering of the mucosa at the site of perforation. The perforation can be closed primarily by placing a U-stitch starting from normal full thickness tissue and then encompassing the tissue proximal to the perforated portion of the mucosa such that it brings it under the full thickness pylorus and allows the site to heal. A piece of omentum can be laid over the myotomy site as well. An incomplete myotomy is usually avoided by visualization of the circular gastric fibers during myotomy. Postoperatively, it is imperative that these infants are kept warm. They are not much different than neonates and may have problems such as apnea or coagulopathy if they become hypothermic. These complications are minimized and better outcomes are achieved with less cost to third party payers when these infants are treated at high volume centers with specialists in pediatric surgery.[19]

Persistent emesis after the procedure is often seen but should progressively improve. It is much more likely in infants that present after a prolonged course since their stomach takes time to return to a normal state from the distended, akinetic state. If this does not improve, an UGI series may be warranted and reconsideration by the operating surgeon as to whether incomplete myotomy should be considered as a cause. In general, postoperative ultrasound is of little value since it will still demonstrate the thickened muscle.

A nonoperative approach with the use of atropine has been reported. One study utilized oral atropine daily until emesis had resolved.[20] Another study used intravenous atropine sequentially increased in dosing until emesis had resolved.[21,22] All studies showed some benefit but there were still many patients that failed and required operative intervention. The patients that did benefit were treated for 1–2 wks in the hospital. Given the extremely low morbidity and mortality with the surgical approach, the authors of one study evaluating atropine discouraged its use given the success of surgery.[22] There may however be some benefit in the future for evaluation of atropine in postoperative emesis or in cases of incomplete myotomy.

The routine preoperative use of a nasogastric tube is not warranted. This has little benefit in ensuring all gastric content is evacuated prior to induction since many become clogged over time and may lead to further electrolyte abnormality.

The addition of antacid into the postoperative management is sometimes beneficial since it may alleviate irritation from concurrent reflux and may help hasten the recovery of the associated gastritis in these patients.

There have been no documented negative long term effects of having pyloric stenosis or undergoing a pyloromyotomy.

REFERENCES

1. Huang LT, Tiao MM, Lee SY, *et al.* (2006) Low plasma nitrite in infantile hypertrophic pyloric stenosis patients. *Dig Dis Sci* **51**(5):869–872.
2. Brouwers AG, Waals-van de Wal CM. (2009) Hypertrophic pyloric stenosis and pulmonary hypertension in a neonate. A common mechanism? *Acta Paediatrica* **98**(6):1064–1065.
3. Everett KV, Capon F, Georgoula C, *et al.* (2008) Linkage of monogenic infantile hypertrophic pyloric stenosis to chromosome 16q24. *Eur J Human Genetics* **16**(9):1151–1154.
4. Dillon PW, Cilley RE. (2000) Lesions of the stomach. In: KW Ashcraft, JP Murphy, RJ Sharp, DL Sigalet, CL Snyder (eds.), *Pediatric Surgery*, pp. 391–405. W.B Saunders Company, Pennsylvania.

5. Osifo DO, Evbuomwan I. (2009) Does exclusive breastfeeding confer protection against infantile hypertrophic pyloric stenosis? A 30 year experience in Benin City, Nigeria. *J Trop Pediatr* **55**(2):132–134.
6. Leaphart CL, Borland K, Kane TD, *et al.* (2008) Hypertrophic pyloric stenosis in newborns younger than 21 days: Remodeling the path of surgical intervention. *J Pediatr Surg* **43**(6):998–1001.
7. Keckler SJ, Ostlie DJ, Holcomb III GW, *et al.* (2008) The progressive development of pyloric stenosis: A role of repeat ultrasound. *Eur J Pediatr Surg* **18**(3):168–170.
8. Tan HL, Blyte A, Kirby CP, *et al.* (2009) Gastric foveolar cell hyperplasia and its role in postoperative vomiting in patients with infantile hypertrophic pyloric stenosis. *Eur J Pediatr Surg* **19**(2):76–78.
9. Lacher M, Schneider K, Dalla Pozza R, *et al.* (2007) Gastric outlet obstruction after long term prostaglandin administration mimicking hypertrophic pyloric stenosis. *Eur J Pediatric Surg* **17**(5):362–364.
10. Banieghbal B. (2009) Rapid correction of metabolic alkalosis in hypertrophic pyloric stenosis with intravenous cimetidine: Preliminary results. *Pediatr Surg Int.* **25**(3):269–271.
11. Ladd AP, Nemeth SA, Kirincich AN, *et al.* (2005) Supraumbilical pyloromyotomy: A unique indication for antimicrobial prophylaxis. *J Pediatr Surg* **40**(6):974–977.
12. Gauderer MW. (2008) Experience with a nonlaparoscopic, transumbilical, intracavitary pyloromyotomy. *J Pediatr Surg* **43**(5):884–888.
13. Sola JE, Neville HL. (2009) Laparoscopic vs open pyloromyotomy: A systematic review and meta-analysis. *J Pediatr Surg* **44**(8):2434–2435.
14. Tander B, Shanti CM, Klein MD. (2009) Access to the hypertrophic pylorus: Does it make a difference to the patient? *Eur J Pediatric Surg* **19**(1):14–16.
15. Hall NJ, Pacilli M, Eaton S, *et al.* (2009) Recovery after open versus laparoscopic pyloromyotomy for pyloric stenosis: A double-blind multicentre randomized controlled trial. *Lancet.* **373**(9661):390–398.
16. Campbell BT, McVay MR, Lerer TJ, *et al.* (2007) Ghosts in the machine: A multi-institutional comparison of laparoscopic and open pyloromyotomy. *J Pediatr Surg* **42**(12):2026–2029.
17. St Peter SD, Holcomb III GW, Calkins CM, *et al.* (2006) Open versus laparoscopic pyloromyotomy for pyloric stenosis: A prospective, randomized trial. *Ann Surg* **244**(3):363–370.
18. St Peter SD, Tsao K, Sharp SW, *et al.* (2008) Predictors of emesis and time to goal intake after pyloromyotomy: Analysis from a prospective trial. *J Pediatr Surg* **43**(11):2038–2041.

19. Safford SD, Pietrobon R, Safford KM, *et al.* (2005) A study of 11,003 patients with hypertrophic pyloric stenosis and the association between surgeon and hospital volume and outcomes. *J Pediatr Surg* **40**(6):967–972.
20. Singh UK, Kumar R, Prasad R. (2005) Oral atropine sulfate for infantile hypertrophic pyloric stenosis. *Indian Pediatric* **42**(5):473–476.
21. Kawahara H, Takama Y, Yoshida H, *et al.* (2005) Medical treatment of infantile hypertrophic pyloric stenosis: Should we always slice the "olive"? *J Pediatr Surg* **40**(12):1848–1851.
22. Meissner PE, Engelmann G, Troeger J, *et al.* (2006) Conservative treatment of infantile hypertrophic pyloric stenosis with intravenous atropine sulfate does not replace pyloromyotomy. *Pediatr Surg Int* **22**(12):1021–1024.

DUODENAL ATRESIA 52

Frederick J. Rescorla

INTRODUCTION

Duodenal atresia represents one of the most common causes of neonatal intestinal obstruction accounting for approximately one in 10,000 live births. More than 50% of affected neonates have associated anomalies with Trisomy 21 occurring in approximately 30% of these children.

PATHOPHYSIOLOGY

Etiology

The etiology of duodenal atresia is felt to be a failure of recanalization of the fetal duodenum. The duodenum is initially in a solid phase and recanalization or vacuolization occurs during the 11th week of gestation. Failure of this recanalization process leads to either a web or a complete atresia. In addition, associated defects, such as annular pancreas, preduodenal portal vein or associated malrotation can lead to obstruction at this site. The pancreas develops from a ventral and dorsal bud with the ventral pancreas normally rotating around the duodenum to the more dorsal location. In annular pancreas the ventral pancreas becomes fixed to the duodenal wall forming a ring like structure around the second portion of the duodenum. In cases of annular pancreas the biliary tree is often abnormal with the bile duct entering proximal or distal to the atresia. Other biliary abnormalities can include biliary atresia which we have seen at our institution as well as choledochal cysts.

Classification

Duodenal stenosis can be related to annular pancreas in the absence of a complete atresia thus leading to a stenosis which may present later in life. A complete atresia is classified as type I, which accounts for more than 90% of all atresias in which a diaphragm occludes the lumen. Within this there is the "windsock" defect in which the membrane dilates and passes distally thus dilating the more distal duodenum and making it somewhat difficult to determine the exact level of the obstruction. This is of particular interest to the surgeon in making sure that the anastomosis is actually proximal and distal to the actual membrane. Type II atresias are connected by a fibrous cord and type III atresia has a gap between the two duodenal segments. The obstruction is classified as preampullary, in which the membrane is proximal to the ampulla of Vater or postampullary accounting for 85% of obstructions in which the membrane is distal to the ampulla of Vater, thus making the emesis green. The bowel distal to the obstruction is decompressed with the exception of the windsock deformity, as noted above, in which the distal bowel is dilated for a variable length from the windsock.

Associated Defects

Over half of the children with duodenal atresia have associated congenital anomalies with approximately 30% having Trisomy 21. Many of these will have associated cardiac defects including a endocardial cushion defect or atrioventricular (AV) canal. Twenty five percent have associated gastrointestinal (GI) anomalies including annular pancreas and malrotation. In addition, nearly half of these children are born prematurely. Approximately 8% have esophageal atresia and TEF.

CLINICAL PRESENTATION

With the advent of increased prenatal ultrasonography, detection of duodenal atresia *in-utero* has increased significantly. In cases with complete obstruction, polyhydramnios occurs in 30% to 80% of cases. Prenatal ultrasound in these cases may detect two fluid filled structures representing the stomach and proximal duodenum. Most of these are detected at the 7th or 8th month of gestation. After birth, the stomach may be noted with a large amount of fluid which is bilious in approximately 85% of the cases due to the postampullary nature of the obstruction. If this is not noted at birth, emesis which again is often bilious, is noted within the first few hours of life in an otherwise healthy child. Abdominal distention is usually not a predominant feature due to the proximal nature and the fact that a large percentage of the stomach empties with emesis.

DIAGNOSIS

Plain abdominal films usually demonstrate the classic double bubble sign with no distal gas. The larger left sided bubble represents the air and fluid filled stomach and the right sided smaller bubble represents the dilated duodenum. The distal bowel is usually gasless. Some institutions perform an upper GI contrast study to rule out malrotation and volvulus, however we usually do not do this at our institution unless air is noted distal to the duodenum. If distal air past the two bubbles is identified an emergent upper GI contrast study should be performed to evaluate for possible malrotation and midgut volvulus.

MANAGEMENT

Initial Management

Emergent surgery is usually not required unless there is concern for malrotation and volvulus. Stabilization with maintenance fluids and further studies are obtained prior to surgery. An echocardiogram is generally performed to evaluate for the associated cardiac defects. In the presence of an AV canal, appropriate cardiology consultation should be obtained prior to repair of the duodenal atresia.

Operative Management

Gastrojejunostomy and duodenojejunostomy have been performed in the past however these techniques are not currently utilized. Gastrojejunostomy is associated with a high incidence of marginal ulceration and bleeding. Duodenojejunostomy left the possibility of a blind loop syndrome as a postoperative complication. Duodenoduodenostomy is the preferred method of reconstruction with the diamond shaped anastomosis the most common procedure currently utilized. Other possibilities include a side-to-side duodenostomy or partial web incision with a Heineke–Mikulicz type duodenoplasty.

If the surgeon should choose for a partial web incision and a Heineke–Mikulicz procedure care should be taken to make sure that the ampulla of Vater is not injured. The ampulla may enter on the web or just proximal or distal and compression of the gallbladder usually allows identification of bile flow into the duodenum and injury can usually be avoided.

The procedure can be performed in an open technique through a right upper quadrant supraumbilical incision or laparoscopically. Upon entry into the abdomen malrotation should be carefully looked for as it is associated in up to 30% of infants and should be corrected at the initial operation. Annular pancreas or preduodenal portal vein can also be indentified at the initial exploration. The hepatic flexure of the colon is mobilized bringing the ascending and transverse colon to the left side thus exposing the entire duodenum. The duodenum is mobilized with a Kocher procedure and the distal duodenum should be mobilized to ensure adequate visualization of the distal bowel.

The intrinsic blockage usually occurs at the junction between the first and second portion of the duodenum in 85% of cases, with a type I membrane, or windsock in 90% of cases. Type II (fibrous cord) represents approximately 1% of cases and type III (complete separation) 7% of total cases. A second associated atresia is present in approximately in 3.5% of cases.

The proximal duodenum is dilated and can be mobilized and brought down to the more distal duodenum. A tapering duodenoplasty has been reported however we have not utilized this at the initial operation as the proximal duodenal dilatation usually resolves after relief of the obstruction. If muscular continuity is noted, there is usually a web or diaphragm or perhaps the "windsock" deformity. The proximal and distal duodenum are opened with the proximal duodenum opened in a transverse direction and the distal in a longitudinal fashion. An interrupted one or two layer anastomosis of 4/0 or 5/0 silk suture or absorbable suture can be utilized for the anastomosis. Many surgeons utilizing a laparoscopic technique, use Nitinol U-clips (Medtronic, Minneapolis, Minnesota) to create the anastomosis. The advantage of the U-clip is that it allows a faster anastomosis without intracorporal suturing in a very small space.

In cases with a preduodenal portal vein, the vein is usually proximal to the obstruction and can be left in place without any further procedure. In cases of annular pancreas the anastomosis should occur from the proximal duodenum to the duodenum distal to the level of the pancreas, with no attempt to divide the pancreas. The incisions in the bowel should be approximately 1.5 cm in length. Once the two ends of the bowel are open it is important to pass a catheter distally and inject saline to evaluate for a distal duodenal or associated jejunoileal atresia. The anesthesiologist advances the oral gastric catheter to ensure that the surgeon can identify it proximally to make sure that they truly have identified and opened the bowel proximal and distal to the atresia. This can be somewhat confusing in cases of the windsock, in which the dilated duodenum (with the windsock within it) gives the appearance of proximal bowel when in fact it is actually distal to the membrane.

If malrotation is encountered the duodenojejunal bands should be taken down with mobilization of the ascending colon to the left side of the abdomen placing the cecum in the left lower quadrant. The appendix is generally removed due to the difficulty in diagnosing appendicitis at a later date should it occur.

POSTOPERATIVE MANAGEMENT

An oral gastric tube is left place to decompress the stomach. The return of bowel function can sometimes take longer than neonates with jejunoileal atresia and this may be due to lack of motility in the dilated duodenum. Normal function through the anastomosis usually occurs by 7–14 days after surgery. If prolonged dysfunction does occur, total parental nutrition may be needed. If bowel function does not return by 3 wks, an upper GI contrast study should be performed to evaluate the anatomy. Some surgeons have utilized a nasal jejunal tube placed at the time of the original operation to allow early postoperative feeding.

Outcomes

The current survival for duodenal atresia is approximately 95%. Complications related to the procedure are very unusual and associated cardiac defects or complications related to prematurity can occasionally lead to significant morbidity and mortality. Late duodenal obstruction after an initial successful procedure is very rare. We have seen several cases of prolonged proximal dilatation with ineffective peristalsis leading to symptoms later in life and there may be a small percentage in need of a proximal tapering procedure at an older age. In performing this procedure an indwelling tube can be advanced into the duodenum and an antimesenteric procedure performed with the stapling device, taking care to avoid narrowing the duodenum.

REFERENCES

1. Bax NM, Ure, van der Zee DC, van Tuijl I. (2001) Laparoscopic duodenoduodenostomy for duodenal atresia. *Surg Endosc* **15**:217.
2. Escobar MA, Ladd AP, Grosfeld JL, *et al.* (2004) Duodenal atresia and stenosis: Long-term follow-up care over 30 years. *J Pediatr Surg* **39**:867.
3. Kimura K, Mukohara N, Nishijuma E, *et al.* (1990) Diamond-shaped anastomosis for duodenal atresia: An experience with 44 patients over 15 years. *J Pediatr Surg* **25**:977.
4. Weber TR, Lewis JE, Mooney D, Connors R. (1986) Duodenal atresia: A comparison of techniques of repair. *J Pediatr Surg* **21**:1133.

JEJUNOILEAL ATRESIA AND STENOSIS

53

Jay L. Grosfeld

INCIDENCE

Jejunoileal atresia (JI) and stenosis is a major cause of neonatal intestinal obstruction. *Atresia* refers to a complete occlusion of the intestinal lumen (95% of cases) and s*tenosis* is a partial intraluminal occlusion, resulting in an incomplete intestinal obstruction (5%). The incidence of JI ranges from one in 330 (United States) and one in 400 (Denmark) live births to one in 1500 live births.[1,2] A higher prevalence is observed in African-American children and among twins. An increased risk of atresia is noted in progeny of mothers using pseudoephedrine, acetaminophen, ergotamine tartrate and caffeine (Cafergot) during pregnancy.[3,4]

Of 387 cases of intestinal atresia and stenosis treated at the Riley Children's Hospital, Indianapolis, IN 194 were jejunoileal, 169 duodenal, and 24 colonic. In JI-atresia, boys and girls were equally affected. The mean birth weight was 2.7 kg (range 0.9 to 4.8 kg), however, ⅓ of infants with jejunal atresia, ¼ with ileal atresia, and >½ of those with multiple atresias were of low birthweight. Trisomy 21 is relatively uncommon in patients with JI-atresia.[5]

ETIOLOGY

Although mucosal atresia is frequently noted in duodenal atresia, JI as a result of epithelial plugging is uncommon. Most JI-atresias are separated by a cordlike segment or a V-shaped mesenteric gap defect and are the result of a late intrauterine mesenteric vascular catastrophe. Frequent clinical instances of intestinal atresia as a result of vascular insults such as volvulus, intussusception, internal hernia, and constriction of the mesentery in a tight gastroschisis or omphalocele defect have been observed. Macroscopic or microscopic intrauterine peritonitis is often noted. Iatrogenic postpartum ileal atresia as a result of umbilical clamping of an occult omphalocele and the occurrence of JI-atresia with infarction of the entire midgut in a tight gastroschisis defect is occasionally seen. Most infants with JI-atresia are full-term babies without associated malformations and have a cord or gap type of atresia. In the 194 patients with JI-atresia or stenosis treated at Riley Children's Hospital, volvulus was detected in 64, malrotation in 32, intussusception in five, internal hernia in two, gastroschisis in 28, and evidence of meconium peritonitis in 24.[5] In rare instances, JI-atresia has been observed to coexist with biliary atresia, duodenal atresia, colon atresia, gastric atresia, Hirschsprung's disease, and arthrogryposis. Hereditary multiple intestinal atresias due to an autosomal recessive transmission have been reported. Instances of familial atresia with renal dysplasia inherited as an autosomal dominant trait and multiple atresias associated with graft-versus-host disease and immunosuppression and cases of multiple atresias with severe immunodeficiency characterized by agammaglobulimemia, B-cell deficiency and impaired T-cell function have rarely been noted.[6–10]

DIAGNOSIS

Clinical Presentation

The pertinent signs of JI-atresia include maternal polyhydramnios, bilious vomiting, abdominal distention, jaundice, and failure to pass meconium on the first day of life. Polyhydramnios (24% of cases) is more common in instances of proximal jejunal atresia. Bilious vomiting is slightly more common in jejunal atresia (84%), whereas abdominal distention is more frequently noted in cases of ileal atresia (98%). Jaundice occurs in 32% with jejunal atresia and 20% with ileal atresia and is associated with an elevation of indirect bilirubin.[1] Although most infants fail to pass meconium in the first 24hrs of life, occasionally meconium and necrotic tissue may be passed per rectum. Proximal jejunal atresia may be associated with upper abdominal distention. More generalized distention usually denotes a low obstruction (e.g. distal small bowel) in which many loops of bowel are filled with air proximal to the level of obstruction. *Intestinal patterning* characterized by visible loops of bowel (occasionally with peristaltic waves) may be noted on the abdominal wall during physical examination. Although distention usually develops 12 to 24 hrs after birth, abdominal distention noted immediately at birth suggests the presence of giant cystic meconium peritonitis.[11,12]

Prenatal Ultrasound Findings

Prenatal ultrasonography in mothers with polyhydramnios has identified small-bowel obstruction associated with atresia, volvulus, and meconium peritonitis. Antenatal diagnosis of small bowel atresia is suspected by the appearance of multiple distended loops of bowel with vigorous peristalsis. Intestinal atresia is also suspected in fetuses with gastroschisis with intestinal dilatation on prenatal ultrasound examination. Although the appearance of echogenic bowel on prenatal ultrasound studies is frequently associated with a gastrointestinal malformation, only 31% of patients with small bowel atresias are diagnosed on prenatal ultrasonography. Abnormalities are more frequently detected when ultrasound scanning is performed later in pregnancy and may be missed if the pregnant mother receives only one scan in the 16th week of gestation. When recognized, the atresia is more often in a proximal location. Prenatal ultrasonography has a relatively poor predictive value for bowel abnormalities and remains a somewhat unreliable method of either detecting or excluding a fetal gastrointestinal malformation. Early studies concerning fetal Magnetic Resonance Imaging (MRI) indicate this may be more accurate than ultrasound in the prenatal diagnosis of bowel atresia.[4]

Radiographic Findings

The diagnosis of JI-atresia is usually confirmed by radiographic examination of the abdomen. Erect and recumbent abdominal radiographs are obtained in each case. Thumb-sized intestinal loops (*rule of thumb*) and air-fluid levels are highly suggestive of neonatal intestinal obstruction. High jejunal atresia may present with a few air-fluid levels and no further gas beyond that point. The more distal the atresia, the greater the number of distended intestinal loops and air-fluid levels seen on the abdominal radiograph. The site of atresia may appear as a larger loop with a significant air-fluid level. Peritoneal calcification is seen in 12% of cases and signifies the presence of meconium peritonitis, a sign of intrauterine intestinal perforation. Rarely, instances of intraluminal calcification (*mummification*) may be observed, suggesting an antenatal volvulus. In giant cystic meconium peritonitis, plain radiographs of the abdomen demonstrate a large air-fluid level in a meconium pseudocyst. This is related to a late intrauterine perforation, resulting in an encapsulated mass (pseudocyst) containing meconium.[12]

The newborn infant rarely demonstrates colonic haustral markings on a plain abdominal radiograph, which may simply show dilated loops of intestine without actually differentiating between the small and large bowel. A barium enema should be performed in each instance of suspected neonatal intestinal obstruction. The first enema the infant receives should be the contrast enema, which serves three purposes: (1) To distinguish between small- and large-bowel distention, (2) To determine if the colon is used or unused (*microcolon*), and (3) To locate the position of the cecum in regard to possible anomalies of intestinal rotation and fixation. The majority of infants with JI-atresia demonstrate a microcolon, which usually limits the obstruction to the distal small intestine. Microcolon is related to the fact that little succus entericus has passed the area of obstruction in the distal fetal small intestine, and the unused colon does not distend (Figure 1). Rarely, however, the colon may appear of normal caliber if the intrauterine vascular catastrophe leading to atresia occurred extremely late in gestation.

There is usually no indication to perform upper gastrointestinal contrast studies in instances of complete obstruction. In cases of intestinal stenosis, however, with an incomplete obstruction this study may prove quite useful.

Differential Diagnosis

Newborns with intestinal obstruction from other causes may present with a clinical picture similar to that of infants with JI-atresia. These include cases of malrotation with or without volvulus, meconium ileus, intestinal duplication, internal hernia, colonic atresia, adynamic ileus related to sepsis, and total colonic aganglionosis. The contrast barium enema often yields valuable information that frequently rules out certain causes of obstruction, particularly colonic atresia and low segment aganglionosis. JI-atresia may coexist with malrotation (10–18%), meconium peritonitis (12%), meconium ileus (9–12%), total colonic aganglionosis and rarely intestinal neuronal dysplasia,

Radiographic findings

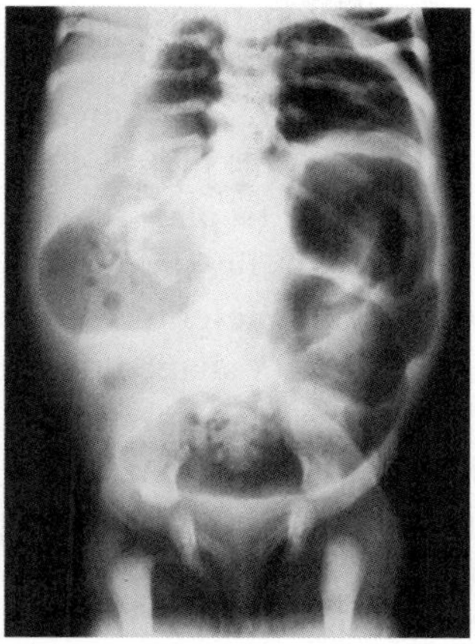

Plain radiograph shows distended bowel loops with A/F levels

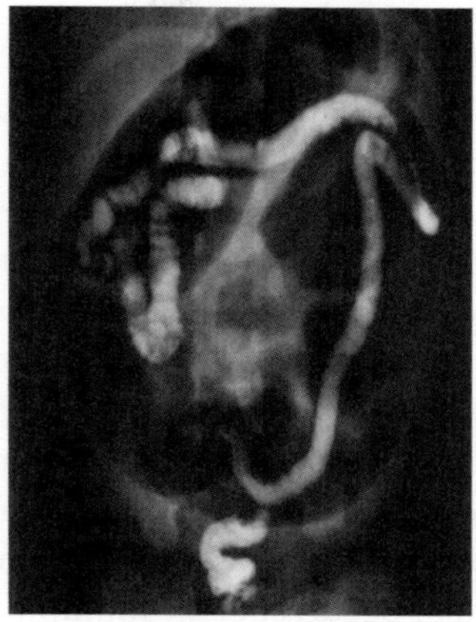

Ba-enema shows, mirocolon, small bowel distension, malrotation with cecum in RUQ

Figure 1.

so that a clear differentiation is not always possible. A careful family history regarding cystic fibrosis may permit preoperative identification of infants with meconium ileus.[1]

Infants with uncomplicated meconium ileus often have dilation of bowel loops of similar size and few, if any, air-fluid levels. The meconium in these patients is extremely viscid and fails to layer out as an air-fluid interface. A *ground-glass appearance* (Neuhauser's sign) or the *soap-bubble sign* of Singleton may be observed in the right lower quadrant and represents viscid meconium mixed with air. Careful evaluation of these patients may avoid an unnecessary operation because at least half of the uncomplicated cases of meconium ileus respond to nonoperative therapy in the form of a diatrizoate (Gastrografin) enema (see Chapter 55) Instances of meconium ileus complicated by atresia, volvulus, or gangrenous bowel require operative intervention, and the appropriate diagnosis is made at the time of laparotomy. Occasionally, instances of colonic atresia may also present with a soap-bubble appearance in the atretic segment on the plain abdominal radiograph.[13,14]

Pathologic Findings

Atresias of the small intestine are equally distributed between jejunum (51%) and the ileum (49%). The atresia is usually single (90%) but may be multiple in 6% to 20% of cases. Multiple atresias more often involve the proximal jejunum. The classification of JI has changed only slightly since the early observations of Louw. Type I referred to a mucosal (septal) atresia with an intact bowel wall and mesentery. Type II has two atretic blind ends connected by a band of fibrous tissue (cord) and an intact mesentery, and type III has the two ends of atretic bowel separated by a gap (V-shaped defect) in the mesentery.[15] Cases of multiple atresias often have foreshortened intestine and are associated with prematurity and a high mortality. At operation, there is a *string*-of-beads or *string-of sausages* appearance. Multiple atresias occur in 14% of cases and as many as 25 separate atresias have been noted. Familial occurrence of multiple atresias affecting the stomach, duodenum, small bowel, and colon may be the expression of a rare autosomal recessive gene associated with an IgM deficiency that eventually is fatal.

Another unusual group of patients with JI-atresia are those with an *apple-peel* or *Christmas-tree* deformity. They present with jejunal atresia near the ligament of Treitz, foreshortened bowel, a large mesenteric gap defect, and the blood supply to the bowel distal to the atresia is precariously supplied in a retrograde fashion by anastomotic arcades from the ileocolic, right colic, or inferior mesenteric artery. Patients with this distinct variation of atresia may have a familial pattern, are often of low birthweight (70%), premature (70%), have malrotation (54%), and an increased number of associated anomalies.[13,14]

Grosfeld *et al.* modified the classification in 1979 to retain the previous nomenclature of Louw, add apple-peel atresia as a special form of type III (IIIb), and consider multiple atresias as type IV (Figure 2). This latter classification has generally been accepted to describe JI-atresias for the past 30 yrs.[16]

MANAGEMENT/TREATMENT

During initial evaluation, the infant is maintained in a warm humidified environment (an Isolette or under an overhead warmer) to avoid hypothermia. An orogastric tube (10 Fr) is passed and the stomach contents are aspirated and presence of bile noted. The tube is placed on drainage to decompress the stomach, and prevent vomiting and further gaseous distention of the obstructed intestine from swallowed air. These precautions also

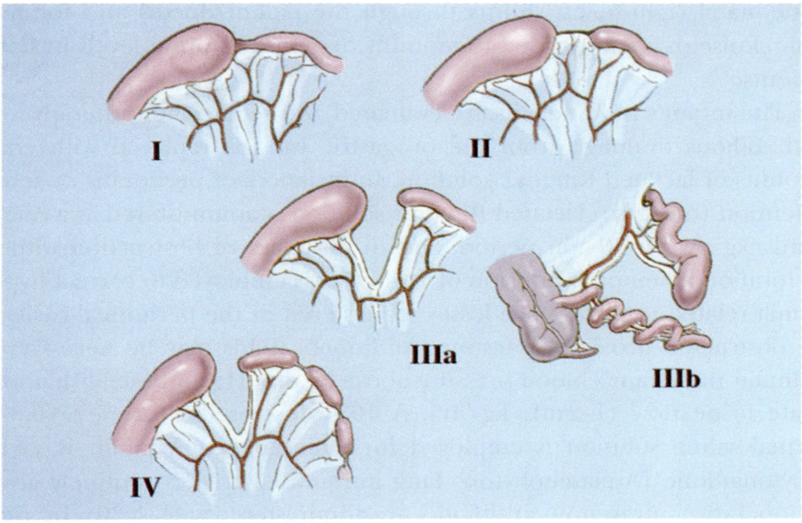

Figure 2. Jejuno-ileal atresia classification.

should be in effect before the infant is evaluated in the radiology department. During transport, the infant should be kept warm and attended by experienced personnel.

The infant's weight is determined, and baseline laboratory data, including complete blood and platelet count, blood urea nitrogen, serum bilirubin, glucose, calcium, pH, blood gas tensions, serum electrolytes, and blood for type and crossmatch are obtained by microtechniques. Urinary volume, specific gravity, and osmolality are measured. The extent of preoperative preparation depends on the delay in diagnosis, the degree of fluid and electrolyte imbalance, severe associated anomalies, and the presence of peritonitis. An intravenous route is established by percutaneous insertion of a short 22 or 24 gauge silicone catheter in the dorsum of the foot or hand. Avoid cutdowns when possible because they are rarely necessary. Percutaneous intravenous central catheter (PICC) lines and central venous catheters used for total parenteral nutrition (TPN) can be inserted percutaneously at a later time if necessary. Routine catheterization of the umbilical vein is avoided because of the increased risk of sepsis. It is used occasionally, however, for short-term exchange transfusion. If the infant has respiratory distress, a percutaneous arterial catheter is inserted into the right radial artery for more accurate PaO_2 monitoring above the level of neonatal right-to-left shunts through the patent ductus and foramen ovale. Pulse oximetry is used to monitor oxygen saturation levels in stable patients.

The infant's fluid deficits are evaluated and replacement therapy initiated. Bilious drainage from the orogastric tube is replaced with equal amounts of lactated Ringer's solution. In instances of peritonitis or severe distention (or both), lactated Ringer's solution is administered at a rate of 20 mL/kg over a 30-min period, and in instances of obstruction without perforation an empiric infusion of 10 mL/kg is employed to correct hypovolemia related to third-space losses sequestered in the peritoneal cavity or the obstructed proximal intestine. Additional fluids may be necessary to maintain the infant's blood pressure above 50 mm Hg and establish appropriate urine flow (1–2 mL/kg/hr). A 10% dextrose in 0.25% or 0.33% normal saline solution is employed for maintenance. Vitamin K_1 oxide (phytonadione [Aquamephyton, 1 mg intramuscularly) is routinely given. Perioperative intravenous antibiotics are administered at least 30 mins prior to surgery (ampicillin 125 mg/kg/day and gentamicin 5 mg/kg/day).

Operating Room Care

After appropriate preparation, the infant is taken to the operating room, and similar precautions concerning transportation and an appropriate thermal environment are observed. The operating room temperature is kept between 75° and 80° F. The patient is placed under a heat lamp on a protected warming blanket, and the limbs are wrapped with soft cotton roll. A small cloth or aluminum lined cap is placed on the baby's head to reduce radiant heat loss. The umbilicus is prepared with a warm iodophor solution and suture ligated after resection of the clamped cord. Patients with bowel obstruction should be intubated while awake to avoid aspiration, and the location of the endotracheal tube should be evaluated by careful auscultation of the chest. A pulse oximeter is useful to monitor oxygen saturation. Monitoring the blood pressure (Doppler), electrocardiogram, pulse rate, and temperature (skin or axillary probe) is routine. Arterial pH and blood gas tensions are acquired as necessary. The anesthetic gases are warmed and humidified to prevent heat loss and drying of the tracheobronchial tree. The abdomen is gently prepared (painted rather than scrubbed) with a warm iodophor (povidone-iodine [Betadine]) solution. Towels are used to drape the abdomen and are held in place with a sterile transparent adhesive iodophor plastic drape which helps maintain body heat. This drape is covered by a pediatric laparotomy sheet with an aperture through which the procedure is carried out.

A right supraumbilical transverse incision allows excellent access to the neonate's peritoneal cavity. A fine-tipped bipolar infant electrocoagulator with fingertip control is used to achieve hemostasis, avoid blood loss and obviate the need for time-consuming clamping and tying during entry. Fluid administration during operation consists of 5 to 10 mL/kg/hr of 5% dextrose in lactated Ringer's solution to replace sequestered tissue fluid losses. Equal volumes of lactated Ringer's solution are administered to replace intraoperative losses from the orogastric tube and any bowel content aspirated during the procedure. Warmed packed red blood cells are transfused if losses are greater than 10% to 15% of the estimated blood volume (80 mL/kg of body weight). Small volume aspiration-collecting systems and close monitoring of sponge weights facilitate these estimates. Blood loss up to 10% to 15% of the estimated blood volume is replaced by infusion of 5% dextrose in lactated Ringer's solution.

Operative Techniques

The operation of choice in JI-atresia and stenosis is related to the pathologic findings and the specific set of circumstances encountered in each case. The decision as to the most appropriate procedure depends on the pathologic type of obstruction (e.g. stenosis or atresias types I, II, IIIa, IIIb, or IV), the presence of malrotation, volvulus, meconium ileus, or variants of meconium peritonitis and the baby's general condition. An additional consideration is in infants with atresia or stenosis associated with gastroschisis or omphalocele, when primary closure of the abdominal wall may present a problem. At operation, the intestine is carefully evaluated, and the proximal and distal ends of the atresia are identified. Gentle evisceration often facilitates inspection. The bowel is carefully inspected so that a complete assessment of the pathologic anatomy is possible. Malrotation, volvulus, or segments of partially resorbed fetal intestine may be noted. A purse-string suture is placed in the distal atretic end of the intestine, and saline (or air) is injected through a 24-gauge venous catheter to rule out an unsuspected distal atretic mucosal membrane or web.[16]

Retention and use of the dilated blind proximal atretic segment of intestine in any type of anastomosis usually results in a functional obstruction.

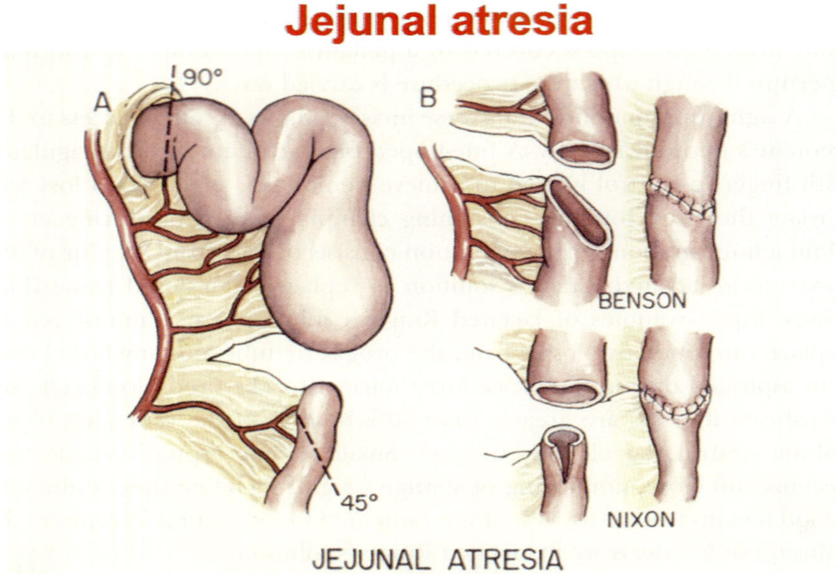

Figure 3. Jejunal atresia repair.

This segment of intestine has ineffective peristalsis and may not allow efficient propulsion following operation. If bowel length is adequate, the proximal dilated atretic segment is resected back to the level where the intestine diameter approaches 1.0 to 1.5 cm (in instances of ileal atresia) or near the ligament of Treitz in instances of proximal jejunal atresia (Figure 3). A Bainbridge infant bowel clamp is applied at a 90° angle on the proximal bowel. A short segment of the distal atretic segment is resected at a 45° angle more distal on the antimesenteric side, and an additional Bainbridge clamp is applied. If there is still a discrepancy in the size of the two lumens, a short antimesenteric incision in the distal atretic intestine alleviates this difference.[17] A two layer interrupted 5–0 silk end-to-oblique anastomosis is then performed (Figure 4). All of the posterior outer layer seromuscular sutures are inserted (usually no more than five) before being tied. The clamps are removed and the crushed tissue trimmed. The posterior inner layer sutures are inserted and brought around anteriorly as an interrupted inverting Connell suture (in-out, out-in) with the knots on the inside. The anastomosis is completed with an outer anterior seromuscular interrupted 5–0 silk Lembert closure. Using 5-0 vicryl or PDS suture for the inner layer and PDS

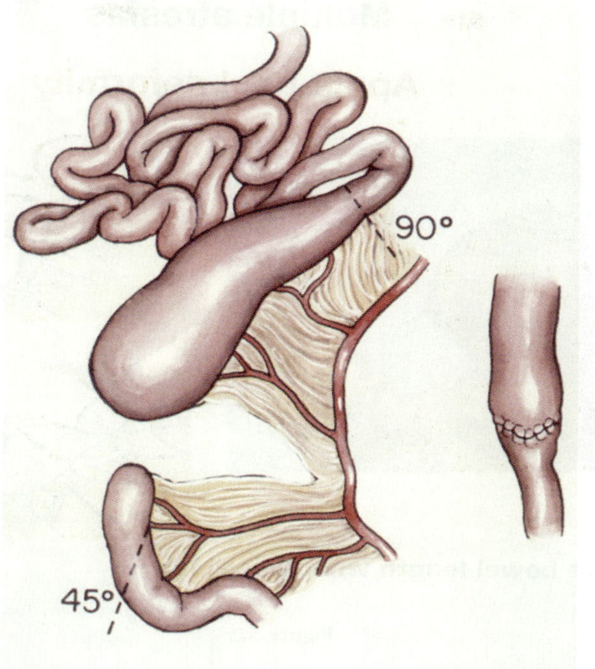

Figure 4. Ileal atresia — end to oblique anastomosis.

for the outer layer can be used as an alternative. Some pediatric surgeons prefer a single layered anastomosis. We have observed a slightly higher leak rate with the single layered technique and stenosis after an interrupted two-layered repair is uncommon. The mesenteric defect is carefully approximated, tucking the longer proximal mesentery to prevent a kink at the anastomosis. An end-to-side ileo-ascending colonic anastomosis may be a reasonable alternative in instances of very distal ileal atresia. The major disadvantage of this procedure however, is bypassing the ileocecal valve. In instances of multiple atresias especially when the bowel length is a problem, an effort is made to preserve as much intestine as possible. Multiple anastomoses may be necessary to accomplish this goal. The decompressed distal atretic segments are usually not dilated and if the lumen is completely patent, resection is unnecessary and a direct anastomosis to the next segment can be performed for type II or III atresias or a transverse enteroplasty for type I mucosal atresias (Figure 5). Intraluminal stenting as a method to

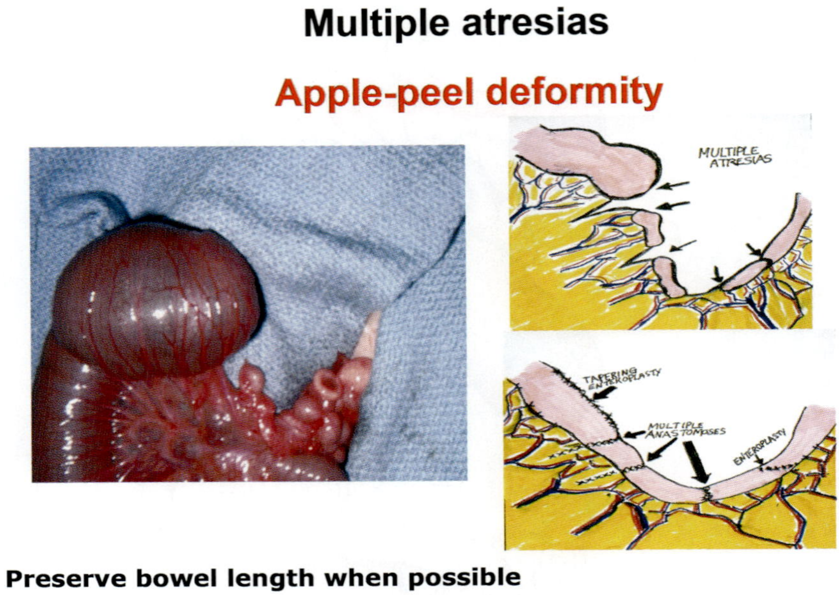

Figure 5.

manage multiple atresias or perforations has been reported however, we have no personal experience with this technique.

Experience has shown that in most cases of proximal jejunal atresia (with adequate length of intestine) resection of the dilated atretic segment near the ligament of Treitz followed by an end-to-oblique anastomosis usually successful. When there is a limited length of remaining intestine (e.g., short gut), an antimesenteric tapering jejunoplasty may be useful.[18] Tapering is accomplished with an autostapling device [US Surgical Corporation, Norwalk, CT] (Figure 6). The most bulbous distal portion of the proximal atretic segment is resected and a 24 to 26 Fr catheter is inserted into the lumen along the mesenteric side. The antimesenteric border of the bowel is then resected between two rows of autostaples up to near the ligament of Treitz. The remaining staple line is oversewn with interrupted 5–0 silk or PDS sutures and the procedure completed by an end-to-oblique anastomosis, as previously described. The dissection and anastomosis are presently performed with the aid of magnifying loupes of

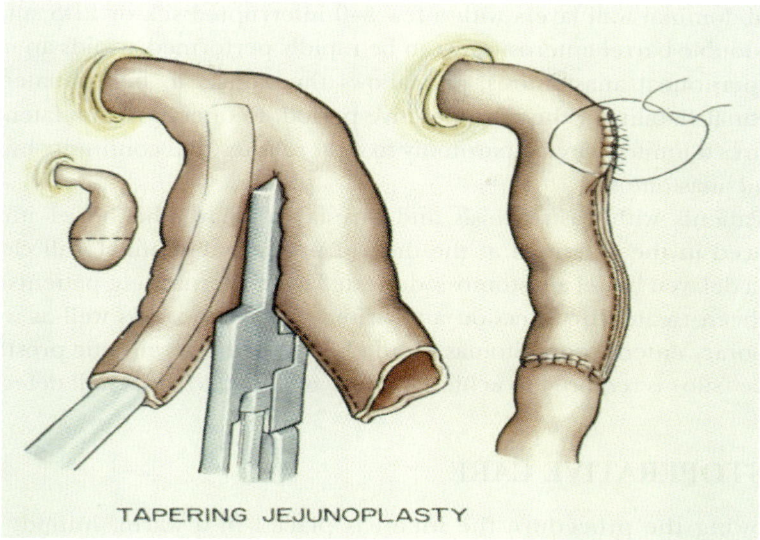

Figure 6. Tapering jejunoplasty.

2.5 to 3 power which allows a much more precise placement of the anastomotic sutures and facilitates the procedure. Intestinal imbrication may also be considered as an effective method to reduce the caliber of distended intestine and restore function.[19] Imbrication preserves the mucosal surface area, but has a tendency to break down with recurrent dilation occurring. The abdominal wall is closed in layers, using continuous 4–0 polyglacten 910 (Vicryl), or PDS on the peritoneum and interrupted inverting 4–0 Vicryl or PDS sutures on the fascial layers. Scarpa's fascia is approximated with a continuous 5–0 Vicryl suture, and the skin edges are approximated with Steri-Strips. A dry sterile dressing is then applied under Op-site adhesive.

Although a primary anastomosis is preferred, it may not be advisable in instances of ileal atresia associated with volvulus when the vascular integrity of the intestine is in question, in severe cases of meconium peritonitis, or in some instances of complicated meconium ileus. In these cases, resection of the atretic ileal segments and exteriorization are carried out. The most expeditious procedure is a side-by-side (modified Mikulicz) double-barrel enterostomy brought out through the wound and fixed to the abdominal wall layers with a few 5–0 interrupted silk or PDS sutures. The double-barrel enterostomy can be rapidly performed, avoids an initial intraperitoneal anastomosis, and allows the stomas to be evaluated for intestinal viability in the postoperative period. Reoperation at a later date requires a limited *target* laparotomy to restore intestinal continuity by end-to-end anastomosis.

Patients with gastroschisis and atresia can have the bowel initially replaced in the abdomen at the time of primary abdominal wall closure with a delayed bowel anastomosis done at 3 wks. Alternatively, patients have also been treated by resection and primary anastomosis as well as with a temporary enterostomy. Stomas should be avoided if a synthetic prosthetic device (silo) is required to achieve closure of the abdominal wall defect.[20,21]

POSTOPERATIVE CARE

Following the procedure the infant is placed in a warm, humid, well-monitored thermoneutral environment. The head of the Isolette/bed is elevated at 30 degrees. Maintenance fluids (10% dextrose in 0.25% or 0.33% normal saline) are administered at 80–100 mL/kg/day. Potassium chloride (2 to 3 mEq/kg/day) is also infused, not in excess of 40 mEq/L. Losses related to orogastric tube drainage are replaced equally with 0.45% normal saline in 5% dextrose and water if the drainage fluid is clear (gastric juice) and by 5% dextrose and water in lactated Ringer's solution if it is green (intestinal drainage). Intravenous infusions should contain vitamins B and C, required for wound healing. Occasionally an additional fluid bolus to counteract excessive third-space losses may be required. A urine output of 40 to 50 mL/kg/day, specific gravity of 1.005 to 1.015, and weight stability usually indicate appropriate hydration. The infant's glucose levels, acid-base balance, and serum bilirubin levels are closely monitored to avoid hypoglycemia, acidosis, and kernicterus. Serum electrolyte values are obtained daily for the first few postoperative days.

Antibiotics are discontinued after 24 hrs except in instances of atresia associated with peritonitis. When the infant has spontaneous bowel motions and the gastric drainage fluid is clear and of minimal volume, the orogastric tube is elevated as a *burp tube*. If no excessive gastric or intestinal reflux occurs, the tube is removed, and clear liquids are initiated (Pedialyte) at 0.5 oz every 3 hrs and advanced in volume, and then a half-strength and finally a full-strength low osmolar small-curd formula (Isomil) is given. The newborn requires 120 calories/kg/day to grow. Lactose intolerance is a frequent problem after major bowel resection, and milk-curd obstruction of the small intestinal anastomosis may occur if a large-curd formula (Similac or Enfamil) is used initially. Malabsorption and diarrhea may be significant in infants with short bowel length, those in whom the ileocecal valve has been resected, and those with multiple atresias or apple-peel atresia. Formulas that contain long-chain fats should be avoided in these patients. Instead, a medium-chain triglyceride or casein hydrolysate diet (Pregestimil) is offered. Occasionally a carbohydrate-free or an easily absorbable elemental diet such as infant Vivonex may also be useful.

If the aforementioned formulas are not tolerated, TPN with a high-calorie (18% glucose, 2.5% amino-acid) infusion is delivered via a PICC line or a centrally placed Silastic (Broviac) catheter tunneled from the chest wall to the subclavian vein, external or internal jugular vein or cephalic vein and advanced into the superior vena cava. This solution delivers 1 calorie/mL of infusate. In addition, 1–2 gm/kg per day of a 10% intravenous fat solution (Intralipid) should be given. This material is isosmolar, supplies free fatty acids, and delivers an additional 1.1 calorie/mL. High doses of intralipid (ie. 3–4 g/kg/day) may result in cholestasis especially in premature patients and should be avoided.[22] Three-omega fatty acid solutions (Omegaven) may obviate this problem. These measures prevent inanition due to protein–calorie malnutrition in cases of prolonged gastrointestinal tract malfunction and allow time for bowel adaptation to occur. Ninety-four of 194 (49%) infants with JI-atresia at Riley Children's Hospital received TPN. During the postoperative period, all infants with JI-atresia undergo a sweat chloride test and cytogenetic testing for the delta F508 gene mutation to rule out cystic fibrosis, which was present in 12.5% of cases. (See Chapter 55)

Morbidity and Mortality

The most common cause of early death in infants with JI-atresia is infection related to pneumonia, peritonitis, or sepsis. The most significant postoperative complications include functional intestinal obstruction at the site of anastomosis and anastomotic leak. Other contributing factors affecting morbidity and mortality include associated anomalies, respiratory distress, prematurity, short-bowel syndrome, and postoperative bowel obstruction owing to volvulus with bowel infarction. In recent years, most reports concerning JI-atresia describe overall survival rates ranging from 80–90% or greater (Table 1). With the advent of sophisticated neonatal intensive care unit (NICU) care, prematurity is much less of an adverse factor than in previous decades. Operative mortality (at 30 days) was 1.5% with three deaths in 194 cases at the Riley Children's Hospital. Death was related to sepsis and multiple organ failure in two infants with meconium peritonitis and in another to sepsis and respiratory failure in a premature infant. However, 21 late deaths occurred from 3 mths to 8 yrs after initial treatment (overall mortality of 12.5%). Deaths were due to sepsis and multiorgan system failure in 10 patients, including five with short bowel syndrome and three cases of atresia associated with gastroschisis. Three patients with short bowel syndrome developed liver failure related to long-term TPN administration. An additional patient with gastroschisis and bronchopulmonary dysplasia died of progressive respiratory failure. One infant with apple-peel atresia succumbed after a septic episode. One anastomotic leak occurred in an infant with ileal atresia and volvulus. All but one patient with multiple atresias, 9 of 11 infants with apple-peel atresia, and 24 of 28 infants associated with gastroschisis survived. A higher mortality persists in

Table 1. Percent survival of jejunoileal atresia.[1]

Author/year	% of Cases
de Lorimier *et al.*, 1969[19]	68
Nixon and Tawes, 1971	62
Louw, 1967[15]	94
Martin and Zerella, 1976	100
Rescorla and Grosfeld, 1985	90
Smith and Glasson, 1989	78
Touloukian, 1993	91
Dalla Vecchia *et al.*, 1998[5]	84
Hou and Zhang, 1999	82
Sweeney *et al.*, 2001	80
Grosfeld, 2006[1]	88

subsets of patients with familial instances of multiple atresias associated with ill-defined immunodeficiency syndromes.

The aggressive use of TPN as adjunctive therapy has significantly improved the outlook for these infants. Excellent long-term outcomes have been observed even in patients with multiple and apple-peel atresias. TPN avoids protein–calorie malnutrition, establishes positive nitrogen balance, and allows for a relatively safe waiting period in instances of JI-atresia associated with anastomotic dysfunction or gastroschisis. This has also been extremely useful in instances of short-bowel syndrome and in infants with temporary exteriorization procedures who have enterostomy dysfunction. After massive bowel resection, TPN maintains the nutritional needs of the infants while allowing appropriate healing and time for adaptation to occur. Short-bowel syndrome is covered extensively elsewhere in this handbook (see Chapter 62).[23–25] Unfortunately, TPN may be associated with severe cholestasis occasionally resulting in progressive liver disease and subsequent hepatic failure. Two deaths at our institution in the past were related to liver failure associated with TPN.

The Bianchi longitudinal lengthening procedure and serial transverse enteroplasty (STEP) procedure devised by Kim and associates are methods that attempt to increase the bowel length in instances of extreme short bowel syndrome (for details see Chapter 62).[23–25] For patients that fail to adapt, an isolated intestinal transplantation procedure may be an alternative treatment pathway. In those babies that do not adapt and develop TPN related liver failure in addition to their short bowel syndrome, a multivisceral organ transplantation procedure may be life-saving (see Chapter 32) Long-term follow-up of infants treated for JI-atresia in the neonatal period is strongly recommended.

REFERENCES

1. Grosfeld, JL. (2006) Jejunoileal atresia. In: JL Grosfeld, JA O'Neill, EW Fonkalsrud, *et al.* (eds.), *Pediatric Surgery*, 6th edition. Mosby-Elsevier, Philadelphia.
2. Louw JH, Barnard CN. (1055) Congenital intestinal atresia: observations on its origin. *Lancet* **2**:1065–1067.
3. Basu R, Burge DM. (2004) The effect of antenatal diagnosis on the management of small bowel atresia. *Pediatr Surg Int* **20**:177–179.
4. Saguintaah M, Couture A, Veyrac C, Baud C. (2002) MRI of the fetal intestinal tract. *Pediatr Radiol* **32**:395–404.

5. Dalla Vecchia L, Grosfeld JL, West KW, *et al.* (1998) Intestinal atresia and stenosis: a 25 year experience with 277 cases. *Arch Surg* **133**:490–496.
6. Fourcade L, Shima H, Miyazaki E, Puri, P. (2001) Multiple gastrointestinal atresias result from disturbed morphogenesis. *Pediatr Surg Int* **17**:361–364.
7. Guttman FN, Braun P, Garance PH, *et al.* (1973) Multiple atresias and a new syndrome of hereditary multiple atresias involving the gastrointestinal tract from stomach to rectum. *J Pediatr Surg* **8**:633–640.
8. Bilodeau A, Prasil O, Cloutier R, *et al.* (2004) Hereditary multiple intestinal atresia: 30 years later. *J Pediatr Surg* **39**:726–730.
9. Moreno LA, Gottrand F, Tvack D, *et al.* (1990) Severe combined immunodeficiency syndrome associated with autosomal recessive familial multiple gastrointestinal atresia. Study of a family. *Am J Med Genet* **37**:143–146.
10. Rothenberg ME, White FV, Chilmonczyk B, Chatila T. (1995) A syndrome involving immunodeficiency and multiple intestinal atresias. *Immunodeficiency* **5**:171–178.
11. Blyth H, Dickson JAS. (1969) Apple-peel syndrome (congenital intestinal atresia): A family study of 7 index patients, *J Med Genet* **6**:275–277.
12. Careskey JM, Grosfeld JL, Weber TR, Malangoni MA. (1982) Giant cystic meconium peritonitis (GCMP): Improved survival based on clinical and laboratory observations, *J Pediatr Surg* **17**:482–489.
13. Festen S, Brevoord JC, Goldhoorn GA, *et al.* (2002) Excellent long-term outcome for survivors of apple peel atresia. *J Pediatr Surg* **37**:61–65.
14. Ros Mar Z, Diez Pardo JA, Ros Miquel M, Benavent I. (1980) Apple-peel small bowel: a review of 12 cases, *Z Kinderchir Grenzgeb* **29**:313–317.
15. Louw JH. (1967) Resection and end-to-end anastomosis in the management of atresia and stenosis of the small bowel. *Surgery* **62**:940–950.
16. Grosfeld JL, Ballantine TVN, Shoemaker R. (1979) Operative management of intestinal atresia and stenosis based on pathologic findings, *J Pediatr Surg* **14**:368–375.
17. Howard ER, Othersen HB. (1973) Proximal jejunoplasty in the treatment of jejunal atresia. *J Pediatr Surg* **8**:685–690.
18. Weber TR, Vane DW, Grosfeld JL. (1982) Tapering enteroplasty in infants with bowel atresia and short gut. *Arch Surg* **117**:684–688.
19. de Lorimier AA, Harrison MR. (1983) Intestinal imbrication in the treatment of atresia. *J Pediatr Surg* **18**:734–737.
20. Molik KA, Gingalewski CA, West KW, *et al.* (2001) Gastroschisis: a plea for risk categorization. *J Pediatr Surg* **36**:51–55.

21. Snyder CL, Miller KA, Sharp RJ, *et al.* (2001) Management of intestinal atresia in patients with gastroschisis. *J Pediatr Surg* **36**:1542–1544.
22. Quiros-Tejeira RE, Ament ME, Reyen L, *et al.* (2004) Long-term parenteral nutritional support and intestinal adaptation in children with short bowel syndrome. a 25 year experience. *J Pediatr* **145**:157–163.
23. Bianchi A. (1999) Experience with intestinal lengthening and tailoring. *Eur J Pediatr Surg* **9**:256–259.
24. Kim HB, Fauza D, Garza J, *et al.* (2003) Serial transverse enteroplasty (STEP): a novel bowel lengthening procedure. *J Pediatr Surg* **38**:425–429.
25. Bueno J, Guiterrez J, Mazariegos GV, *et al.* (2001) Analysis of patients with longitudinal lengthening procedure referred for intestinal transplantation. *J Pediatr Surg* **36**:178–183.

MALROTATION 54

Kristen A. Zeller and Frederick J. Rescorla

CLINICAL PRESENTATION

The hallmark presentation of malrotation that of bilious emesis in the newborn is always a surgical emergency until proven otherwise. The onset of symptoms in the newborn is typically acute. Bilious emesis is the most common presenting symptom, but others include coffee ground emesis, abdominal distention, pain, and bloody stools. Approximately half of patients with malrotation present in the newborn period, and a majority present within the first year of life. Although less common, malrotation may be diagnosed in older children and adults, often after an evaluation for vague abdominal complaints such as pain, feeding intolerance, malabsorption, intermittent vomiting, chronic diarrhea, or failure to thrive. Malrotation may be diagnosed incidentally when imaging studies are obtained for other purposes, such as a Computed Tomography (CT) scan of the abdomen and pelvis for trauma. At the opposite end of the spectrum, malrotation may present *in utero*, resulting in prenatal volvulus and atresias or even fetal demise.

PATHOPHYSIOLOGY

Incidence

The true incidence of malrotation is unknown. The term "malrotation" actually represents a spectrum of disorders of intestinal rotation, some of which may remain asymptomatic. Although malrotation is commonly reported to have an incidence of 1 in 500 live births, the incidence of clinically significant cases is estimated to be approximately one in 6,000 patients. For patients who present in the neonatal period, there is a 2:1 male predominance and an equal incidence in males and females who present beyond 1 yr of age. Malrotation may also present in combination with a variety of other anomalies. By definition, patients with gastroschisis and omphalocele are also malrotated, as the intestines do not properly return to the peritoneal cavity and therefore fail to undergo the normal embryological fixation of the root of the mesentery. Most patients with congenital diaphragmatic hernia have malrotation due to displacement of the intestines into the chest. Patients with complex congenital heart disease and heterotaxy are also at higher risk for coexistent malrotation.

Embryology

An understanding of normal embryologic development is essential in the comprehension of malrotation. During the fourth week of development, the midgut is a straight tube which derives its blood supply from the superior mesenteric artery (SMA). Physiologic herniation of the midgut through the umbilical ring occurs at about 6 wks. During this time, the bowel grows in length and undergoes a counter-clockwise 270° rotation around the axis of the SMA. Upon completion of the rotation, the fourth portion of the duodenum moves into the left upper quadrant and fixes itself to the retroperitoneum, configuring the characteristic "C-loop". At 10 wks of gestation the intestinal loop returns to the abdominal cavity. Normally, the proximal prearterial limb returns first. As the distal limb (colon) becomes intraabdominal, it moves over the SMA, taking its position to the right of the artery for a 270° counter-clockwise arc. Attachment of the mesentery to the retroperitoneum occurs during the fourth and fifth months of gestation. This results in a broad-based mesentery that extends from the left upper quadrant to the right lower quadrant. A failure of this 270° counter-clockwise rotation will result in a spectrum of anomalies: nonrotation, incomplete rotation, reverse rotation, incomplete fixation, and mesocolic hernias.

Classification

Malrotation actually denotes a spectrum of disorders of embryologic rotation and fixation. These may be broadly categorized as nonrotation, incomplete rotation, and reverse rotation.

Nonrotation: This is characterized by a counter-clockwise rotation of only 180° caused by the distal cecocolic limb entering the abdomen first rather than last. The duodenum descends to the right of the SMA and the cecum is found in the pelvis or left iliac region. This is typically asymptomatic, but a narrow-based mesentery still predisposes to the possibility of volvulus.

Incomplete rotation: This is the classically described malrotation, in which duodenal obstruction is caused by Ladd's bands or volvulus. The duodenum lacks 90° and the cecocolic loop lacks 180° of the normal 270° counter-clockwise rotation.

Reverse rotation: Rather than a 270° counter-clockwise rotation, the bowel makes a 90° clockwise turn upon returning to the peritoneal cavity. This results in the transverse colon lying underneath the duodenum and SMA. This may be associated with partial mesenteric arterial, venous, and lymphatic obstruction. This is found in only 4% of cases.

In the mildest form of this spectrum, rotation occurs normally but there is incomplete fixation of the mesentery to the retroperitoneum. This results in a mobile cecum, subhepatic cecum, or a retrocecal appendix. Increased mobility of the cecum may predispose this portion of the bowel to segmental volvulus.

Mesocolic hernias, also called paraduodenal hernias, result from entrapment of the small bowel behind the mesocolon related to faulty intestinal rotation. A right mesocolic hernia is caused by failure of the prearterial limb to rotate around the SMA, trapping the small bowel in the mesentery of the ascending colon. A left mesocolic hernia results from rotation of the prearterial limb to the left and entrapment of the small bowel in the mesentery of the descending colon.

DIAGNOSIS

The diagnosis of malrotation is based on clinical findings and radiographic imaging. For a newborn presenting with bilious emesis, the initial diagnostic test of choice is a supine and decubitus abdominal radiograph. Findings may range from a normal bowel gas pattern to an obstructive pattern, characterized by dilated loops with air-fluid levels. Some may demonstrate gastric and duodenal distention with a relative paucity of distal bowel gas. Others may have a "double bubble", indicating an obstruction at the level of the duodenum. A characteristic finding in the setting of acute midgut volvulus is a nearly gasless abdomen with a central mass effect. Although not diagnostic, plain films suggestive of volvulus in the clinical setting of a newborn with bilious emesis and an acute abdomen may provide all the information necessary to proceed to the operating room. Most often the presentation is merely suggestive of malrotation, and an emergent upper gastrointestinal (GI) contrast study performed under fluoroscopy by an experienced radiologist is the test of choice for making a definitive diagnosis. In cases of malrotation with midgut volvulus, the contrast will end abruptly with a "bird's beak" in the second or third portion of the duodenum. Four findings characteristic of malrotation without volvulus on the upper GI include displacement of the ligament of Treitz such that it does not cross the midline nor ascend to the level of the gastric antrum, abnormal position of proximal jejunal loops in the right upper quadrant, deformity of the duodenum demonstrating a "bird's beak", "corkscrew", or "coiled" configuration, and incomplete duodenal obstruction, usually at the third portion. Delayed films may demonstrate opacification of the cecum in an abnormal location. Occasionally a contrast enema may be needed to fully understand the anatomy. Abnormal cecal position alone, as demonstrated by delayed upper GI images or contrast enema, is not diagnostic of malrotation. Demonstration of an abnormally positioned ligament of Treitz is necessary for the radiographic diagnosis of malrotation.

Ultrasound has also been found to be helpful in the diagnosis of malrotation. The position of the SMA in relation to the superior mesenteric vein is typically constant — the artery should be anterior and to the left of the vein. Reversal of this orientation is strongly suggestive of malrotation. Also, a "whirlpool sign" identified by ultrasound is indicative of malrotation with a midgut volvulus.

SURGICAL MANAGEMENT

The acuity of presentation dictates the speed with which the patient is taken to the operating room upon diagnosis. For a newborn with the acute onset of bilious emesis, the baby is emergently taken to the operating room, with simultaneous initiation of resuscitative efforts. Impending ischemia of the midgut due to volvulus demands prompt surgical correction. For the older child or adult with chronic symptoms and a diagnosis of malrotation without volvulus, plans for surgical intervention may be made on a semi-elective basis after thoughtful discussion with the patient about their symptoms and the correlation with the radiologic findings.

Operative correction of malrotation as described by Dr. William E. Ladd in 1936 includes counter-clockwise detorsion of the midgut, lysis of the duodenal bands (aka "Ladd's bands"), broadening the base of the mesentery, and appendectomy. The patient is explored through a limited right upper quadrant transverse incision. The initial maneuver performed is a quick evisceration of the bowel to evaluate for midgut volvulus and assess the viability of the intestines. A thorough examination is performed to identify areas of intestinal ischemia or infarction as well as other anomalies such as intestinal atresia. A volvulus, if present, will be identified at the root of the small bowel mesentery. Torsion occurs in a clockwise rotation along the axis of the SMA. Reduction is accomplished by careful counterclockwise rotation of the intestines, relieving both the mesenteric vascular compromise and the closed-loop intestinal obstruction. After the volvulus is addressed and the bowel has had time to reperfuse, necrotic segments of bowel may require resection. Resection is limited to clearly necrotic intestine so that bowel length may be preserved. Creation of an anastomosis vs. an enterostomy is performed as is suitable to the pathology encountered. A second-look laparotomy may also be indicated if sizable lengths of bowel exhibit marginal viability, and utilizing in these cases the "clip and drop" technique of resecting clearly necrotic portions and leaving the marginal bowel closed with clips until a repeat operative evaluation in 24–48 hrs. As short bowel syndrome and subsequent intestinal failure may result from aggressive bowel resections, care should be taken to ensure that no more intestine is resected than is necessary. In some cases, the entire midgut may be found to be frankly necrotic. This finding will necessitate prompt and honest discussions with family, as in most cases this is an unsurvivable situation. The options include comfort measures, which may be the most compassionate treatment available, or consideration of resection with total parenteral nutritional support and subsequent small intestinal transplantation.

After the volvulus is addressed, the next step in management is relief of duodenal compression. Ladd's bands, the peritoneal attachments of the cecum which distort and obstruct the duodenum, must be carefully divided. A generous Kocher maneuver is performed, resulting in anterior, lateral, and posterior mobilization of the duodenum throughout its length. Care is taken to stay close to the duodenum throughout the mobilization to minimize the risk of violating the thin midgut mesentery. Approximately 10% of patients with malrotation also have an associated duodenal stenosis or web, so luminal patency must also be confirmed. If there is any question, this may ruled out by passage of a nasogastric tube through the duodenum and into the jejunum. Next, the base of the mesentery is broadened by incising the peritoneal adhesions that fuse the mesentery to itself. This allows the cecum to be placed in the left lower quadrant and the duodenum aligned down the right paracolic gutter.

Because this positions the appendix in an abnormal location, a patient with surgically treated malrotation would have an atypical presentation of appendicitis. To avoid this possibility, Ladd routinely performed an appendectomy as part of the operation. A standard or inversion appendectomy may be performed. Upon completion of the appendectomy, the viscera are returned to the peritoneal cavity. The right colon is placed in the left paracolic gutter and the duodenum in the right gutter. The duodenum and ileocecal valve are therefore positioned as far apart as possible. While returning the bowel to the abdominal cavity, care is taken to ensure the mesentery remains flat. Some have also proposed fixation of the colon to the left paracolic gutter to help minimize the risk of future volvulus, but there is no data to demonstrate that this is effective.

This operation is typically performed as an open procedure, although there are techniques reported for performing the procedure laparoscopically. There remains debate as to whether the laparoscopic approach equals the open technique.

POSTOPERATIVE MANAGEMENT

Due to the extensive manipulation of the bowel and its mesentery, it is common for patients to have a prolonged postoperative adynamic ileus. A nasogastric tube is recommended for decompression until the return of bowel function. Adequate intravenous access for hydration is necessary. If peripheral access is inadequate or unreliable, a central line may be required. Antibiotics beyond the perioperative period are not necessary unless extensive bowel necrosis or perforation was encountered during the operation. If intestinal length is inadequate to support full enteral nutrition postoperatively, long-term parenteral hyperalimentation may be necessary.

Outcomes

Most patients who undergo surgery for malrotation do well. Survival with resolution of symptoms can be expected for a majority of patients. Mortality rates for operative cases of malrotation range from 3–9%. For those with malrotation but no midgut volvulus, the associated mortality is only 1%. In contrast, the risk of intestinal necrosis requiring resection for those who present with volvulus is 15–30%, and the risk of death approaches 50%. Early deaths are attributed to sepsis and multi-organ system failure, while late deaths result from complications of intestinal failure. The risk of recurrent volvulus cannot be eliminated by a Ladd's procedure. All patients with malrotation carry a lifelong risk of volvulus, although it is greatly minimized after a Ladd procedure is performed. Adhesive bowel obstruction is a more likely postoperative complication.

REFERENCES

1. Bass KD, Rothenberg SS, Chang JH. (1998) Laparoscopic Ladd's procedure in infants with malrotation. *J Pediatr Surg* **33**:279.
2. Mehall JR, *et al.* (2002) Management of typical and atypical intestinal malrotation. *J Pediatr Surg* **37**:1169.
3. Durkin ET, Lund DP, Shaaban AF, Schurr MJ, Weber SM. (2008) Age-related differences in diagnosis and morbidity of intestinal malrotation. *J Am Coll Surg* **206**:658–662.

Distal Bowel Obstruction

MECONIUM ILEUS 55

Frederick J. Rescorla

CLINICAL PRESENTATION

Meconium ileus occurs as a result of abnormally thickened meconium creating a neonatal intestinal obstruction in the terminal ileum. It is generally classified as simple or complicated. In simple meconium ileus, the thick meconium creates a mechanical obstruction within the dilated ileum with associated inspissated pellets of meconium in the distal ileum. These neonates present within the first 1–2 days of life with bilious emesis, abdominal distention and failure to pass meconium. The ileum is distended with the thick abnormal meconium. They often appear normal at delivery but develop abdominal distention over the first 24–48 hrs as swallowed air, initial feedings and intestinal secretions lead to distention of the more proximal small bowel. This is then followed by bilious emesis.

Complicated meconium ileus occurs when the dilated ileal segment undergoes an *in utero* event such as twisting of the dilated ileum or perforation leading to atresia, volvulus, meconium peritonitis or giant cystic meconium peritonitis. Many of these neonates, particularly those with meconium peritonitis and giant cystic meconium peritonitis, often manifest evidence of a bowel obstruction at birth with abdominal distention and bilious gastric aspirate. Neonates with atresia and volvulus usually develop abdominal distention within the first 24 hrs of life.

CYSTIC FIBROSIS AND PATHOPHYSIOLOGY OF MECONIUM ILEUS

The association of inspissated meconium with abnormalities of the pancreas were first described in 1905 and in 1936 the term cystic fibrosis (CF) was introduced. Subsequent studies demonstrated that the abnormal nature of the meconium is due to abnormal mucus production and an abnormal concentrating process of the meconium in the duodenum and proximal small bowel. The resultant meconium ileus is the earliest manifestation of CF.

CF is the most common potentially lethal genetic defect affecting caucasians. It is an autosomal recessive disease with a 5–6% carrier rate affecting approximately 1:1,150 to 1:2,500 live births. The incidence is much lower in African–American and Hispanic populations. The CF gene was localized to the seventh chromosome in 1989. Mutations in the CF transmembrane conductance regulator gene (CFTR) leads to CF. Over 1,000 mutations have been discovered however the most common mutation is the ΔF508 which is responsible for approximately 70% of defective CFTR alleles and 90% of cases of CF in the United States.

The clinical manifestations of CF primarily affect the gastrointestinal and respiratory systems and are related to mucosal obstruction of the exocrine glands. Meconium ileus is the first manifestation of CF in approximately 15–20% of children. In affected families with an affected child with meconium ileus the incidence of subsequent children with meconium ileus is as high as 40% whereas the usual rate with two carrier parents would be 25%. Pulmonary symptoms related to abnormal thick tenacious secretions which obstruct the distal airway and are associated with recurrent infection. The predominant gastrointestinal feature is abnormal pancreatic secretions with pancreatic exocrine insufficiency creating the need for enzyme supplementation. The pancreas progressively develops chronic fibrosis. Rectal prolapse and gallbladder (acalculous and calculous) disease are other gastrointestinal manifestations. Boys with CF are usually infertile due to glandular obstruction of the vas deferens *in utero* leading to involution of the wolfian duct and vas deferens.

DIAGNOSIS AND INITIAL MANAGEMENT

Prenatal ultrasound may demonstrate a hyperechoic mass with dilated small bowel although this has not been shown to be a highly sensitive or specific test. In cases of meconium peritonitis or giant cystic meconium peritonitis, abdominal ascites may offer a clue to prenatal intestinal perforation.

Simple Meconium Ileus

Neonates with simple meconium ileus usually present at 24–48 hrs of age with signs and symptoms of a distal mechanical bowel obstruction. Initial management should include oral gastric decompression, intravenous fluids, laboratory evaluation and broad spectrum antibiotics. The initial differential diagnosis includes Hirschsprung's disease, ileal and colonic atresia, small left colon syndrome, meconium plug syndrome and sepsis.

Two view (supine and decubitis) abdominal films are the first diagnostic study and usually demonstrates dilated bowel often without air fluid levels since the meconium is very thick not allowing an air fluid interface. The air mixed with the thick stool can create a ground glass appearance. If this is noted a contrast enema is indicated (see therapy below).

Complicated Meconium Ileus

Neonates with ileal atresia usually develop abdominal distention within 24 hrs of birth with signs of a distal bowel obstruction. Plain radiographs usually reveal one or two very dilated loops of ileum and the radiographic appearance may not be distinguishable from other etiologies such as colonic atresia or Hirschsprung's disease. A barium enema is the next diagnostic procedure and will reveal a small caliber, microcolon, and if contrast refluxes into the distal ileum, this will also be of small caliber.

Neonates with volvulus or meconium peritonitis are usually noted with distention at birth. Plain films in cases of volvulus demonstrate a very dilated loop. A barium enema reveals a microcolon and is useful to the surgeon to exclude a second distal blockage. Prenatal volvulus with ischemia and perforation leads to meconium peritonitis which may include adhesive meconium peritonitis, meconium ascites or giant cystic meconium peritonitis. Patients with meconium peritonitis frequently develop calcification throughout the abdominal cavity and linear calcifications are often seen with giant cystic meconium peritonitis. These later cases often have a giant pseudocyst that may fill with air shortly after birth with the cavity so large that it is often relatively easy to distinguish from a loop of bowel. If the proximal perforation seals the films may demonstrate minimal bowel gas with evidence of ascites. In general there is no role for non-operative management in neonates with complicated meconium ileus, although there are rare cases with evidence of calcification on radiographs without signs or symptoms of a bowel obstruction in which intestinal continuity has been restored.

NONOPERATIVE MANAGEMENT (SIMPLE MECONIUM ILEUS)

Helen Noblet in 1969 described four neonates with simple meconium ileus successfully treated with full strength Gastrografin enemas, a hyperosmolar (1900 mOsm/L) solution of diatrizoate meglumine with an added wetting agent, 0.1% polysorbate 80 (Tween 80). Three of these children required two enemas and they also all received N-acetylcysteine by oral gastric tube for five days (10% solution, 5 mL). Dr. Noblet's initial criteria for performing the enemas are still relevant today: Adequate intravenous fluid replacement to correct any deficit as well as fluid given postprocedure to allow for the hyperosmolar nature of the Gastrografin; radiographs that demonstrate no volvulus, atresia, perforation, or peritonitis; and, an initial diagnostic enema to exclude other causes of obstruction which also demonstrates the obstructive meconium in the terminal ileum. Most radiologists currently use either dilute Gastrografin or some other agent to perform this procedure. Extreme care must be taken if the agent is hyperosmolar compared with serum. Complications of Gastrografin have included perforation, necrotizing enterocolitis, shock and death.

A summary report of the use of Gastrografin revealed a success rate of 55% with a 9.6% incidence of perforation. A survey of the Society for Pediatric Radiology noted a success rate of 62% with a perforation of 2.75 %. This later study noted a higher success rate with Gastrografin vs. none Gastrografin agents, however there were no differences in success rates of different osmolar contrast concentrations reflected as the contrast: serum osmolality ratio. This later observation would tend to support the use of near isotonic contrast to avoid the hemodynamic disturbance associated with hyperosmolar contrast agents. This study also noted the highest success when the dilated ileum was filled with contrast. At our institution we frequently use N-acetylcysteine per OG tube started after the initial enema. The neonates typically starts passing bowel movements and the obstruction resolves over the next 24 hrs. If the obstruction does not resolve and if the child is clinically stable, a repeat enema (one or two) may be useful.

OPERATIVE MANAGEMENT

Neonates with uncomplicated meconium ileus which have failed therapeutic enemas, and all neonates with complicated meconium ileus require operative intervention. This was generally a fatal condition until 1948 when Hiatt and Wilson described success with enterotomy and irrigation of the obstructing meconium pellets. The morbidity and mortality associated with operative intervention in children with CF lead to subsequent procedures which were designed to relieve the obstruction and allow postoperative irrigation to clear the obstruction with the advantage of needing a limited, secondary procedure or none at all.

Gross in 1953 used resection of the dilated segment of bowel with a Mikulicz enterostomy. A Mikulicz crushing clamp could then be placed through the two limbs to create an anastomosis below the level of the *fascia* and Gross described later extraperitoneal stoma closure, often at the bed side. Bishop and Koop in 1957 described resection of the dilated ileal segment and a proximal end to distal side ileal anastomosis with distal ostomy. This procedure minimized contamination, allowed an anastomosis between appropriately sized bowel and provided access to the distal bowel for decompression, also allowing bed side closure of the stoma. Most of these stomas did however require operative closure. Santulli and Blanc reported resection with a side-to-end anastomosis and proximal enterostomy. Swenson in 1962 reported resection with primary anastomosis, however this was not widely utilized due to concerns of an anastomic leak. Unfortunately all of these procedures had the disadvantage of an ileal resection. They did however improve the survival of these infants with meconium ileus at a time prior to advances in pediatric anesthesiology and intensive care units.

O'Neal in 1970 reported the use of a tube enterostomy placed at the junction of the proximal distended bowel and distal decompreseed small bowel with the thick meconium pellets which would then allow postoperative irrigation and eliminated the need for a second procedure. Enterotomy with irrigation as originally described by Hiatt and Wilson became popular in the 80's and this is currently the treatment of choice for uncomplicated meconium ileus that fails nonoperative management. Sutures are placed on the antimeseteric wall of the ileum and an enterotomy created. It is often very difficult to remove the very thickened meconium and this usually requires a combination of manual evacuation and irrigation. At our hospital we generally use a saline irrigation to simply break up the thick meconium and pellets and remove this through the enterotomy however others utilize contrast agents or 4% N-acetyl cysteine. The appendix has also been used to instill irrigation solutions and evacuate the meconium however this does require the ability to break up the meconium pellets and thick meconium and pass it into the colon, which is often of relatively small caliber in these children and can be somewhat difficult. It is imperative for the surgeon to insure that the thickened meconium is cleared so that there will be no need for a second procedure or postoperative irrigations as postoperative enemas in the presence of an enterotomy would include some risk of perforation.

Newborns with complicated meconium ileus require operative intervention. In cases of ileal atresia and volvulus, resection of the dilated bowel and removal of the inspissated meconium along with a primary end-to-end or end-oblique anastomosis is usually possible. Most authors recommend resecting 10–15 cm of the dilated bowel in cases of atresia as this segment is often atonic if left in place.

Management of meconium peritonitis and giant cystic meconium peritonitis can be quite difficult. In addition, if operative repair is delayed this occasionally can be become infected. An approach should be undertaken which attempts to preserve as much bowel as possible. If a safe anastomosis cannot be performed, then a proximal enterostomy is utilized with subsequent ostomy take down approximately 6 wks later. A contrast enema must be performed prior to ostomy closure to evaluate the colon and, if possible, terminal ileum. If this ostomy is proximal total parenteral nutrition (TPN) is usually required.

POSTOPERATIVE MANAGEMENT

Neonates who are successfully treated with contrast enemas can usually start on feedings once the signs of bowel obstruction resolve usually within 24 hrs. Those undergoing operative decompression with enterotomy can be started on feeds once there is evidence of return of bowel function. If most of the thick meconium has been removed, regular feeds with enzyme supplementation can usually be utilized. Neonates with ileal atresia not infrequently require TPN for seven to fourteen days until bowel function returns and children with meconium peritonitis or giant cystic meconium peritonitis may require TPN for a longer time period.

Postoperative testing to confirm CF should be performed in all children. An elevated sweat chloride determination is the definitive test for CF. This is however difficult to perform in newborns as they often do not yield adequate sample size. Genetic testing for CF is also determined at many institutions. In general 100% of children with simple meconium ileus have CF although rarely neonates with pancreatic insufficiency from other causes may present with meconium ileus. Neonates with meconium peritonitis have a 15–50% incidence of CF. Within the entire population of neonates with ileal atresia, approximately 15% have CF and this is often evident at the index operation with the hard pellets noted within the distal bowel and very thick meconium in the dilated segment.

Postoperative management with a multi-disciplinary team including those skilled in enzyme supplements and management of the associated pulmonary problems is essential in these young children. At most institutions, the pediatric pulmonary and gastroenterology physicians along with specialized dieticians are active in the management of these children.

LONG-TERM COMPLICATIONS

Distal Intestinal Obstruction Syndrome

Mechanical intestinal obstruction from thickened bowel contents after the neonatal period was initially termed meconium ileus equivalent. This was later termed the more accurate Distal Intestinal Obstruction Syndrome (DIOS) which is currently utilized. Precipitating events for the development of this syndrome include cessation or decrease in enzyme therapy as well as inadequate fluid replacement, particularly during warm weather. Clinical presentation usually includes crampy abdominal pain with decreased stool frequency and sometimes nausea, vomiting and a mass of the right lower quadrant. Plain radiographs generally demonstrate a large colonic load of fecal material. DIOS usually responds to nonoperative therapy such as the use of Miralax, stool softeners and enemas. Occassionally a radiologic enema with agents designed to promote evacuation similar to that of meconium ileus are needed.

Other Related Disorders: Rectal Prolapse, Gallbladder Disease and Hernias

Rectal prolapse can occur in 11–30% of children with CF. This usually responds to nonoperative management with stool softeners. Rarely it may require injection of the rectal wall with a sclerosing agent or rectopexy.

Children with CF have an increased incidence of gallstones as well as biliary dyskinesia and not infrequently require cholecystectomy. Children with CF have been report with an increased incidence of inguinal hernia and hydroceles, with a rate as high as 15% compared with a 3.5–5% incidence in other children. It should be noted by the surgeon that the vas deferens is absent in boys with CF and the surgeon should be aware of this at the time of hernia repair.

REFERENCES

1. Rescorla FJ, Grosfeld JL. (1993) Contemporary management of meconium ileus. *World J Surg* **17**:381.
2. Bishop HC, Koop CE. (1957) Management of meconium ileus: Resection, Rous-en-Y anastomosis and ileostomy irrigation with pancreatic enzymes. *Ann Surg* **145**:410.
3. Del Pin CA, Czyrko C, Ziegler MM, *et al.* (1992) Management and survival of meconium ileus, a 30 year review. *Ann Surg* **215**:179–185.
4. Noblett HR. (1969) Treatment of uncomplicated meconium ileus by Gastrografin enema: A preliminary report. *J Pediatr Surg* **4**:190–197.
5. O'Neill JA, Grosfeld JL, Boles ET, Jr, *et al.* (1970) Surgical treatment of meconium ileus, *Am J Surg* **119**:99–105.
6. Rescorla FJ, Grosfeld J, West KJ, *et al.* (1989) Changing patterns of treatment and survival in neonates with meconium ileus, *Arch Surg* **124**:837–840.
7. Rommens JM, Iannazzi MC, Kerem B, *et al.* (1989) Identification of cystic fibrosis gene: Chromosome walking and jumping. *Science* **245**:1059–1065.
8. Santulli TV, Blanc WA. (1961) Congenital atresia of the intestine: Pathogenesis and treatment. *Ann Surg* **154**:939–948.

COLONIC ATRESIA 56

Alan P. Ladd

CLINICAL PRESENTATION

The presentation of infants with colonic atresia often occurs within the first 72 hrs of life. Clinical symptoms will include abdominal distension and failure to pass meconium, with later presenting symptoms including refusal of feedings and bilious emesis. These symptoms often occur much later than those associated with more proximal obstruction from jejunoileal atresias. Preliminary evaluation often includes abdominal radiographs that note diffuse intestinal distension and often a largely dilated piece of intestine within the mid-abdomen with air-fluid levels. Over two-thirds of these children will be of full-term gestation, with the remaining premature infants often of near-term gestational development. Gender association with this intestinal anomaly shows a near equal prevalence between the genders, with a 4:3 male to female ratio.[1] Up to 20% of the noted infants will have gastroschisis as a readily apparent anomaly; however, the occurrence of concurrent colonic atresia may not be immediately apparent.

PATHOPHYSIOLOGY

Incidence

Colonic atresia occurs in roughly 1 in 60,000 live births and accounts for less than 10% of all gastrointestinal atresias. A clear discernable etiology to the formation of colonic atresia has yet to be elucidated, but the current presiding theory is that of intrauterine vascular obstruction. As the presentation is often phenotypically identical to the varied presentations of jejunoileal atresias, the etiologic mechanism is felt to be similar through mesenteric vascular obstruction felt to be secondary to an internal hernia, volvulus, intussusception or fascial compression related to gastroschisis. Alternate theories of possible intrinsic vascular emboli with origination from the placenta, fetal infection with varicella, or a global intestinal malformative process, that would account for cases of multiple concurrent intestinal atresias, have been put forth.[1,2]

Pathology/Classification

The classification of colonic atresia follows the standard classification of intestinal atresia, as modified by Grosfeld *et al.* (See Chapter 54 Jejunoileal Atresia).[3] Type I represent a mucosal web with outer identification of a luminal transition zone based on the marked diameter change of the contiguous intestine. Type II is represented by an atretic segment of intestine bridging the proximal and distal segments in relation to the atresia; whereas, Type IIIa atresias have no continuity of the associated intestine and are marked by a defect within that mesentery. Type IV is associated with numerous segmental atresias, occasionally incorporating more proximal processes of jejunoileal atresia.

In the largest review of this disorder by Etensel *et al.*, the majority (60.4%) of cases were identified as type IIIa defects, with all other types also represented: Type I, 15%; type II, 14%; and type IV, 10%. Though specificity as to the actual location of represented defects is not clear in most published reports, the majority of cases appear to involve the right colon vs. the left colon at a ratio of 3:1. Additionally, concurrent small intestinal atretic processes are found in roughly 16%.[1]

Unlike cases of duodenal and jejunoileal atresia, the concurrent presence of prematurity is less frequent in cases of colonic atresia, occurring in approximately one-third of cases. The presence of associated anomalies in newborns with colonic atresia occurs in approximately 47%. The greatest association lies in the presence of other concurrent gastrointestinal anomalies, including additional intestinal atresias in 16.5% and intestinal malrotation in 16%. The presence of gastroschisis among patients with colonic atresia occurs in 18%. Two rare cases of choledochal cysts and colonic atresias have also been reported. Concurrent findings of other anomalies of cardiac lesions or musculoskeletal anomalies are quite rare among these children.[1]

The concurrent presence of Hirschsprung's disease has also been recorded in the presence of colonic atresia. Accumulation of data from reviews of colonic atresia has noted only 27 cases of Hirschsprung's disease among 260 patients with colonic atresia, for an incidence of approximately 10% of cases, a number most likely overestimating the true incidence.[1]

DIAGNOSIS

As with all instances of suspected intestinal obstruction of the newborn, the initial study of choice will often be the abdominal radiograph. Based on this study, the occasional appearance of disproportionate distension of the distal gastrointestinal tract may signify an obstructive process within the colon. Findings of significantly distended intestine with a marked air-fluid level may also denote a colonic atresia process. Based upon the clinical suspicion and findings of the abdominal radiograph, a contrasted enema study is often chosen as the study of choice in the determination of an actual obstructive process and discern among diagnoses of colonic atresia, meconium ileus, small left colon, or more proximal ileal atresia. Disuse atrophy of the distal intestinal segment should be evident along with the pronounced cutoff of the proximal gastrointestinal segment. Associated findings on the contrasted enema study may suggest the concurrent presence of intestinal malrotation.

The presence of a concurrent colonic atresia with the presentation of gastroschisis may be easily noted. But on occasions it may be difficult to decipher, based upon the amount of inflammatory suppuration present on the mesentery and eviscerated intestine. Suspected cases may require a contrasted enema, even following prior operative repair of the abdominal wall defect, in order to clearly delineate the colonic anatomy.

SURGICAL MANAGEMENT

The management of colonic atresia lies solely with surgery. Though historical reports often tout the improved survival of this condition with a staged approach to treatment, with the use of a temporary diverting colostomy as the primary management, most contemporary reports denote the safety and feasibility of a primary anastomosis at the time of diagnosis.[1,2,4] In cases of colonic atresia associated with gastroschisis, the majority of authors have favored the initial formation of an end colostomy and staged repair.

Given the notation of anomalous innervation and vascularity to the distal-most and more proximal portions of the intestinal atresia process, recommendations are for the resection of the bulbous proximal portion of the atresia and a partial resection of the distal end of the atresia, leaving a widely patent, spatulated distal end for anastomosis. It is essential that patency of the distal colon is confirmed prior to attempting anastomosis, excluding concurrent atresias or stenosis of the distal colon segment. Concurrent evaluation of the entire intestinal tract at the time of initial operative intervention should be performed to exclude concurrent abnormalities in intestinal rotation, malrotation, or proximal jejunoileal atresia.

With a small but finite risk of associated Hirschsprung's disease present in children with colonic atresia, it is recommended that distal colonic biopsy be performed to exclude this associated anomaly. Recommendations are for frozen section analysis of the distal colon at the time of any primary anastomosis to avoid anastomotic complications from a distal functional obstructive process. The concurrent diagnosis of Hirschsprung's disease may be approached by either primary or staged pull-through techniques, based upon the surgeon's preference.

POSTOPERATIVE CONSIDERATIONS

Outcomes from the correction of colonic atresia are quite favorable. Areas of major impact on patient morbidity from operative correction lie on aspects of delay in diagnosis and treatment, technical errors, nutritional depletion, sepsis, or associated anomalies. Little data is present on the individual impact of these precedent conditions on survival, aside from delay in treatment. Those infants with time of diagnosis and intervention of greater than 72 hrs have a historical mortality rate of 45%, as compared to a 25% mortality among children undergoing earlier intervention.[2] The ultimate quality of life and morbidity associated with the repair of colonic atresia is often more reflective of the outcomes from any associated condition. Contemporary follow-up of patients with colonic atresia have noted a survival that often approaches 90–100%. Infants with associated congenital anomalies and low birth weights of less than 2 kg have the greatest levels of mortality that approach 55%.

Patients with intestinal failure from either short bowel syndrome from associated proximal intestinal atresia or from functional obstructive enteropathy are often faced with the greatest morbidity as these children require parenteral nutrition prior to intestinal adaptation or need for intestinal lengthening procedures or transplantation.

In general, infants with colonic atresia will eventually tolerate enteral nutrition despite early requirements for parenteral nutrition; most will transition to full enteral feedings. As suggested by outcomes data by Piper *et al.*, children with colonic atresia often transit from parenteral nutrition to full enteral nutrition on an average of 1 wk. Greater variation is seen when infants have other associated congenital anomalies or aspects of short bowel syndrome.

REFERENCES

1. Etensel B, Temir G, Karkiner A, *et al.* (2005) Atresia of the colon. *J Pediatr Surg* **40**:1258–1268.
2. Dassinger M, Jackson R, Smith S. (2009) Management of colonic atresia with primary resection and anastomosis. *Pediatr Surg Int* **25**:579–582.
3. Grosfeld JL, Ballantine RV, Shoemaker R. (1979) Operative management of intestinal atresia and stenosis based on pathologic findings. *J Pediatr Surg* **14**:368–375.
4. Piper HG, Alesbury J, Waterford SD, *et al.* (2008) Intestinal atresias: Factors affecting clinical outcomes. *J Pediatr Surg* **43**:1244–1248.

HIRSCHSPRUNG'S DISEASE 57

Robert T. Russell and Alan P. Ladd

INTRODUCTION

Harald Hirschsprung, a Danish pediatrician, presented the classic description of the disease that carries his name to the Pediatric Congress in Berlin in 1886. Since then, our current understanding of the pathology, pathophysiology, genetics, and our ability to successfully treat these patients has come a long way. Hirschsprung's disease (HD) characteristically occurs in otherwise healthy full-term infants. The incidence of HD ranges from 1 in 4,400 to 1 in 7,000 live births with a male to female ratio of 4:1 in classic HD.[1]

The usual presentation of HD in the newborn involves a delayed passage of meconium, constipation, abdominal distention, poor feeding, and/or emesis. Beyond the newborn period, children may present with constipation, abdominal distention, and failure to thrive. Furthermore, patients with HD may also present with a clinical picture of enterocolitis including a history of constipation followed by explosive diarrhea, fever, and distention. Physical examination often demonstrates abdominal distention that has worsened since birth. Rectal examination may reveal a tight anal sphincter and decompression with digital rectal examination or a soft catheter may reveal explosive production of stool. Other diagnoses that must be considered in the newborn period along with HD are meconium ileus, distal small bowel atresia, low imperforate anus, small left colon syndrome, meconium plug syndrome, and functional constipation.

PATHOPHYSIOLOGY

HD can be attributed to cellular and molecular abnormalities in the development of the enteric nervous system and incomplete migration of neural crest cells. The intestine contains three neuronal plexuses: the submucosal plexus (Meissner's), the intermuscular myenteric (Auerbach's), and a smaller mucosal plexus. Each plexus contains an integrated neuronal network that aids in controlling intestinal absorption, secretion, blood flow, and motility. In HD, normal intestinal motility is compromised due to the absence of ganglion cells in the submucosal and myenteric plexus. In conjunction with the absence of ganglion cells seen in HD, cholinergic hyper-innervation, inadequate distribution of nitric oxide synthetase, and abnormalities in intestinal cells of Cajal have also been associated with HD.[2–4]

The gross features of HD vary widely with the duration of the disease and length of intestine involved. As the infant ages, the proximal ganglionic segment of bowel hypertrophies, well defined tenia are lost, and a transition zone of variable length from ganglionic to aganglionic intestine will develop. Histologically, the absence of ganglion cells in the distal submucosal and intermuscular myenteric plexus is the hallmark of the disease. Associated hypertrophic nerve fibers extending into the submucosa may be identified by the pathologist with special acetylcholinesterase staining.

Aganglionosis is classically limited to the rectosigmoid region in approximately 75% of cases. Long-segment HD, which describes additional aganglionosis of the descending colon, splenic flexure, and/or transverse colon, occurs in approximately 15% of cases. Other rare forms of HD including total colonic aganglionosis, acquired, and ultrashort HD, have been described and comprise a small proportion of the HD population.[5]

HD is usually an isolated disorder of healthy, full-term infants, however strong genetic associations have been elucidated and several associated congenital anomalies have been recognized. Genetic studies have isolated at least 10 mutations in different genes associated with its development. The more commonly identified genetic mutations include the *RET* gene, *EDNRB* gene, and the *END3* gene. Many polymorphisms have been described specific to the *RET* proto-oncogene, several of which are associated with particular HD phenotypes. HD has been associated with other genetic abnormalities; specifically, Trisomy 21 (Down syndrome) has been reported to occur in 4–16% of children with HD.[6] Other less frequent associations include atrio and ventriculoseptal defects, congenital central hypoventilation syndrome, multiple endocrine neoplasia type II, neurofibromatosis, Waardenburg's syndrome, and anorectal malformations.

DIAGNOSIS

In patients with suspected distal obstruction, imaging should begin with supine and lateral decubitus abdominal radiographs. These will usually demonstrate distended loops of intestine and may show a relative paucity of air in the rectum. Rarely, free intraperitoneal air will be seen on abdominal radiographs representing perforation of the proximal bowel from HD. This is more common with long-segment involvement.

The next step in evaluation should be a contrast enema, which can elucidate other causes of distal intestinal obstruction from HD. Water soluble contrast should be utilized for the enema for two purposes: this will avoid barium peritonitis in the unlikely event there is occult perforation and high-osmotic, water soluble contrast is more effective in relieving an obstruction secondary to meconium. Classic enema findings in HD demonstrate a narrow, spastic distal colorectal segment with a dilated proximal segment. Most commonly, this transition zone is located in the rectosigmoid colon. Other findings on the contrast enema that may suggest HD include a rectosigmoid index (the ratio of rectal diameter/ sigmoid diameter) of less than 1.0 and retention of barium on a 24-hr postevacuation film. Contrast enemas have a sensitivity between 65–80% and a specificity of 65–100%.[7–9]

The gold standard for the diagnosis of HD is rectal biopsy. Most commonly, these are performed as partial thickness, suction rectal biopsies which can be performed at the bedside or in the clinic. The recommended biopsy is obtained 2 cm or more above the dentate line so as to avoid the rectal transition zone, within 2 cm of the dentate line, in which the presence of ganglion cells is variable. The reported sensitivity and specificity of rectal suction biopsy are >90% and >95%, respectively. When diagnosis cannot be made by suction rectal biopsy, a full thickness, posterior, rectal wall biopsy should be obtained in the operating room. This may be required for older children with suspected HD when it may be difficult to obtain an adequate specimen of submucosal tissue for pathologic diagnosis.

In patients with suspected enterocolitis based on presenting symptoms and physical exam, the diagnostic algorithm will be different. These patients should have abdominal radiographs to characterize their bowel gas pattern, but contrast enema should be avoided due to the risk of perforation. These patients may require aggressive fluid resuscitation based on their presenting hemodynamic status with initial boluses of 20 mL/kg of normal saline and continuation of intravenous fluids at one and a half maintenance until resuscitated based on adequate urine output. Due to the fact that enterocolitis is believed to be the result of intestinal stasis, bacterial overgrowth, and systemic illness due to bacterial translocation, broad spectrum antibiotics (i.e. piperacillin/tazobactam or cefoxitin along with flagyl) should be initiated along with coverage for *C. difficile.* In addition, treatment should include a regimen of decompression and irrigation of the rectum and distal colon with a rectal tube to decompress the colon above the transition zone. This can be performed at the bedside with a 20–24 french foley catheter (based on the child's size). Initially on placement of the catheter above the sphincter, there may an impressive evacuation of air and liquid stool. Once the air and stool are evacuated, saline irrigation through the tube in 10–20 mL aliquots can be performed up to volumes of 20 mL/kg. This irrigation should be allowed to passively drain after each aliquot of saline is instilled. Typically, decompression/irrigations will be performed every 6 hrs until there is improvement in the patient's distention on physical exam, when it can then be tapered to once or twice daily. If the bowel cannot be successfully decompressed with washouts, the patient will require a diverting enterostomy just proximal to the transition zone, proven by intraoperative biopsy.

SURGICAL MANAGEMENT

Surgical approaches for HD are usually undertaken after the diagnosis has been definitively established by suction or open rectal biopsy. Historically, a two- or three-staged repair was performed. The principles for effective surgical treatment for HD include resection of the aganglionic portion of bowel, identification of normal proximal bowel for creation of a colostomy or an enteroanal anastomosis while preserving fecal continence, urinary function, and sexual function. The most commonly used operations for HD were developed by Swenson, Duhamel, and Soave and are described below.[10–12]

The transanal pull-through without intraabdominal dissection (endorectal Soave pull through) described by de la Torre and Langer has become the predominant approach.[13,14] A self-supporting retractor or a series of sutures are placed to retract the anal verge. A circumferential mucosal incision is made approximately 0.5 to 1 cm above the dentate line to avoid the anal sphincter complex that lies in this location. Traction sutures are then placed on the mucosal–submucosal tube and dissection is continued submucosally within the rectal wall, dividing vessels as they enter the rectum. Once dissection is carried up to the level of the peritoneum, full thickness rectum is incorporated into the dissection and the posterior muscular rectal cuff is divided to prevent constriction of the pull-through segment by the outer cuff. Once the suspected transition zone is reached, biopsies are sent to determine the level at which there is normally innervated bowel. Once this is confirmed, the colon is divided just proximal to the apparent transition zone and the coloanal anastomosis is completed. Another variation of this procedure described by Georgeson in 1995 is the laparoscopic-assisted transanal endorectal pull-through (LATEP).[15] This technique utilizes initial laparoscopy to biopsy the region of the transition zone, identified based on change of intestinal caliber, and additional division of the colonic mesentery of the involved distal segment of bowel. The transanal dissection then proceeds as described previously. Contraindications to a primary pull-through during the neonatal period are severe enterocolitis, massive proximal dilatation, inability to determine the transition zone, and significant medical comorbid conditions.

Since Duhamel's initial description of his operation for HD in1956, there have been many modifications to his technique. The Duhamel procedure consists of the preservation of a distal portion of aganglionic rectum, a retrorectal dissection to facilitate the pull-through and anastomosis of ganglionated proximal intestine to the backwall of the native colon immediately proximal to the dentate line. This procedure is usually performed in infants between 3 to 6 mths of age. Abdominal exploration is performed to mobilize the proximal colon and to resect the distal aganglionic bowel to the level of the peritoneal reflection. Retrorectal blunt dissection is performed to create a plane through which the proximal bowel can be pulled through. The proximal colon is then marked with multiple sutures for orientation to prevent torsion of the bowel. The surgeon then proceeds to the perineum where the posterior rectum is incised via a full thickness curvilinear, 180° incision approximately 1 cm above the dentate line. This posterior rectal incision connects the aganglionic rectum with the retrorectal space through which the functional proximal bowel can be tunneled. The lumen of the neorectum is then opened and sutured in an end to side fashion with the native rectum.

A GIA or EndoGIA stapler is then utilized to complete the side-to-side anastomosis between the neorectum (pull-through segment) and native rectum from both a transanal approach (distal to proximal) and an abdominal approach (proximal to distal).

The Swenson procedure has been used less frequently due to increased incidence of injury to nerves controlling genitourinary function. The operation is essentially a low anterior resection of the rectum followed by end to end anastomosis of the pulled through bowel to the everted rectal cuff, at a level 1–2 cm above the dentate line.

Although most pediatric surgeons no longer use a diverting colostomy or ileostomy routinely, there are still indications in appropriately selected patients. Children presenting with severe enterocolitis that do not promptly respond to resuscitation, IV antibiotics, and decompression should undergo a proximal diversion. Although rare, any patient presenting with perforation secondary to HD should undergo repair of the perforation and proximal diversion. A definitive procedure can be performed after the diagnosis has been confirmed and the child has recovered. Furthermore, some children present late and have a massively dilated proximal colon due to HD. This will compromise the surgeon's ability to safely perform a pull-through as a one-step procedure. If the proximal bowel is unable to be decompressed with enemas or bowel management, these patients require colostomy or ileostomy to adequately decompress the proximal bowel.

POSTOPERATIVE CONSIDERATIONS

Most children with HD have a good outcome following surgical treatment, but there are several commonly encountered postoperative problems that include ongoing obstructive symptoms, incontinence, and enterocolitis. Obstructive symptoms may take the form of abdominal distention, vomiting, and/or severe constipation and may present early or late in the postoperative period. The most common etiologies of persistent postoperative obstructive symptoms are mechanical obstruction from stricture formation, recurrent or residual aganglionosis, motility disorder, or functional megacolon from stool-holding behavior. First, confirmation is made of the original pathology to confirm ganglion cells were present within the pull-through segment of intestine. Next, it is imperative to perform a rectal biopsy to determine whether there are normal ganglion cells present in the reconstructed (pull-through) segment. If there are not, these children should undergo a repeat pull-through. If there is not a concern for persistent aganglionosis, investigation as to the etiology of the obstruction should include a barium enema to rule out a stenosis or obstructive etiology. This will discern if there is an anastomotic stenosis or stricture that may be dilated or warrant a redo pull-through. If repeat biopsy shows ganglion cells and there is no anatomical etiology for persistent obstruction, a motility work-up should be pursued. If focal abnormalities are found, consideration should be given for resection or repeat pull-through using normal bowel. If the motility disorder is diffuse, a bowel management regimen and/or prokinetic agents may be used. A bowel management regimen may consist of a stimulant laxative (i.e. senna) or an osmotic laxative (i.e. polyethylene glycol) to achieve one to two stools daily. This will need to be adjusted based on the individual patient's response and titrated to achieve the desired effect.

Enterocolitis may be a presenting feature of Hirschsprung's disease, but it also may occur postoperatively. The clinical features of enterocolitis are fever, abdominal distention, and diarrhea. The frequency of this occurrence postoperatively is difficult to exactly estimate due to its broad definition, but published data quote an incidence of 5–42%. There are mechanical issues specific to the different surgical procedures that can increase the likelihood of enterocolitis. For example, a dilated rectal pouch after a Duhamel can cause stasis of stool and an inadequately split cuff after a Soave can lead a functional obstruction, both increasing the likelihood of postpull-through enterocolitis. Treatment should be similar to that detailed above with IV fluids, IV antibiotics, and saline irrigation with decompression. Once the patient's enterocolitis has been treated effectively, there must be consideration as to the etiology of enterocolitis. Repeat rectal biopsy must be performed to rule out incorrect reconstruction with an aganglionic segment or pull-through of the transition zone. Finally, anatomical reasons for slow transit or stasis of stool should be considered which can be assessed with a contrast enema once the enterocolitis has been treated.

Few complications have a greater impact on the patient's quality of life than incontinence. The reported incontinence rates after pull-through are 3–8%, but this is often an underreported postoperative sequelae. With gaining popularity of the endorectal pull-through, there was concern for a potential increase in incontinence due to the greater amount of retraction on the anal sphincters during dissection and anastomosis. However, postoperative manometric studies comparing transabdominal and perineal approaches demonstrate similar postoperative resting anal pressure, stool frequency, and loss or absence of the anorectal inhibitory reflex.[16]

Close postoperative follow-up is essential for these patients. A 2- to 3-wk postoperative visit will allow assessment of the anastomosis and initial dilation via digital rectal examination in clinic. This will also allow for the opportunity to educate caregivers on the signs and symptoms of enterocolitis in the postoperative period. Persistent fever, abdominal distention, obstipation, and/or explosive diarrhea should be warning signs for entercolitis which should prompt caregivers to seek immediate medical attention. Additional follow-up should be every 3 mths after the initial clinic visit for the first year and then yearly surveillance unless problems arise.

REFERENCES

1. Orr J, Scobie W. (1983) Presentation and incidence of Hirschsprung's disease. *BMJ* **287**:1671.
2. Vizi ES, Zseli J, Kontor E, *et al.* (1990) Characteristics of cholinergic neuroeffector transmission of ganglionic and aganglionic colon in Hirschsprung's disease. *Gut* **31**:1046–1050.
3. Kusafuka T, Puri P. (1997) Altered mRNA expression of the neuronal nitric oxide synthase gene in Hirschsprung's disease. *J Pediatr Surg* **32**:1054–1058.
4. Vanderwinden JM, Rumessen JJ, Liu H, *et al.* (1996) Interstitial cells of Cajal in human colon and in Hirschsprung's disease. *Gastroenterology* **111**:901–910.
5. Tietelbaum DH, Cilley RE, Sherman NJ, *et al.* (2000) A decade of experience with primary pull-through for Hirschsprung disease in the newborn period: A multicenter analysis of outcomes. *Annals of Surgery* **232**:372–380.
6. Amiel J, Sproat-Emison E, Garcia-Barcelo M, *et al.* (2008) Hirschsprung disease, associated syndromes and genetics: A review. *J Med Genet* **45**:1–14.
7. Rosenfield NS, Ablow RC, Markowitz RI, *et al.* (1984) Hirschsprung disease: Accuracy of the barium enema examination. *Radiology* **150**:393–400.
8. Jamieson DH, Dundas SE, Belushi SA, *et al.* (2004) Does the transition zone reliably delineate aganglionic bowel in Hirschsprung's disease? *Pediatr Radiol* **34**:811–815.
9. Proctor ML, Traubici J, Langer JC, *et al.* (2003) Correlation between radiographic transition zone and level of aganglionosis in Hirschsprung's disease: Implications for surgical approach. *J Pediatr Surg* **38**:775–778.
10. Swenson O, Bill AH. (1948) Resection of rectum and rectosigmoid with preservation of the sphincter for benign spastic lesions producing megacolon. *Surgery* **24**:212–220.

11. Duhamel B. (1956) Une nouvelle operation pour le megacolon congenital: L'abaissement retro-rectal et trans-anal du colon et son application possible au traitement de quelques autres malformations. *Presse Med* **64**:2249–2250.
12. Soave F. (1964) A new surgical technique for treatment of Hirschsprung's disease. *Surgery* **56**:1007–1014.
13. Langer JC, Minkes RK, Mazzioti MV, *et al.* (1999) Transanal one-stage Soave procedure for infants with Hirschsprung's disease. *J Pediatr Surg* **34**:148–151.
14. De la Torre-Mondragon L, Ortega-Salgado JA. (1998) Transanal endorectal pull-through for Hirschsprung's disease. *J Pediatr Surg* **33**:1283–1286.
15. Georgeson KE, Fuenfer MM, Hardin WD. (1995) Primary laparoscopic pull-through for Hirschsprung's disease in infants and children. *J Pediatr Surg* **30**:1017–1022.
16. Hollwarth ME, Rivosecchi M, Scleef J, *et al.* (2002) The role of transanal endorectal pull-through in the treatment of Hirschsprung's disease: A multi-center experience. *Pediatr Surg Int* **18**:344–348.

ANORECTAL MALFORMATIONS

58

Alan P. Ladd

CLINICAL PRESENTATION

The newborn findings of an anorectal malformation (ARM) are often dictated by the severity of the anomaly and the gender of the child. Often it is external inspection that allows for the initial recognition of a developmental anomaly of the rectum. If not recognized with early newborn assessment, the timing of presentation may vary from its recognition early in life related to the absence or paucity of meconium passage in the newborn-period to delayed identification of a rectal fistula with incomplete meconium or stool evacuation and associated constipation, abdominal distension, or eventual anorexia.

A thorough perineal examination of the male or female infant will often discern the nature and severity of the ARM. Recognition of incorrect rectal formation is often aided by an observational period for assessment of meconium passage. The surgeon should patiently allow up to 24 hrs for the development of appropriate intraintestinal and –rectal pressure for the passage of meconium through any fistulous connection present. In male children, this will often allow for the identification of a perineal fistula vs. a communication with the urethra or bladder neck, through passage of meconium in the urine.[1] Corresponding presentations in female infants will allow for either the presentation of a perineal or vestibular fistula, within the posterior aspect of the vaginal introitus, or a single perineal opening for the passage of stool and urine that depicts a cloacal anomaly.

Complete physical examination of the newborn, in addition to the perineum, will help to identify associated anomalies that may impact the child's wellbeing and thus the timing of reconstructive interventions. Identification of a posterior sacral mass or presacral mass with gluteal malformation may depict the concurrent presence of a myelomeningocele or presacral tumor. Associated findings of an incompletely formed sacrum or flat bottom may also imply the presence of a lower vertebral anomaly or sacral malformation that may also coincide with the presence of a spinal anomaly or tethered cord. Cardiac evaluation and assessment of physiologic stability will help to identify patients with concurrent cardiac anomalies and its impact on the general care of the infant and timing of reconstruction. Other aspects of the physical examination should include passage of a nasogastric tube to exclude the presence of an associated esophageal atresia and assessment for radial limb anomalies, all potential manifestations of the VACTERL (Vertebral, Anal, Cardiac, TracheoEsophageal, Renal, Limb (radial)) association.

PATHOPHYSIOLOGY

Embryology

The etiology of ARMs remains unknown. Other than the rare familial predisposition for these anomalies noted in successive generations, ARMs tend to be isolated anomalies from abnormal embryologic development. The common theories in ARMs lie with the premise of incomplete separation of the urogenital cavity and the anorectal cavity during their normal developmental separation at 6 to 7wks of gestation. Failure of normal septation of these cavities promotes the formation of abnormal external openings and maintained fistulous connections with the break down of the cloacal membrane at 7wks' gestation.[2,3]

Classification

A generalized estimate as to the frequency of presentation of ARMs is 1 in 5000 live births. The classification for these anomalies is largely based on the gender of the newborn/infant. Each gender may have variants of imperforate anus without an associated fistula, with the level of the rectum either residing below the coccyx or above. Pure rectal atresia with an associated rectal membrane is also found in both genders, as well as variants in which the fistula externalizes on the perineum, as a perineal fistula.

Higher, more complex forms of imperforate anus are defined by the level of the fistulous opening/connection. In females, the fistula may be to the vestibule, just inside the introitus. Higher fistulous openings in female infants are designated as cloacal anomalies with variable distances of the common urogenital and anorectal channel. For male infants, higher fistulous openings are to variable locations along the distal urinary tract, thus forming rectourethral fistulas anywhere along the urethra, including high communications to the bulbar and prostatic urethra, or even higher more complex formations to the bladder neck as rectovesical fistulas.

The most common malformation of anorectal development in female children is the rectovestibular fistula. Higher malformations in males are more common with the rectrourethral fistula being predominant. Lack of any rectal fistula formation in the presence of pure rectal atresia is estimated to occur in only 5% of these malformations, with a significant correlation to the simultaneous presence of Trisomy 21.[1]

Pathology

In addition to the failed formation of the hindgut with this disorder, the formation of the associated sphincteric complex within the perineal body is often affected. This sphincteric complex forms as a compilation of voluntary striated muscles of the external sphincter and the involuntary smooth muscle of the internal sphincter. With development of an ARM, the contribution of muscle to the striated component of the sphincter will vary from a near normal complex to little discernable muscle, thus affecting ultimate future continence. With the additional lack of alignment in the formation of the anus and its appropriate consolidation with the forming rectum, there is a lack of formation of a true anal canal. This additionally impacts future continence from the absence, and thus lack of sensation, to this discriminate area of the anoderm. The development of ARMs has the additional, variable impact on overall proprioception of the rectal canal, often leaving the patient with an incomplete sensation of rectal distension, needed for proper continence.[1]

Associated Malformations

The prevalence of associated conditions in infants with ARMs approaches 60%.[4] Higher malformations, that imply a more abnormal result from embryologic formation, are more often associated with other abnormalities.

Up to one-third of patients with ARMs have associated cardiac anomalies, ranging from the more prevalent atrial septal defects and patent ductus arteriosis, to more rare ventricular septal defects and transposition of the great arteries.[4,5] Given this high prevalence, initial evaluation of the newborn with discovered ARM should undergo immediate clinical assessment for abnormal cardiovascular physiology, as well as an immediate echocardiogram. Findings from this evaluation will help to appropriately time surgical intervention for the ARM.

Concurrent urologic anomalies are most prevalent among the associated conditions with ARM. This is explained by the shared embryologic origin of the anomaly with the formation of ARMs. Up to one-half of patents with ARMs will have associated urologic abnormalities, with vesicoureteric reflux being most common.[6,7] Findings of renal agenesis and dysplasia are also common, and can be depicted on prenatal ultrasound studies. In male infants, cryptorchidism, bifid scrotum and hypospadias can occur.[8] Gynecologic anomalies including atresia of the cervix, vaginal atresia and development of paired hemivagina with associated hemiuterus may all present initially as hydrocolpos, and may require radiologic and surgical interrogation in order to discern the actual anatomic anomaly.[1] Gastrointestinal anomalies may also be present with anomalies of tracheal and esophageal formation being present in 10% of cases.[5] Concurrent presence of duodenal atresia has also been reported in up to 2%.

DIAGNOSIS AND MANAGEMENT

Once an ARM is suspected, a thorough physical examination should be performed. The presence of meconium and the location of its passage, often will then discern the nature of the ARM. A perineal, vestibular, and urethral opening of an ARM should be evident, with the latter presenting with meconium in the urine over the initial 24-hr period of observation. During this time of initial evaluation and observation, the child should be left as nothing by mouth with an orogastric tube for decompression and placed on intravenous fluids with additional intravenous antibiotic coverage with ampicillin and gentamicin. This would be the optimal time to evaluate for any associated conditions that might impact the care of the child, especially identification of cardiac anomalies with an echocardiogram.

If there is no presence of a fistula or meconium passage, a cross-table lateral radiograph of the pelvis with the child in the prone position is obtained, in an attempt to discern the level of the distal rectum. The relationship of the distal rectum to the tip of the coccyx will then aid in the discernment of the severity of the malformation and the intended treatment (Figures 1 and 2).[1] Based on the findings of this evaluation, either primary repair of the malformation is attempted in the newborn period, or the child undergoes colonic diversion and delayed reconstruction. Clinical instability of the newborn related to additional comorbid conditions will favor a plan of delayed reconstruction. Under this latter setting, perineal or vestibular fistulas may be simply dilated to accommodate appropriate passage of stool and obviate the need of a diverting colostomy. In female newborns, perineal examination may reveal a single opening that drains urine and stool. This represents a cloacal anomaly and should undergo primary diversion, delaying reconstruction until a full urologic evaluation has occurred.

OPERATIVE CONSIDERATIONS

In the event that the patient requires formation of an ostomy, the position of the ostomy must be such that it would not interfere with future

Algorithm for the treatment of a male newborn with an anorectal malformation. PSARP, posterior sagittal anorectoplasty. Used by permission ( )

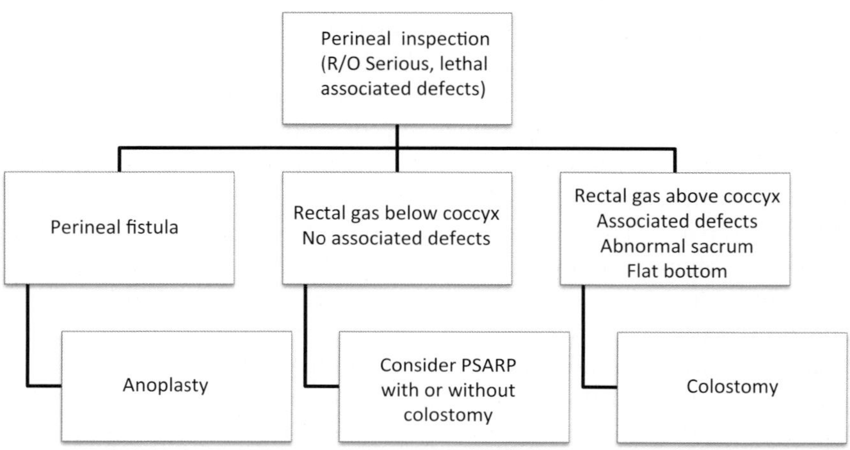

Figure 1. Newborn male — anorectal malformation.

Algorithm for the treatment of a female newborn with an anorectal malformation. *Depending on the experience of the surgeon and general condition of the patient. Used by permission ( )

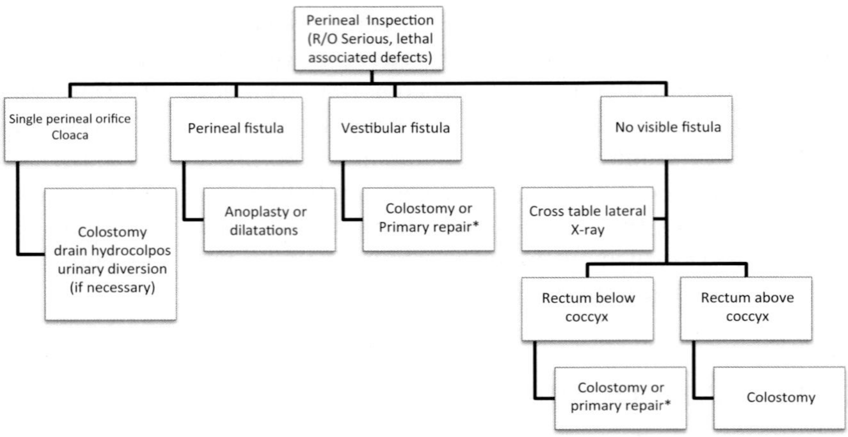

Figure 2. Newborn female — anorectal malformation.

reconstruction efforts. The most common location for diversion will be at the descending colon–sigmoid colon junction. By utilizing this location and positioning the ostomy as proximal as possible to the descending colon, the lateral colon peritoneal attachments will prevent stoma prolapse. The redundancy of the sigmoid colon should also allow for reconstruction without interference of the distal stoma. In cases of complex cloacal anomalies, a more proximal site of colostomy formation may be required so that distal segments of the colon may not only be used for rectal reconstruction but also for the construction of a neovagina in complex repairs. The colostomy is approached through a left lower quadrant oblique incision, incorporating the region of the midpoint between the umbilicus and iliac crest, for appropriate stoma appliance fit. The proximal colostomy and distal mucous fistula should be completely separated and positioned at the ends of the laparotomy incision to minimize distal fecal flow that would allow urinary tract contamination. Additional efforts should allow for evacuation of meconium from the distal segment at the initial operation. The presence of the mucous fistula not only allows for decompression of the distal rectal segment, but also a route for contrasted study of the distal rectal segment and discernment of the level of fistulous communication.

During the formation of a colostomy in a female patient, every effort should be attempted to decompress any evident hydrocolpos. This may involve direct leveling vaginostomy formation for larger collections or placement of a transabdominal catheter into the fluid collection, verifying drainage of each hemivagina, if present.[1] Additional assessment of the distal urinary tract should be performed at the initial operation to discern if appropriate bladder evacuation is present. Atresia or stenosis of the common channel in cloacal anomalies will require a formation of a vesicostomy for appropriate urinary diversion. Assessment of the length of the cloacal common channel with endoscopy will allow for appropriate planning with future reconstruction attempts.

All anomalies of ARM may be approached by the posterior sagittal approach as popularized by Pena, in deliberate attempt to avoid injury to pudendal nerve innervation of the sphincteric complex and pelvic floor. Additional utility of an abdominal approach by either open or laparoscopic techniques may be required in the reconstruction of cloacal anomalies and for visualization and division of a bladder neck fistula in male patients. The majority of reconstructions are performed in the prone position with the pelvis elevated. In all cases, a foley catheter should be inserted to aid in identification of and in avoidance of injury to the urethra. Perineal stimulation is essential for evaluating the location of the sphincteric complex.

In cases with a perineal fistula, the timing of surgery is best within the first 48 hrs, when the meconium remains sterile in nature. This technique can be accomplished without the need of proximal colonic diversion, and merely protected with prophylactic antibiotic coverage.[1] In the situation where the reconstruction must be delayed for clinical reasons, primary reconstruction may also be performed; however, the use of parenteral nutrition and delayed oral feedings for 1 wk are recommended to avoid perineal infection and failure of the reconstruction. Similar considerations can be made for females with vestibular fistulas who are amenable to early, primary reconstruction. For vestibular fistulas, the dissection in maintained within the perineal body and through the anal dimple, without need to open the posterior perineum. Tedious dissection of the fistula from the posterior vaginal wall is required in order to split the often long and thin common wall, prior to full rectal mobilization. Rectoanal anastomosis incorporates reapproximation of the muscle complex with the rectal wall under a slight amount of tension, to avoid future mucosal extrophy or prolapse.

The tenets of repair of higher ARMs lie in maintaining the entire dissection within the midline. This will allow for the least damage to the lateral innervation of the muscular complex or to the vascular supply. Appropriate visualization may be accomplished through extension of the posterior incision to the level of the sacrum. Once the rectum is identified, incision of the investing fascia of the rectum and division of the lateral blood supply to the rectum is required for appropriate mobilization for final anastomosis, basing the distal rectal blood supply on the intramuscular blood supply of the rectal wall.[1] Division of fistulous connections requires tedious dissection to avoid entrance into the urethra or bladder and formal closure of the urinary side of the fistula with fine, absorbable suture. Final reconstruction places the rectum within the muscle complex that includes the sphincter mechanism.

The repair of cloacal anomalies intends to accomplish the achievement of fecal continence, urinary control and sexual function. Proper identification of the anatomic variations of the rectum, vagina and urinary tract is essential prior to final operative planning. Endoscopic interrogation of each of these components is required for proper mapping of the pertinent anatomy, often at a setting separate from that of final reconstruction. Determination of the length of the common channel is important to preparing the patient for aspects of the reconstruction. Those channels less than 3 cm usually allow for reconstruction to be accomplished merely through a posterior sagittal approach, whereas, those with longer channels often require additional laparotomy for appropriate reconstruction. The correction of this anomaly should incorporate expertise in urologic reconstruction and often done in conjunction with pediatric urologic specialists. For this procedure, the rectum is separated from the vagina in a fashion similar to that for vestibular fistulas. Urogenital mobilization is then utilized for the advancement of the vagina and bladder towards the perineum for reconstruction. Cloacas with longer channels (approximately 40% of cases) will require more complex reconstruction, often with the need for separate distal vaginal replacement with the use of a rectal or small intestine segment of intestine.

POSTOPERATIVE CONSIDERATIONS

Management

Prophylactic antibiotic coverage is often maintained for the first 48 hrs usually with a second generation cephalosporin or ampicillin and

Table 1. Anal dilatation program.

Patient age	Hegar dilator
1–4 mths	Size no. 12
4–8 mths	Size no. 13
8–12 mths	Size no. 14
1–3 yrs	Size no. 15
3–12 yrs	Size no. 16
>12 yrs	Size no. 17

Used with permission ( )

aminoglycoside antibiotics. Initiation of oral feedings may resume with return of bowel function for those cases requiring laparotomy or within 24 hrs if a total posterior approach was accomplished. In cases of a rectourethral fistula, the foley should be maintained in position for a minimum of 7 days as a stent for urethral healing.

In order to avoid future anal stenosis, a dilation program is initiated in all patients at 2–3 wks of surgery to avoid anal stricture. Hegar dilators are used to sound the rectum and dilation is performed twice a day. Advancement in dilator size is continued by one increment per week, until the desired dilator size is accomplished (Table 1). Colostomy closure in those with staged procedures may be accomplished once appropriate rectal size has been achieved with rectal dilations. Rectal dilations are often tapered over the course of the first 3 mths. As per Pena's protocol, dilations are then performed once a day for 1 mth, twice a week for 1 mth and then continued weekly for the next 3 mths time span.[1] A constipating diet may aid in reducing the frequency of stooling postoperatively and the development of perineal excoriation. Vigilance in perineal care is maintained immediately following colostomy takedown with the application of barrier creams or ointments to avoid immediate perineal excoriation.

Complications

The most common complication from anorectal reconstruction lies in the development of infection. Though superficial infections may be managed appropriately with early initiation of parenteral antibiotics, severe infections that may result in wound dehiscence or rectal stricture are more complicated. Fecal diversion with colostomy formation must be strongly considered in these cases in attempts to preserve a primary reconstruction and avoid surgery for cases of dehiscence. Additional aspects that impact postoperative complications are rectal segment ischemia and suture line tension, each of which is best addressed with appropriate attention to operative technique at the time of reconstruction.

Rectal strictures, or vaginal strictures in the case of cloacal repairs, are often the result of contamination and infection, ischemia, and/or tension. The anal dilation program should avoid minor anal strictures related to wound healing. More severe, intractable strictures could reflect underlying ischemia. The development of long-segment stenosis or obstruction from the development of acquired atresia will require reoperative management for reconstruction.

The development of rectal prolapse should be an infrequent occurrence with proper operative technique. Prolapse should be limited by the posterior tacking of the rectal wall to the levator muscle complex during closure, tapering of the rectum as deemed necessary, and performance of the anoplasty under a small degree of tension to allow for minor rectal retraction.[1] Clinically significant prolapse is often depicted by excess mucous production, anal excoriation or skin ulceration. Significant rectal prolapse may require formal rectopexy to the levator muscular complex or sacrum. More minor degrees of prolapse may often be treated through resection or trimming of the involved segment with limited revision anoplasty, again performed under slight tension.

Injuries to the urologic tract in male patients should be rare if appropriate technique is utilized. Preoperative distal colostogram should be utilized to correctly identify involved structures in the malformation. Clear delineation of the distal fistula should be noted prior to operative planning in all cases other than the more rare pure rectal atresias. High-variant fistulas to the bladder neck place the nearby structures of the ureters, seminal vesicles, vas deferens, and bladder neck at greater risk if the anatomy is not apparent during reconstruction.

Ultimate continence for children with ARMs is largely related to the severity of the malformation. Those children with lower lesions often have better voluntary control of bowel movements with less soilage than those with higher defects. Total continence with voluntary bowel movements and lack of soiling is 88% in those children with perineal fistulas, 64% in females with vestibular fistulas, 22% in boys with prostatic fistulas and 7% in those with bladder neck fistulas.[1] Continence may be reflected by the early results of function after final reconstruction. Those children with one to three bowel movements per day with no interim soiling will have the best outcomes.[1]

Pseudocontinence maybe achieved by 6–7 yrs of age if the child remains without voluntary control of defecation. Creation of a continent appendicostomy allows the family and child to develop a regimen of antegrade colonic washouts on a daily basis that provides perineal cleanliness over 24 hrs. The associated operation for the appendicostomy (Malone procedure or Malone antegrade colonic enema (MACE)) allows for the creation of a catheterizable channel between the skin and cecum. This conduit is most often constructed from the appendix, but if not available, a tubularized portion of cecal wall may be utilized. The attainment of pseudocontinence then lies in the titration of colonic irrigation volume to achieve a complete washout. The technique is initiated with approximately 10 mL/kg of tap water flushes up to a liter, with additional volume or addition of polyethylene glycol to the irrigation until soiling episodes are eliminated.

Urologic problems in children with noncloacal, ARMs is rare. Girls with cloacal malformations may require urinary catheterization based on the anatomic variant. Girls with a shorter common channel require intermittent catheterization or continent diversion in up to 28%; whereas, those with a longer common channel have lessor function and require catheterization or diversion in 70–80%.[1]

REFERENCES

1. Pena A, Levitt MA. (2006) Anorectal malformations. In: JL Grosfeld, JA O'Neill Jr, EW Fonkalsrud, AG Coran (eds.), *Pediatric Surgery*, 6th edition, pp. 1566–1589. Mosby Inc, Philadelphia.
2. de Vries PA, Friedland GW. (1974) The staged sequential development of an anus and rectum in human embryos and fetuses. *J Pediatr Surg* **9**:755–769.
3. Stephens FD. (1988) Embryology of the cloaca and embryogenesis of anorectal malformations. *Birth Defects Orig Artic Ser* **24**:177–209.
4. Boocock GR, Donnai D. (1987) Anorectal malformation: Familial aspects and associated anomalies. *Arch Dis Child* **62**:576–579.
5. Greenwood RD, Rosenthal A, Nadas AS. (1975) Cardiovascular malformations associated with imperforate anus. *J Pediatr* **86**:576–579.
6. McLorie GA, Sheldon CA, Fleisher M, Churchill BM. (1987) The genitourinary system in patients with imperforate anus. *J Pediatr Surg* **22**:1100–1104.

7. Partridge JP, Gough MH. (1961) Congenital abnormalities of the anus and rectum. *Br J Surg* **49**:37–50.
8. Hoekstra WJ, Scholtmeijer RJ, Molenoar JC, *et al.* (1983) Urogenital tract abnormalities associated with congenital anorectal anomalies. *J Urol* **130**:962–963.

Miscellaneous

GASTROESOPHAGEAL REFLUX 59

Mark S. Chaet

CLINICAL PRESENTATION

Gastroesophageal reflux disease (GERD) can be observed at any age. The incidence of GERD is difficult to accurately state. However, the management of GERD is an important and time-consuming part of a pediatric surgeon's practice.

GERD presents either with overt emesis, esophageal irritation, or complications of gastric contents into the tracheobronchial tree. Infants and children can have severe emesis to result in poor weight gain or failure to thrive. Patients with esophageal irritation have symptoms ranging from discomfort and poor feeding to injury of the mucosa resulting in bleeding, ulceration or stricture formation. Children who present with *silent reflux* have episodes of apnea, laryngospasm or pulmonary infections from gastric contents that reach the level of the epiglottis and spill over into the tracheobronchial tree. Typically the first step of treatment is medical management with acid reduction and gastric motility agents. If these agents provide limited or temporary improvements of signs and/or symptoms of GERD, surgical management is indicated.

Many children with GERD have associated anomalies. This disease is seen commonly in children with developmental delay, cardiac anomalies, esophageal atresia and congenital diaphragmatic hernia. The evaluation and treatment of these children present additional challenges for the medical and surgical team.

PATHOPHYSIOLOGY

It is completely normal for infants to have some degree of gastroesophageal reflux during the first 6 mths of life. Generally the frequency and volume of the infant's emesis decreases during this period of time. There are several changes that occur during infancy that are responsible for the typical resolution of significant GER. First, the lower esophageal sphincter (LES) matures and begins to act as an effective physiologic valve. Second, the esophagus grows in length creating a greater amount intraabdominal conduit and contributes to the formation of the angle of His creating a second physiologic valve to prevent GERD. Finally, as children grow they eat in more upright positions and ingest more solid or thickened foodstuffs. Both physiologic and anatomic disturbances to these developments can result in GERD. It is important to note, however, that some degree of reflux is normal and surgical treatment is indicated to address the complications of GERD.

The most common anatomic findings which contribute to GERD include hiatal hernia, absent angle of His and a shortened intraabdominal esophagus. Physiologic causes include medications (specifically their affect upon the LES), poor esophageal/gastric motility and poorly functioning LES.

DIAGNOSIS

The diagnosis of GERD with clinically significant vomiting is fairly straightforward. The families of these children can describe the frequency and volume of the emesis as well as report on the child's weight gain. It is important to separate infants with emesis into those with anatomic anomalies (pyloric stenosis, duodenal web, esophageal stricture) and GERD. This can be accomplished with a barium esophagram/upper gastrointestinal series (UGI). If there are no anatomic abnormalities and the barium passes into the small bowel reasonably quickly then no further work-up is necessary. If there is delay in the passage of the barium, a radionuclide emptying scan should be obtained in order to better define the degree of delay. In cases of significant delayed gastric emptying a pyloromyotomy or pyloroplasty should be considered in addition to the gastric fundoplication.

Infants and children with *silent* GERD will have a history of apnea, coughing or pulmonary infections. Some may even present with worsening or refractory asthma. Confirmation of GERD can be accomplished in several ways. Some of the studies useful for evaluation of GERD include contrast esophagrams/UGI, upper endoscopy, scintigraphy and esophageal pH measurement. The gold standard study for diagnosis is an upper endoscopy with a biopsy demonstrating esophagitis. In most cases this requires general anesthesia and cessation of medications used to reduce gastric acid production. General anesthesia is also typically used during bronchoscopy and the finding of lipid-laden macrophages is diagnostically accurate for GERD with pulmonary aspiration. Although these two approaches are more invasive than the other studies listed, the results are quite definitive. An UGI study with contrast may demonstrate frank reflux to the upper esophagus quickly proving significant GERD. The absence of such a finding, however, does not exclude the diagnosis of reflux. Similarly, a few episodes of GER into the lower or mid-esophagus does not equate with significant reflux disease. If the child is not able to take the contrast orally, a nasogastric tube may be used to fill the stomach but it should be pulled back for the study as to avoid interfering with the LES and giving misleading results. A delayed view of the stomach is a reasonable measure of normal gastric emptying but it is difficult to quantify the meaning of delayed progress of the contrast through the pylorus. Scintigraphy can be used to identify reflux, pulmonary aspiration of gastric contents, as well as delayed gastric emptying. The accuracy of the former two findings is helpful but there are no clear definitions for delayed gastric emptying in children as there are for adults. A pH probe or Bravo capsule can also be useful. Once again cessation of medications used to reduce acid production is necessary prior to testing. Which mode of investigation or combination of studies to choose will depend upon the patients' presentation and findings during the diagnostic evaluation (Figure 1).

SURGICAL MANAGEMENT

There are several common types of gastric fundoplications: the Nissen, Thal, Toupet, and Dor. The technique that is chosen will depend upon the surgeon's preference as well as the child's presenting medical issues (Table 1). Laparoscopic gastric fundoplication has become the standard approach for surgical management of GERD. Whether a complete (360°) or partial (270°) wrap is done will depend upon the surgeon's preference in most cases. The author generally favors a complete 360° wrap and that is the technique described below.

The child is placed under general anesthesia with endotracheal intubation in the supine position. Infants and toddlers are positioned at the far

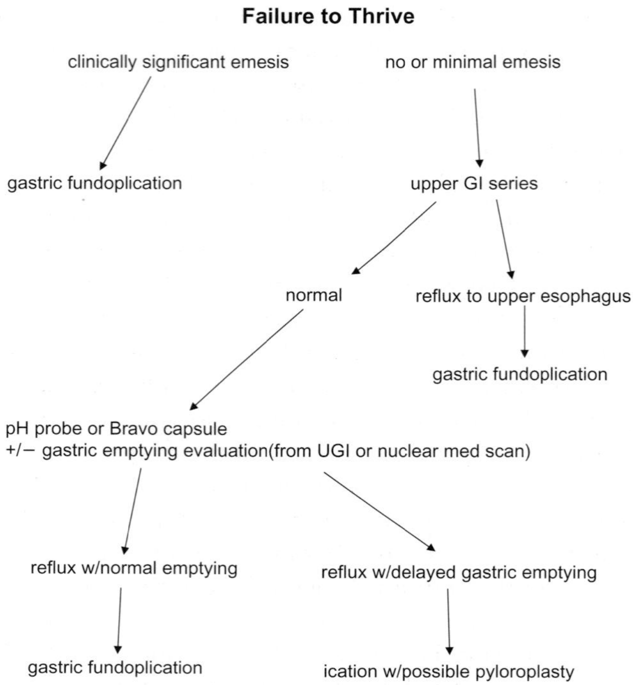

Figure 1. Work-up for FTT leading to gastric fundoplication.

Table 1. Types of gastric fundoplications and indications.

Type	Description	Indication
Nissen	360° wrap	Most commonly used technique
Thal	270° anterior wrap	For abnormal esophageal motility or surgeon preference
Toupet	270° posterior wrap	For abnormal esophageal motility or surgeon preference
Dor	180° anterior wrap	After Heller myotomy(achalasia)
Collis–Nissen	360° wrap with gastroplasty	Foreshortened esophagus
Belsey	270° anterior wrap (thoracic approach)	Surgeon preference

end of the table. Larger children may be placed in a modified lithotomy position to allow the surgeon to stand in between the legs if preferred. The surgeon stands on the child's right side or at the foot of the table. All trochar sites are treated with local anesthetic prior to incision. Initial entry into the abdominal cavity is accomplished through an open technique at the umbilical scar. Once the abdomen is insufflated, a 5 mm trochar and 30° or 45°telescope is introduced to allow placement of the remaining ports. One 5 mm port is placed in the site of the gastrostomy tube if one is in the treatment plan. Another 5 mm port is placed in the right upper quadrant near the liver edge one third of the way between the midline and the anterior axillary line. Finally, a 3 m or 5 mm is placed in the right lower quadrant to allow entry of the liver retractor. Occasionally, an additional (fifth) port is helpful for applying traction to the stomach during dissection at the hiatus. In most cases, however, four access points for instrument entry are all that is required. The anterior esophageal hiatus is assessed and the gastro-hepatic membrane is divided. By retracting the esophagus to the left side of the midline, the peritoneum over the right diaphragmatic crus is visualized and incised. Transoral placement of a bougie may aide in the retroesophageal dissection. Care is taken to maintain a fully transverse plane of blunt dissection as to avoid entry into the mediastinum. Identification of the posterior vagus nerve during this dissection is important in order to preserve this structure. If a hiatal hernia is present it should be repaired with interrupted nonabsorbable braided suture. At this point the two most cephlad short gastric vessels can be divided although this is not routinely necessary. This can be accomplished from an anterior approach to the left upper quadrant or by delivering the fundus behind the esophagus and addressing the vessels with the wrap being held in place. It is important that the portion of stomach that is brought posterior to the esophagus be under minimal tension before the wrap is secured. With the fundus free and the bougie in place, a 360° wrap can be completed. Two or three interrupted nonabsorbable braided sutures are placed from the stomach left of the esophagus to the portion of fundus delivered posterior to the esophagus. Some surgeons include the anterior esophagus in the uppermost suture to avoid slipping of the wrap. Alternatively, securing the wrap to the right portion of the diaphragmatic crus with two separate sutures is also effective. The bougie is then removed and the liver retractor withdrawn. If gastrostomy tube is not planned an anterior gastropexy can be completed with a single nonabsorbable braided suture from the anterior stomach to the anterior abdominal wall near the site of the left uppermost trochar. Many surgeons omit this step, but if it is done care must be taken to avoid creating traction on the wrap during the gastropexy.

If a gastrostomy tube is necessary, a grasper is used to secure the site on the anterior stomach near the greater curve. Above the gastrostomy tube site (trochar) a large suture needle on 0 or number 1 monofilament suture is passed through the abdominal wall, anterior stomach wall and back out the abdominal wall. This is repeated below the gastrostomy tube site. With these two sutures in place the grasper is released and the trochar removed. A vascular introducer needle is placed through the trochar tract into the stomach to allow placement of a wire into the stomach. Sequential dilators are passed over the wire up to 24 Fr. A balloon secured button type gastrostomy device is then placed over the wire. Once the balloon is inflated the abdominal stay sutures are secured over a Silastic disk. As an alternative, a more open technique can also be completed. Once the stomach is controlled with the 5 mm grasper the trochar site skin incision is enlarged to allow direct visualization of the *fascia*. The stomach is then sutured directly to the *fascia* and a tube inserted through a gastrostomy incision.

After a final visual evaluation of the operative area the insufflation is released and trochars are removed. Each fascial defect is closed with absorbable suture. Skin closure can be completed with absorbable suture or a skin adhesive.

Open gastric fundoplication can be completed through an upper midline incision or a saber incision across the upper abdomen. The former is considerably more common and is described below. The skin is incised from just below the xiphoid process to a point superior to the umbilical ring. Once the peritoneal cavity is accessed the diaphragmatic attachments to the left lobe of the liver are divide. This will allow retraction of the left lobe of the liver to the right if the child's midline and exposure of the esophageal hiatus.

A plane of dissection around the esophagus is completed and care taken to identify and protect the anterior and posterior vagus nerves. The hiatus posterior to the esophagus is evaluated for a hiatal hernia and repaired with interrupted sutures if one is found. The upper short gastric vessels are ligated and divided freeing up the fundus of the stomach. The fundus is then delivered posterior to the esophagus and a bougie placed from mouth to stomach. The 360° wrap is then completed. Two or three interrupted nonabsorbable sutures are placed from the stomach left of the esophagus to the portion of fundus delivered posterior to the esophagus.

Some surgeons include the anterior esophagus in the uppermost suture to avoid slipping of the wrap. Alternatively, securing the wrap to the right portion of the diaphragmatic crus with two separate sutures is also effective. The bougie is then removed and the liver retractor withdrawn. If a gastrostomy tube is needed, a Stamm technique (see Gastrostomy Chapter 61) is used. In the absence of a gastrostomy an anterior gastropexy can be completed with a single nonabsorbable suture from the anterior stomach to the anterior abdominal wall. A nasogastric tube should be place prior to closure of the abdomen. The left lobe of the liver is placed back into its normal position and the midline wound closed.

POSTOPERATIVE MANAGEMENT

For a laparoscopic fundoplication without a gastrostomy tube a nasogastric tube is kept in place overnight. Once removed the child is started on clear liquids and advances to a soft diet. Most of these children will be discharged 1 day after their surgery. If a gastrostomy tube is placed an additional day is often required to get feedings to an adequate level. This is usually due to the child's comorbidities that contributed to requiring a gastrostomy tube rather than the technique of tube placement. The tube can be left to drain by gravity for 12–24 hrs prior to starting feeds. In smaller children it is often advantageous to begin with continuous feeding and work towards bolus feeds through outpatient management. The family should return to the office in 5 days to have the gastrostomy tube sutures removed. Periodic visits to the office thereafter are based upon the child's tolerance to feedings and need for gastrostomy tube changes.

In children that have undergone open gastric fundoplication, nasogastric or gastrostomy tubes are left to drain by suction or gravity respectively for 2–4 days. Feeds are begun when signs that the postoperative ileus has resolved. Careful evaluation of the child's fluid and electrolyte status are especially important in these cases. A typical hospital stay of 5–7 days after surgery can be expected.

COMPLICATIONS

The most common problems in the early postoperative period are intolerance to bolus feeding and dysphagia. It is not unusual to witness gagging after feeds in response to rapid gastric distention. Occasionally children may experience a rapid emptying of the gastric contents into the small intestine. This described dumping syndrome presents with abdominal discomfort and diarrhea. The majority of these issues are usually corrected by trying smaller volumes of feeds or continuous feedings. A much more serious postoperative complication is gas bloat syndrome. Since the laparoscopic approach allows most children to be discharged 1 day after surgery the parents must be carefully educated on the presentation and urgency of gas bloat syndrome. Less commonly, the fundoplication could be too tight or the wrapped segment too long. If a symptomatic narrowing of the distal wrap persists beyond the perioperative period dilations or even laparoscopic exploration is indicated.

It is not unusual for the fundoplication to loosen over time as the child grows. This is seen more commonly in children whom continue to wretch or gag during feedings. Additionally there may be some cephlad migration of the wrap. The decision to reoperate should be based upon the child's symptoms of GERD rather than in response to radiologic findings. Reoperations through a laparoscopic approach are usually successful and should be attempted in the majority of cases.

Pulmonary complications such as postoperative pneumonia and pneumothorax are occasionally seen. Rare complications of intestinal or gastric perforations have also been reported. As with all abdominal procedures there is an expected incidence of intestinal obstruction and wound infection. Both of these complications should be seen less commonly when a laparoscopic approach is completed.

NONSURGICAL THERAPY

Some children may present with reasonable indications for surgical treatment of GERD but not be appropriate surgical candidates for a variety of reasons. The most common reason for this situation is poor nutritional condition. In other cases comorbidities may make the child a poor candidate for general anesthesia. Most surgeons feel that after the third reoperation for GERD a fourth is not indicated, as its success is unlikely. Finally, the surgeon may have to face parents that fully refuse any surgical intervention. In all of these cases nonsurgical therapies should be investigated and used. Medications that should be used include acid reducing agents (H2 blockers, proton pump inhibitors) and motility agents (metoclopramide, erythromycin, azithromycin). Nutritional support can be administered through postpyloric continuous tube feedings, either gasto-jejunal or naso-jejunal. These therapies may be used as a bridge to surgery or as palliative care.

Miscellaneous

GASTROSTOMY 60

Mark S. Chaet

INTRODUCTION

In all pediatric surgery practices there is a collection of patients and procedures that require expertise in the placement and management of gastric access devices. Children that require gastrostomy tubes vary in their presentation age from neonates to young adults. The majority will have associated medical problems that will impact upon the preoperative evaluation, intraoperative technique and long-term management of the access devices.

INDICATIONS

The most common use for a gastrostomy is for nutritional support. These children present either with failure to thrive or studies that demonstrate aspiration of orally fed liquids and solids. This may be due to either neurological disease or anatomical anomalies. Other children might require gastrostomy placement due to problems related to the esophagus. Early placement of gastrostomy tubes in infants with esophageal atresia is necessary. Infants and children with esophageal stricture (congenital or acquired) are managed with gastrostomy feedings and access for guided dilations. In a rare number of children access through the gastrostomy is necessary for the administration of medications that will not be taken orally. Table 1 lists some of the more common situations that might require gastrostomy placement in infants, toddlers and adolescents.

Table 1. Typical reasons for gastrostomy tube placement by age of presentation.

Neonates	
	Failure to thrive
	Oropharyngeal incoordination (oral aspiration)
	Esophageal atresia
	Intestinal atresia
	Craniofacial anomalies (cleft palate)
	Neurological injury (IVH)
	Pulmonary insufficiency (BPD)
Toddlers	
	Failure to thrive
	Esophageal injury (caustic ingestion, battery injury)
	Medication administration (cystic fibrosis, HIV, organ transplant)
	Neurological injury (cerebral palsy, traumatic brain injury, CNS tumor)
Adolescents	
	Neurological injury (cerebral palsy, traumatic brain injury, CNS tumor)
	Poor oral intake (eating disorders)
	Esophageal injury (caustic ingestion, battery injury)
	Medication administration (cystic fibrosis, HIV, organ transplant)

SURGICAL OPTIONS

Access to the stomach can be accomplished operatively through an open procedure (Stamm technique) or by a laparoscopic approach. The open procedure is typically completed through a midline incision and the gastrostomy tube placed through a separate stab incision. Once access to the abdominal cavity is gained, the stomach is delivered through the wound. A site is chosen near the greater curvature that will allow delivery of the gastrostomy to the skin site without tension. Two purse string sutures are placed followed by creation of a gastrostomy at the center of the purse strings. A Pezzer or mushroom-tip catheter is placed into the stomach and the two sutures secured in a fashion to invert the gastric entry site. The other end of the catheter is then passed through the abdominal wall. The stomach is secured to the anterior abdominal wall with four quadrant sutures. An exit site suture is then placed at the skin to anchor the tube. The midline incision is closed and both wounds are dressed. A much less common option for gastrostomy tube construction is the Janeway procedure. This procedure involves creating a gastric tube from the greater curvature or anterior gastric wall. The open end is matured as an ostomy, which is intended to be continent. As one might expect, the Janeway gastrostomy presents with additional possible complications and complicated care issues that have made it an unpopular option.

Laparoscopic placement of a gastrostomy tube is completed through two access ports. Open entry through the umbilicus allows placement of a 5 mm trochar for insufflation and access for the 30° or 45° telescope. A second 5 mm trochar is placed at the site of the gastrostomy tube. A grasper is used to secure the site on the anterior stomach near the greater curve. Above the gastrostomy tube site (trochar) a large suture needle on 0 or number 1 monofilament suture is passed through the abdominal wall, anterior stomach wall and back out the abdominal wall. This is repeated below the gastrostomy tube site. With these two sutures in place the grasper is released and the trochar removed. A vascular introducer needle is placed through the trochar tract into the stomach to allow placement of a wire into the stomach. Sequential dilators are passed over the wire up to 24 Fr. A balloon-secured button-type gastrostomy device is then placed over the wire. Once the balloon is inflated the abdominal stay sutures are secure over a Silastic disc. As an alternative, a more open technique can also be completed. Once the stomach is controlled with the 5 mm grasper the trochar site skin incision is enlarged to allow direct visualization of the *fascia*. The stomach is then sutured directly to the *fascia* and a tube inserted through a gastrostomy incision. After a final visual evaluation of the operative area, the insufflation is released and umbilical trochar is removed. The fascial defect is closed with absorbable suture. Skin closure can be completed with absorbable suture or a skin adhesive.

Another gastrostomy placement technique available to the surgeon is the percutaneous/endoscopic route (PEG tube). The first percutaneous endoscopic gastrostomy performed on a child was in 1979 at *Rainbow Babies and Children's Hospital* of Cleveland by Michael W. L. Gauderer, pediatric surgeon, and Jeffrey Ponskey, endoscopist. Here the stomach is accessed with a flexible endoscope large enough to have a working port for a endoscopic snare. The endoscope is passed into the stomach and the stomach is insufflated. By visualizing the endoscope's light through the abdominal wall an area on the anterior gastric wall is chosen for the tube placement. The stomach is then accessed with a sheathed needle. Once a looped string is passed through the sheath it is grasped endoscopically with the snare and brought out through the mouth. The PEG tube is then attached to the string and the tube is pulled through the abdominal wall until the inner disc is secured at the gastric wall. The device is held in place with a Silastic disc, T-bar or bolster which effectively closes the space between the stomach and abdominal walls. Care must be taken to assure that there are no organs or tissues caught between the stomach and the anterior abdominal wall.

POSTOPERATIVE MANAGEMENT

The tube can be left to drain by gravity for 12–24 hrs prior to starting feeds. In smaller children it is often advantageous to begin with continuous feeding and work towards bolus feeds through outpatient management. If the tube was placed laparoscopically, the sutures are removed 5 to 7 days after surgery. Periodic visits to the office thereafter are based upon the child's tolerance to feedings and need for gastrostomy tube changes. Most families will request a button-type device and if this was not used initially then a change in the office can be completed in approximately 2 mths, thus giving the gastrostomy tube tract a chance to mature.

The daily care of the gastrostomy tube is an important topic to discuss with the child's family. The tube must be flushed after use to avoid occlusion from formula or medication. The skin around the site should be cleaned daily using soapy water or alcohol. Many parents have reported seeing more granulation tissue when hydrogen peroxide is used for cleaning.

The caregivers must also be informed that the gastrostomy tube site will close very rapidly once the tube is dislodged so timely replacement (within a few hours) is important.

TYPES OF GASTROSTOMY DEVICES

The classic gastrostomy tubes were either Pezzer or Malecot catheters placed with the Stamm technique. Most families today become familiar with skin level appliances and will request these as either primary or replacement devices. There are two types of skin level tubes as well as several commercial brands. The most common device is secured in place by inflating an internal balloon with water. The second type is held in place with a flexible flange, which is inserted in an elongated configuration. Once in position the internal rod or suture/bolster (depending upon the brand) is removed allowing the flange to expand into position.

PEG tubes typically have a Silastic disc that resides within the stomach and secures the device against the bolster on the skin. Repeat endoscopy can be used for tube removal by cutting and retrieving the disc. Alternatively, the tube can be pulled at the skin until it is delivered through the gastrostomy tract or it separates from the catheter. In older children it should pass uneventfully through the gastrointestinal tract.

COMPLICATIONS/FOLLOW-UP

There are very few complications associated with matured gastrostomy tube sites. The most common, however, is the development of granulation tissue at the skin around the device. This is best treated with weekly applications of silver nitrate and daily cleaning with alcohol. In some instances the granulation tissue grows to such an extent that excision with the electric cautery is necessary. Another problem associated with gastrostomy tubes is infection. The organisms responsible are usually skin flora, which respond to topical and parenteral antibiotics but a fungal infection must also be considered.

Accidental removal of the tube occurs more frequently with some children than in others, but it will certainly occur at some point. The tract closes rapidly so the caretaker should know how to replace the device effectively. If the tube is dislodged before the first scheduled device change then it may be wise to have the gastrostomy tube replaced by medical personnel. A radiologic contrast study should be completed if the replacement is difficult or gastric contents are not easily withdrawn from the device.

Gastric outlet obstruction can occur if the gastrostomy tube tip migrates to the pylorus. This complication is easily corrected once it is recognized and can be avoided by using a skin level button-type device rather than a tube. Children may also present with small bowel obstructions due to internal hernias created by gastrostomy tube placement. This requires operative therapy if early decompression through the gastrostomy tube is unsuccessful.

Once the gastrostomy device is no longer needed it can be removed in the office. If the tract persists and gastric contents continue to leak through the ostomy over the course of 2 to 3 wks, an operative closure is necessary. This is a relatively simple procedure that requires general anesthesia and an overnight hospital stay.

NECROTIZING ENTEROCOLITIS

61

Hayden Stagg and Danny Little

CLINICAL PRESENTATION

Necrotizing enterocolitis (NEC) is the most common surgical emergency in newborns. The mortality from NEC is approximately 25% which is greater than the cumulative mortality of all other congenital anomalies of the gastrointestinal (GI) tract. This disorder is seen primarily in premature infants, particularly in those weighing less than 1000 g with equal incidence between males and females. NEC onset is inversely proportional to gestational age with onset after 3–4 wks for infants born <28 wks and after 3–4 days for term infants. Geographic and temporal variations have been noted with clustered cases leading to concern over "NEC" outbreaks in the neonatal intensive care unit (NICU).

Currently more babies are born at the limits of prematurity. Subsequently, the incidence of NEC is increasing. When an infant develops abdominal distention, intolerance to enteral feeds, and potentially hematochezia, the infant is placed on a "NEC watch". This clinical change will usually prompt a surgery consult. Examination will reveal a distended, tender abdomen. Although the entire GI tract can be involved, NEC is most prominent in the jejunum, ileum, and right colon. Abdominal discoloration and induration are often present. Intestinal loops may be palpable through the abdominal wall. Swelling of the abdominal contents may lead to diaphragmatic elevation and respiratory embarrassment.

Bowel sounds may not be present, but this is not a reliable finding. The severity of NEC may be staged using the Modified Bell's Staging Criteria (Table 1). These criteria, originally proposed in 1978 and redefined in 1982, are based on systemic, intestinal, and radiologic signs.

In severe cases, systemic signs including apnea, decreased urine output, acid-base imbalance, thermal instability, respiratory failure, and cardiovascular collapse are present. Over the course of a few hours, an infant with NEC may rapidly deteriorate. In this scenario, the "feeding and growing" preemie is transformed into a severely ill patient, requiring hemodynamic support with vasoactive medications and advanced ventilator support including the use of the high frequency oscillatory ventilator (HFOV).

There is a similar group of infants with symptoms and signs comparable to those with NEC. Pneumoperitoneum is noted on plain film and an isolated intestinal perforation is ultimately found on exploration. This condition is often associated with indomethacin administration prescribed to close the patent ductus arteriosus. Whether this represents a milder variant along the NEC spectrum or a separate disease process remains debatable.

PATHOPHYSIOLOGY

The pathophysiology of NEC is not completely understood. Although multiple risk factors have been attributed, prematurity remains the most important. A central role for mucosal ischemia leading to cellular injury, apoptosis, and loss of gut barrier has been proposed. The preterm GI tract is characterized by a paucity of cellular and humoral immunity, decreased gastric secretion, impaired regulation of blood flow, incomplete innervation, decreased motility, and immature intestinal epithelium. The preemie is inherently predisposed to developing NEC with even minor insults. The triad of enteral feeding, ischemia, and infection will usually be present with NEC.

The role of feeding in the development of NEC is complex; however several main factors come into play. First, the preterm GI tract is lined with immature epithelium with decreased absorptive capacity. Also, there is decreased motility. These combined forces lead to stasis of bowel contents, bacterial overgrowth, and eventual tissue damage. Early feedings don't necessarily predispose the infant to NEC. In fact, small enteral feedings of human milk (combined with parenteral feedings to achieve full nutrition) may stimulate gut maturation and mucosal integrity. This can be

Table 1. Modified Bell's classification of NEC.

	Stage I	Stage II	Stage III
Physiologic signs	Temperature instability, apnea, bradycardia, lethargy	Metabolic acidosis thrombocytopenia	Neutropenia, DIC, sepsis, cardiovascular collapse
Physical signs	Feeding intolerance, increased residuals, mild abdominal distension, bilious emesis	Bloody stools, moderate abdominal tenderness/distension, mild discoloration, palpable mass	Diffuse peritonitis, severe abdominal tenderness, distension and discoloration, palpable right lower quadrant mass
Radiograpic signs	Mild ileus	Moderate to severe ileus, fixed loops of bowel, pneumatosis intestinalis	Pneumoperitonum, portal venous gas

augmented by initiating low-volume hypo-osmolar "tropic feeds" over 7 to 10 days. Enteral increases should be no more than 20 cal/kg/day. The osmolarity of enteral feedings has been linked with the development of NEC. Hyper-osmolar feeds have been proposed to shift fluid from the intravascular space to the intraluminal space, thus decreasing intestinal blood flow. Formula (when compared with breast milk) has a significantly higher incidence of NEC. This may be attributed to formula not containing many of the protective agents found in breast milk such as gut trophic hormones, components of both cellular and humoral immunity, and probiotic factors. It is important to note however that some infants, most notably very low birth weight infants, will develop NEC without being fed.

Ischemia is central to the pathophysiology of NEC. Several factors can cause ischemia in the premature infant. During times of physiological stress, adrenergic system influences the redistribution of blood to the developing brain and heart and away from the splanchnic bed. Bowel ischemia ensues. Congenital heart defects, in particular PDA, causes decreased intestinal blood flow by shunting systemic flow. Also, indomethacin has the deleterious effect of restricting intestinal blood flow, thus exacerbating NEC. Premature infants exposed to cocaine *in utero* are at increased risk of NEC, mainly due to cocaine's vasoconstrictive effects. Lipopolysaccharide (LPS or endotoxin) produced in gram-negative septicemia causes hypotension, shock, and further exacerbates intestinal ischemia.

Bowel ischemia leads to mucosal injury and interruption of the gut barrier. With stasis of the colonized intestinal tract, bacterial overgrowth occurs, leading to invasion through the injured mucosa. A wide variety of organisms have been associated with NEC including the common organisms *Klebsiella pneumoniae, Escherichia coli,* clostridia, coagulase-negative staphylococci, and rotavirus. As poor perfusion, bacterial overgrowth, and subsequently transmural necrosis occurs, NEC develops as the final endpoint of these processes along with the systemic manifestation of septic shock.

Currently, the role of ischemia-reperfusion injury is under investigation. During reperfusion, enzymatic reactions catalyzed by xanthine oxidase lead to the formation of reactive oxygen species. These free radicals cause cellular damage and lead to increased intestinal permeability. This has been confirmed by administering the xanthine oxidase inhibitor allopurinol which decreases the incidence of NEC. Also various inflammatory mediators, including platelet activating factor, tumor necrosis factor, and several of the interleukins have been shown to play important roles in the pathogenesis of NEC.

DIAGNOSTIC STUDIES

Initial plain films may be normal or reveal a paralytic ileus (Figure 1). During the first 48 hrs of the NEC watch, scheduled radiographs are obtained every 6 to 8 hrs. As mucosal integrity is lost, hydrogen gas penetrates this inner layer revealing pneumatosis intestinalis on X-ray. Transverse pneumatosis in the submucosa is often described as "bubbly gas" (Figure 2) which can be mistaken for fecal matter or meconium mixed with air, yet linear, subserosal pneumatosis is a sure sign of NEC. The precise location of NEC is difficult to determine from plain films.

As pneumatosis extends into the portal circulation, linear branching radiolucencies may be seen over the liver (Figure 3). Portal venous air notes disease progression and is associated with higher incidence of bowel

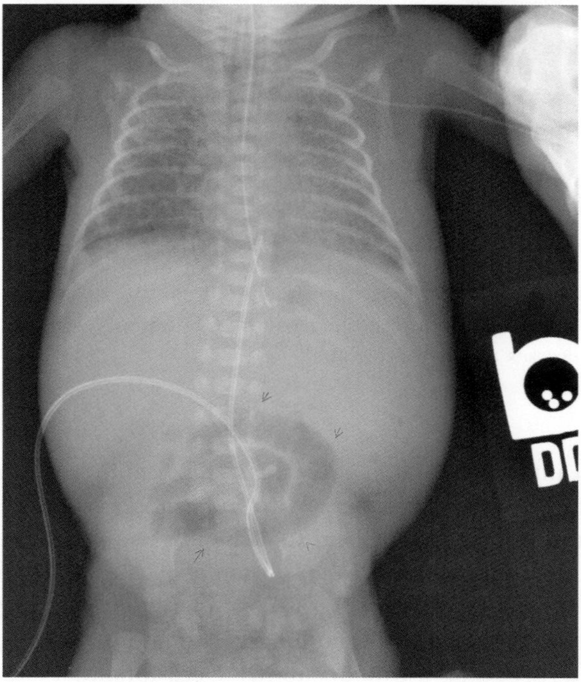

Figure 1. Initial KUB in a 750 g infant girl on a "NEC watch" demonstrating an ileus. She had previously been tolerating enteral drip feeds. Two days later she developed free air and underwent exploration with resection of necrotic ileum and ileostomy creation.

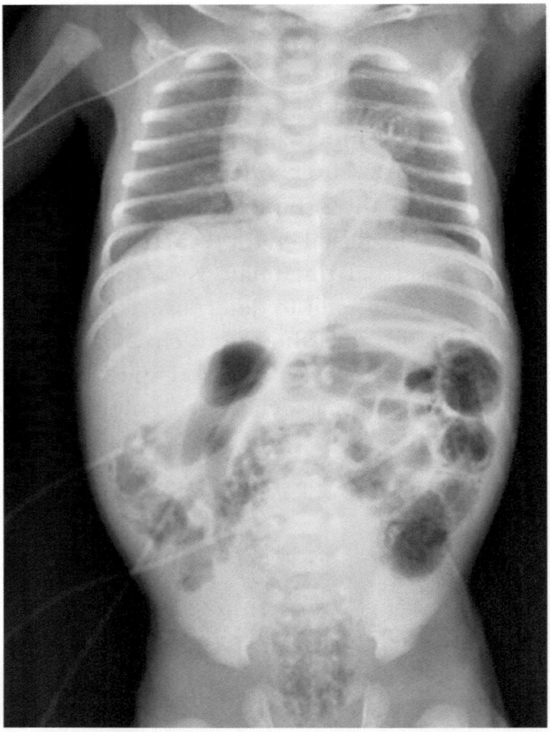

Figure 2. Typical "bubbly gas" appearance in an infant who has developed pneumatosis intestinalis scattered across the abdomen. Note the right sided picc catheter crosses the mediastinum.

necrosis and ultimately higher mortality. This finding may be difficult to see on desktop imaging programs. With full thickness bowel injury, pneumoperitoneum will be seen. Given that small amounts of free air may be missed on supine radiograph, the importance of diligent review of the left lateral decubitus X-ray cannot be overstated (Figures 4a and 4b). Cross table lateral views may also compliment the supine view, but they are harder to interpret than a true decubitus. Occasionally, a large amount of free air may be seen in the central portion of the abdomen and is referred to as the "football sign" (Figure 5). The finding of "free air" necessitates surgical intervention. Sonography with color Doppler may show increased bowel wall echogenicity, portal venous gas, and bowel necrosis. Additional

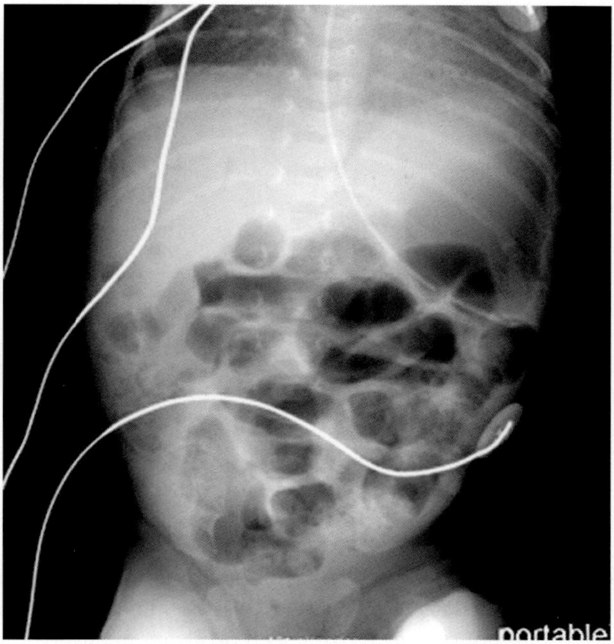

Figure 3. KUB taken following clinical deterioration on "NEC watch". Note the linear pneumatosis along the right side of the abdomen. Additionally, portal venous gas is present. The appearance of portal venous gas can sometimes be difficult to visualize on commonly used desktop programs.

imaging with contrast studies or computed tomography are not indicated given they require patient transport, risk temperature instability, and generally do not add to the clinical picture.

Occasionally an infant with NEC will be noted to have dilated, tubular loops of bowel that do not change on subsequent radiographs. When this pattern does not evolve over 24 hrs, the bowel is considered "fixed". Surgery is then recommended to remove an expected necrotic intestinal segment.

MEDICAL TREATMENT

The diagnosis of NEC is being established earlier allowing quicker implementation of medical therapy. In the right clinical scenario, the practitioner

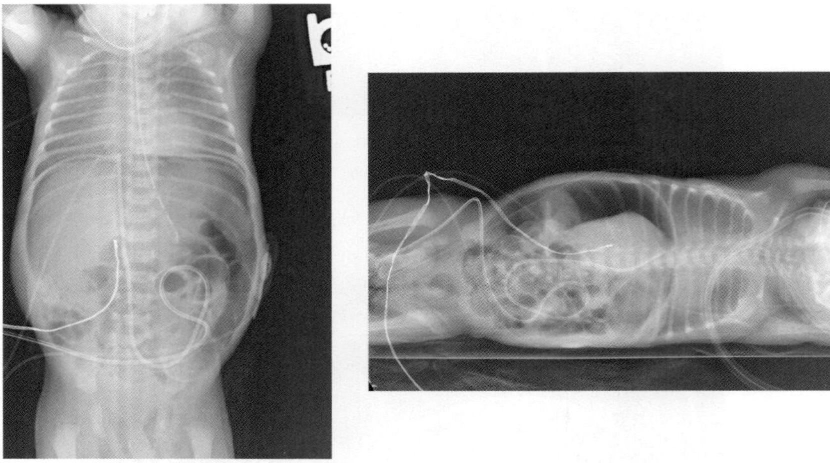

(a) (b)

Figure 4. (a) This KUB shows free air that layers out anterior to the bowel. The inexperienced observer may miss this finding. The importance of a left lateral decubitus cannot be overstated. (b) Here we see the same child in the decubitus view. The large amount of free air is easily seen overlying the liver.

should not wait for the development of pneumatosis before beginning therapy. Enteral feeds are discontinued immediately, and an oral–gastric tube is placed, often producing bilious aspirates. Broad spectrum antibiotics are initiated. Ampicillin, gentamicin, and clindamycin remain a common regimen, although newer agents may be substituted. Parenteral nutrition should be ordered. Of note, similar configuration may be seen with early sepsis, but fortunately both diseases are initially treated similarly. Families should be alerted to the infant's significant clinical change, invited to visit at the bedside, and notified that surgery is a possibility. Given that many of these infants are in "feeding and growing mode" a family visit at bedside can greatly facilitate their understanding of the severity of the situation.

The initial request for a surgery consult is usually associated with pending laboratory and radiological tests. There are several duties that the house office must complete in caring for these patients (Table 2). Leukocytosis, hyponatremia, and thrombocytopenia are common. Metabolic acidosis may be seen on blood gas measurements. It is crucial that the house officer verifies the administration of sodium bicarbonate as its use may lead

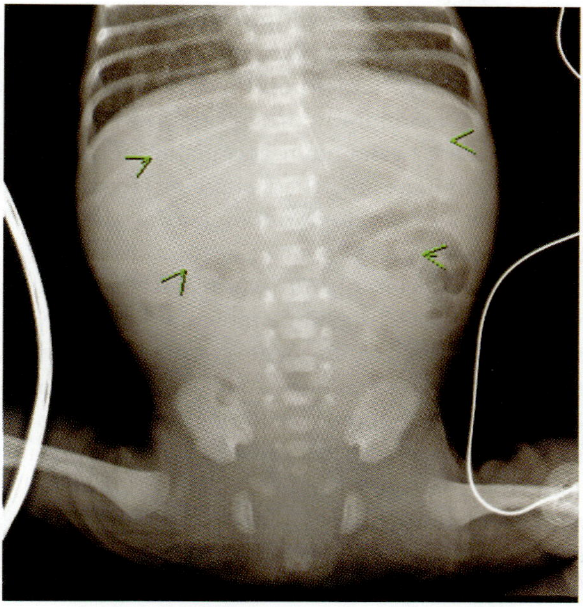

Figure 5. Referred to as the "football sign", free air has collected along the central portion of the abdomen.

Table 2. Checklist for the house officer.

(1)	Serial physical exams, documented in the patient's chart, every 6 to 8 hrs during the first 48 hrs.
(2)	Timely review of X-rays. Do not wait for the "official" report to be dictated.
(3)	Follow-up on labs, including complete blood count, chemistry panel, blood gases, and C reactive protein.
(4)	Bedside discussion with neonatology team.
(5)	Notify family that the surgery service is involved.
(6)	Update senior resident and staff with any clinical deterioration.

to artificially improved blood gases and a false sense of security. The house officer should follow the lab trend over time. Neutropenia is an ominous sign.

Intubation and mechanical ventilation may be required along with isotonic volume resuscitation with crystalloid or colloid. Ventilator strategies on the conventional ventilator are similar to ventilator techniques in the adult units where respiratory rate and pressure settings (or tidal volume) are used to control ventilation and FIO_2 and PEEP are adjusted to improve oxygenation. However, management on the HFOV will likely be foreign to the house officer. Not uncommonly, these patients will require a high mean airway pressure and FIO_2 to maintain acceptable pO_2. Ventilation on the HFOV is controlled with adjusting the Delta P or Hertz. Worsening ventilation with increasing pCO_2 is treated with increasing the Delta P or decreasing the Hertz frequency.

Most infants who deteriorate and require surgery will do so within the first 48 hrs with some cases needing immediate operative intervention. Intestinal perforation occurs in up to 30% of infants. If this level of illness is not met, then a period of bowel rest and antibiotic administration for 10–14 days is generally recommended. Premature cessation of therapy may lead to recurrence of symptoms. Not uncommonly disappearance of bowel air may be mistaken for clinical improvement. Abdominal girth may be measured. With true clinical improvement abdominal girth and gaseous intestinal distention will subside together. Subsequently oral feeds are resumed. With the success of medical therapy, one must remember the possibility of a developing intestinal stricture as the injured bowel heals. Typically this will be diagnosed with a barium enema (BE) obtained 4–6 wks following initial treatment.

SURGICAL TREATMENT

Traditionally, up to 50% of those diagnosed with NEC will require surgery. Pneumoperitoneum is the only absolute indication for surgery. Yet, several other findings may prompt a surgeon to consider operative intervention (Table 3). These include portal venous gas, fixed intestinal loop, and cellulitis of the abdominal wall. Increase in disease intensity despite

Table 3. Indications for surgical management.

Absolute	Pneumoperitoneum
Relative	Clinical deterioration despite maximal medical therapy
	Fixed intestinal loop
	Portal venous gas
	Positive paracentesis
	Peritonitis

maximal medical support may warrant exploration, even in the absence of free air. Goals of surgical management include resection of necrotic bowel, removal of contamination, and preservation of bowel length.

When a decision to operate has been made, the house officer should ensure adequate blood products are ordered including at least 20 mL/kg of packed red blood cells, fresh frozen plasma, and platelets. Intravenous antibiotics should be continued and adjusted based on renal function. Parental consent should discuss all possibilities including isolated perforation to NEC totalis. Anesthesia should be notified to discuss where the operation will occur.

Real dangers exist when transporting these infants to the operating room. The distance lends itself to patient hypothermia which will contribute to bleeding during the case. Additionally, the endotracheal tube can easily become dislodged en route, especially when the HFOV is used with its "fixed" tubing circuit length. For theses reasons, many surgeons prefer to bring the operating room to the child in the NICU. Apart from inferior lighting, the benefit of a well planned operation in the NICU generally outweighs any negatives.

The infant is approached through a low right transverse incision well away from the brittle neonatal liver. The three most likely findings include: isolated perforation or localized NEC, multiple areas of necrosis with adequate remaining length, or NEC totalis. Isolated disease will be treated with resection of necrotic bowel. The remaining proximal bowel will be brought out as an ostomy, and the distal bowel may be brought out as a mucus fistula. Alternatively, surgical clips can control the distal segment that is then left *in situ*. Later when ostomy takedown is considered, complete distal intestinal patency can then be studied with a BE that refluxes up to the level of the clips. Stomas are not without complications including retraction, stenosis, ischemia, and parastomal hernia. These findings have led some to recommend primary anastomosis in stable infants with limited NEC.

Occasionally exploration will reveal multiple areas of necrosis, scattered throughout the bowel. Viability of the challenged bowel is questioned. Bowel perfusion may be assessed with gross appearance, Doppler examination of the distal mesentery, and/or wood's lamp examination of the bowel following intravenous fluoroscein administration. Multiple strategies exist, but the safest is to resect obviously necrotic areas, "clip and drop" the remaining intestinal segments, and plan for a second look procedure in 24–48 hrs.

Approximately 10% of patients will have NEC totalis. Typical findings include pan-necrosis from the ligament of Trietz to the right colon. There are no good surgical options. Candid discussion with family preoperatively is essential. Further intraoperative discussion is also advisable. NEC totalis is uniformly associated with short bowel syndrome and high mortality. Traditionally, many surgeons would proceed with abdominal closure and recommend comfort care for the infant. Death can usually be expected within 24 hrs. With the advancement in isolated intestinal and multivisceral transplantation, the ethics of this approach are less clear, owing that a fraction of these unfortunate cases may be salvaged. Intraoperative discussion with the family is recommended. Understandably, many families will request full support and thus the necrotic bowel is excised, proximal diversion is created, and gastrostomy placed. A tunneled central venous line will need to be placed for long-term parenteral nutrition. This procedure may be done later when infection has subsided.

In unstable or very low birth weight infants, bedside peritoneal drainage should be considered. In this technique, a right lower abdominal incision is created, abdominal cavity irrigated, and a Penrose drain advanced (Figure 6). Peritoneal drainage is clearly useful as a temporizing procedure, allowing initial decompression and stabilization. With further resuscitation a formal laparotomy may safely be planned. In select group of patients, primary peritoneal drainage may be definitive with no additional procedure required. However, in multiple published series, the majority of patients still require open laparotomy. Recent evaluations have shown no clear benefit for peritoneal drainage over formal exploration.

RESOLUTION OF NEC

Most infants with NEC will require a NEC watch for 7–14 days and not require surgery. NEC infants will require longer hospitalization than matched infants without NEC. Survivors experience a 25% long-term sequelae related to the GI tract (Table 4). Problems encountered during recovery or convalescence from NEC include malabsorption, recurrent disease, persistent low grade inflammation and bleeding, and continual consumptive physiology with thrombocytopenia. Continued low grade bleeding may indicate smoldering disease and possible subclinical stenosis. A BE is warranted. Additionally, a BE is routinely obtained before

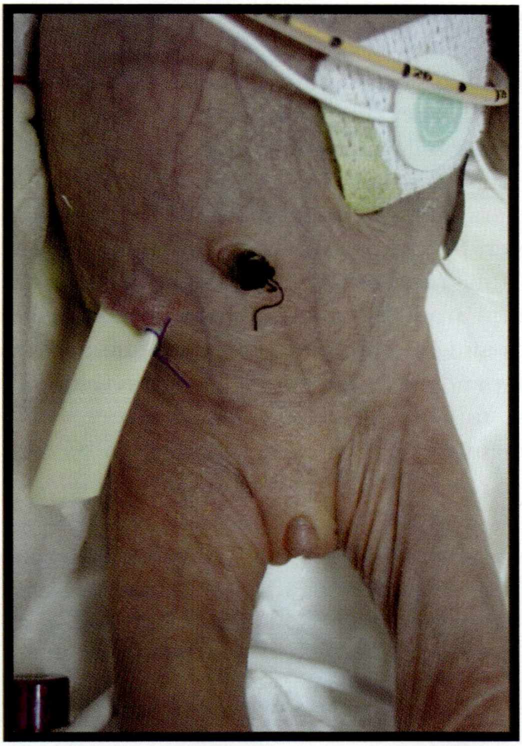

Figure 6. Postoperative view of a 650 g infant girl who developed NEC with rapid clinical deterioration. 1/4 inch Penrose drain was placed at bedside allowing the child to stabilize before definitive exploration. Note the subumbilical approach used in order to avoid the liver and potential catastrophic bleeding.

Table 4. Long-term complications following NEC.

Short bowel syndrome
Intestinal strictures
Cholestatic liver disease
Neurodevelopmental complications
Intestinal malabsorption
Anastomosis ulceration
Recurrent NEC

ostomy reversal. If a colonic stricture is discovered, this should be excised during ostomy takedown (Figure 7). Of note, strictures may be managed with balloon dilatation although this approach is not commonly used in neonates. Generally speaking, the infant is ready for his ostomy to be reversed 6 to 8 wks following creation. This generally coincides with a weight greater than 2 kg and an expected discharge within a few weeks. If the infant is tolerating full enteral feeds, the infant could be discharged and return later for takedown. Less common complications include enterocolic fistulas and enterocysts. Recently, several reports have commented on neurodevelopmental outcomes. In the National Institute of Child Health and Human Development studies, NEC has been found to be an independent predictor of neurodevelopmental morbidity. Unfortunately, only 50% of infants surviving NEC have normal neurodevelopment.

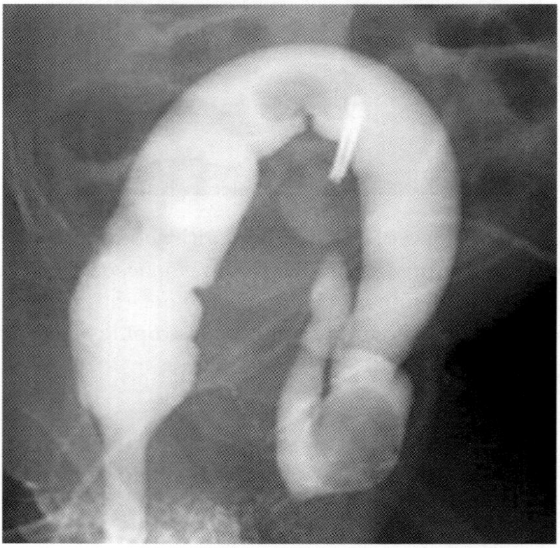

Figure 7. This child underwent exploration at 860g for perforated ileum and right colon. The barium exam pictured is 2 mths following surgery. The two clips seen were placed across the distal bowel during initial exploration. Note the inability to advance contrast past the upper sigmoid colon. A lengthy stricture involving the transverse and descending colon was identified during surgery.

REFERENCES

1. Hintz SR, Kendrick DE, Stoll BJ. (2005) Neurodevelopmental and growth outcomes of extremely low birth weight infants after necrotizing enterocolitis. *Pediatrics* **115**:696–703.
2. Kim SS, Albanese CT. (2006) Necrotizing enterocolitis. In: JL Grosfeld, JA O'Neill, AG Coran, EW Fonkalsrud (eds.), *Pediatric Surgery*, 6th edition, pp. 1427–1452. Mosby, St Louis, MO.
3. Ladd AP, Rescorla FJ, West KW. (1998) Long-term follow-up after bowel resection for necrotizing enterocolitis: Factors affecting outcome. *J Pediatr Surg* **33**:967–972.
4. Moss RL, Dimmitt RA, Barnhart DC, *et al.* (2006) Laparotomy versus peritoneal drainage for necrotizing enterocolitis and perforation. *N Engl J Med* **25**: 2225–2234.

Miscellaneous

SHORT BOWEL SYNDROME 62

James C.Y. Dunn

CLINICAL PRESENTATION

The clinical finding of malabsorption after the extensive loss of the small intestine is known as short bowel syndrome. This occurs most frequently in neonates, with 20% occurring beyond the neonatal period.[1] In the pediatric population, the main causes of short bowel syndrome are necrotizing enterocolitis, meconium ileus, gastroschisis, intestinal atresia, and midgut volvulus. Trauma, ischemic vascular disease, adhesive obstruction, long-segment Hirschsprung's disease, and Crohn's disease can also lead to short bowel syndrome.

EPIDEMIOLOGY

Incidence

The reported incidence of short bowel syndrome is 5 in 1,000,000 population per year.[1] In neonates, the incidence of short bowel syndrome is 1 in 4,000 live births, with much greater risk in premature infants as compared to term infants. In extremely low birth-weight infants, the incidence of short bowel syndrome is over 1%.

Classification

Patients can be divided into three categories based on the anatomy of the residual intestine. The first category of patients has lost only small bowel but their entire large bowel is intact. The intestinal continuity is restored with enteroenterostomy. The second category of patients has lost both small and large bowel, and the small bowel is anastomosed to the large bowel. The last category of patients has extensive small and large bowel loss, resulting in high output jejunostomy. These patients are the most difficult to manage and have the highest mortality.

It has been suggested that 15 cm of the small intestine with an ileocecal valve or 40 cm of the small intestine without an ileocecal valve is needed for survival.[2] This is an over simplification because the prognosis also depends on the underlying etiology, the age of the patient, and the function of the remaining intestine. Nevertheless, the length of the remaining intestine is a strong predictor of outcome in patients with short bowel syndrome. At 30 wks of gestation, the length of the small intestine is only half of that at 40 wks of gestation. The length of the small intestine is 200–300 cm in full-term newborns, depending on the method of measurement and the size of the infant. The intestine continues to grow in length, and at 18 mths of age, the length of the small intestine doubles that at birth. Because the length of the intestine increases with age of the patient, it is important to document patients' remaining intestine not only by the absolute length but also by the percent of expected length. Short bowel syndrome generally occurs when over 60% of the small intestine is lost, and the mortality increases significantly when more than 90% of the small intestine is lost.

PATHOPHYSIOLOGY

Significant metabolic derangements can occur in short bowel syndrome. With the loss of small intestine, the stomach secretes more acidic fluid into the intestinal tract due to hypergastrinemia. The loss of jejunum decreases carbohydrate digestion and absorption due to the loss of enzymes and transporters on enterocytes' brush border. Cholecystokinin and secretin production by the jejunum is also impaired, leading to altered pancreaticobiliary secretions and poor fat and protein absorption. If there is adequate ileum present, the loss is better tolerated because the ileum can adapt and compensate for the loss of the jejunum. The loss of ileum results in the malabsorption of vitamin B12, fat-soluble vitamins A, D, E, K, and bile salts. In contrast, the jejunum is unable to assume these functions and diarrhea results from the large volume of water, electrolytes, and bile salts that pass into the colon. The absence of an ileocecal valve allows bacteria to reflux into the small bowel and results in bacterial overgrowth. The increased absorption of oxalates by the colon can lead to the formation of renal calculi.

MANAGEMENT

Nutritional Support

Before parenteral nutrition became available, patients with short bowel syndrome faced over 90% chance of mortality. In contrast, the overall mortality of patients with short bowel syndrome is less than 20% at 1 yr in more recent series. Home parenteral nutrition programs have been successful in maintaining these patients long term. In addition to providing nutrients, excess fluid and electrolyte loss needs to be replaced, and electrolytes and trace mineral and vitamins are monitored weekly. The long-term use of parenteral nutrition, however, is expensive. Approximately 40,000 patients annually receive total parenteral nutrition in the United States. At an estimated cost of $200,000 per patient each year, this translates into eight billion dollars to support patients on total parenteral nutrition in the United States each year.

When the gastrointestinal function returns after intestinal loss, it is important to restart enteral nutrition as early as possible. Enteral feeding is associated with less cholestatic problems and is trophic to the small bowel. This is often accomplished with a gastrostomy tube so that continuous, slow feeding into the shorten bowel can be done to optimize nutrient absorption. The infants should still receive some oral feeding to avoid oral aversion that frequently develops in these patients. An elemental formula is often employed because of better absorption compared to standard formula, although it has higher osmolality and maybe less trophic to the small bowel. The patient's stool output should be monitored for reducing substances and undigested fat as an index of adequate absorption.

Intestinal Rehabilitation

After the loss of the small intestine, the remaining intestine undergoes compensatory hyperplasia and hypertrophy that occurs over the ensuing months to years. For some patients, the adaptation will eventually allow patients with short bowel syndrome to be weaned from parenteral nutrition.

It has been shown that specialized therapy for short bowel syndrome at rehabilitation centers may reduce or eliminate the need for parenteral nutrition by optimize the health of the remnant intestine and enhancing bowel adaptation.[3] A variety of pharmacotherapy may be helpful in patients with short bowel syndrome. Acid reducing agents such as histamine-2 receptor blocker is useful to minimize the effects of hypergastrinemia in short bowel syndrome. Anti-motility agents including loperamide and diphenoxylate increase transit time to enhance nutrient and fluid absorption. A potential side effect of these agents is bacterial overgrowth, which can be treated with metronidazole. In the absence of ileum, the excess bile salts that enter the colon can be sequestered by cholestyramine. For patients with high-output jejunostomies, the somatostatin analogue octreotide may be considered to suppress gastrointestinal secretions.

A multitude of growth factors have been used to enhance intestinal adaptation, mostly in the experimental setting. The first trial to use growth factors in the treatment of patients with short bowel syndrome employed glutamine and growth hormone. Glutamine is an amino acid needed by enterocytes, and growth hormone produces generalized anabolic effects as well as specific transport effects. Although the results from the initial trial using glutamine and growth hormone were encouraging, subsequent randomized, prospective trials did not demonstrate a clear benefit. Other hormones, including epidermal growth factor, insulin-like growth factor 1, glucagons-like peptide 2, and hepatocyte growth factor are currently being evaluated in preclinical and clinical trials.

SURGICAL PROCEDURES

A few surgical procedures designed to increase the transit time have been described. A short segment of the small intestine can be reversed and anastomosed to restore continuity. Similarly, a segment of the colon may be interposed between the small intestines to slow down transit. Other anatomical arrangements to achieve the same goal are to create a recirculating loop of small intestine and to add intestinal intussusception valves. All of these procedures have only been reported anecdotally, and a potential problem with these approaches is bacterial overgrowth that may result from the stasis of the enteric content. These procedures have been largely abandoned.

The small intestine is often dilated in patients with short bowel syndrome. This is in part due to the adaptive response but can also be caused

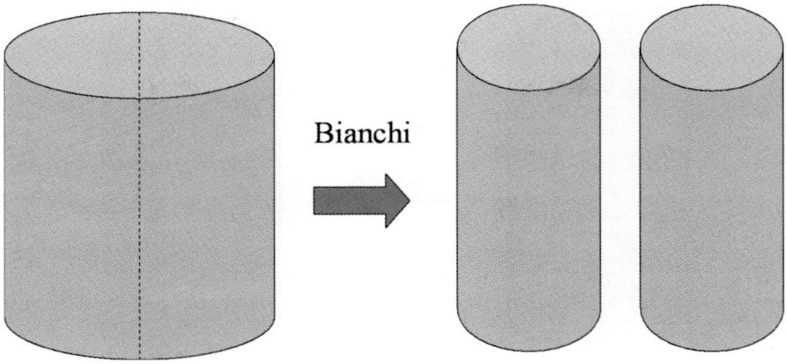

Figure 1. Bianchi procedure. The dashed line indicates the direction of the intestinal division with a stapler.

by distal obstruction from a stenotic segment or an anastomotic stricture. Tapering of the dilated intestine is performed to decrease the stasis and bacterial overgrowth in dilated segments of the intestine. This can be done by folding in the anti-mesentery side of the dilated intestine with sutures, but the sutures may become undone with time. An alternative approach is to remove the anti-mesentery side of the dilated intestine to achieve a narrower lumen. The disadvantage of such an approach is the resultant decrease in the absorptive area. A clever way to decrease the luminal diameter while preserving the intestinal surface area is intestinal lengthening. This was first described by Bianchi, who divided the dilated intestine longitudinally to form two narrower intestinal segments, each based on one half of the mesentery blood supply (Figure 1). The two segments can then be anastomosed to end up with a longer but narrower intestinal segment. The long-term results from the Bianchi procedure have been mixed.[4] While some patients appeared to have benefited and were weaned from parenteral nutrition, many continued with the need for parenteral nutrition. No prospective, randomized trials have been done with the Bianchi procedure. More recently, another intestinal lengthening procedure, serial transverse enteroplasty (STEP), was described.[5] Instead of longitudinal division, the dilated intestine is divided by repeated application of a stapler that partially transects the intestine transversely (Figure 2). This approach also preserves the intestinal surface area and achieves a longer zig-zag channel that is narrower in diameter. A prospective registry of patients who have undergone the STEP procedure is being used to follow the long-term

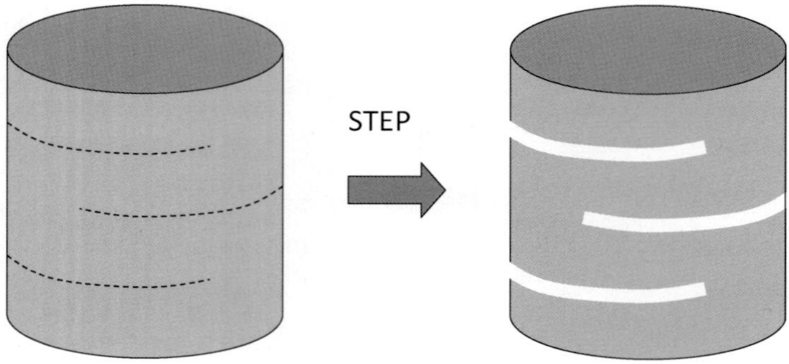

Figure 2. STEP procedure. The dashed line indicates the direction of the intestinal division with multiple applications of a stapler.

fate of these patients. Another method to lengthen the intestine in short bowel syndrome is based on the tissue expander concept often used in surgery. By applying a gradual axial force to an intestinal segment, one can increase the length of the intestine in an animal model of short bowel syndrome.[6]

Intestinal transplantation, often done together with liver transplantation, may be considered in patients with short bowel syndrome. This is usually reserved for patients who developed liver failure as a consequence of parenteral nutrition toxicity and in patients who had nearly exhausted their central venous access. Although the outcome following intestinal transplantation is improving, it is still limited by complications of immunosuppression and donor availability.

COMPLICATIONS

Central Venous Catheter Infection and Thrombosis

Due to its high osmolality, parenteral nutrition is usually infused through an indwelling central venous catheter. The most common complication associated with the use of a central venous catheter is blood stream infection. Gram-positive organism is responsible for the majority cases of blood stream infections, and this often can be treated with a course of intravenous antibiotics. When Gram-negative or fungal infection develops, the central venous catheter will need to be removed to clear the blood stream infection. A more significant complication associated with the use of a central venous catheter is venous thrombosis. Swelling and edema of the affected extremity will usually resolve once the catheter is removed, and anti-coagulation is generally recommended for deep venous thrombosis. The thrombosed vein may recanalize later, but often it will no longer be possible to reuse the vein for central venous catheter placement. Repeated thrombotic events will limit the available routes of central venous access, and this would be an indication to proceed with a transplantation evaluation.

Parenteral Nutrition Associated Liver Disease

Although parenteral nutrition provides adequate calories to patients with short bowel syndrome, its long-term use is associated with cholestatic liver disease, especially in infants. This may progress to liver cirrhosis, and it accounts for one-third of long-term deaths in patients with short bowel syndrome. The exact etiology of parenteral nutrition associated liver disease is yet to be determined, but it appears that the intralipid used to provide the fatty acids is at least partially responsible. Intralipid is a fat emulsion derived from soybean and contains omega-6 fatty acid. It has been customary to provide 3–4 g/kg/day of fat to infants with short bowel syndrome. In experimental animals, omega-6 fatty acid induces cholestasis, which can be reversed by giving omega-3 fatty acid. Omega-3 fatty acid is a principle component of fish oil. Although not approved for routine use in the United States, omega-3 fatty acid given at 1 g/kg/day appears to reverse the cholestasis caused by parenteral nutrition in recently reported clinical series.[7]

OUTCOME

The mortality of patients with short bowel syndrome has continued to decline over the last few decades. In large centers where multidisciplinary teams can offer a comprehensive intestinal rehabilitation program, more than 80% of the patients are now expected to survive. With innovative therapies on the horizon, it is anticipated that nearly all patients with short bowel syndrome can survive without the need for transplantation in the future. Therapies that will restore the intestinal function in patients with short bowel syndrome so that they may eat a normal diet will be the ultimate goal.

REFERENCES

1. Wales PW, Christison-Lagay ER. (2010) Short bowel syndrome: Epidemiology and etiology. *Semin Pediatr Surg.* **19**:3–9.
2. Wilmore DW. (1972) Factors correlating with a successful outcome following extensive intestinal resection in newborn infants. *J Pediatr* **80**:88–95.
3. Byrne TA, Wilmore DW, Iyer K, *et al.* (2005). Growth hormone, glutamine, and an optimal diet reduces parenteral nutrition in patients with short bowel syndrome: a prospective, randomized, placebo-controlled, double-blind clinical trial. *Ann Surg* **242**:655–661.
4. Bianchi A. (1999) Experience with longitudinal intestinal lengthening and tailoring. *Eur J Pediatr Surg* **9**:256–259.
5. Javid PJ, Kim HB, Duggan CP, Jaksic T. (2005) Serial transverse enteroplasty is associated with successful short-term outcomes in infants with short bowel syndrome. *J Pediatr Surg* **40**:1019–1023.
6. Chang PC, Mendoza J, Park J, Lam MM, Wu B, Atkinson JB, Dunn JC. (2006) Sustainability of mechanically lengthened bowel in rats. *J Pediatr Surg* **41**:2019–2022.
7. de Meijer VE, Gura KM, Le HD, Meisel JA, Puder M. (2009) Fish oil-based lipid emulsions prevent and reverse parenteral nutrition-associated liver disease: The Boston experience. *JPEN J Parenter Enteral Nutr* **33**:541–547.

Miscellaneous

INTUSSUSCEPTION 63

Corey Tomlinson, John M. Draus Jr. and Bryan J. Dicken

INTRODUCTION

Intussusception was recognized and operative management proposed in 1674 by Paul Barbette. However, intussusception remained almost universally fatal until the introduction of pneumatic reduction in the 1800s. In 1864, David Greig suggested the use of hand bellows, which successfully reduced four of five intussusceptions with the air passing readily into the bowel "...with great relief to the child". Greig is credited with the first strict criteria for clinical diagnosis: "obstinate vomiting...obstinate constipation...paroxysms of pain...hard tumor in the abdomen, and...passage of blood per anus." In 1905, Hirschsprung reported 107 cases treated with hydrostatic reduction with a mortality of only 23% — a drastic improvement over the previously reported 90% mortality.

CLINICAL PRESENTATION

The presence of two classic symptoms, abdominal pain with vomiting, and two classic signs, abdominal mass with rectal bleeding, helps make the diagnosis of intussusception. The average lead-time is 24 hours. The triad of intermittent colicky abdominal pain, vomiting, and bloody stools is encountered in only 20–40% of cases. At least two of these findings are present in approximately 60% of patients. The most common (85%) symptom of intussusception is sudden onset of severe, colicky abdominal pain.

The child will respond to pain by cessation of activity and by drawing the legs into the chest.

The abdominal mass of intussusception is described as "sausage like". It is most often palpated in the right upper quadrant and may extend to the epigastrium. The mass may be slightly tender and is best appreciated when the child is lying quietly between attacks of pain. What may be more impressive is an empty right lower quadrant — called Dance's sign. Blood per rectum occurs in 32–61% of cases. A rectal examination may reveal either occult blood or frankly bloody, foul smelling stool, described as "currant jelly". In addition to bloody stools, diarrhea may occur in up to 30% of patients.

An important subset of patients presents with lethargy and unresponsiveness. One study demonstrated that in 17% of cases, one or more neurological symptoms were present leading to the recommendation that intussusception be considered in any child presenting with lethargy, hypotonia and/or sudden alterations of consciousness, even in the absence of the classic symptoms. Conservative management is successful less frequently and surgical complications arise more frequently in the toxic-appearing child.

PATHOPHYSIOLOGY

Incidence

After pyloric stenosis, intussusception is the most common cause of bowel obstruction in children, with annual hospitalization rates of 56/100,000 children. Intussusception is seen most frequently between the ages of 5 and 9 months, with 67% of cases occurring in the first year of life. The disease can occur at any age, with 10–25% occurring after age two. Neonatal and preterm infant intussusception is a rare phenomenon.

Pathology

The pathogenesis of intussusception involves the prolapse of an intestinal segment into an immediately adjacent segment of bowel. Peristaltic waves propagate the proximal invaginated bowel segment, the *intussusceptum*, into the distal bowel lumen, the *intussuscipiens*. With further propagation, the mesenteric vessels are pulled into the distal bowel lumen leading to local bowel edema and venous congestion. With time, the static portion of bowel begins to weep mucus and blood, leading to "red currant jelly stool". As the process continues, the high venous pressure and congested bowel limits arterial in-flow and necrosis, perforation, and death results if left untreated.

Types of Intussusception

Fixed vs. Transient

Intussusception may be classified as either fixed or transient. Fixed intussusceptions represent the majority (80%), and all require intervention. Spontaneous reduction of intussusception occurs in 20% of cases. Included in this group are children in whom parents have reported prior similar symptoms, and patients are found at laparotomy to have an already reduced segment, albeit bruised and edematous. Eighty-six percent of these intussusceptions involve only the small bowel. Transient intussusception may be encountered with gastroenteritis as the bowel can be inflamed, full of mucus, hyperactive and have mesenteric lymphadenitis. Asymptomatic patients with incidental radiologic intussusception should be managed conservatively.

Idiopathic

When no pathologic lead point (PLP) can be identified, 90% of the intussusceptions occur in the ileocolic area. The majority are due to thickened mucosa, mesentery, or lymphoid tissue. Children have considerably more lymphoid tissue than adults. When an infectious disorder is contracted, the distal ileum can become inflamed and enlarged. This lymphoid hyperplasia has been suggested as the lead point in the pathogenesis of idiopathic intussusception. This disorder was once believed to occur more often in the spring and autumn when rates of viral infection are highest, although it now appears to have no variations with seasonal changes or peaks in upper respiratory infections. Primary nonenteric adenovirus infection contributes to childhood intussusception, as does acute primary HHV-6, HHV-7 and EBV infections. Rotavirus vaccine has also been implicated in idiopathic intussusception. These vaccines were found to have the greatest risk in the first 3–14 days after receipt of the first dose in infants older than 3 mths. The original vaccines were subsequently removed from the market and have been replaced.

Pathologic lead point

An important consideration is the presence of a PLP. Adult intussusception differs from that of children in that a majority of adult causes have a PLP, where as the majority of childhood causes do not. The incidence of a PLP causing intussusception in children ranges from 5% to 14 %, with 97% of the PLP's discovered during surgical intervention. Two types of PLP have been identified: single lesions or diffuse gastrointestinal abnormalities, with Meckel's diverticulum as the single most common cause. Other less commonly reported causes of PLP are polyps, duplications, periapendicitis, appendiceal stump, appendiceal mucocele, suture lines, lymphoid hyperplasia, ectopic pancreas, trauma, benign tumors (adenoma, leiomyoma, carcinoid, neurofibroma, hemangioma), and malignant tumors (lymphoma, sarcoma, leukemia). Diseases that cause bowel wall thickening or disordered motility include: Henoch–Schonlein purpura, cystic fibrosis, celiac disease, hemophilia, neutropenic colitis, Hirschsprung's enterocolitis, Peutz–Jeghers syndrome and familial polyposis.

A PLP occurs in less than 4% of children <2 yrs of age, but can occur in up to one third of patients after 2 yrs old. The most significant clue to a PLP is the presence of an underlying disease that may predispose the patient to intussusception. Four important factors that may be associated with the presence of a PLP include an ileocolic intussusception, an older child, the association of a long duration of symptoms with weight loss, and recurrent intussusception. Two thirds of PLPs may be identified at ultrasonography with a 40% chance of diagnosing a PLP on contrast enema. Air enema has a lower rate of detection at only 11%.

Postoperative

Intussusception may develop during the postoperative course of a patient who has undergone a laparotomy with extensive bowel handling and packing. These patients may present with a small bowel obstruction (SBO). It is estimated that this type of intussusception accounts for 5–10% of all postoperative SBO. The intussusception frequently occurs in the more proximal small bowel, and its diagnosis requires a high clinical suspicion.

Anatomic types

The most common type of intussusception is ileocolic, followed by the ileoileocolic. This variation starts as an ileoileal intussusception that invaginates into the cecum and subsequently into the colon. Forty percent of ileoileocolic intussusceptions have a PLP as an underlying cause. These intussusceptions are often characterized by a complete SBO and are more difficult to reduce, with a 25% success rate with barium enema (BE). Other less common variations include appendicocolic, cecocolic, and colocolic. These types are almost invariably associated with a PLP. The jejunojejunal and ileoileal intussusceptions, seen in the postoperative period, are infrequently related to a PLP.

Intussusception around tubes

Intussusception has occurred with gastrojejunostomy and nasojejunal tubes, leading to an antegrade intussusception at the end of the nasojejunal tube. This results in a high-grade SBO. The diagnosis is made with US and treatment is by removing, replacing, or converting the tube to a gastrostomy or nasogastric tube with seldom need for surgical intervention. Retrograde jejunoduodenogastric intussusceptions occur when gastrostomy tubes migrate by gastric peristalsis through the pylorus and into the duodenum or jejunum leading to painless, bilious vomiting, with high grade SBO.

DIAGNOSIS

Plain Films

The accuracy of abdominal radiographs (AXR) in diagnosing intussusception is roughly 50%. The role is therefore limited, and perhaps best used to exclude the presence of free air, which would preclude performance of contrast enema. The absence of bowel gas in the ascending colon is one of the most specific signs of intussusception seen on plain films. Two findings can exclude idiopathic ileocolic intussusception: an AXR filled with gas throughout and a colon completely outlined with stool. Characteristic signs on AXR include the meniscus sign and the target sign. A target sign on AXR consists of concentric circles of fat density, similar in appearance to a doughnut, visualized to the right of the spine and is caused by layers of peritoneal fat surrounding and within the intussusception alternating with layers of mucosa and muscle. The presence of a curvilinear mass within the course of the colon, particularly in the transverse colon just beyond the hepatic flexure, is nearly pathognomic of intussusception.

Ultrasound

Abdominal ultrasound (US) is a pillar in the diagnosis of intussusception. US has a sensitivity of 98–100% and a specificity of 88–100%. A graded compression examination along the entire course of the colon, as well as each of the upper and lower quadrants, is performed to indentify the intussusception and to ascertain vascular perfusion. The characteristic US appearance is that of a 3–5 cm mass (target sign) usually found just deep to the anterior abdominal wall. A hyperechoic tubular structure covered on each side by a hypoechoic rim can also be seen and is called the pseudo-kidney. Doppler studies may be used to identify the presence of ischemia and to predict the reducibility of the intussusception by enema. Ominous signs include a thick peripheral hypoechoic rim of the intussusceptum, free intraperitoneal fluid, fluid trapped within the intussusceptum, enlarged mesenteric lymph nodes within the intussusception, a PLP, and absence of blood flow in the intussusceptum on Doppler interrogation.

Contrast Enema

All children should have surgical consultation prior to enema to assess for peritoneal signs and for postreduction management. Prior to US, BE was considered the gold standard for the diagnosis of intussusception. Successful reduction of an ileocolic intussusception via a contrast enema is traditionally defined by the absence of a filling defect in the colon, in addition to reflux of contrast into the terminal ileum (TI). Failure to demonstrate reflux into the TI, even in the setting of no filling defects in the colon has served as an indication for either repeating a contrast enema or operative exploration. Reflux of contrast into the TI may be difficult to achieve even after successful reduction because of edema of the valve caused by venous congestion. It is has recently been demonstrated that patients who undergo reduction of ileocolic intussusception without residual defects in the colon, but in whom reflux of contrast into the ileum is not demonstrated, may be considered for nonoperative management, assuming they become asymptomatic after the procedure. Treatment of patients with overnight observation can help avoid repeat enemas or surgical exploration.

MANAGEMENT

When the diagnosis of intussusception is confirmed, options for definitive treatment include medical management, radiologic reduction, and operative intervention. Radiologic hydrostatic or air enemas are often first attempted in a stable patient prior to proceeding to a laparoscopy or laparotomy.

Medical

Under specific conditions, intussusceptions caused by PLP's of the diffuse thickened bowel wall variety can be treated with steroids before, along with, and/or after radiologic reduction attempts. Treatment of lymphoid hyperplasia and Henoch–Schonlein purpura in this fashion has been reported. This conservative approach must be used cautiously and under the guise of a surgical team.

Radiologic Management

The overriding principle of radiologic reduction is that the patient must be volume resuscitated and have stable vital signs. If instability or shock is present, then urgent operative intervention must be employed. Free air or signs of peritonitis should be considered contraindications to radiologic reduction. Relative contraindications to enemas include symptoms >24 hours, and ultrasonography findings of intestinal ischemia or trapped fluid.

Four techniques of nonoperative radiologic reduction are commonly used: Pneumatic reduction with fluoroscopic guidance, pneumatic reduction with US guidance, hydrostatic reduction with US guidance, and hydrostatic reduction with fluoroscopic guidance. Successful fluoroscopic reduction varies widely, but averages 84%. Recently there has been a trend from hydrostatic to pneumatic reduction techniques with increasing use of US. This technique has the clear advantage of avoiding radiation exposure, providing more information than fluoroscopic techniques, high accuracy and reliability for monitoring the reduction process, visualizes all components of the intussusception including the postreduction edematous ileocecal valve, and can more easily identify PLPs. Its main disadvantage is less experience with pneumatic reduction under US guidance.

Hydrostatic barium enema vs. Pneumatic air enema

The main advantage of hydrostatic reduction is the vast experience and familiarity with the contrast agent and the use of fluoroscopy by most radiologists. It is simple, safe and efficacious. The disadvantage of barium is that if perforation occurs, patients tend to have longer colonic tears, increased peritoneal contamination, and rapid fluid shifts when hypertonic water-soluble agents are used. Several factors are predictive of a possible BE perforation: age younger than 6 months, symptoms present for 72 hours, and complete SBO.

Pneumatic reduction has gained wide acceptance because of several factors; it is easy to perform, can be done quickly, is less messy, delivers less radiation, is more comfortable, and results in similar perforation rates with less peritoneal contamination. Its main disadvantage is the lack of experience with pneumatic reduction under US guidance. Additional disadvantages include the passage of air into the TI without reduction of the intussusception and possible tension pneumoperitoneum in the event of perforation. The pneumatic technique starts with a low pressure (50 mm Hg) and slowly increases the pressure as necessary, never exceeding 110 to 120 mm Hg. Several studies have demonstrated the rates of success with air enema are higher than with liquid enema reduction.

After successful radiologic reduction, the child should be admitted for observation. A small percentage of patients (0.5–15%) will have a recurrence of the intussusception, usually within 24 hours but sometimes after days or weeks. Even after reduction by laparotomy, the recurrence rate is 1–5%. If the success of enema reduction remains doubtful, if pain recurs, or both, a repeat US is a valuable adjunct. Once a child has been symptom free, resumes normal activity and is tolerating a diet, discharge may occur.

Techniques to Improve Reduction Rates

The use of glucagon, steroids, sedation, and smooth muscle relaxation to improving reduction rates has been studied. To date, the literature provides no clear benefit, and their utility remains controversial. Transabdominal manipulation however, has been shown to improve the success rates of reduction.

Delayed repeat enema

Historically, it was standard practice that immediate operative intervention was required if an intussusception was irreducible by enema techniques. At surgery, however, 10% were spontaneously reduced and another 40% were easily reduced manually. These findings imply that many intussusceptions are reduced by nonoperative means. Although success with enema reduction has been shown to decline as duration of symptoms increases, repeat enema is both safe and effective in recurrent intussusception as long as the child remains clinically stable.

The use of delayed repeat enema was initiated based upon guidelines from Toronto, which suggests the duration of symptoms should be less than 36 hours, temperature less than 38°C, pulse less than 150/min, intussusception moves on enema, patient becomes asymptomatic, and an interval of 2 to 4 hours between attempts is appropriate and safe. The success rate of the delayed repeat enema was 60% and reduction was achieved in 9 of 10 patients on the first repeat attempt. Children may benefit from additional, nonsurgical reduction attempts at referral centers, unless absolute contraindications are present.

Perforations Postenema

Perforations caused by hydrostatic enema usually result in large colonic tears. Barium perforations often leave a solidified stool mixture in the peritoneum. Patients perforated with barium had longer anesthetic times, more often required bowel resection, and had increased morbidity and a longer hospital stay than did those perforated with air. In contrast, when a pneumatic enema perforation occurs, the rent is smaller and the peritoneal contamination is much less and easier to evacuate. Rarely, tension pneumoperitoneum can occur after pneumatic perforation, and urgent needle aspiration may be necessary. This is best done in the midline, above the umbilicus, with an 18-gauge needle.

Surgical Management

Surgical reduction is required in 6–61% of children, including patients with failed enema reduction, those with a PLP, or in patients with contraindications to enema reduction. The surgical approach involves a transverse incision overlying the palpable mass. The operative reduction involves constant, slow, squeezing motions in a retrograde direction through the wall of the intussuscipiens without interruption. Serosal tears may occur. Tears that are long or deep may require suture plication. If the reduction continues to progress, regardless of tears, one should cautiously "press on". When the intussusception fails to reduce, one should consider resection with primary repair.

The viability of every intussusceptum should always be inspected and is often quite blue, congested, bruised, and may have questionable viability. Time and a warm lap sponge will almost always return the bowel to its natural pink color. When considering reduction, one must weigh the risks of perforation and contamination against a successful reduction. However, successful reduction of necrotic bowel will likely lead to smaller segmental resection. If manual reduction has been successfully completed, it is prudent to check for a PLP, most commonly from a Meckel diverticulum or distal ileal neoplasm.

Laparoscopy is now an established modality in the treatment of intussusception. Its role is not clearly defined, and its use depends on the surgeon's laparoscopic skills. The reported conversion rate for a laparoscopic intussusception reduction to an open procedure varies from 12.5–50%. Nevertheless, laparoscopic reduction has been used successfully for children with uncomplicated intussusception, uniformly improving the length of hospital stay and decreases time to full feeding.

The approach requires the reduction of the bowel with a squeezing action using atraumatic bowel graspers with counter traction, using a continuous pulling technique. This technique can be used safely in patients with no signs of perforation, peritonitis, or hemodynamically instability. The laparoscopic technique should be considered as the initial approach in pediatric patients with irreducible intussusception, regardless of age, who present within 1.5 days of the onset of symptoms. After successful reduction, the surgeon must carefully examine the intestine to ensure bowel health. In addition, the surgeon must be diligent in searching for a PLP, as recurrence is common if the PLP is not diagnosed. Neither the number of previous episodes of intussusception nor the level of the intussusceptum appears to increase the risk of conversion to open procedure. A PLP however, is a risk factor for conversion. A recent report has suggested combining laparoscopic reduction with hydrostatic enema, to limit the traction on the bowel.

REFERENCES

1. Guo JZ, Ma XY, Zhou QH. (1986) Results of air pressure enema reduction of intussusception: 6,396 cases in 13 years. *J Pediatr Surg* **21**:1201.
2. Harrington, L, *et al.* (1998) Ultrasonographic and clinical predictors of intussusception. *J Pediatr* **132**:836–839.
3. Kaiser AD, Applegate KE, Ladd AP. (2007) Current success in the treatment of intussusception in children. *Surgery* **142**:469–475; discussion 475.
4. Shekherdimian S, *et al.* (2009) Contrast enema for pediatric intussusception: is reflux into the terminal ileum necessary for complete reduction? *J Pediatr Surg* **44**:247–249; discussion 249–250.
5. Bailey KA, Wales PW, Gerstle JT. (2007) Laparoscopic versus open reduction of intussusception in children: A single-institution comparative experience. *J Pediatr Surg* **42**:845–848.

Miscellaneous

MECKEL'S DIVERTICULUM 64

Ali Cadili, John M. Draus Jr. and Bryan J. Dicken

INTRODUCTION

Meckel's diverticulum is the most common congenital anomaly of the gastrointestinal tract, occurring in about 2% of the population. This diverticulum is typically located in the terminal ileum within 100 cm of the ileocecal valve. Clinicians frequently allude to the rule of two's when discussing Meckel's diverticulum: 2% of the population, 2 feet from the ileocecal valve, 2 inches in length, twice as common in males as in females, symptomatic in 2%, and may contain two types of heterotopic tissue — gastric and pancreatic. Meckel's diverticulum is a vestigial remnant of the omphalomesenteric duct. It is a true, congenital, diverticulum comprised of all three normal layers of the intestinal wall.

An understanding of the embryology of a Meckel's diverticulum is important in appreciating the breadth of possible presentations and complications arising from this entity. At 3 weeks gestation, the embryonic yolk sac communicates with the gastrointestinal tract through a vitelline duct. This duct normally disappears during the eighth week of gestation; just around the time the functioning placenta begins to replace the yolk sac as the primary source of delivering nutrients to the developing fetus. Failure of the duct to involute may result in one of several manifestations including cysts, a fibrous band connecting the intestine to the umbilicus, umbilical sinuses, complete persistence as an omphaloileal fistula, or a discrete Meckel's diverticulum.

CLINICAL PRESENTATION

Most cases of Meckel's diverticulum are asymptomatic. When symptoms do occur, however, they usually result from either ectopic tissue or remnant bands. Symptoms are more likely to occur in children less than 10 years of age, males, and patients with long diverticula that have a narrow base.

The most common symptom attributed to Meckel's diverticulum is gastrointestinal bleeding, occurring in more than 50% of symptomatic cases. Most bleeding diverticula (approximately 90%) contain ectopic gastric mucosa. The bleeding originates from the ileal mucosa adjacent to the diverticulum rather than the diverticulum itself. This mucosa is exposed to the ulcerogenic effects of the acid produced from the heterotopic gastric mucosa located within the diverticulum. Children typically present with hematochezia in a bleeding Meckel's whereas adults mostly present with melena. Although *Helicobacter pylori* infection has been associated with gastroduodenal ulcers and bleeding, it has not been found to play a significant role in bleeding from a Meckel's diverticulum.

Adults with Meckel's diverticulum most commonly present with gastrointestinal obstruction. Gastrointestinal obstruction accounts for about 40% of the complications arising from Meckel's diverticulum in adults. Obstruction in the setting of Meckel's diverticulum may arise secondary to bowel loops, which may become entrapped around a remnant band connecting the diverticulum to the umbilicus. Alternatively, a bowel volvulus may arise around the band. Obstruction may occur secondary to inflammation of the diverticulum (diverticulitis), or the diverticulum may act as a lead point for an intussusception. Finally, Meckel's diverticulum may be found within inguinal or femoral hernias where incarceration may produce intestinal obstruction; hernias containing a Meckel's diverticulum are referred to as Littre's hernias.

Inflammation of a Meckel's diverticulum occurs in about 20% of symptomatic cases. This is thought to occur through a mechanism similar to that of acute appendicitis; namely, luminal obstruction that results in distention, bacterial overgrowth, and wall compromise. Meckel's diverticulitis is clinically indistinguishable from acute appendicitis. In fact, it is thought to account for approximately 16% of cases of negative appendectomies. In some cases, Meckel's diverticulitis may be complicated by perforation, either localized with abscess formation or free flowing, or fistula formation. In some instances, Meckel's diverticulitis may be complicated by perforation or fistula formation. The incidence of cancer in a Meckel's diverticulum has been reported in 0.5 to 3.2% in symptomatic cases. Of these cases, more than one third have been found to harbor a carcinoid-type tumor. Other forms of cancer found in Meckel's diverticulum include adenocarcinomas, sarcomas, and lymphomas.

Umbilical symptoms from this disease result from a spectrum of abnormalities revolving around the incomplete involution of the embryonic vitelline duct. These variants of Meckel's diverticulum manifest as either a completely patent omphalomesenteric tract or a blind-ending sinus pouch. A completely patent tract may present as a draining enterocutaneous fistula, prolapsed bowel into the umbilical opening (which may in turn lead to obstruction and/or strangulation), and/or an umbilical abscess.

DIAGNOSIS

The majority of cases of Meckel's diverticulum are diagnosed in symptomatic patients. Fewer than 10% of symptomatic cases are successfully diagnosed on preoperative evaluation. A firm diagnosis based on clinical grounds cannot usually be made since the manifestations of complicated Meckel's diverticulum (such as bleeding, obstruction, perforation, and inflammation) are clinically indistinguishable from other underlying etiologies.

Plain radiography may be useful in evaluating complications of Meckel's diverticulum such as perforation or obstruction. However, this modality lacks the sensitivity and specificity to either diagnose a Meckel's diverticulum or distinguish it from other underlying causes. It is useful, however, as a first-line test in the evaluation of patients with gastrointestinal symptoms. Small bowel contrast studies, such as small bowel follow-through and enteroclysis, are generally the most specific means of preoperatively diagnosing a Meckel's diverticulum. Studies assessing the efficacy of these modalities, however, have found their sensitivity in detecting Meckel's diverticulum to fall below 50%. There is evidence that small bowel contrast studies are more accurate in detecting Meckel's diverticulum in adults than they are in children. While abdominal ultrasound is useful in the diagnosis of Meckel's diverticulitis and intussusception, it has not been found to be accurate in diagnosing the underlying diverticulum.

Computed Tomography (CT) and Magnetic Resonance Imaging (MRI) are helpful in investigating the patient presenting with acute abdominal signs and symptoms. Not only will these studies accurately identify acute complications (such as perforation or inflammation), they are excellent modalities for ruling out other possible diagnoses such as appendicitis. Their utility in specifically diagnosing Meckel's diverticulum is limited.

About 60% of cases of Meckel's diverticulum contain ectopic mucosa and 60% of these are gastric mucosa. Other types of heterotopic mucosa include pancreatic, duodenal, colonic, hepatobiliary. Most symptomatic cases of Meckel's diverticulum have been found to contain ectopic gastric mucosa. Overall, about 50% of cases of Meckel's diverticulum harboring ectopic gastric mucosa will go on to produce symptoms. These symptoms include diverticulitis, gastrointestinal bleeding, gastrointestinal obstruction, fistulization, and umbilical symptoms. Ectopic gastric mucosa is diagnosed in the preoperative period by a technetium 99m pertechnetate scan (Meckel scan). This nuclear medicine imaging test relies on the affinity of technetium 99m pertechnetate for gastric mucosa. The sensitivity of a Meckel's scan is from 50 to 91%. As mentioned earlier, other types of ectopic tissue have been localized to Meckel's diverticulae although they have shown no affinity for nuclear medicine scans.

Angiography is another localizing study but should be limited to cases where the patient acutely presents with significant gastrointestinal hemorrhage. The reason for this is multifold. First, angiography is an invasive test and the information obtained can be acquired using less invasive techniques such as CT angiography or MR angiography. Second, angiography requires relatively brisk bleeding (at a rate of at least 0.5 mL/min) in order to effectively localize the site of hemorrhage. Third, angiography is unique among imaging tests in that it carries the possibility of therapeutic intervention.

Another useful test for the localization of gastrointestinal bleeding is a technetium 99m tagged red blood cell scan. This method requires a bleeding rate of no less than 0.1mL/min to effectively localize the source of gastrointestinal hemorrhage. This modality has been found to be more sensitive but less specific than angiography in localizing the source of gastrointestinal hemorrhage. Images obtained more than 2 hrs after the injection of the labeled erythrocytes are much less accurate in localizing the source of hemorrhage. This is likely because the moving blood within the intestine tends to confound the localization effort.

The choice of imaging study should be guided by the patient's clinical presentation and the immediate complication at hand rather than the desire to confirm or rule out a Meckel's diverticulum as the underlying pathology. In cases requiring urgent surgical intervention, there is no advantage to be gained from the preoperative identification of a Meckel's diverticulum.

The differential diagnosis of Meckel's diverticulum is extensive and depends largely upon the patient's clinical presentation. The patient presenting with abdominal pain, tenderness, and elevated white blood count should be evaluated for acute appendicitis. In older adult patients, the possibility of acute diverticulitis originating from a redundant sigmoid colon should also be considered. In the patient presenting with visceral perforation (heralded by acute abdominal pain, tenderness, and free air under the diaphragm on an upright chest radiograph) the foremost differential would be a perforated duodenal ulcer. Perforation of another part of the gastrointestinal tract secondary to volvulus, intussusceptions, or obstruction should also be considered. Other important differential diagnoses for Meckel's diverticulum include inflammatory bowel disease, neoplasm, and polyps.

MANAGEMENT

Treatment depends on the presentation and the patient's clinical status. In patients presenting with acute gastrointestinal bleeding, the foremost priority in management should be assuring the patient's airway, breathing, and hemodynamic status. A nasogastric tube may be useful for ruling out a brisk upper gastrointestinal source of hemorrhage. Examination of the anus and a digital rectal examination are important in confirming/ruling out the presence of anal canal pathology or rectal polyps. The first diagnostic modality to be used is usually a colonoscopy although this is much less likely to be useful in localizing the source in the setting of acute brisk bleeding. The next diagnostic step may be a tagged red blood cell scan. Although this modality is not therapeutic, it may successfully localize the source of hemorrhage and help direct a subsequent surgical resection.

Conventional angiography is another option for patients with nonlocalized, ongoing bleeding. This modality carries diagnostic as well as therapeutic capabilities through gelfoam or coil embolization. However, complications of such procedures have been shown to occur in approximately 9.3% of cases. The complication of significant bowel ischemia necessitating subsequent surgical resection has been reported to occur in up to one third of cases. However, the recent introduction of microcatheters and newer embolization techniques, have led to the virtual abrogation of major ischemic complications.

The most appropriate surgical procedure for a symptomatic Meckel's diverticulum is segmental ileal resection to include both the diverticulum and the opposing ileal mucosa. Alternatively, simple diverticulectomy may be employed; however, this is not the preferred approach, and should not be used in cases of bleeding, tumor, or presence of concomitant ileal ulceration or inflammation. An uncomplicated Meckel's diverticulum discovered incidentally on imaging studies is not an indication for surgery. Controversy still exists regarding the management of an intraoperatively discovered incidental Meckel's diverticulum. The traditional surgical view has been to avoid the routine resection of Meckel's diverticulae found incidentally. It has long been believed that the risk of developing subsequent symptoms from such diverticulae is so low that the complications from the surgery itself outweigh this risk.

This traditional view has been challenged by data concerning the natural history of incidental Meckel's diverticulae. The lifetime risk of complications requiring surgical intervention from incidental Meckel's was reported to be 6.4%. The risk of morbidity from such intervention was found to be 19% while the risk of mortality was 1.5%. In contrast, the rate of morbidity following removal of incidentally discovered Meckel's diverticula was 4% with a 1% risk of mortality. Based on this information, routine prophylactic surgery for Meckel's diverticulae seems justifiable.

In an effort to reconcile these opposing views, some have advocated the prophylactic resection of only those diverticulae that exhibit features rendering them at higher risk for symptom development. Data from retrospective series indicate that patients less than 50 years of age, of male gender, with diverticulae greater than 2 cm in size, and ectopic gastric mucosa are more likely to be produce symptoms. The finding of an ulcer crater or thickening upon the palpation of the small bowel wall adjacent to and opposite the Meckel's diverticulum may be a factor favoring resection. This approach is not based on any firm evidence, however, and should therefore be considered in the context of the particular situation at hand. Where appropriate, a simple diverticulectomy is the preferred approach.

Ultimately, the decision of whether or not to resect an incidentally discovered Meckel's diverticulum is a clinical judgment that should be tailored to the circumstances of the case at hand. For example, a patient who is hemodynamically unstable and/or has undergone a complicated operative procedure should not be burdened with an additional resection that is not completely necessary.

REFERENCES

1. Rossini P, Gourtsoyiannis N, Bezzi M, *et al.* (1996) Meckel's diverticulum: Imaging diagnosis, *AJR Am J Roentgenol* **166:** 567–573.
2. Snyder CL. (2007) Current management of umbilical abnormalities and related anomalies. *Sem Ped Surg* **16**: 41–49.
3. Thurley PD, Halliday KE, Somers JM, Al-Daraji WI, Ilyas M, Broderick NJ. (2009) Radiological features of Meckel's diverticulum and its complications. *Clin Radiol* **64**: 109–118.
4. Park JJ, Wolff BG, Tollefson MK, *et al.* (2005) Meckel diverticulum: The mayo clinic experience with 1476 patients (1950–2002). *Ann Surg* **241**: 529–533.

Miscellaneous

ACUTE APPENDICITIS 65

Donald A. Plumley

INTRODUCTION

Abdominal pain is a common presenting complaint in a children's emergency department and often results in pediatric surgery consultation. Because acute appendicitis is a more frequent cause of abdominal pain, appendectomy is the most common intraabdominal surgical procedure in children. The ability to identify, diagnose and treat this problem in an expeditious and cost-effective fashion is expected of the pediatric surgical consultant. Prompt and accurate diagnosis reduces the significant morbidity and cost associated with a misdiagnosis. Despite technologic advances, primarily in imaging, diagnosis still requires a skilled clinician who is able and willing to perform a thorough and detailed history and physical examination. Appendicitis remains an enigma, a seemingly simple disease that despite our best efforts remains the most commonly misdiagnosed surgical condition.

PATHOPHYSIOLOGY

Epidemiology

Acute appendicitis is the most common surgical emergency in children younger than 15 yrs of age with over 70,000 cases reported annually in the United States. Although appendicitis can occur at any age, the peak incidence is in the 10–19 yr old age group (23.3 cases/10,000 populations per year).

There is a slight preponderance in males, and a 7% lifetime risk of developing appendicitis. Perforation rates are variable and may approach one third of children treated at children's hospitals. This may be a reflection of unequal access to care with a higher perforation rate in certain ethnicities and socioeconomic classes.

Etiology/Pathophysiology

The appendix is a true cecal diverticulum that arises at the convergence of the taenia coli. The appendicular artery, a branch of the ileocolic artery, is found in the mesoappendix that courses posterior to the ileocecal junction. The appendix and cecum form as a single anatomic unit of the midgut between the 8th and 12th weeks of gestation. The appendix can vary considerably in size and position and it is this variability in anatomic lie that contributes to the broad spectrum of symptoms at presentation. The base of the appendix arises in the right lower quadrant but the tip can extend to the pelvis, right upper quadrant, retrocecal region, and even retroperitoneum.

The appendix is a blind ending lymphoid lined structure that drains into the cecum via a small lumen. Obstruction of this lumen results in appendiceal distension, inflammation and eventual perforation of this structure. Obstruction in the pediatric population is most commonly a result of lymphoid hyperplasia, with peak incidence in childhood through young adulthood. This peak coincides with maximal lymphoid tissue in the appendix. Other causes of obstruction include fecalith, carcinoid, parasites, foreign body and Crohn's disease.

Wangensteen described the pathophysiolgy and resultant signs and symptoms of appendicits in an animal model with obstruction of the appenidcular orifice. Luminal obstruction leads to the distension of the appendix that is associated with generalized abdominal pain via the T10 dermatome, nausea and anorexia. As intraluminal pressure continues to increase, the appendix becomes engorged and edematous. This is the result of lymphatic and venous obstruction. The tissue then becomes ischemic, with localized pain and a resultant leukocytosis. Left untreated, the tissue will infarct, become gangrenous and perforate.

Whether the appendix is a vestigial structure or plays an immunologic role is debated. Fortunately, there appears to be no adverse effect of its surgical removal.

CLINICAL PRESENTATION

A careful and detailed clinical history is the first step in the evaluation of a child with suspected appendicitis. Pain is the most common and consistent presenting complaint in patients with acute appendicitis. A classic presentation is generalized abdominal pain that precedes nausea and vomiting. Typically, pain localizes to the right lower quadrant over a period of 8–12 hrs. The pain continues to worsen over the next 12–24 hrs, with rupture occurring 24–48 hrs after the onset of symptoms. This time course can be altered by antibiotic administration, steroids and co morbidities. Development of symptoms can also be prolonged by a pelvic or retrocecal location. Unfortunately, many pediatric patients fail to present with the classic symptoms described above.

Pain should be qualified with location, duration, severity, type (cramp, stab, and ache), migration and previous similar episodes. A history of pulmonary, genitourinary, and gynecologic problems should also be obtained, since these can often mimic appendicitis.

Anorexia, nausea and vomiting often occur shortly after the onset of pain. These are relatively nonspecific findings in children with abdominal pain and need to be considered with other elements of the history. Fever is usually only low grade, high spiking fevers are more commonly seen with perforation, pneumonia or urinary tract infections (UTIs). Less reliable complaints include diarrhea, constipation and urinary symptoms. These findings can all be associated with appendicitis, but the interpretation of a constellation of symptoms along with a thorough physical exam will confirm the diagnosis in a good percentage of children.

Physical Exam

Physical examination in a child presenting with abdominal pain is of great importance in the diagnosis of acute appendicitis. Often, in uncomplicated cases, examination coupled with a detailed history is all that is needed to make the diagnosis. In more complex cases, the examination serves to guide prudent ordering of laboratory tests and images. Examination of a child requires patience, perseverance and practice. Its importance in the diagnostic armamentarium however cannot be underestimated.

Examination of a child should start as one enters the room. One should speak in a quiet friendly voice and observe the child surreptitiously.

Complete an entire history before approaching the child. The patient should be observed in a parent's arms or bed as well as in an active state. Examination of the abdomen begins with light tapping in each quadrant and is followed by a percussion exam to localize and qualify the severity of pain. It is common practice to start the exam in a quadrant where there is no pain/discomfort and to finish in the painful quadrant. Finally, deep palpation of each quadrant is performed to better define areas of tenderness, mass or referred pain from the left to right (Rovsing's sign.) A quiet conversation about an age appropriate subject will often distract the patient and allow for a more accurate exam.

The examination concludes with an attempt to reproduce the pain by coughing, jumping, shaking or heel strike. In difficult cases, I will check for a psoas sign(right lower-quadrant pain that is produced with extension of the hip while the patient is lying on their left side) and an obturator sign(pain elicited by flexion and medial rotation of the hip.) Rectal or pelvic examinations are rarely if ever indicated. Toddlers with significant stranger anxiety may never allow a good exam, but a second exam or one after the child has fallen asleep can sometimes be helpful.

Laboratory Test

There is no single specific laboratory test that is specific for the diagnosis of acute appendicitis. Results of some laboratory tests along with the history and physical exam however can help confirm the diagnosis.

A urinalysis often will show a high specific gravity and elevated ketones secondary to poor oral intake, nausea, vomiting and anorexia. Pyuria is more suggestive of an UTI or pyleonephritis while hematuria is more suggestive of infection or renal calculi. A few leukocytes or microscopic hematuria can be a sign of ureteral or bladder irritation by an inflamed appendix. A beta-HCG should also be performed in all girls that have reached menarche to rule out pregnancy.

A complete blood count (CBC) with differential should be obtained, as the white blood cell count in acute appendicitis is usually mildly elevated. A low leukocyte count is suggestive of viral illness while a significant leukocytosis is commonly seen with pulmonary and urinary infections or perforated appendix. A differential with a left shift of increased polymorphonuclear lymphocytes and band forms should be noted. Leukocytosis with a left shift is independently associated with appendicitis in children.

C-reactive protein has been used by some centers but does not add much to the diagnostic specificity of a CBC and differential. Electrolytes and liver function tests are only ordered if the child has been chronically ill or appear profoundly dehydrated. Unfortunately, there is no single serum marker that is specific for acute appendicitis.

Imaging

In patients with a history and physical examination consistent with acute appendicitis no imaging is required. Imaging is useful only in cases where the diagnosis is unclear based on the clinical presentation. In an attempt to limit cost, resource utilization, and radiation exposure, only the imaging modalities that are necessary to complete the diagnosis are obtained.

Plain films are sometimes useful in the evaluation of patients with a chronic course or where the diagnosis is more consistent with other etiologies of abdominal pain. A plain film series can demonstrate obstruction, ileus or constipation. Plain films are useful in the identification of 90% of kidney stones but rarely facilitate visualization of a fecalith.

Ultrasound is helpful in diagnosing appendicitis in children, but availability, quality and accuracy are variable. Ultrasound findings that are consistent with acute appendicitis include an appendiceal width greater than 6 mm, localized pain, noncompressibility and free fluid. Advanced cases of perforation will demonstrate a phlegmon or abscess. Ultrasound also is very useful in girls to evaluate for any underlying gynecologic pathology.

Computed Tomography (CT) scan has high sensitivity and specificity for the diagnosis of acute appendicitis. It is widely utilized and provides a quick and thorough evaluation of the abdomen and pelvis. CT scan findings in acute appendicitis include a thickened wall, fat stranding, fecalith, phlegmon, or abscess. Appendicitis cannot be excluded if the appendix is not visualized, especially with a short duration of symptoms and minimal inflammation. Unfortunately, this modality is often used as a screening test and administers a significant radiation dose that may increase a child's lifetime cancer risk. Most clinical pathways and studies by pediatric surgeons have looked at diagnostic models that limit the use of CT scan to select cases.

The diagnostic algorithm for abdominal pain (Figure 1) reserves CT scan for cases with an indeterminate diagnosis after a thorough history, physical exam, laboratory and ultrasound findings.

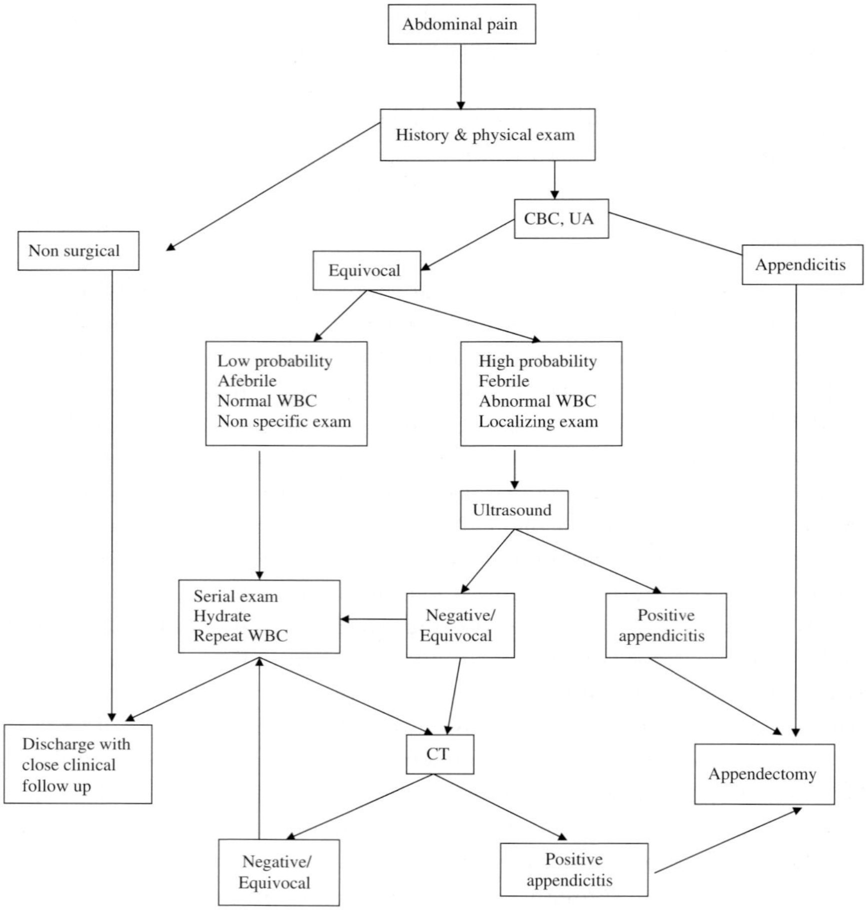

Figure 1. Diagnostic algorithm for abdominal pain.

MANAGEMENT

Treatment for acute appendicitis is fairly straightforward once the diagnosis has been established. The method and timing of appendectomy can vary, but the ultimate goal of appendiceal extirpation is curative.

The child should be hydrated and receive preoperative antibiotics prior to the operating room. A second generation cephalosporin usually suffices, unless the child is toxic. In such an instance, broad spectrum antibiotics can be used. The operative approach can vary and is often institutional or user dependent. Outcomes between open appendectomy and one performed laparasocpically are minimal. The length of surgery, length of stay, return to baseline activity, and complication rates vary little in the hands of skilled surgeons.

Open appendectomies have been performed for over 100 years and can be safely performed in patients of any age. The benefits of open appendectomy over the laparoscopic approach include minimal resource utilization, less expense, single small incision in young thin patients and ease of performance. An open appendectomy is performed through a transverse or oblique skin incision with utilization of a muscle splitting technique. The peritoneum is carefully opened and the appendix is located. Usually the appendix can be identified by palpation and gentle blunt dissection, followed by mobilization into the operative field. The mesoappendix is ligated and divided. The appendix is then ligated and the stump cauterized. Traditionally the stump is inverted with a purse string or Z stitch, this however is not necessary. The muscle layers are approximated with dissolvable suture, and the skin is closed in a subcuticular fashion. A drain is rarely indicated.

Laparascopic appendectomy can be safely performed in children of any age and size. The benefits of laparoscopy are small incisions and excellent visualization of other organs (especially pelvic structures in girls). Laparoscopic appendectomy can be performed through 1–3 ports. Traditionally, an umbilical port, a left lower quadrant port and suprapubic port are placed. The appendix is mobilized, and the mesoappendix is divided with an endo-GIA stapler, harmonic scalpel or electrocautery. The appendix is then amputated with another load of the endo-GIA stapler or by placement of an endoloop.

Postoperative care is similar with either approach. In uncomplicated cases no further antibiotics are administered, diet is resumed and pain can be adequately controlled with parenteral narcotics or nonsteroidal anti-inflammatory drugs. Children are usually discharged within 24 hrs.

Perforated appendicitis is treated with broad spectrum antibiotic. Traditionally, ampicillin, gentamicin and clindamycin or metronidazole is administered while other institutions advocate single drug therapy or early conversion to oral antibiotics. The duration of intravenous antibiotics varies and again is institutional dependent. Five full days of antibiotics are adequate if the patient is afebrile, ambulating and tolerating a regular diet. If the child remains febrile or develops an ileus, the antibiotics are continued. If symptoms persist, a complication should be suspected. Diet is resumed as bowel function returns, and activity is encouraged.

Patients with a long duration of symptoms (>7 days), or those who have a palpable abdominal mass or abscess by preoperative imaging can be treated with nonoperative medical management. These children are started on broad spectrum antibiotics and if significant, abscess cavities are drained by the surgeon or Interventional Radiology. These children then undergo an interval appendectomy 6–8 wks later (Figure 2).

Differential Diagnosis

The differential diagnosis for acute appendicitis is quite extensive. Abdominal pain is a common presenting symptom in children, but acute appendicitis accounts for only a small percentage of these patients. Common causes of abdominal pain in children can be classified as gastrointestinal, urologic,

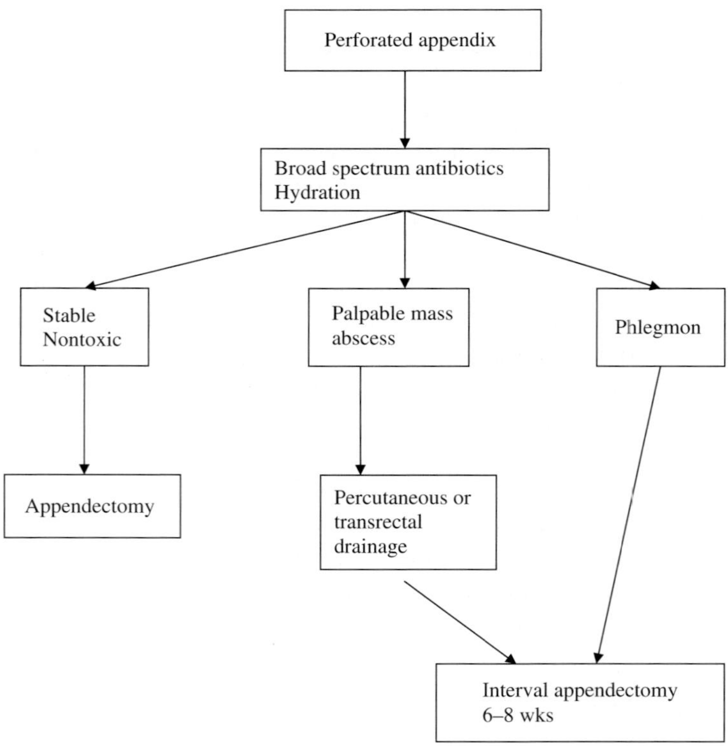

Figure 2. Diagnostic algorithm for perforated appendix.

gynecologic and pulmonary (Table 1). Metabolic, congenital, and malignant etiologies are rarely encountered. The diagnosis may be confirmed prior to surgery but is often may not identified until the time of the operation. If a normal appendix is encountered, other etiologies of pain should be considered. One should inspect the mesentery (lymph nodes), ileum (inflammation, Meckel's) and ovaries (torsion, tumor, cyst).

COMPLICATIONS

Complications are rarely encountered with straightforward acute appendicitis, adding to the challenge of an accurate and prompt diagnosis. The

Table1. Differential diagnosis for abdominal pain.

Gastrointestinal
Gastroenteritis
Mesenteric adenitis
Meckel's diverticulitis
Torsion omentum
Crohns disease
Typhlitis
Constipation
Intussusception
Urologic
Pyelonephritis
Urinary calculi
Urinary tract infection
Gynecologic
Ovarian cyst
Mittelschmerz
Ovarian torsion
Ovarian tumor
Pelvic inflammatory disease
Ectopic pregnancy
Pulmonary
Pneumonia
Pleurisy
Pleural effusion

complication rate does become significant in children that have a perforation. While fever and feeding intolerance are fairly common in the early postoperative course following perforation of the appendix, these symptoms usually resolve by the third to fourth postoperative day. If fever persists, an abscess should be considered. In most cases, an abscess can be treated by CT or ultrasound guided drainage. If feeding intolerance continues, plain films should be obtained to rule out a small bowel obstruction. Intrabdominal or pelvic abscess occurs in about 5% of perforated appendicitis patients, while adhesive small bowel obstruction is much less common. Wound infections are also rare, occurring in less than 5% of cases. Mortality is rarely seen and is usually related to underlying co morbidities.

REFERENCES

1. Silen W. (2005) *Cope's Early Diagnosis of the Acute Abdomen.* Oxford University Press, London.
2. Wangensteen OH, Bowers WF. (1937). Significance of the obstructive factor in the genesis of acute appendicitis. *Arch Surg* **34**:496–526.
3. Ponsky TA, Huang ZJ, Kittle K, Eichelberger MR, Gilbert JC, Brody F, Newman KD. (2004) Hospital and patient level characteristics and the risk of appendiceal rupture and negative appendectomy in children. *JAMA* **292**:1977–1982.
4. Kosloske AM, Love CL, Rohrer JE, Goldthorn JF, Lacey SR. (2004) The diagnosis of appendicitis in children: Outcomes of a strategy based on pediatric surgery evaluation. *Pediatrics* **113**:29–34.
5. Pena BM, Cook EF, Mandl KD. (2004) Selective imaging strategies for the diagnosis of appendicitis in children. *Pediatrics* **113**:24–28.

INFLAMMATORY BOWEL DISEASE

66

Evan R. Kokoska

BACKGROUND

The worldwide prevalence of inflammatory bowel disease (IBD) is approximately 2 million people and the incidence is 1 in 1000 Western country inhabitants. Presentation is not uncommon (15–25%) in childhood and the usual onset is during the second and third decades. Crohn's disease (CD) is more frequent than ulcerative colitis (UC) with a slight male preponderance.

It is well reported that many affected children have a genetic component such that a child with a known IBD family member may be predisposed to either UC or CD. IBD is more common among families with northern European or Jewish ethnicity. In addition to a genetic susceptibility, environmental factors may have a role. While cigarette smoking is a risk factor for CD, it appears to be protective for UC. However, cigarette smoking does not seem to have a role in children. Infectious pathogens (such as *Yersinia* species, *E. coli*, *Listeria*, etc.) may elicit or contribute to ongoing gut inflammation in CD. While the exact etiology of IBD is unclear, there exists an interplay involving a genetic defect in underlying immune function which is associated with an excessive gut reaction to normal microflora.

DIAGNOSIS

Children with IBD typically present with abdominal pain, diarrhea, perianal disease, weight loss, and growth delay. The diagnosis of IBD involves endoscopic assessment of the gut with histological tissue examination. Laboratory work can be helpful. C-reactive protein and erythrocyte sedimentation rate (ESR) elevation, anemia, leukocytosis, and thrombocytosis have a high sensitivity (when normal, can rule out the disease) for IBD. Serology testing, in contrast, has a high specificity (when abnormal, can rule in the disease). The sensitivity and specificity of perinuclear anti-neutrophile cytoplasm antibodies (pANCA) for UC are 55% and 89%, respectively, while, for CD, anti-*Saccharomyces cerevisiae* antibodies (ACSA) has a sensitivity and specificity of 37% and 97%, respectively.

Differentiating UC and CD is largely dependent upon disease location. For this reason, all patients warrant complete gastrointestinal (GI) tract evaluation. This should include esophagogastroduodenoscopy (EGD), colonoscopy with ileal intubation, and radiographic small bowel (SB) assessment. SB imaging can be done with a SB follow-through (less common), computed tomographic (CT) enteroclysis, or magnetic resonance (MR) enteroclysis (as MR machines become faster). In older symptomatic children, in whom endoscopy of the terminal ileum is normal or difficult, examination of the SB mucosa with wireless capsule endoscopy can also be helpful. Capsule endoscopy should be preceded, however, by SB imaging to rule out a stricture.

Crohn's Disease and Ulcerative Colitis

CD generally presents in an insidious fashion with abdominal pain, weight loss, and malaise. Inflammation is transmural and pan-enteric, can occur from the mouth to the anus, and commonly has focal disease and "skip" lesions. Oral ulcers and peri-anal disease are common in CD. Disease can be localized to the ileocecum (50–60%), colon only (25–30%) or SB only (15–20%). Isolated jejunal and ileal disease (10%) is more common in children. The rectum is usually spared. Extra-intestinal symptoms associated with CD include arthritis and primary sclerosing cholangitis. The transmural nature of CD commonly leads to regional complications such as fistulae, abscesses, and strictures. Endoscopic characteristics of CD range from aphthous ulcers limited to the mucosa to longitudinal deep ulceration with pseudopolyps. On biopsy, granulomas are seen 50% of the time.

Children with UC commonly present with bloody diarrhea and tenesmus and the differential diagnosis should include infectious colitis. The inflammation associated with UC is limited to the mucosa, usually starts in the rectum (at the dentate line) with continuous proximal extension. Perianal disease is rare in children with UC. In addition, the diagnosis of UC should include the exclusion of SB disease and the absence of granulomas on microscopic tissue evaluation.

Indeterminant Colitis

The diagnosis of UC vs. CD is difficult 10–15% of the time and currently indeterminant colitis (IC) is considered to be a subgroup of pediatric IBD. IC can present with pain, bleeding, diarrhea, and weight loss. IC is characterized by an early age of onset (within the first several years of life), endoscopic features of colonic erosions and ulcers, and overlapping histologic features of CD and UC. While the rectum is usually spared, IC is associated with a rapid progression to pancolitis. Currently, most authors believe UC and CD may not be two distinct diseases but rather represent two ends of a clinical spectrum.

MEDICAL TREATMENT OF IBD

Medical treatments of IBD target both the induction of and maintenance of disease. Sulfasalazine and 5-aminosalicylates (5-ASA) are locally effective anti-inflammatory agents useful for induction during mild flares and maintenance therapy for UC. Corticosteroids have highly effective anti-inflammatory activity and provide excellent control for moderate to severe CD and UC. Chronic use, however, is undesirable in children due to attendant toxicities and growth retardation.

Immunomodulators (azathioprine and 6-mercaptopurine (6-MP)) cause immunosuppression in large part through the induction of lymphocyte apoptosis. Immunomodulators are very effective in long term maintenance of both CD and UC. The addition of 6-MP to corticosteroids in children with CD helps to decrease the overall steroid need and improve remission. Adverse effects include pancreatitis, leukopenia, and elevated liver function tests.

Infliximab (Remicade), a biological agent, is a monoclonal antibody that binds tumor necrosis factor-alpha (TNF-α), an important proinflammatory cytokine believed to be involved in both UC and CD. Infliximab promotes significant mucosal healing which has a dramatic effect upon symptoms lasting approximately 8 wks. It is useful for the induction and maintenance of active and fistulizing CD. The role of infliximab in children with UC is currently limited. Infliximab has also been shown to help control extra-intestinal CD symptoms including arthritis and pyoderma gangrenosum. Its use has been associated with the occurrence of rare but fatal hepatosplenic T-cell lymphoma.

SURGICAL INTERVENTION

Operative Treatment of CD — Small Bowel

In pediatric CD, the likelihood of surgery is 30% and 50% after 3 and 5 yrs, respectively. The major indication for the operative management of CD is medically refractory acute disease (perforation and/or abdominal abscess) or chronic disease (stricture or internal fistula). Resection should be limited to grossly diseased bowel only with the goal of the preservation of as much SB length as possible. Recurrent CD is the rule rather than the exception. Endoscopic evidence of recurrent disease at the resection site is seen 72% of the time after 1 yr. However, children with CD can have a fairly prolonged symptom free interval (up to 4 yrs) following SB and ileocecal resections. Stricturoplasty, most commonly a Heineke–Mikulicz, in the absence of intestinal perforation or abdominal sepsis, may have a selective role for the treatment of duodenal, focal enteric or anastomotic strictures.

Operative Treatment of CD and ID — Colon

Similar to Crohn's SB disease, the indication for colectomy for either CD or ID is failed medical management. For limited disease, segmental resection is recommended. However, patients and families should be counseled that resection of grossly diseased colon only is associated with a high rate of recurrent disease in the remaining colon. As compared to SB resection, the symptom free interval after segmental colonic resections is much shorter (up to 1 yr). For children with more generalized colonic disease, the recommended operation is a subtotal colectomy with ileorectal anastomosis, with the goal of preserving anorectal continence. In patients with severe peri-anal disease or a lead pipe rectum, temporary ileal diversion (6–12 mths) can be helpful.

Treatment of CD — Perianal Disease

Over half of children with CD have signs of perianal disease. Adequate diagnosis involves an exam under anesthesia and anoscopy. MRI with contrast can be useful to assess the extent of perirectal disease. In general, initial conservative treatment is recommended as aggressive operative management may cause outcomes (such as anal incontinence) that are worse than the disease itself. Initial medical treatment includes warm sitz baths and fiber products. Antibiotics (metronidazole or ciprofloxacin; 6–8 wk courses) may be helpful but recurrence is common after discontinuance. Immunomodulators and infliximab have also been shown useful for pediatric perianal CD.

Excision of skin tags and hemorrhoids in children with CD may lead to chronic nonhealing ulcers. Thus, local treatment is indicated with the exception of bleeding or a malignant concern. Perineal abscesses and perianal fistulae can arise from either cryptoglandular areas or an anal canal fissure or ulcer. Simple incision and drainage of anorectal abscesses will usually allow for resolution of the inflammatory process. Antibiotics should also be employed in cases of buttock cellulitis. Children with normal continence and simple fistulae (such as intersphincteric or low trans-sphincteric) can be managed with fistulectomy.

In children with high complex fistulae, placement of a noncutting seton (such as a vessel loop) will establish drainage and prevent a potential abscess. Chronic fistulae in the absence of significant proctitis can be treated with rectal mucosal advancement flaps, with or without proximal diversion. Anovaginal or rectovaginal fistulae can also be managed with transanal flap advancements, with a 60–80% success rate. Persistent failure of all other methods necessitates permanent ileostomy with or without proctectomy.

Operative Treatment of UC — Colon and Rectum

Proctocolectomy (PC) is curative in patients with UC. In the pediatric population, indications for PC include acute disease (toxic megacolon, bleeding, or perforation) and symptomatic disease refractory to medical management. Mucosal dysplasia is rarely an issue for the pediatric patient but should be considered for adolescents with prolonged disease. The risk of colorectal cancer in patients with UC is 2%, 8%, and 18% after 10, 20, and 30 yrs, respectively.

In most cases, children with UC are on moderate to high doses of steroids. With acute operative indications, most surgeons recommend total abdominal colectomy with ileostomy and a Hartmann's pouch. Intestinal continuity is then restored 3–6 mths later with or without a temporary loop ileostomy. In cases of chronic disease or dysplasia, ileal pouch anal anastomosis (IPAA) can be safely done in the same stage as total PC.

Long term outcome following PC with IPAA appears to be independent upon the type of pouch, type of anastomosis (stapled vs. hand-sewn), or number of stages. Thus, operative technique should be dependent upon the comfort level of the surgeon. Acutely (first 2 yrs), straight pouches have a significantly higher frequency of stooling while J pouches have a higher incidence of pouchitis. It has been clearly shown that an operative experience exceeding several hundred cases is associated with a significantly lower complication rate.

While IC is not a contra-indication for PC with IPAA, this procedure should *not* be implemented in children with clear signs of CD (such as aphthous ulceration, rectal sparing, or granuloma formation). During the operation, meticulous SB inspection for evidence of CD (such as fat wrapping, inflammatory skip lesions, and hyperemia) is critical. Crohn's colitis usually recurs and will eventually lead to pouch failure.

The overall complication rate following initial resection and the reconstructive stage in children with UC is high (30–60%). Early complications are commonly associated with pouch tension, ischemia, or torsion, and include ileoanal separation (2–6%), pouch fistula (5–10%), pelvic abscess (6–12%), and anal stricture (2–15%). Anal stricture or narrowing is a common early cause of pouch dysfunction but is usually amendable to serial dilation (either digital or balloon). Strictures refractory to either medical treatment or repeated dilations may require an advancement flap anoplasty.

Adhesive SB obstruction, related to the resection and/or ileostomy, occurs 15–30% of the time following PC with IPAA. Stool continence generally improves markedly in the first 12 mths and the majority of patients are continent by 24 mths. However, in the long term, the cumulative rate of pouch failure is 15% at 10–15 yrs.

Pouchitis occurs 20–50% of the time following PC with IPAA for UC and is recurrent or chronic 5–15% of the time. Signs and symptoms of pouchitis are crampy pain, tenesmus, frequency (+/− bloody stools), and endoscopic and histologic evidence of inflammation. It is important to rule out infectious causes such as *C. difficile* or cytomegalovirus (CMV). Initial treatment includes antibiotics (ciprofloxacin or metronidazole; 2–4 wk courses) and probiotics. Recurrence is common (up to 60%) requiring an additional antibiotic course. Chronic pouchitis can be treated with topical 5-ASA agents, 6-MP, or infliximab. Recurrent pouchitis, while an uncommon cause of pouch failure, seems to be an important predictor of CD.

Despite the absence of preoperative clinical features (radiographic, endoscopic, and histologic) of CD, up to 15% of patients, in experienced centers, develop signs of CD. These signs include chronic pouchitis, recurrent pelvic abscesses, perineal disease, or strictures. Patients with signs of CD generally have a very good response to infliximab therapy and 60–70% of the time can maintain a pouch long term. However, the other third eventually require pouch excision with permanent ileostomy.

REFERENCES

1. Hugot, *et al.* (2007) Inflammatory bowel diseases: The pediatric gastroenterologist's perspective. *Pediatr Radiol* **37**:1065–1070.
2. Alexander F. (2007) Complications of ileal pouch anal anastomosis. *Sem Pediatr Surg* **12**:200–204.
3. Strong SA. (2007) Perianal Crohn's disease. *Sem Pediatr Surg* **16**:185–193.
4. Markowitz J. (2008) Current treatment of inflammatory bowel disease in children. *Dig Liver Dis* **40**:16–21.
5. Romano C, *et al.* (2008) Indeterminant colitis: A distinctive clinical pattern of inflammatory bowel disease in children. *Pediatrics* **22**:e1278–e1281.
6. RIBD Working Group. (2008) Refractory inflammatory bowel disease in children. *J Pediatr Gastroenterol Nutr* **47**:266–272.
7. Ba'ath ME, *et al.* (2007) Surgical management of inflammatory bowel disease. *Arch Dis Child* **92**:312–316.

Miscellaneous

POLYPOID DISEASES 67

Evan R. Kokoska

BENIGN POLYPS

Children with benign polyps generally present with hematochezia, pain, prolapse, or a nonreducible intussusception and are found in 1% of all school aged children. The most common cause of rectal bleeding in children is lymphoid polyps (15%) or juvenile polyps (80%).

Lymphoid Polyps

Lymphoid polyps are usually flat or nonpedunculated and on a microscopic level composed of prominent submucosal lymphoid tissue or Peyer's patches. The natural history is spontaneous regression and resection is only indicated in the setting of bleeding or a bowel obstruction.

Isolated Juvenile Polyps

Isolated juvenile polyps may be up to several centimeters in diameter and commonly have an ulcerated surface. The polyps are made up of either retention or inflammatory tissue and many times appear to be a mucosal reaction to an inflammatory process. The polyps are either solitary (50%) or few (3–5; 40–50%) in number and frequently found in the rectosigmoid region. Recommended treatment of symptomatic isolated polyps is either endoscopic excision or, when large, segmental bowel resection. The remainder of the small bowel and colon should also be inspected to rule-out any synchronous polyps.

HAMARTOMATOUS CONDITIONS WITH MALIGNANT POTENTIAL

Juvenile Polyposis Syndromes

Isolated juvenile polyps are defined as less than five in total number and felt to be nonmalignant. In contrast to children with isolated polyps, children with juvenile polyposis syndromes demonstrate polyps either throughout the entire gastrointestinal (GI) tract or confined to the colon and rectum. While the lesions are technically hamartomas, patients have a significantly increased risk of colorectal cancer (CRC). This is felt to be secondary to chronic inflammation and eventual mucosal dysplastic or adenomatous changes.

Diffuse juvenile polyposis (DJP) of infancy is a nonfamilial condition characterized by extensive polyposis throughout the entire GI tract. Infants present with bleeding, small bowel obstruction, intussusception, and protein losing enteropathy. The condition is almost universally fatal during the first several years of life and operative treatment is generally supportive. DJP is an autosomal dominant (AD) disease in which the juvenile polyps are confined to the colon and rectum. Patients have a 50% lifetime risk of the development of CRC. Juvenile polyposis coli (JPC) is also AD and most children have either a family history or 50–100 polyps throughout the GI tract. For both DJP and JPC, there is debate regarding whether total proctocolectomy (PC) with endorectal pull-through (ERPT) is warranted. At minimum, close endoscopic surveillance (at least biennially — every other year) is recommended.

Peutz–Jeghers Syndrome (PJS)

Peutz–Jeghers Syndrome (PJS) is an AD inherited condition characterized by melanotic spots on the buccal mucosa and lips and intestinal polyposis. The polyps are encountered in the small intestine (55%), stomach and duodenum (30%), and colorectum (15%). The lesions are pedunculated and made up of smooth muscle (of the muscularis mucosa) arborization. Presentation varies depending upon polyp location. Younger patients usually present with small intestinal obstruction or intussusception. Other morbidity includes abdominal pain, hematochezia, and colonic prolapse.

Similar to patients with juvenile polyposis, patients have a significantly increased (13 fold) risk of death from a GI cancer, felt in part to be due to malignant transformation. Almost 50% of patients with PJS die from cancer by age 57 yrs and the cumulative risk of cancer development is 93% in patients aged 15–64 yrs. Treatment should include an aggressive screening and biopsy program (at least biennially) as well as comprehensive genetic counseling.

ADENOMATOUS POLYPOSIS SYNDROMES WITH MALIGNANT POTENTIAL

Adenomatous polyps, with the potential for malignant degeneration, constitute 3% of all pediatric polyps. Of all patients with CRC, 5–10% is associated with a clear genetic syndrome. The diagnosis of familial adenomatous polyposis (FAP), an AD disorder, is made by visualizing numerous colonic adenomas (at least 5 but usually over 100), evidence of other polyps throughout the GI tract, and a family history. Patients usually present in the second and third decades of life with pain or bleeding. All of these patients develop CRC at a mean age of 39 yrs. Malignant changes are demonstrated 7% and 15% of the time by the age of 20 and 25 yrs, respectively. The genetic basis of FAP is loss of the tumor suppressor gene adenomatous polyposis coli (APC) at chromosome 5q. Diagnosis can be further suggested by slit lamp exam demonstrating congenital hypertrophy of the retinal pigment epithelium and usually can be confirmed with genetic testing.

Patients with FAP can have noncolonic adenomas in the duodenum (60–90%), ileum (10–25%) and stomach (5%) and also have a significantly increased risk of thyroid cancer and hepatoblastoma. Desmoid tumors, or diffuse mesenteric fibromatosis, occur up to 20% of the time following colectomy and can have substantial morbidity due to obstruction or constriction of the intestines, blood vessels, and ureters.

Phenotypic variants associated with FAP (or an APC germline mutation) include Gardner syndrome and Turcot syndrome. Patients with Gardner syndrome also have skull and mandible osteomas (80%), epidermal inclusion cysts (35%), and dental abnormalities. Turcot syndrome is associated with concomitant brain tumors (gliomas, ependymomas, and medulloblastomas).

Attenuated adenomatous polyposis coli (AAPC) is also associated with an APC gene mutation. AAPC is characterized by fewer and more proximal polyps (<30) and a later presentation. MYH-associated polyposis (MAP) is an autosomal recessive (AR) polyposis syndrome. In MAP, the genetic perturbation involves the MUTYH gene on chromosome 1 which encodes for a deoxyribonucleic acid (DNA) repair enzyme.

MANAGEMENT

In children with known FAP, screening for hepatoblastoma with alpha-fetoprotein (AFP) should be done to age 5 yrs. Annual to biennial flexible sigmoidoscopy should be started by age 10–12 yrs. Medical treatment of the adenomatous polyposis syndromes is limited. Nonsteroidal anti-inflammatory drugs (NSAIDs) may decrease the number of polyps but do not overall affect the management. The progression of desmoid tumors may decrease with the use of anti-estrogen therapy (Tamoxifen) and NSAIDs (Sulindac).

Surgery for FAP is usually delayed until the late teenage years unless biopsies demonstrate advanced histologic features. Most authors recommend PC before the age of 25 yrs. While some have advocated rectal sparing operations in cases with minimal rectal adenomas, total abdominal colectomy, mucosal proctectomy, and ERPT is the preferred management. In part this is based upon observations that following a total abdominal colectomy and ileorectal anastomosis, 44% of patients require subsequent rectal treatment. Patients with preserved rectum develop cancer 10% and 30% of the time by ages 50 and 60 yrs, respectively.

Intestinal continuity can be restored with either an ileal J-pouch or straight ileal-anal anastomosis, depending upon surgeon experience and patient anatomy. Pouchitis, a common complication following PC for ulcerative colitis, occurs less frequently (15–20%) in patients with FAP. In patients with favorable anatomy (minimal tension or pouch ischemia), a "protective" loop ileostomy may not be necessary. Laparoscopic assistance, especially for colonic mobilization, has been well described.

Postoperative complications include wound infection, anastomotic dehiscence or leak, injury to the ureters, prostate, bladder, and ejaculatory dysfunction. Following either a J-pouch or ileo-anal anastomosis, incontinence of gas and stool is common for the first 2 yrs. This complication can be reduced but probably not negated by minimizing the stretching of the sphincteric complex during the rectal mucosectomy. Anti-motility agents (Imodium and Lomotil) and fiber may be helpful during this postoperative phase. The goal after 2 yrs is bowel control with 6–8 semi-formed stools a day. This typical postoperative course should be explained when counseling families.

Families with FAP and the other familial syndromes should be referred for genetic counseling. In addition, it is *critical* that patients be educated on the need for lifelong cancer surveillance, even after a PC with ERPT. Esophagogastroduodenoscopy (EGD) and endoscopic pouch visualization with ablation of any remaining ileal polyps is still necessary. It is believed that the increased cellular proliferation within the efferent loop of ileal pouches is associated with an increased risk of adenomas and cancer. Ileal pouch cancer has been reported and the long term incidence of pouch adenomas is up to 60%.

HEREDITARY NONPOLYPOSIS COLORECTAL CANCER (HNPCC)

Hereditary nonpolyposis colorectal cancer (HNPCC), or Lynch syndrome, is characterized by the early onset of CRC, with a familial association, in the absence of colonic or rectal adenomas. The Amsterdam criteria for a family with HNPCC is three affected individuals across two generations with at least one individual as a first degree relative of the other two and a diagnosis before the age of 50 yrs. The lifetime risk of CRC with HNPCC is 60–80%. Lynch syndrome 1 is limited to the colon while Lynch syndrome 2 is also associated with other extracolonic cancers (such as endometrial, ovarian, stomach, pancreatic, etc.). Any child presenting with CRC in the absence of a polyposis syndrome warrants a familial genetic investigation for HNPCC.

REFERENCES

1. Wehbi M, *et al.* (2009) Familial adenomatous polyposis. Emedicine. Retrieved January 5, 2010, from http://emedicine.medscape.com/article/175377-overview.

2. Shalkow J, *et al.* (2009) Colorectal tumors. Emedicine. Retrieved January 5, 2010, from http://emedicine.medscape.com/article/993370-overview.
3. Mukherjee S, *et al.* (2009) Peutz–Jeghers syndrome. Emedicine. Retrieved January 5, 2010, from http://emedicine.medscape.com/article/182006-overview.
4. Tajika M, *et al.* (2009) Prevalence of adenomas and carcinomas in the ileal pouch after proctocolectomy in patients with familial adenomatous polyposis. *J Gastrointest Surg* **13**:1266–1273.

FISTULA-IN-ANO 68

Brian Duffy

INTRODUCTION

Fistula-in-ano (FIA) is an abnormal communication between the anus and the perianal skin. The purpose of this chapter is to outline a brief history, define the pathophysiology, review the clinical presentation, and discuss the approach to surgical management. This chapter will focus mainly on the infant population. Acquired FIA in this age group arises predominantly from a perianal abscess (PA) in the absence of underlying systemic disease. The management of perianal fistula in the setting of inflammatory bowel disease will be covered in another chapter in this handbook. Our understanding of FIA is incomplete and treatment is still controversial. We will investigate some of the controversy, then propose a reasonable and practical approach to surgical management.

Although PA and FIA have been recognized for hundreds of years, we do not know the exact underlying etiology. Several hypotheses have been proposed, but none have been reliably proven with scientific data. In 1880, Herrmann and Desfosses proposed that FIA arises from infection of the small anal glands.[1] In 1956, Eisenhammer suggested that PA arises from infection of these glands within the intersphincteric space, and that FIA can be a natural sequela of this infection.[1] In 1961, Parks postulated that cystic dilation of the anal glands was a necessary precursor to infection, but that individual susceptibility to infection is dependent upon the number, depth, and configuration of the glands.[1] In 1980, Shafik proposed that entrapment of migratory cells from the urogenital sinus during development of the perineum leads to ectopic epithelium which may perpetuate subsequent infection.[1] Although there is no unifying theory, the consensus in the literature is that PA and FIA arise primarily from infection of the anal glands and that treatment should target the infection and the fistula tract.

PATHOPHYSIOLOGY

Incidence

Perianal disease is relatively common for the pediatric practitioner. Since many of the available studies regarding PA and FIA focus on adults, the exact frequency is difficult to quantify for infants and children. In some large series looking at FIA, between 0.5% and 4.3% are children.[2] In the pediatric population, the overwhelming majority of affected infants are male. Additionally, the disease process presents before 1 yr of age in 57–86% of cases.[2] In one review, FIA is reported to occur in infants less than 1 yr of age in up to 96% of cases.[3] For reasons that are not completely understood, FIA is much less common in female infants.[4] Despite the difference in frequency, treatment follows the same algorithm.

Classification

Anal fistulas can be classified by the Park's Classification which includes four types: intersphincteric, transsphincteric, suprasphincteric, and extrasphincteric. Despite this traditional classification system in adults and the adherence to Goodsall's Rule, infantile FIA are different from those found in adults. Most FIA in infants are of the simple intersphincteric type and form a direct trajectory between the anal crypts of Morgagni, located at the dentate line, and the perianal skin. In the pediatric literature, FIA have also been characterized as simple, low, and direct.[5] Complex and high fistulas are generally not seen in infants and children unless there are other predisposing factors such as immunocompromise or inflammatory bowel disease.[1] As a result, FIA in infants is usually amenable to simple fistulotomy with no major concern for damage to the anal sphincter muscle complex.

Pathology

FIA occurs predominantly in male infants and is preceded by PA in the majority of cases.[1–2,5] Identification of specific etiologic factors is rare. FIA can occur around the entire circumference of the anus, but is most common at the 3 o'clock and 9 o'clock positions.[6] While there is agreement that most chronic FIA are preceded by PA, the rate of development of FIA after PA drainage is reported with wide variation in the literature, ranging from relatively low at 13%[5] to as high as 28–85% of cases.[2] Furthermore, fistulotomy or fistulectomy may lead to a recurrence in 0–68% of cases.[2] As a result of this wide variation, there has been difficulty in defining a standard approach for surgical management.

Although there is no adequate explanation for the male predominance, Fitzgerald suggested that excess androgen stimulation causes formation of abnormal anal glands which predispose to infection and fistula formation.[1,5] Shafer proposed a developmental anomaly that includes a focally irregular and thick dentate line with deep crypts that retain bacteria and thereby predispose to infection.[5] Histologic evaluation of the fistula tracts has revealed various epithelial linings including squamous, columnar, and transitional epithelium, as well as granulation tissue, none of which have provided any insight into the underlying etiology. Understanding the pathophysiology and natural course of these lesions may help to better delineate optimum management.

Microbiology

Since most FIA are preceded by PA, the microbiology of the offending organisms is worthy of note. As with the difference in frequency of FIA between males and females, the bacterial flora also differs markedly between the two populations. Enteric organisms, namely *Escherichia coli*, are predominantly cultured from males. Skin organisms, such as *Staphylococcus aureus*, are predominant in females.[1,5] Moreover, infants with abscess from enteric organisms are more likely to develop a fistula than those with skin flora.[5] These differences in microbiology appear to reflect the source of bacteria and may help explain the difference in frequency of FIA between males and females. Nevertheless, since the specific organism is usually not known at the initial clinical setting, antibiotic therapy should be empiric and cover a broad spectrum.

CLINICAL PRESENTATION

Infants with FIA present across a broad clinical spectrum. Subtle constitutional signs include fever, fussiness, and discomfort during bowel movements. On examination, there are usually subtle signs of inflammation, including perianal erythema and/or induration. Practitioners may notice a small opening in the skin which may represent the fistula tract. Since the skin can epithelialize and heal quickly, the fistula orifice is not always readily apparent. Depending on the situation and the extent of the disease process at presentation, there may be an associated pustule or abscess, with or without spontaneous drainage through the skin. If an abscess and fistula tract are present, pus may drain directly into the anal canal and can sometimes be expressed from the anus with manual pressure to the perianal skin.

PA and FIA are usually localized problems. Only rarely do they present as a severe or fulminant soft tissue infection with overwhelming signs of sepsis. Depending upon the initial and subsequent management of these problems, the occurrence of an abscess or fistula may follow a relapsing and remitting course. Antibiotic therapy +/− surgical drainage may solve the acute problem, but the abscess or fistula is prone to recurrence. Parents need to be counseled about the possibility of recurrence so that they have appropriate expectations.

While most cases in infants occur without specific etiologic factors, frequent recurrence or unusual clinical circumstances should raise the possibility of other systemic diseases. In one case series, children older than 2 yrs of age were most at risk for these systemic problems, including specifically Crohn's disease, diabetes mellitus, leukemia, and neutropenia.[4] Other predisposing factors include trauma, radiation, ulcerative colitis, tuberculosis, lymphogranuloma venereum, and HIV infection.[4,7] Sexual abuse should also be considered when a child presents with FIA without a history of PA or other predisposing factors.[4] Clinicians need to be aware of these other predisposing factors so that they can recommend the appropriate evaluation and treatment.

SURGICAL MANAGEMENT

Although PA and FIA are seemingly trivial problems, they can be a nuisance to both parents and clinicians. Optimum surgical management for PA and FIA is controversial. While there are many opinions regarding appropriate treatment based on anecdote, personal bias, and clinical experience, some of the key questions that clinicians have tried to answer are:

(1) Is a perianal abscess best treated with antibiotic therapy or drainage?
(2) Should exploration for FIA be done at the initial incision and drainage?
(3) Is fistulotomy necessary? If so, when is the appropriate timing?
(4) What is the natural course of FIA with nonoperative management?

Our goal for this handbook is to briefly outline some of the controversy, then present a practical approach for dealing with these clinical questions.

Of note, when the literature is reviewed, fistulotomy and fistulectomy are often used interchangeably. In infants, fistulotomy is the treatment of choice when needed. It is performed by placing a lacrimal duct probe through the external opening in the perianal skin along the length of the fistula tract and through the internal opening within the anal canal. Once the tract is demonstrated, the surgeon opens the fistula over the probe along its entire length, usually with the bovie electrocautery. Curettage of the epithelial lining or granulation tissue within the fistula tract is recommended to promote healing and decrease the risk of recurrence. The wound is left open to heal by secondary intention and parents are provided with instructions for local wound care.

Standard treatment for PA consists of antibiotic therapy +/− incision and drainage. Smaller abscesses can be treated with antibiotic therapy only. Larger abscesses often require incision and drainage. In the largest series to date looking at infants with perianal abscess, nonsurgical treatment with antibiotic is associated with a significantly lower rate of fistula formation than incision and drainage.[8] As there are no size criteria in the literature to guide the decision for incision and drainage, the decision is based entirely on clinical judgment.

Since an abscess can arise from a developing fistula, some clinicians have proposed exploring for and treating the fistula with a fistulotomy at the time of the initial incision and drainage. Shafer *et al.* found that the recurrence rate for PA was reduced from 15% to 0% by performing a fistulotomy at the time of primary treatment.[9] Additionally, Murthi *et. al.* found that careful search for a coexisting fistula at the time of inital incision and drainage reduces recurrence rates for perianal abscess.[9] Although these studies show a benefit some clinicians are opposed to this approach.

Opponents argue that the rate of fistula formation after incision and drainage of an abscess is low and that probing the area may actually create a false passage that can lead to fistula formation.[5,10] Furthermore, looking for and treating a fistula poses the risk of injury to the anal sphincter and requires general anesthesia. In support of a conservative approach, Watanabe *et al.* report that two-third of children with abscess do not develop FIA. Of the children who later develop FIA, almost half have no evidence of fistula recurrence with nonoperative management.[6] Similar conclusions were drawn by Serour *et al.* who found that the low rate of FIA after needle aspiration makes incision of the abscess with the concomitant search for a fistula unnecessary.[11] These results tend to support a more conservative approach to PA and FIA in infants. Using this approach, a fistula that develops after abscess drainage can be treated later as a separate entity.

While fistulotomy is acceptable treatment for infants with an established fistula tract, observation alone is also acceptable and poses less risk. Based on some surgeons' clinical experience, FIA are observed to follow a time-limited course that may allow for spontaneous closure without the need for surgical intervention. Rosen *et al.* found that 77% of their male infant cohort developed fistulas after incision and drainage, but all fistulas subsequently healed with nonoperative management over a period of observation lasting 6 +/– 4 mths. Age range at the time of resolution was 10 +/– 3.5 mths.[12] Advantages of this approach include no risk of damage to the anal sphincter as well as the cost savings from general anesthesia and surgical intervention. Despite this study, many authors argue that there are a significant percentage of patients who will ultimately require a fistulotomy and that not all patients can be treated by the nonoperative approach.[13] Proponents in this group maintain that surgical management with fistulotomy is low risk and can help resolve the problem expeditiously. Based on these studies, we conclude that observation for FIA is an acceptable alternative, with operative management reserved for a select population of infants refractory to spontaneous fistula closure.

In reviewing the literature, the treatment options for PA and FIA are relatively simple, but the management should be individualized to the patient and family. In summary, small abscesses can usually be treated with antibiotic alone. Large abscesses or abscesses that are persistent despite an appropriate course of antibiotic therapy warrant incision and drainage. Based on the premise of *primum non nocere*, we do not recommend routinely probing for or treating FIA by fistulotomy at the time of the initial incision and drainage procedure. If the FIA is obvious at the initial drainage procedure or there are frequent recurrent abscesses in the same location, we recommend fistulostomy. If the FIA is relatively asymptomatic, we recommend a period of observation with nonoperative management. Fistulotomy should be reserved for infants who fail a reasonable course of non-operative management.

COMPLICATIONS & RECURRENCE

No major long-term complications have been reported in infants after fistulostomy. Long-term follow-up is scarce, but follow-up has been reported by Festen and van Harten for children over a range of 1–24 yrs of age.[2] All children 3 years of age and older were continent for feces. Two children with prior fistulotomy had temporary soiling that resolved. One child had constipation and the other child had nocturnal incontinence.[2] Late recurrences of FIA were rare, and most healed spontaneously without the need for surgical intervantion.

Overall, as few as 1/3 of infants develop FIA after initial incision and drainage of a perianal abscess.[6] Nonoperative management can be an effective strategy as long as the parents are amenable and cooperative. Some infants ultimately require fistulotomy which is safe and effective. Recurrence rates for FIA are reported to be low.[14] Children at increased risk for recurrence include older children, those with purulent drainage at the time of fistulotomy, and those with prior abscesses.[14] Overall, good clinical judgment and proper surgical technique can help minimize complications and recurrence.

REFERENCES

1. Al-Salem AH, Qaisaruddin S, Qureshi SS. (1996) Perianal abscess and fistula-in-ano in infancy and childhood: A clinicopathological study. *Pediatr Pathol Lab M* **16**:755–764.
2. Festen C, van Harten H. (1998) Perianal abscess and fistula-in-ano in infants. *J Pediatr Surg* **33**:711–713.
3. Deodhar J, Khan AR. (2010) Fistula-in-Ano. *eMedicine Pediatrics.*

4. Lahoti SL, McNeese MC, McClain N, Girardet R. (2002) Two cases of anal fistula in girls evaluated for sexual abuse. *J Pediatr Surg* **37**:132–133.
5. Nix P, Stringer MD. (1997) Perianal sepsis in children. *Brit J Surg* **84**:819–821.
6. Watanabe Y, Todani T, Yamamoto S. (1998) Conservative management of fistula-in-ano in infants. *Pediatr Surg Int* **13**:274–276.
7. Grant HW. (1999) Patterns of presentation of human immunodeficiency virus type I infected children to the pediatric surgeon. *J Pediatr Surg* **34**:251–254.
8. Christison-Lagay ER, Hall JF, Wales PW, Bailey K, Terluk A, Goldstein AM, Ein SH, Masiakos PT. (2007) Nonoperative management of perianal abscess in infants is associated with decreased risk for fistula formation. *Pediatrics* **120**:548–552.
9. Murthi GS, Okoye BO, Spicer RD, Cusick EL, Noblett HR. (2002) Perianal abscess in childhood. *Pediatr Surg Int* **18**:689–691.
10. Macdonald A, Wilson-Storey D, Munro F. (2003) Treatment of perianal abscess and fistula-in-ano in children. *Brit J Surg* **90**:220–221.
11. Serour F, Gorenstein A. (2006) Characteristics of perianal abscess and fistula-in-ano in healthy children. *World J Surg* **30**:467–472.
12. Rosen NG, Gibbs DL, Soffer SZ, Hong A, Sher M, Pena A. (2000) The nonoperative management of fistula-in-ano. *J Pediatr Surg* **35**:938–939.
13. Oh JT, Han A, Han SJ, Choi SH, Hwang EH. (2001) Fistula-in-ano in infants: Is nonoperative management effective? *J Pediatr Surg* **36**:1367–1369.
14. Novotny NM, Mann MJS, Rescorla FJ. (2008) Fistula-in-ano in infants: Who recurs? *Pediatr Surg Int* **24**:1197–1199.

Section 8:
Liver, Biliary Tree & Pancreas

BILIARY ATRESIA 69

Danielle Hsu and James C. Y. Dunn

CLINICAL PRESENTATION

Most infants with biliary atresia are full term with a low to normal birth weight. Clinical features usually include jaundice, pale stools, and dark urine by 4 to 6 wks of age in an otherwise healthy infant. Depending on the extent of biliary obstruction at the time of diagnosis, portal hypertension can be present with resultant hepatosplenomegaly. Rarely, cases present with coagulopathy secondary to vitamin K malabsorption and deficiency.

PATHOPHYSIOLOGY

Incidence

Biliary atresia is a rare disease with an incidence of approximately 1:5,000 to 1:18,000 live births. It is more common in Asia and the Pacific region than in the rest of the world. Females are affected slightly more frequently than males (female-to-male ration of 1.7).[1,2]

Classification

Two forms of biliary atresia are described. The more common perinatal or postnatal form of biliary atresia accounts for approximately 80–90% of cases, is characterized by an initial jaundice-free period, and is not associated with congenital anomalies. The fetal or embryonic form is characterized by early cholestasis without a jaundice-free period. This type accounts for 10–20% of cases of biliary atresia and has a high frequency of associated malformations such as asplenia or polysplenia, situs inversus, cardiac anomalies, the absence of the inferior vena cava, portal vein anomalies, intestinal malrotation, annular pancreas, Kartagener's syndrome, polycystic kidneys, and cleft palate. Biliary atresia splenic malformation syndrome describes the clustering of biliary atresia with polysplenia or asplenia, abdominal situs inversus, intestinal malrotation, positional abnormalities of the portal vein and hepatic artery, and cardiovascular defects. There are three common anatomic variants of biliary atresia:

Type I — Distal ducts obliterate, leaving patent proximal extrahepatic ducts above the level of the cystic duct-common duct junction (6%)

Type II — Proximal ducts obliterate, sparing the gallbladder, cystic duct, and common bile duct (11%)

Type III — Obliteration of entire extrahepatic ductal system and gallbladder (85–90%)

Pathology

Biliary atresia is a sclerosing inflammatory process affecting previously formed bile ducts. The etiology is unknown, but there is a growing belief that biliary atresia is not a single disease but the result of processes ending in a common final inflammatory pathway targeting and destroying the extrahepatic bile ducts. Theories on the pathogenesis of biliary atresia focus on immune-mediated ductal injury, a viral agent as an inflammatory trigger, and genetic predisposition or defects in morphogenesis. Other proposed mechanisms include exposure to toxin and defects in prenatal circulation leading to ductal ischemia.

Biliary atresia is not an inherited disorder as it uncommonly recurs in families and is rarely concordant in twins.[3] Patients may however have a genetic predisposition to an aberrant immune response to viral or toxin exposure, or mutations in genes regulating bile duct morphogenesis. The fetal form of disease in particular is thought to be caused by defective morphogenesis of the biliary tree due to its common association with other congenital anomalies. Recently Hayashida *et al.* and Kobayashi *et al.* suggested maternal microchimerism as a potential causative factor in which maternal cells could elicit an immune response in the fetus similar to graft-vs.-host disease.[4,5] Other genes under investigation include CFC1, JAGGED1, and alpha-1-antitrypsin heterozygosity.[6–8] A murine model of biliary atresia can be induced by neonatal inoculation with reovirus, rotavirus, and cytomegalovirus leading to strong interest in the possible role of viral infection in the pathogenesis of human disease[9–12]; however, studies looking for evidence of viral pathogens in patients with biliary atresia have been inconclusive.[2,3] An inflammatory component both in humans and murine models has been repeatedly demonstrated. Lymphocytic infiltration into the connective tissue of the porta hepatis and into bile duct epithelial cells is seen in patients with biliary atresia, and proinflammatory cytokines such as interferon-gamma, interleukin (IL)-2, IL-12, and tumor necrosis factor (TNF)-alpha have been shown to be prominent in livers with biliary atresia.[13,14] Although data are strongly suggestive of an inflammatory component, the exact pathogenesis and trigger are unknown, as is the mechanism by which immune cells induce biliary damage.

DIAGNOSIS/WORK-UP

Infants with biliary atresia have persistent, progressive jaundice, which may initially be confused with physiological jaundice or breast milk jaundice. The diagnosis of biliary atresia can be challenging because there are multiple causes of neonatal cholestasis (Table 1). Physiological jaundice typically lasts 2–3 days in normal term babies, while breast milk jaundice can last up to 4 wks. However, in biliary atresia most of the bilirubin is conjugated whereas in physiological and breast milk jaundice the serum bilirubin is mainly unconjugated. Current guidelines by the North American Society for Pediatric Gastroenterology, Hepatology, and Nutrition recommend that an evaluation for cholestasis should be performed in any infant with jaundice at the 2-wk well child visit. Evaluation of breast fed infants may be delayed until 3 wks of age if they have no history of dark urine, pale stools, have a normal physical examination, and can be reliably monitored.[15] The stool of infants with biliary atresia is acholic, and the urine is dark. By 4 wks, the liver becomes large and firm. Splenomegaly may develop by 6 wks. Ascites with prominent abdominal veins is evidence of portal hypertension associated with advanced liver disease, however does not usually occur until after 6 mths. Currently there is no good screening test, although recently, Taiwan has been using stool color charts distributed to parents to identify when stools are pale and hasten referral.[16] Diagnosis

Table 1. Differential diagnosis of neonatal cholestasis.

Infectious
Viral: cytomegalovirus, rubella, herpes virus, hepatitis (A, B, C, D, and E), toxoplasmosis, syphilis, adenovirus, enterovirus, reovirus, HIV, parvovirus, coxsackievirus B, echovirus 14,19
Bacterial: sepsis, urinary tract infection, syphilis, tuberculosis
Metabolic/Genetic
Alagille syndrome
A1AT deficiency
Cystic fibrosis
Disorders of glucose metabolism: galactosemia, tyrosinemia, fructosemia, glycogen storage disease type IV
Disorders of amino acid metabolism: tyrosinemia
Hypothyroidism
Progressive familial intrahepatic cholestasis (Byler's disease)
Anatomic or obstructive cholestatic disorders
Choledochal cyst
Bile duct stenosis or stricture
Sclerosing cholangitis of the newborn
Biliary atresia (intrahepatic, extrahepatic, hypoplasia)
Inspissated bile plug syndrome
Bile duct compression by tumor or mass
Miscellaneous
Parenteral alimentation cholestasis
Drugs

of biliary atresia is made based on a combination of serum tests, radiographic studies, and liver histology (Figure 1).

Liver function tests typically demonstrate a rise in conjugated bilirubin, alkaline phosphatase, and a striking increase of gamma glutamyl transferase with mild to moderate elevation of serum transaminases. A conjugated bilirubin level that represents more than 20% of the total bilirubin concentration should be considered abnormal. In the early stages, prothrombin time and albumin are usually normal. Abdominal ultrasound after a 4 hr fast may show an absent or contracted gallbladder. Or it may demonstrate the presence of the fibrotic remnant of the extrahepatic biliary tree which appears

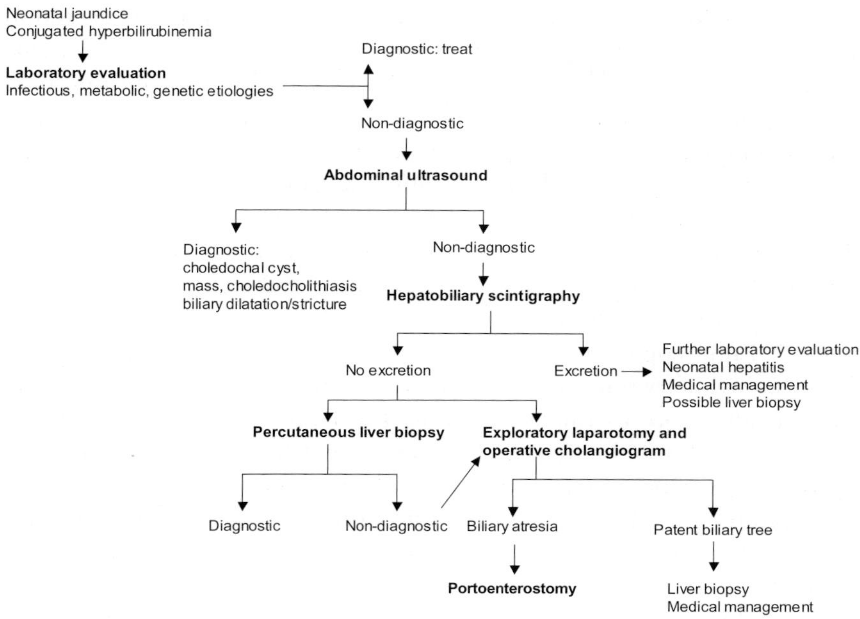

Figure 1. Algorithm for the evaluation of neonatal jaundice.

as a triangular or tubular-shaped density immediately cranial to the portal vein bifurcation (triangular cord sign). Intrahepatic bile ducts rarely become dilated except late in the disease when cysts known as bile lakes may be present. The presence of a gallbladder, however, does not rule out biliary atresia.

Hepatobiliary scintigraphy can be helpful in differentiating biliary atresia from other causes of conjugated hyperbilirubinemia. If the administered radioisotope appears in the intestine, complete biliary obstruction can be excluded. Improved sensitivity and specificity have been reported if the patient is premedicated with oral phenobarbital (5 mg/kg daily) for 5 days to induce hepatic microsomal enzymes and increase hepatocyte processing of the radionuclide. Infants with primary hepatocellular disorders typically have impaired hepatocyte uptake of the radionuclide, whereas infants with biliary atresia have prompt uptake but no excretion into the gut. Delayed imaging is performed at 4 to 6 hrs and at 24 hrs when earlier biliary excretion is not visualized. Sensitivity of this exam is high.

Specificity is lower however, ranging from 40–75% as reduced excretion into the intestine is also seen in children with severe intrahepatic cholestasis such as Alagille's syndrome. The lack of excretion into the intestine, however, does not establish the diagnosis of biliary atresia. A recent study demonstrated an increase in specificity to 90% with the addition of single photon emission computed tomography 4 to 6 hrs postinjection of tracer without premedication with phenobarbital.[17] Magnetic resonance cholangiography allows visualization of the biliary tract and has become another helpful tool in diagnosing biliary atresia. In initial studies, negative and positive predictive values range from 91–100% and 75–96%, respectively.[18,19] Endoscopic retrograde cholangiopancreatography can be used to visualize the biliary tract. This is a technically difficult study in infants however and therefore is usually only found at large centers. The duodenal tube test, performed often in Japanese and Chinese centers, passes a nasoduodenal tube into the third part of the duodenum to enable continuous aspiration to identify bile. Identification of bile avoids the need for surgery, whereas lack of bile in intestinal secretions is suggestive of biliary atresia.[20]

Liver histology obtained by percutaneous biopsy shows portal tract fibrosis, cholestasis and proliferation of biliary ductules. Other neonatal liver diseases with similar clinical presentations such as alpha-1-antitrypsin deficiency and other forms of neonatal hepatitis must be excluded. Liver biopsy samples taken before 6 wks of age may not have typical histological features, and therefore biopsies might need to be repeated.[21] While liver biopsy may establish other causes of jaundice, there are no pathologic features that will make the definitive diagnosis of biliary atresia. Radiographic studies and hepatobiliary scintigraphy are helpful, but surgical exploration and cholangiography remain the gold standard of diagnosis, particularly in cases where the above studies are inconclusive.

MANAGEMENT

In patients in whom biliary atresia is suspected based on previous work-up, exploratory laparotomy and operative cholangiogram is the next step. Preoperatively infants are given vitamin K (1 mg/kg) to minimize vitamin K deficient coagulopathy. The patient is placed in the supine position. A right subcostal incision is made to expose the porta hepatis. The liver and extrahepatic biliary tree are examined, after which the gallbladder is catheterized for intraoperative cholangiogram. If the biliary tree is patent and intact, a wedge liver biopsy if often performed and the procedure concluded.

If the diagnosis of biliary atresia is confirmed with cholangiogram, the surgeon proceeds with hepatic portoenterostomy, first described by Morio Kasai in the 1950s. The remnant of the gallbladder is mobilized from the liver bed. The hepatoduodenal ligament is incised, the cystic artery is ligated and the hepatic artery is identified. Dissection is continued along the atretic hepatic ducts to the hilum of the liver. For type I and II biliary atresia, deep portal dissection is not required and a Roux-en-Y hepaticojejunostomy is performed. For type III biliary atresia, complete excision of the atretic extrahepatic bile ducts above the level of portal vein bifurcation is required. Bile ductules are reported in a central zone and two lateral zones in the portal plate. More satisfactory bile flow is achieved with dissection of the two lateral zones in addition to the central zone. A 40-cm Roux limb of jejunum is anastomosed to the porta hepatis using fine, interrupted, absorbable sutures. A closed suction drain is placed in the foramen of Winslow and the abdomen is closed.

Modifications to the original Kasai procedure have been described. The Roux limb can be exteriorized as a double-barreled stoma to allow for the daily quantification of bile output with closure 1 to 2 mths later. However, this technique is rarely used due to the risk of postoperative complications including dehydration and electrolyte abnormalities, as well as the requirement to refeed the bile drainage. An anti-reflux valve formed by intussuscepting a portion of the Roux limb upon itself has also been described to prevent cholangitis. However, this technique has largely been abandoned due to questionable efficacy in preventing cholangitis as well as the risk for obstruction.[22] Recently, laparoscopic, and robotic surgeries have been utilized to perform hepatic portoenterostomy. However, the long-term efficacy of these techniques in establishing bile drainage has not yet been validated.[23,24] Therefore the open technique currently remains the standard of care.

POSTOPERATIVE CONSIDERATIONS

Management

Broad-spectrum antibiotics are generally administered until the patient is tolerating an oral diet, at which point the patient is switched to prophylactic oral antibiotics for 12 mths. Ursodeoxycholic acid may be effective in optimizing bile flow, and is administered when patients are tolerating a diet at many centers, although data are conflicting. Corticosteroids are often used postoperatively to improve bile flow and decrease rates of postoperative cholangitis, which most likely arises from an ascending infection in the setting of impaired bile drainage. Steroids may attenuate the inflammatory response associated with biliary atresia through their immunological and anti-inflammatory effects, in addition to increasing bile flow by induction of canalicular electrolyte transport.[25] The role of corticosteroids however remains controversial, and a definitive clinical advantage has not been established. Limitations of existing studies include lack of an established dosing regimen or tapering schedule, and mostly retrospective or nonrandomized data. A large prospective, multicenter, placebo controlled trial of high-dose steroids following hepatic portoenterostomy is currently in progress through the Biliary Atresia Research Consortium.[1]

Complications/Morbidity

Immediate complications include wound infection, bleeding, and anastomotic leaks. One of the most important complications is cholangitis. It occurs in approximately 50% of patients during the first 2 yrs after surgery. More than half of these patients have their first episode within the first 6 mths and 90% within the first year.[26] Multiple pathogens have been implicated including *Escherichia coli, Klebsiella, Psuedomonas, Staphylococcus, Enterobacter, Streptococcus faecalis, Bacteroides, Clostridia, and Candida.* Cholangitis must be suspected if the child has fever, acholic stools, elevated liver function tests, abdominal pain, pruritis, or shoulder pain. Infants with recurrent cholangitis should be evaluated for anatomic obstruction within the Roux limb via ultrasound or hepatobiliary scintigraphy. Repeated episodes of cholangitis worsen the prognosis of patients with biliary atresia, and recurrent, intractable cholangitis is an indication for liver transplantation.

Long-term complications include fat malabsorption and malnutrition leading to fat-soluble vitamin deficiency. If the child has steatorrhea, providing 40–60% of the fat as medium chain triglycerides can be helpful.[27] Infants with biliary atresia often have increased resting energy expenditure and impaired protein metabolism compared with normal infants. Positive nitrogen balance should be maintained and the diet should be supplemented with fat-soluble vitamins (vitamin A, D, E, and K). To prevent malnutrition, achievement of 110–160% of the recommended daily energy intake is recommended, which may require the use of supplemental nocturnal enteral feedings. Portal hypertension develops in the majority of patients with biliary atresia after portoenterostomy. Approximately 50% of all survivors aged 5 yrs have esophageal varices. Variceal hemorrhage is directly related to poor initial bile drainage and increases with native liver survival.[28,29] Other complications of portal hypertension include ascites, hypersplenism, and hepatopulmonary syndrome. Portal hypertension and its sequelae are best treated with liver transplantation. Long-term survival with a cirrhotic native liver is a risk factor for the development of malignancy such as hepatocellular carcinoma, hepatoblastoma, or cholangiocarcinoma. The risk and prevalence are unknown, however patients should undergo regular screening with ultrasound and alpha fetoprotein levels.

Outcomes

Eventually, 60–70% of patients undergoing Kasai portoenterostomy require liver transplantation or succumb to the disease due to progressive liver failure. Survival with the native liver after Kasai portoenterostomy is 30–40% of patients at 10 yrs.[29,30] Biliary atresia is the most common indication for liver transplantation in children accounting for almost 50% of pediatric liver transplants in the United States. Prognostic factors of the success of the Kasai procedure include the anatomy of the extrahepatic biliary remnant, age at Kasai procedure, occurrence of postoperative cholangitis, presence of cirrhosis, experience of the hospital in management of biliary atresia patients, size of ductules in portal plate, and presence of liver fibrosis at the time of surgery.

Data from Japan demonstrate an advantage when operating on infants younger than 30 days, no difference in outcome in those operated on between 30 and 90 days, and significant disadvantage for those operated on later than 90 days.[31] If done within first 3 mths of life, hepatoportoenterostomy can restore bile flow from the liver to intestine in 40–80% of patients. However, even in infants older than 100 days, Davenport *et al.* published a 5- and 10-yr actuarial survival with native liver of 40–45%.[30] Although the majority of patients eventually require liver transplantation, hepatic portoenterostomy remains an important bridge to transplantation in patients with biliary atresia.

REFERENCES

1. Sokol RJ, Shepherd RW, Superina R, *et al.* (2007) Screening and outcomes in biliary atresia: Summary of a National Institutes of Health workshop. *Hepatology* **46**:566–581.
2. Mieli-Vergani G, Vergani D. (2009) Biliary atresia. *Semin Immunopathol* **31**:371–381.
3. Hartley JL, Davenport M, Kelly DA. (2009) Biliary atresia. *Lancet* **374**:1704–1713.
4. Hayashida M, Nishimoto Y, Matsuura T, *et al.* (2007) The evidence of maternal microchimerism in biliary atresia using fluorescent in situ hybridization. *J Pediatr Surg* **42**:2097–2101.
5. Kobayashi H, Tamatani T, Tamura T, *et al.* (2007) Maternal microchimerism in biliary atresia. *J Pediatr Surg* **42**:987–991; discussion 991.
6. Davit-Spraul A, Baussan C, Hermeziu B, *et al.* (2008) CFC1 gene involvement in biliary atresia with polysplenia syndrome. *J Pediatr Gastroenterol Nutr* **46**:111–112.
7. Kohsaka T, Yuan ZR, Guo SX, *et al.* (2002) The significance of human jagged 1 mutations detected in severe cases of extrahepatic biliary atresia. *Hepatology* **36**:904–912.
8. Campbell KM, Arya G, Ryckman FC, *et al.* (2007) High prevalence of alpha-1-antitrypsin heterozygosity in children with chronic liver disease. *J Pediatr Gastroenterol Nutr* **44**:99–103.
9. Riepenhoff-Talty M, Schaekel K, Clark HF, *et al.* (1993) Group A rotaviruses produce extrahepatic biliary obstruction in orally inoculated newborn mice. *Pediatr Res* **33**:394–399.
10. Allen SR, Jafri M, Donnelly B, *et al.* (2007) Effect of rotavirus strain on the murine model of biliary atresia. *J Virol* **81**:1671–1679.
11. Szavay PO, Leonhardt J, Czech-Schmidt G, and Petersen C. (2002) The role of reovirus type 3 infection in an established murine model for biliary atresia. *Eur J Pediatr Surg* **12**:248–250.
12. Hsu HY, Chang MH, Ni YH, Huang SF. (2001) Cytomegalovirus infection and proinflammatory cytokine activation modulate the surface immune determinant expression and immunogenicity of cultured murine extrahepatic bile duct epithelial cells. *Clin Exp Immunol* **126**:84–91.
13. Mack CL, Falta MT, Sullivan AK, *et al.* (2007) Oligoclonal expansions of CD4+ and CD8+ T-cells in the target organ of patients with biliary atresia. *Gastroenterology* **133**:278–287.

14. Davenport M, Gonde C, Redkar R, *et al.* (2001) Immunohistochemistry of the liver and biliary tree in extrahepatic biliary atresia. *J Pediatr Surg* **36**:1017–1025.
15. Moyer V, Freese DK, Whitington PF, *et al.* (2004) Guideline for the evaluation of cholestatic jaundice in infants: recommendations of the North American Society for Pediatric Gastroenterology, Hepatology and Nutrition. *J Pediatr Gastroenterol Nutr* **39**:115–128.
16. Hsiao CH, Chang MH, Chen HL, *et al.* (2008) Universal screening for biliary atresia using an infant stool color card in Taiwan. *Hepatology* **47**:1233–1240.
17. Sevilla A, Howman-Giles R, Saleh H, *et al.* (2007) Hepatobiliary scintigraphy with SPECT in infancy. *Clin Nucl Med* **32**:16–23.
18. Han SJ, Kim MJ, Han A, *et al.* (2002) Magnetic resonance cholangiography for the diagnosis of biliary atresia. *J Pediatr Surg* **37**:599–604.
19. Norton KI, Glass RB, Kogan D, *et al.* (2002) MR cholangiography in the evaluation of neonatal cholestasis: Initial results. *Radiology* **222**:687–691.
20. Larrosa-Haro A, Caro-Lopez AM, Coello-Ramirez P, *et al.* (2001) Duodenal tube test in the diagnosis of biliary atresia. *J Pediatr Gastroenterol Nutr* **32:**311–315.
21. Azar G, Beneck D, Lane B, *et al.* (2002) Atypical morphologic presentation of biliary atresia and value of serial liver biopsies. *J Pediatr Gastroenterol Nutr* **34**:212–215.
22. Ogasawara Y, Yamataka A, Tsukamoto K, *et al.* (2003) The intussusception antireflux valve is ineffective for preventing cholangitis in biliary atresia: a prospective study. *J Pediatr Surg* **38**:1826–1829.
23. Dutta S, Woo R, Albanese CT. (2007) Minimal access portoenterostomy: Advantages and disadvantages of standard laparoscopic and robotic techniques. *J Laparoendosc Adv Surg Tech A* **17**:258–264.
24. Esteves E, Clemente Neto E, Ottaiano Neto M, *et al.* (2002) Laparoscopic Kasai portoenterostomy for biliary atresia. *Pediatr Surg Int* **18**:737–740.
25. Alvaro D, Gigliozzi A, Marucci L, *et al.* (2002) Corticosteroids modulate the secretory processes of the rat intrahepatic biliary epithelium. *Gastroenterology* **122**:1058–1069.
26. Bassett MD, Murray KF. (2008) Biliary atresia: Recent progress. *J Clin Gastroenterol* **42**:720–729.
27. Beath SV, Booth IW, and Kelly DA. (1993) Nutritional support in liver disease. *Arch Dis Child* **69**:545–547.
28. Miga D, Sokol RJ, Mackenzie T, *et al.* (2001) Survival after first esophageal variceal hemorrhage in patients with biliary atresia. *J Pediatr* **139**:291–296.

29. van Heurn LW, Saing H, Tam PK. (2004) Portoenterostomy for biliary atresia: Long-term survival and prognosis after esophageal variceal bleeding. *J Pediatr Surg* **39**:6–9.

30. Davenport M, Puricelli V, Farrant P, *et al.* (2004) The outcome of the older (> or = 100 days) infant with biliary atresia. *J Pediatr Surg* **39**:575–581.

31. Nio M, Ohi R, Miyano T, *et al.* (2003) Five- and 10-year survival rates after surgery for biliary atresia: A report from the Japanese Biliary Atresia Registry. *J Pediatr Surg* **38**:997–1000.

CYSTIC DISORDERS OF THE BILE DUCTS (CHOLEDOCHAL CYSTS)

70

David T. Schindel and Sarah C. Oltmann

CLASSIFICATION/INCIDENCE

A therapy-based classification scheme was originally proposed by Alonso-Lej *et al.* in 1959, and later modified by Todani *et al.* in 1977.[1] (Figure 1) Documented incidence is roughly 1 in 13,000 in the United States, while Asian populations have rates as high as 1 in 1,000 described.[2] Females are three times more commonly affected than males.[3] Although considered a congenital disorder, only a fourth of patients are diagnosed before 1 yr of age.

Type Ia, Ib, Ic
Solitary, extrahepatic fusiform or cystic dilatation of the common bile duct are the most prevalent form, found in 85% to 90% of patients.[3] The right hepatic, left hepatic and intrahepatic ducts are normal. The gallbladder typically inserts into the cystic dilatation.

Type II
A single diverticulum of the common bile duct is found in 2.6% of patients with cystic disorders.[3] The remaining intra and extrahepatic ducts are normal in these instances.

Type III
A cystic dilatation of the bile duct which is typically intraduodenal, but may also be intrapancreatic. Often referred to as a choledochocele, and found

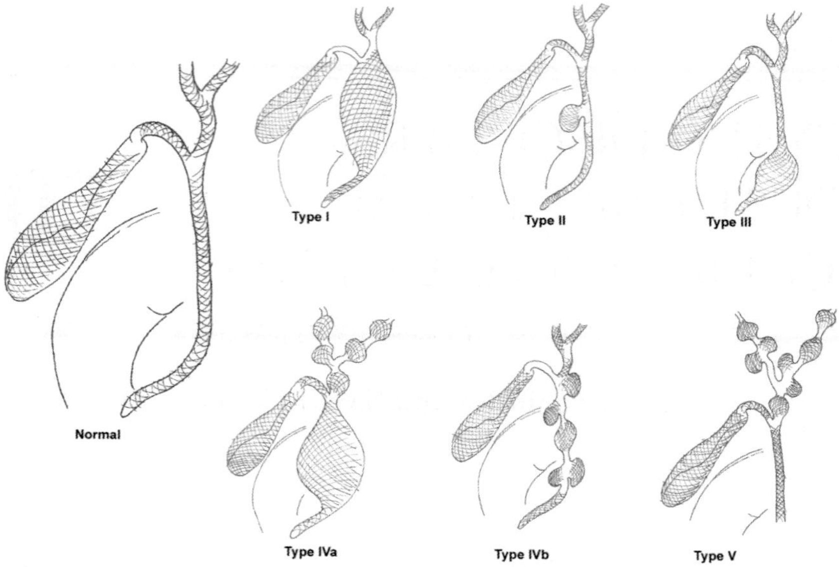

Figure 1. Choledochal Cyst Classification System.

in 4% of patients.[3] This anomaly can either involve the confluence of the common bile duct and the main pancreatic duct, or involve that portion of the duct below a normal main pancreatic and common bile duct junction. The intrahepatic ducts are unremarkable.

Types IVa/IVb

Type IVa is described as multiple fusiform extrahepatic and intrahepatic cysts. Type IVb consists of multiple extrahepatic cysts only, with a normal intrahepatic biliary tree. Type IV anomalies are found in 13% of patients.[3]

Type V

Single or multiple intrahepatic cysts characterize this type found in 1% of patients.[3] The extrahepatic biliary tree is unremarkable. This is also referred to as Caroli's disease or Caroli's syndrome. Caroli's disease generally affects the larger, main intrahepatic ducts of a specific hepatic segment, and occurs sporadically. Caroli's syndrome is a more serious manifestation, as it is more often diffuse, and can affect any portion of the intrahepatic biliary tree. It is associated with congenital hepatic fibrosis, and recurrent cholangitis. Caroli's syndrome is also inherited in an autosomal recessive manner, and has been associated with autosomal recessive polycystic kidney disease.

PATHOPHYSIOLOGY

Initially considered a developmental anomaly, evidence suggests that a degenerative pathology is a more likely explanation. These hypotheses have some form of "obstruction" of the duct as a central theme. The most commonly quoted theory as put forth by Babbitt in 1969 describes the association of a cystic bile duct dilatation with an anomalous pancreatic junction which has a long common channel greater than or equal to 15 mm.[4] "A long common channel" is found in 57% to 96% of cases.[3] This common channel can allow the reflux of pancreatic secretions into the bile ducts resulting in ductal inflammation, and subsequent ectasia and dilatation. Other researchers have suggested that abnormal function of the sphincter of Oddi might also predispose to pancreatic reflux into the bile ducts, causing a similar scenario of bile duct damage and subsequent dilatation.[5] Kusunoki *et al.* in 1988 demonstrated high levels of retroviral RNA in the biliary tissue of patients with cystic dilatations of the bile ducts when compared to normal controls.[6] These researchers hypothesized that a viral infection and resultant oligoganglionosis of the bile ducts might be an explanation for the obstructive fibrosis commonly found at the inferior portions of the bile ducts in patients having a choledochal cyst. While a complete understanding of the etiology of choledochal cysts remains elusive, patients having an anomalous pancreaticobiliary communication are 50 times more likely to have bile duct cancer then those without the anomaly.[4]

CLINICAL PRESENTATION

In newborns, choledochal cysts most commonly present with jaundice as a singular finding. The diagnosis is often made during an evaluation for jaundice and acholic stools. However a palpable abdominal mass with or without jaundice may be noted. Increasingly, choledochal cysts are perinatally identified by fetal imaging. Initial manifestations of bile duct cysts are less common in older children. In such cases, right upper quadrant pain, jaundice, acute pancreatitis or cholangitis are typically found. In a series of 35 children, Goon *et al.* found that 47% of the patients having a choledochal cyst presented with abdominal pain, 47% presented with a palpable abdominal mass and 69% were jaundice at initial presentation.[7] Only 6% had all three symptoms. While uncommon, spontaneous perforation of the bile duct usually occurs in children less than 2 yrs of age. This complication of a choledochal cyst is typically characterized with abdominal pain, vomiting and abdominal distention. Colicky abdominal pain, often associated with a fatty meal, is often the dominant compliant in children over 1 yr of age.[8]

DIAGNOSIS

Patients who present with jaundice, abdominal distention or pain are often referred for laboratory evaluation. While no specific laboratory study determines the diagnosis of a choledochal cyst, a hepatic profile is usually suggestive of obstructive jaundice. Serum amylase/lipase elevation may also be present. Pancreatic inflammation is often associated with the passage of a choledochal stone or debris which can form as a result of bile stasis within the cyst. Several authors report increasing numbers of choledochal cyst being diagnosed at the time of routine prenatal screening ultrasound.[9]

Postnatally, ultrasonography (US) is currently the screening study of choice due to the widespread availability of this noninvasive and inexpensive modality. US is capable of demonstrating the size, shape, and location of the cyst. In addition, US will accurately determine the presence of choledocholithiasis, the extent of intrahepatic ductal dilatation, and the degree of pancreatic inflammation. Some cite the disadvantage of US is that it does not accurately visualize the pancreaticobiliary junction.[10] However, the author utilizes US as a singular modality in preparation for surgery. In addition to US, routine intraoperative cholangiography (IOC) is used to further evaluate the anatomy of the cyst and duct including the pancreaticobiliary junction. Computed Tomography (CT) or Magnetic Resonance Imaging (MRI) are superior to US for more clearly documenting anatomical details of a choledochal cyst.[10] Endoscopic retrograde choledochopancreatography (ERCP) most accurately evalutes the pancreaticobiliary communication and has been used in both infants and older children. However, ERCP requires a general anesthetic and the information obtained duplicates what can be achieved through IOC. While MRI can be useful, it often requires sedation to achieve appropriate views. In the author's opinion, these modalities are best suited for when the diagnosis is in doubt, or when a mass or anatomical anomaly is suggested by US. It is the author's practice to use CT to further evaluate the intrahepatic anatomy of type IV and V cysts.

Percutaneous transhepatic cholangiography (PTC) is not necessary for the diagnosis or preoperative assessment of a choledochal cyst. However, biliary duct drainage by PTC might be indicated in the rare patient ill from progressive obstructive jaundice, hepatic failure or cholangitis secondary to a choledochal cyst. Routine IV cholangiography and hepatobiliary nuclear scintigraphy are not indicated diagnostic modalities.

SURGICAL MANAGEMENT

Definitive surgical repair of a choledochal cyst should be performed on an elective basis. While no optimal timing for repair from time of diagnosis exists, most authors recommend early excision, even in newborns.[9] This approach seemingly results in fewer adverse complications. When a child presents with acute pancreatic or hepatic disorders, appropriate medical therapy should be instituted in effort to reverse the inflammatory or obstructive process. Intravenous antibiotics that cover enteric organisms are appropriate if infectious complications are noted. In patients with hepatic dysfunction, a coagulopathy is often noted. Such patients may require correction with the administration of vitamin K or fresh frozen plasma. Rarely, these adverse conditions cannot be reversed with appropriate medical therapy and urgent PTC or ERCP to decompress the bile ducts should be considered.

Since 1970, cyst excision with Roux-en-Y-choledochojejunostomy or Roux-en-Y-hepaticojejunostomy has been the preferred procedure.[11] Previous authors have reported a 10% to 15% risk of cancer development in the cyst if left *in situ*.[12] Roux-en-Y reconstruction has been associated with lower rates of postoperative cholangitis when compared to other methods of bile duct reconstruction.[11]

A right upper quadrant, subcostal incision is the most common approach to the choledochal cyst and choledochocele. Both laparoscopic and robotic approaches have been described.[13] However, these techniques are technically challenging and are not widely utilized or accepted as standard approaches. At the author's institution, robotic choledochal cyst excision and Roux-en-Y hepaticojejunostomy has been performed. The degrees of movement with the robotic arms, in addition to the excellent view of the operative field might offer distinct advantages over traditional laparoscopic approach as the cyst is dissected from the porta hepatis. However, the lack of tactile feed-back with current robotic technology remains problematic. From the author's perspective, additional experience is needed to determine the efficacy of these approaches before they can be widely recommended.

The author begins the procedure by performing an intraoperative cholangiogram via a catheter placed into the gallbladder. The cholangiogram delineates both the intra and extrahepatic duct anatomy. Defining the pancreaticobiliary duct junction facilitates complete resection of the distal portion of the cyst, while avoiding injury to the pancreatic duct. After the cholangiogram, a liver biopsy is performed to assess the degree of liver injury induced by cholestasis. The gallbladder is then dissected free from the gallbladder fossa. The cystic artery is divided leaving the cystic duct and gallbladder in continuity with the cyst to be excised. For the vastly more common type I cyst, dissection is carried onto the anterior surface of the cyst or common bile duct, dividing the peritoneal reflection to expose the regional anatomy. The portal vein is then mobilized from the medial and posterior aspects of the cyst. Once the distal extent of the cyst has been identified, the common bile duct is then divided and sutured closed taking care to avoid the underlying pancreatic duct or a common channel duct below the confluents of the pancreatic duct. One method felt helpful to avoid injury to the pancreatic duct, yet insure complete excision of the distal extension of the cyst, is to perform a cystotomy and view the anatomy from within the cyst. Opening the cyst also allows any debris within the cavity to be flushed from the distal common channel and pancreatic ducts. The cyst, having been divided distally, is then elevated which simplifies proximal dissection. The transition from abnormal cyst to normal caliber common hepatic duct is then identified, and the duct divided. At the hepatic hilum, dissection beyond the confluence of both hepatic ducts may be necessary to complete cyst excision.

If the pericystic inflammation obscures the anatomy, making the risk of blood loss or injury to the portal vein considerable, a technique described by Lilly should be considered.[11] With this maneuver, the anterior cyst wall is incised transversely. A plane of dissection is then developed establishing an intramural separation of the thick inner lining of the cyst from the thinner outer layer which directly overlies the portal vein. This intramural plane is then extended caudad and cephalad until normal common bile duct and hepatic duct dimensions are identified. The cyst is then excised, and the distal common bile duct is sutured closed.

Once cyst excision is completed, the author prefers a 40 cm long, retrocolic Roux-en-Y limb for bile duct reconstruction. In the author's experience, the choledochoenteric anastomosis is typically best fashioned end-to-side using an absorbable monofilament suture. A hilar hepaticojejunostomy, as proposed by Stringer *et al.*, allows for a wide, choledochoenteric reconstruction which may reduce the incidence of anastomotic stricture.[14] If cyst excision beyond the hepatic duct confluence is necessary, each hepatic duct is anastomosed separately to the Roux-en-Y limb in a end to side manner. Anastomotic stenting is not typically necessary. The author favors an intestinal stapler to construct the Roux-en-Y enteroenterostomy in a side-to-side manner. A side-to-side anastomosis using an intestinal stapler insures that the anastomosis is broad and therefore, at least theoretically, less likely to stricture upon healing. The reconstruction is oriented in an antegrade fashion, which may also improve Roux-en-Y emptying and thereby reduce the incidence of cholangitis as a result of the reflux of enteric contents. Some authors advocate the use of an intussuscepted, full thickness valve to prevent reflux of enteric contents into the bile ducts, thereby reducing postoperative cholangitis.[15] However, it is the author's experience that with an appropriately constructed Roux-en-Y limb of at least 20 cm or greater in length, this is not necessary.

Routine right upper quadrant drainage is not felt to be necessary by the author and, in fact, may increase the likelihood of a leak. However, selective drain placement when there is concern for the integrity of the anastomosis is a prudent choice.

For type II cysts, cyst excision flush to the common bile duct is performed. Primary closure over a T-tube is the preferred method of reconstruction. However, a Roux-en-Y choledochojejunal anastomosis can be similarly fashioned.

Type IVb cysts are best managed with excision and Roux-en-Y hepaticojejunostomy, similarly to type I. With type IVa cysts, the extrahepatic portion of the anomaly is also managed with excision and Roux-en-Y hepaticojejunostomy. For type IVa patients with diffuse intrahepatic disease, liver transplantation may be the most appropriate method for management. However, a portion of intrahepatic lesions are unilobar making them amendable for lobectomy with Roux-en-Y hepaticojejunostomy bile duct reconstruction. Unilobar, type V cysts can be managed with lobectomy alone, but bilateral lesions typically will ultimately require hepatic transplantation.

Choledochoceles (type III) are best approached in an individual manner. Malignant transformation of type III cysts is reportedly low and many, if not most, are managed without complete excision.[3] A cyst located in the head of the pancreas may be dissected from the surrounding tissue and completely excised, but the risk of bleeding and injury to the pancreatic duct is considerable. In the author's experience, a cholangiogram performed via the gallbladder typically defines the pertinent anatomy. A duodenotomy is then performed, and the ampulla identified. The ampulla may be cannulated and a transduodenal cholangiogram performed in addition. Often the cyst is located just proximal to the ampulla, and abuts the lumen of the duodenum. A transduodenal partial or complete excision of the cyst may be possible if anatomy is favorable. However, sphincteroplasty, allowing internal drainage of the cyst into the duodenum thereby relieving the obstruction, is often the most appropriate therapy. A Whipple procedure should only be considered in those cases complicated by severe, complex, obstructive disease which is not amendable to other methods.

POSTOPERATIVE CONSIDERATIONS

Management/Complications

Typically, patients remain NPO with a nasogastric tube placed to low intermittent suction until bowel function resumes. Empiric antibiotics are continued for 24 hrs postoperation. Postoperative bleeding is uncommon if operative hemostasis was meticulous. Coagulation parameters should be assessed as needed, and corrected as necessary. If a right upper quadrant drain was left postoperatively, drain output is typically followed for 48–72 hrs and then removed if noted to be nonbilious.

Bile leakage from the choledochoenterostomy occurs in a minority of patients, and is best managed conservatively by placement of an ultrasound or CT guided drain, when clinically relevant. A bile collection, resultant from a leaking anastomosis, is typically confined subhepatically and is heralded by jaundice, right upper quadrant pain and, perhaps, fever. The drain is placed to closed bulb suction and oral feeds resumed. Antibiotics are given until clinical concerns for cholangitis have resolved. Most commonly, the leakage stops within 2 wks postoperation.

Gentle dissection of the distal choledochal cyst and avoidance of the pancreatic duct reduces the risk of postoperative pancreatitis. Pancreatitis may be more common following the operative treatment of choledochoceles, and should be managed conservatively, as symptoms typically subside following resolution of papillary edema within a few days. An injury to the pancreatic duct, and resultant obstruction, is a major complication resulting in the potential for a chronic fistula and/or pancreatitis.[16]

Acholia, worsening jaundice and/or worsening elevation of liver function tests in the early postoperative period suggest obstruction of the cholodochoenteric anastomosis. Most commonly this is due to edema which resolves within the first week of surgery. Initiating IV antibiotics during this period to cover enteric organisms is appropriate. If findings are persistent or worsening, and intrahepatic ducts are dilated on US, PTC should be considered to evaluate the anastomosis and provide intrahepatic biliary decompression as appropriate. Reoperation is typically necessary to correct the problem.

Follow-up

In the late postoperative period, jaundice, elevations of liver function tests, right upper quadrant pain and/or fever may herald a cholodochoenteric anastomotic stricture. Such strictures may present at any point in the future following a seemingly complete cyst excision and successful reconstruction. Often the stricture is localized at the anastomosis and may be amendable to resection and reanastomosis. These strictures are thought to be secondary to local ischemia at the site of anastomosis, and as a result, emphasis should be placed on using a scalpel to incise and transect the proximal duct. Bile duct cancer may also present initially as a stricture at the anastomosis and should be considered in the operative plan. Often, decompressive PTC is necessary to stabilize and improve hepatic synthetic function prior to reoperation.

Bile duct cancer development from choledochal cysts is a well-reported concern.[3] The tumor's pathophysiology is felt secondary to mucosal damage induced by bile stagnation and activated pancreatic enzymes. When presented with a patient with previous partial excision of a choledochal cyst, reoperation to complete the excision is appropriate, with the exception of partially excised choledochoceles (type III). Mucosal damage induced by episodes of cholangitis or as a result of bile stagnation, such as in the case of a cholodochoenteric anastomosic stricture, may also induce malignant change. Therefore, clinically relevant strictures should be addressed by reconstruction upon presentation.

Calculi occurring in the common channel or intrapancreatic ducts following resection of choledochal cysts have been reported.[16] Such calculi might be induced by debris caused by stagnation of bile within the choledochal cyst. Such pancreaticolithiasis is best diagnosed by ERCP and treated by endoscopic or transduodenal sphinterotomy.

Little data exists in the current literature to outline an optimal algorithm for the long term follow-up of patients having had choldedochal cyst excision and hepaticojejunostomy. Because of the risk of anastomosic stricture, and the development of bile duct cancer despite complete cyst excision, yearly follow-up with US and liver function tests seems appropriate.

REFERENCES

1. Todani T, Watanabe Y, Narusue M, *et al.* (1977) Congenital bile duct cysts: Classification, operative procedures and review of thirty-seven cases including cancer arising from the choledochal cyst. *Am J Surg* **134**:263.
2. Hays DM, Goodman GN, Snyder WH, *et al.* (1969) Congenital cystic dilatation of the bile ducts. *Arch Surg* **98**:457.
3. de Vries JS, de Vries S, Aronson DC, *et al.* (2002) Choledochal cysts: Age of presentation, symptoms, and late complications related to Todani's classification. *J Pediatr Surg* **37**:1568.
4. Babbitt DP. (1969) Congenital choledochal cysts: New etiological concept based on anomalous relationships of the common bile duct and the pancreatic bulb. *Ann Radiol* **12**:231.
5. Narita H, Hashimoto T, Suzuki T, *et al.* (1990) Clinical and experimental studies on the activation mechanism of pancreatic enzymes refluxing into the biliary tract with an anomalous pancreatico-biliary ductal junction. *J Jpn Soc Pediatr Surg* **26**:609.
6. Kusunoki M, Saitoh N, Yamamura T, *et al.* (1988) Choledochal cysts. Oligoganglionosis in the narrow portion of the choledochus. *Ann Surg* **123**:984.
7. Goon HK, Tai A, Samad SA. (1992) Congenital bile duct dilatation: Review of 35 cases. *Pediatr Surg Int* **7**:332.
8. Singhavejsakul J, Ukarapol N. (2008) Choledochal cysts in children: Epidemiology and outcomes. *World J Surg* **32**:1385–13888.
9. Foo DC, Wong KK, Lan LC, *et al.* (2009) Impact of prenatal diagnosis on choledochal cysts and the benefits of early excision. *J Paediatr Child Health* **45**:28–30.
10. Chavhan GB, Babyn PS, Manson D, *et al.* (2008) Pediatric MR cholangiopancreatography: Principles, technique, and clinical applications. *Radiographics* **28**:1951–1962.
11. Lilly JR. (1978) Total Excision of choledochal cyst. *Surg Gynecol Obstet* **146**:254.
12. Ishibashi T, Kasahara K, Yasuda Y, *et al.* (1997) Malignant change in the biliary tract after excision of choledochal cyst. *Br J Surg* **84**:1687–1691.

13. Kang CM, Chi HS, Kim JY, *et al.* (2007) A case of robot-assisted excision of choledochal cyst-hepaticojejunostomy, and extracorporeal Roux-en-y anastomosis using the da Vinci surgical system. *Surg Laparosc Endosc Percutan Tech* **17**:538–541.
14. Stringer MD. (2007) Wide hilar hepaticojejunostomy: The optimum method of reconstruction after choledochal cyst excision. *Pediatr Surg Int* **23**:529–532.
15. Saeki M, Nakano M, Hagane K, *et al.* (1991) Effectiveness of an intussusceptive antireflux valve to prevent ascending cholangitis after hepatic portojejunostomy in biliary atresia. *J Pediatr Surg* **26**:800.
16. Komuro H, Makino SI, Yasuda Y, *et al.* (2001) Pancreatic complications in choledochal cyst and their surgical outcomes. *World J Surg* **25**:1519–1523.

LIVER CYSTS AND ABSCESSES

71

Mauricio A. Escobar

LIVER ABSCESSES

Clinical Presentation

Children with liver abscesses typically have nonspecific signs and symptoms. The diagnosis of a liver abscess is difficult to establish from the clinical picture alone. Patients commonly manifest fever, lethargy, vomiting, hepatomegaly, and abdominal pain and tenderness. The classic symptoms of fever, right upper quadrant tenderness, and jaundice are only present in approximately 10% of patients. Neonates typically have nonspecific signs and symptoms related to sepsis. Children with amebic hepatic abscesses typically present with high fevers and tender hepatomegaly.

Pathophysiology

Neonatal liver abscess is a rare entity with less than 100 reported cases in the literature. There are larger case series for older children. The average age of presentation is 7–10 yrs, and there may be a slight male predominance. Risk factors include bacteremia, umbilical vein catheterization, central venous catheters with parenteral nutrition infusions, necrotizing enterocolitis, hepatic trauma, appendicitis, cholecystitis, ovarian cyst, prematurity, and history of previous surgery. Newborn very-low-birth-weight preterm infants are at greater risk of developing liver abscess due to the decreased adherence and chemotaxis of their neutrophils.

Pediatric liver abscesses are often, but not always, associated with immunosuppression. They have been described with disorders of innate immunity, malignancies, Crohn's disease, diabetes mellitus, and abdominal sepsis. Hepatic abscesses are strongly associated with chronic granulomatous disease (CGD), a rare immunologic disorder characterized by defective phagocyte oxidase activity resulting from diminished function of reduced nicotinamide adenine dinucleotide phosphate oxidase.

Liver abscesses in children may be bacterial (pyogenic), fungal, parasitic, or viral in origin. Pyogenic abscesses may develop through multiple routes including the biliary system, systemic circulation (hepatic artery or venous system), portal circulation, or via direct spread from contiguous structures. Liver abscesses may be acquired from breast milk when there is lymphangitis of the breast from the mother. While staphylococcus is the offending organism in this setting, most neonatal cases of pyogenic abscess result from gram negative bacteremia through the portal vein. However, most pyogenic abscesses in infants and children occur due to systemic bactermia with *Staphylococcus aureus*.

Rarer causes of liver abscesses in neonates have also been reported. They may be associated with listeriosis, congenital tuberculosis, and congenital syphilis. Fungal liver abscesses (most commonly from *Candida albicans*) occur most frequently in individuals with prolonged antibiotic exposure or compromised immune systems. Amebic liver abscess in neonates is extremely uncommon (see Figure 1). An abscess is termed *cryptogenic* when no identifiable etiologic agent is recovered from the culture.

Pyogenic abscesses can be found in any part of the liver. The majority of abscesses are found in the posterior portion of the right lobe, and this is thought to be due to the pattern of portal venous flow. However, multiple liver abscesses are also found, and they may involve other organs as well.

Diagnosis/Work-up

Labs may show leukocytosis, elevated liver enzymes, erythrocyte sedimentation rate, or raised C-reactive protein. Abdominal ultrasound (U/S) or Computed Tomography (CT) of the abdomen is necessary to confirm the diagnosis. Whenever possible, liver abscess cultures should be obtained. Serology is useful for the diagnosis of amebiasis.

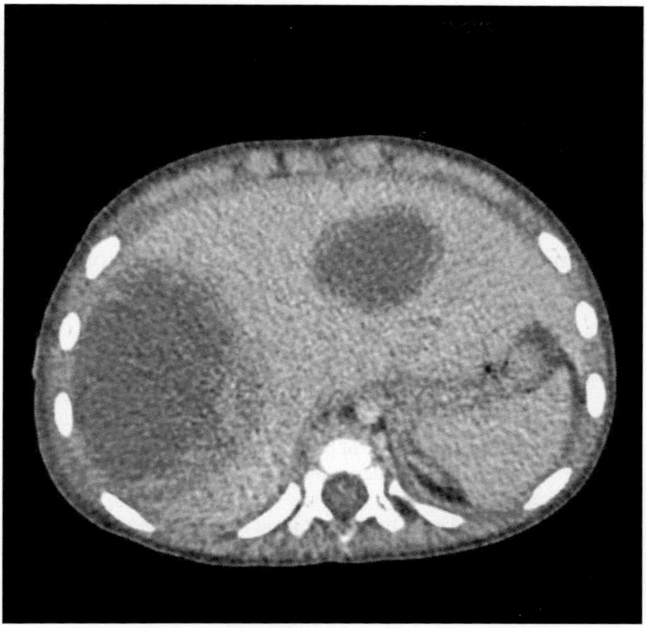

Figure 1. CT scan of a 16-mth old boy with liver abscesses secondary to amebiasis treated with percutaneous drainage and metronidazole.

Management

Treatment of pediatric hepatic abscesses consists of multiple systemic antibiotics with percutaneous drainage with interventional radiology of macroscopic abscess collections. Volume resuscitation is critical before any intervention is entertained. Patients may require admission to the neonatal or pediatric intensive care units for closer monitoring. Surgical drainage is recommended with abscess rupture on presentation, multiloculated abscesses not amenable to percutaneous drainage, incomplete percutaneous drainage, or if there is a known surgical pathology in the abdomen (appendicitis, etc.). While an open approach is the gold standard, laparoscopy has been successfully utilized in draining these abscesses. Drains are typically left in place.

If multiple microabscesses of the liver are noted, then therapy is antimicrobials alone. Antibiotics are tailored to the specific offending organism and are usually continued from 4–6 wks. It is recommended to continue antibiotics following drainage for at least 2 wks. Hepatic amebiasis is treated with metronidazole and percutaneous drainage if risk of rupture is assessed.

Postoperative Considerations

Drains are typically removed when a predetermined set of criteria set forth by the surgeon and/or interventional radiologist is achieved. Typically, the drain output quantity and quality is monitored, and the

Algorithm for Liver Abscess

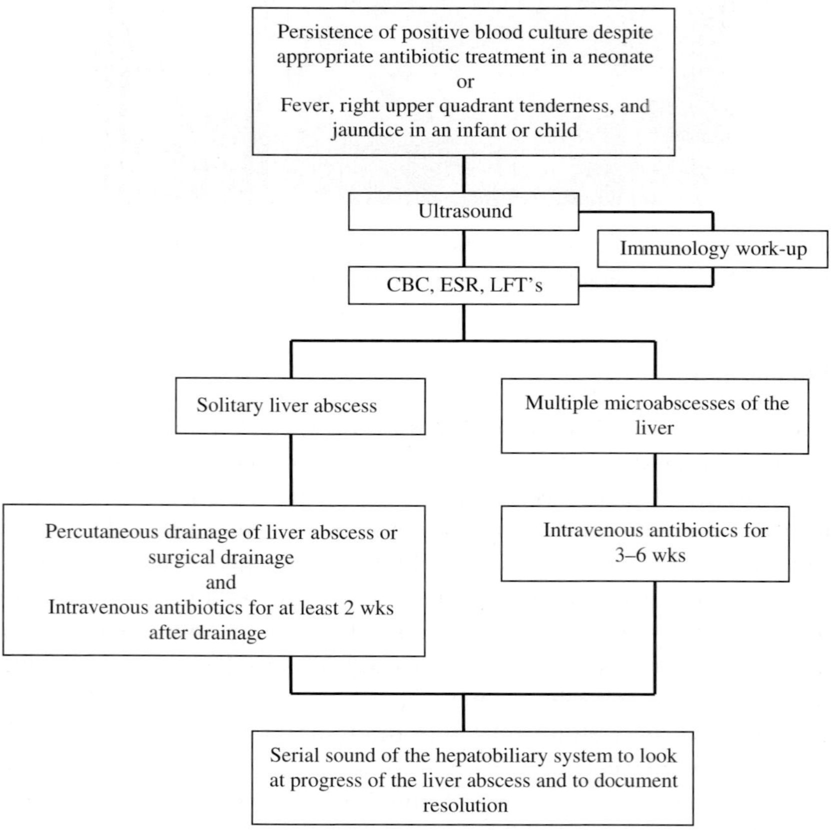

Adapted from Tan *et al.*

drain is removed when the output is less than 10–30 mL/day. Serial ultrasounds or CT's are useful adjuncts to determine the resolution of the liver abscess in both neonates and older children. Antibiotics are continued as noted above. Patients may be released from the hospital with central venous access and drains if the family is capable to complete convalescence at home. Careful follow-up is mandatory until all signs of abscess are gone.

Pyogenic neonatal liver abscess is uniformly fatal if untreated. Complications include bacteremia and rupture of the abscess into the peritoneal cavity. Patients may have concomitant abscesses elsewhere (empyema, cerebral, etc.). Although the prognosis for pyogenic liver abscess has improved dramatically, mortality may still be as high as 50% in neonates with complications. Long-term complications have also been reported including hemobilia and portal vein thrombosis. Hemobilia is diagnosed and treated with angiography. Portal vein thrombosis in adults is typically treated with anticoagulation, but no clear body of literature exists in neonates. Bilomas may also occur that may require drainage and/or endoscopic retrograde cholangiography (ERCP) and stenting or surgery.

SOLITARY LIVER CYSTS

Clinical Presentation

Liver cysts may be detected prenatally or postnatally. Prenatal diagnosis is made with ultrasonography. Postnatal imaging (U/S, CT, or Magnetic Resonance Imaging [MRI]) is required to further evaluate the cyst. The presence and characteristics of the cyst dictate management.

Cysts detected postnatally present in a variety of ways. Most simple cysts are asymptomatic unless large, and are incidental findings on imaging for an unrelated problem. The most common complaints are abdominal distension and/or mass, feeding difficulties, abdominal pain, and duodenal obstruction. A variety of complications have been reported in association with congenital cysts, including rupture with subsequent peritonitis, infection, and sometimes jaundice. Patients may present with complications of related disease, such as respiratory distress or hemoptysis from pulmonary hydatid disease. The series from Boston Children's Hospital of congenital solitary nonparasitic cysts of the liver noted two thirds of cysts were incidental findings at autopsy.

Pathophysiology

Simple cysts account for most of the prenatally detected and postnatally diagnosed solitary lesions. They are more common in females. Simple cysts are generally thought to arise from aberrant bile ducts or from intrahepatic peribiliary glands. Simple cysts are typically unilocular and may be completely intrahepatic, partially extrahepatic, or pedunculated. The presence of septa raises the suspicion of other pathologies.

The differential diagnosis of a solitary liver cyst in a child is myriad. These include:

(1) Congenital
  Simple
  Mesenchymal hamartoma
  Intrahepatic choledochal cyst
  Ciliated hepatic foregut cyst
  Epidermoid cyst
  Lymphangioma
(2) Acquired
  Parasitic (hydatid)
    Hydatid disease is a parasitic infestation by a tapeworm of the genus
  Echinococcus.
  Posttraumatic
  Neoplastic: cystadenoma, sarcoma, teratoma
  Biliary cysts (biliary atresia post-Kasai, traumatic)
  Abscess (see above).

Diagnosis/Work-up

Ultrasound is the mainstay of diagnosis. An MRI or CT is indicated if the cyst appears complex (i.e. septations). Anything other than a small unilocular smooth-walled anechoic cyst demands further imaging. MRI is useful for differentiating cystic tumors such as mesenchymal hamartomas. CT is the best test for the differentiation of hydatid from amebic and pyogenic cysts in the liver. The indirect hemagglutination test and the enzyme-linked immunosorbent assay (ELISA) may be useful in diagnosing hydatid disease. The Casoni intradermal skin test is now largely abandoned because of its low sensitivity, low accuracy, and potential for severe local allergic reaction.

Management

Asymptomatic simple cysts are monitored with serial ultrasonography. Intervention is warranted if there is progressive enlargement, symptoms, or the diagnosis is in question. Total surgical excision (usually by anatomic resection) is the best treatment for two reasons. First, it eliminates recurrence. Second, the procedure is curative in the event that the lesion is not a simple cyst (i.e. a mesenchymal hamartoma, etc.). If complete resection is too hazardous, acceptable alternatives include aspiration, sclerotherapy, and laparoscopic excision or fenestration, provided the

Algorithm for Solitary Liver Cyst

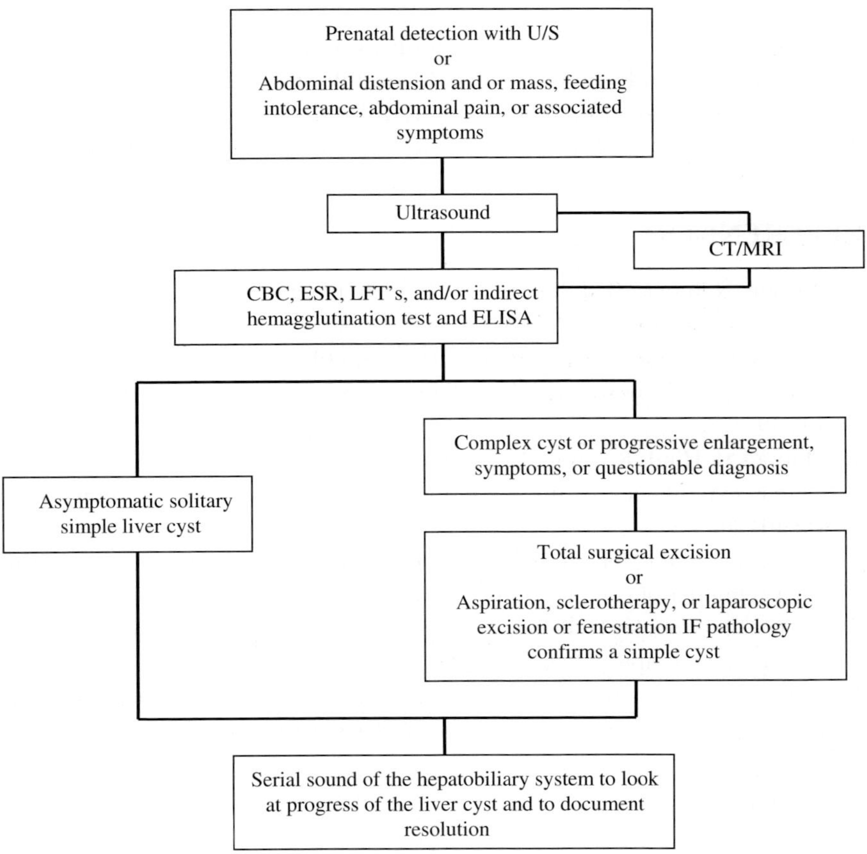

pathology confirms a simple cyst. Complex cysts should be treated with complete excision whenever possible to eliminate future malignant potential.

Choledochal cysts are discussed elsewhere. Intrahepatic choledochal cysts not safely amenable to resection can be treated by wide cystoenterostomy. Patients with polycystic liver disease, Caroli's disease, congenital hepatic fibrosis, and biliary atresia are not discussed in this chapter. Hydatid cysts are treated by surgical excision with or without chemotherapy. Spillage of the cyst can result in a life-threatening anaphylactic reaction. Interventional radiology techniques have also arisen that are promising.

Postoperative Considerations

Recurrence is the most common complication following incomplete excisions or aspiration. Fistulas may also form. Bilomas may also occur if there is biliary communication. These may require drainage and/or ERCP and stenting or surgery. Follow-up is dictated by the pathology of the liver cyst.

REFERENCES

1. Awasthy N, Juneja M, Talukdar B, *et al.* (2007) Hemobilia complicating a liver abscess. *J Trop Pediatr* **53:**278–279.
2. Donovan MJ, Kozakewich H, Perez-Atayde A. (1995) Solitary nonparasitic cysts of the liver: The Boston children's hospital experience. *Pediatr Pathol Lab Med* **15:**419–428.
3. Muorah M, Hinds R, Verma A, *et al.* (2006) Liver abscesses in children: A single center experience in the developed world. *J Pediatr Gastroenterol Nutr* **42:**201–206.
4. Rao S, Solaymani-Mohammadi S, Petri Jr, WA, Parker S. (2009) Hepatic amebiasis: A reminder of complications. *Curr Opin Pediatr* **21:**145–149.
5. Rogers TN, Woodley H, Ramsden W, *et al.* (2007) Solitary liver cysts in children: Not always so simple. *J Pediatr Surg* **42:**333–339.
6. Tan NWH, Sriram B, Tan-Kendrick APA. (2005) Neonatal hepatic abscess in preterm infants: A rare entity? *Ann Acad Med Singapore* **34:**558–564.

GALLBLADDER DISEASE IN CHILDREN 72

Frederick J. Rescorla

The incidence of gallbladder disease in children has increased significantly over the past several decades. This has included both cholelithiasis as well as biliary dyskinesia, however over the past 10 yrs, biliary dyskinesia has surpassed cholelithiasis as the most common indication for cholecystectomy in children. Gallbladder disease however is still much less frequent in children compared with adults. In adults 12% of women and 4% of men over 40 yrs of age have cholelithiasis, whereas only 0.13% to 0.22% of children have gallstones. The rise in cholelithiasis in children is primarily related to nonhemolytic conditions including the use of total parenteral nutrition (TPN), stasis and sepsis and other factors related to prematurity, as well as use of oral contraceptives, obesity, cystic fibrosis, pregnancy, and previous ileal resection.

Acalculous Gallbladder Disease

Acalculous gallbladder disease can include hydrops of the gallbladder, acalculous cholecystitis, gallbladder polyps and biliary dyskinesia. Biliary dyskinesia will be discussed as a separate section.

Hydrops is noted with massive distention of the gallbladder in the absence of stones and is often associated with Kawaski's Disease. This is usually associated with transient obstruction of the cystic duct, as well as increased mucous production by the gallbladder. Conservative management is usually recommended and antibiotics may be indicated for sepsis or fever. If significant pain with ongoing gallbladder distention or gallbladder necrosis occurs cholecystectomy may be indicated.

Acalculous cholecystitis often occurs in the setting of sepsis, burns or other significant trauma with associated dehydration, hypotension and lack of bowel function. TPN is often utilized in these children and may be associated with decreased gallbladder contractility and progressive distention, stasis and potential infection. Ultrasound is very useful to follow for gallbladder wall thickening, as well as pericholecystic fluid.

Polyps are an unusual finding in children. They are often associated with gallstones and may be due to excessive accumulation of cholesterol within the epithelial lining leading to polyps. Most are cholesterol polyps. In the adult population where they are more common, polyps less than 1 cm. in size are usually treated with observation only, whereas larger polyps may have the ability to develop into adenocarcinoma.

Biliary Dyskinesia

This disorder was initially termed cystic duct syndrome in 1963 and in 1975 early studies demonstrating crystals or bacteria in the duodenal bile reported cure rates of over 90% with cholecystectomy in affected patients. A subsequent study in 1986 by Brugg noted patients with bile crystals had gallbladder ejection fractions of 25.9% +/– 14.8% with all having cholecystitis on pathologic examination whereas those with no bile crystals had ejection fractions of 60.3% +/– 23.3%.

Abnormal emptying of the gallbladder identified by a low gallbladder ejection fraction on hepatobiliary scintigraphy scan was first identified as the cause for chronic abdominal pain in adults in the 1980's and termed gallbladder or biliary dyskinesia. The relief of abdominal pain with cholecystectomy in adults with poor gallbladder ejection fractions was noted with many reports noting a success rate between 60–85%. Some reported higher success rates in patients in which the final pathology demonstrated inflammatory changes within the gallbladder, as well as those with a very low ejection fraction (<15%) compared to a borderline low ejection fraction. This was recognized as an increasing cause of abdominal pain in children in the mid 1990's and many centers reported alleviation of symptoms in children with biliary dyskinesia after removal of the gallbladder. This is currently being diagnosed with increased frequency in children with chronic abdominal pain and has surpassed cholelithiasis as the most common indication for cholecystectomy in children. The incidence of biliary dyskinesia in Kansas City reported by Holcomb was 2% in the time period between 1990 and 1998. A subsequent review at a children's hospital during the period 1998–2003 reported that 58% of the children undergoing cholecystectomy had biliary dyskinesia. This later is also reflective of our experience at Riley Hospital for Children over the past 10 yrs.

Nonhemolytic Cholelithiasis

Gallstones have been identified in neonates and infants who have received TPN and some studies have demonstrated that up to 43% of children receiving long term TPN developed gallstones. It is likely due to the changes in bile composition related to either the amino acid infusion or the lack of enteral feeding while on TPN. Lack of enteral feeding leads to poor gallbladder contractility and reduced enterohepatic circulation of bile. Many neonates receive short term TPN for uncomplicated gastroschisis and intestinal atresia and very few of these infants develop gallstones. Other factors suspected of contributing to the development of gallstones in neonates include sepsis, dehydration, furosemide therapy, short bowel syndrome and ileal resection related to necrotizing enterocolitis. Although stones in adolescents and adults are primarily cholesterol stones, those in younger children are usually calcium carbonate and black pigment stones.

The etiology of gallstones in older children includes obesity, which is increasing at an alarming rate among adolescents within the United States. Other causes include oral contraceptive use, cystic fibrosis, pregnancy and a history of previous ileal resection. It has also been noted in patients undergoing cardiac transplantation and patients who have undergone previous extracorporeal oxygenation. Among children with cholelithiasis, cholesterol gallstones have surpassed that of hemolytic disease as the leading cause of cholelithiasis in children under 18 yrs of age. The primary symptom is usually abdominal pain and the classic history of fatty food intolerance is often not noted.

Hemolytic Cholelithiasis

Hemolytic cholelithiasis remains a common cause for gallstones in children related primarily to sickle cell disease as well as hereditary spherocytosis and thalassemia. The incidence of gallstones in sickle cell disease patients appears to be age dependent with 50% of patients developing gallstones by 20 yrs of age. Gallbladder sludge is frequently noted in patients with sickle cell disease and elective cholecystectomy is often recommended in the presence of sludge with or without stones. This is based on some studies demonstrating that as many as 65% of patients with sludge eventually develop stones.

The presence of cholelithiasis in hereditary spherocytosis ranges from 43–63% and again is dependent on the duration of the disease process and the rate of hemolysis. A recent study from our institution in patients undergoing laparoscopic splenectomy noted that the incidence of gallstones was 27% in children less than 10 yrs of age and 56% in those greater than 10 yrs of age ($p < 0.05$). Due to this association, gallbladder ultrasound is recommended prior to elective splenectomy to determine the need for concomitant cholecystectomy. Prophylactic cholecystectomy in children without stones undergoing splenectomy, however is not indicated. Thalassemia major represents another group of children at risk for cholelithiasis, although the incidence has decreased due to the routine administration hypertransfusion regimens.

CLINICAL PRESENTATION

Gallbladder disease in infants is often due to an associated condition such as the use of TPN, history of ileal resection related to necrotizing enterocolitis or gastroschisis, prematurity, or prolonged fasting for another condition often with TPN. In many of these infants receiving TPN, the onset of jaundice related to cholestasis occurs prior to the identification of gallstones.

Gallstones that occur between infancy and adolescence are usually calcium bilirubinate stones with calcium carbonate and cholesterol. The diagnosis is sometimes difficult in these young children. Clinical presentation of acute cholecystitis is often associated with pain, nausea, vomiting, and right upper quadrant pain. Chronic cholecystitis with cholelithiasis is more common than acute cholecystitis and the symptoms and physical examination in adolescents with gallbladder disease are usually related to nausea, vomiting, intermittent abdominal pain, as well as intolerance to fatty foods. Several studies have demonstrated that the pain is less well localized than in adult series.

Patients with biliary dyskinesia frequently present with chronic abdominal pain, some with right upper quadrant but others with periumbilical pain or mid epigastric pain. It is often associated with intolerance to fatty foods, nausea, vomiting, and occasionally constipation and weight loss. The nonspecific nature of the symptoms results in many of those children undergoing extensive workups including CT scans prior to a determination of the gallbladder ejection fracture.

Choledocholithiasis and Gallstone Pancreatitis

Occasionally children will present with common hepatic and common bile duct stones leading to obstruction with jaundice or gallstone pancreatitis. At Riley Hospital for Children we have most commonly seen this in children with sickle cell disease or hereditary spherocytosis but occasionally as the first symptom in nonhemolytic gallstones. In some children with hereditary spherocytosis it has been the initial presenting symptom. In the absence of pancreatitis the options are: Initial endoscopic retrograde cholangiopancreatography (ERCP) with stone extraction; laparoscopic cholecystectomy with cholangiography, and common duct flushing in an attempt to remove the stone; or laparoscopic or open common duct exploration if stones remain by cholangiogram at time of cholecystectomy. If the stone cannot be extracted as time of laparoscopic cholecystectomy the surgeon can simply close and utilize postoperative ERCP with stone removal, although this has the slight risk that if stone removal is not possible a subsequent open procedure would be necessary. The preferred method at our institution is preoperative ERCP with endoscopic retrieval and sphincterotomy. We are however fortunate to have a very experienced group of gastroenterologists skilled at this procedure. Laparoscopic cholecystectomy is usually performed 1 or 2 days after stone extraction.

In patients with gallstone pancreatitis, appropriate supportive care is necessary in an attempt to allow resolution of the pancreatitis. Occasionally emergent ERCP is necessary if obstructive jaundice is also present. After the pancreatitis has resolved, elective cholecystectomy is performed prior to discharge. In these situations, an intraoperative cholangiogram is usually performed to evaluate for the residual presence of choledocholithiasis. A preoperative ultrasound can often identify signs of choledocholithiasis such as a dilated duct.

DIAGNOSIS

Abdominal ultrasound is the most frequently used modality to detect the presence of cholelithiasis. It is also effective in determining common bile duct or common hepatic duct dilatation, as well as thickening of the gallbladder wall with acute cholecystitis and other abnormalities associated with the pancreas. Scintigraphy with technetium-99M-labeled iminodiacetic acid demonstrates nonvisualization of the gallbladder in the presence of acute cholecystitis. Nonvisualization may also occur in some fasting patients or in association with severe illness or sometimes in the presence of TPN thus yielding a false positive result.

The cholecystokinin (CCK) — stimulated ejection fraction scintigraphy has been utilized since 1981. It has been shown to be 80–90% sensitive in identifying patients with biliary dyskinesia. Most centers report a gallbladder ejection fraction of less than 35% as abnormal. The reliability of the CCK stimulated ejection fraction predicting success with cholecystectomy has been questioned in several studies. In a retrospective evaluation of the review of 38 patients in our institution, a CCK stimulated ejection fraction of less than 15% predicted successful outcome as did nausea associated with abdominal pain. As noted in the discussion of choledocholithiasis, ERCP is often useful in select situations to remove common duct stones.

NONSURGICAL TREATMENT

In the 1980's and 90's oral dissolution therapy with bile salts and extracorporeal shock wave lithotripsy both became popular in adults however, both had limited success. Lithotripsy had the down side of frequent treatments, as well as high cost and a 50% risk of recurrence within 5 yrs. In a similar fashion, dissolution therapy required prolonged treatment and had a very high recurrence rate. Undoubtedly the introduction of laparoscopic cholecystectomy in the late 1980's and the loss of the major morbidity and mortality associated with open cholecystectomy markedly affected the treatment paradigm for gallbladder disease.

Infants and young children, below the age of two or three, often develop gallstones related to TPN in association with fasting and often ileal resection. In many of these children with the onset of enteral feeds and a reduction or elimination of TPN, there has been noted gallstone resolution and therefore a 6–12 mth period of observation is reasonable in the absence of symptoms.

SURGICAL MANAGEMENT

Indications for Cholecystectomy

The four major complications associated with cholelithiasis include cholecystitis, jaundice, cholangitis, and biliary pancreatitis. The presence of symptoms associated with stones is generally considered an adequate indication for cholecystectomy. One of the primary reasons to proceed is to prevent the occurrence of cholecystitis, jaundice, cholangitis or gallstone pancreatitis. These later two conditions can be associated with significant morbidity and even mortality. Although abdominal pain with stones, that being symptomatic chronic cholelithiasis, is perhaps the most common indication for cholecystectomy, chronic cholecystitis, jaundice related to common duct stones and biliary pancreatitis are being seen with increasing frequency.

In patients diagnosed with biliary dyskinesia, the presence of pain with a low gallbladder ejection fraction is usually an adequate indication to proceed with cholecystectomy. One rationale for the more liberal use of laparoscopic cholecystectomy in these patients is to avoid the morbidity and cost of further diagnostic studies such as ERCP or magnetic resonance cholangiopancreatography (MRCP). Laparoscopic cholecystectomy in experienced hands is a very safe procedure and is thus recommended by pediatric and adult gastroenterologists prior to proceeding to more advanced studies in these studies.

Preparation

Most children require no special preparation, however patients with sickle cell disease have a significant risk for postoperative complications such as sickle crisis and acute chest syndrome and have been the subject of several studies to decrease the complication rate. Based on multicenter studies of sickle cell patients, most hematologists recommend transfusion of affected children to a hemoglobin of 10 gm/dL preoperatively, whereas prior recommendations were to transfuse until the hemoglobin S-fraction was less than 30–35%. Despite this, acute chest syndrome is still possible and meticulous attention should be made to fine details of patient care, including adequate perioperative and postoperative fluid hydration and pulse oximetry monitoring. Patients with acute cholecystectomy are generally treated with intravenous fluids and antibiotics followed by laparoscopic cholecystectomy a few days later during the same admission.

Cholecystectomy

The laparoscopic approach for cholelithiasis in adults was introduced in the late 80's and introduced in children in the early 1990's and has since become the standard for gallbladder removal. Approximately 90% of the cholecystectomies in children are performed laparoscopically. The patient is positioned in the supine position with the video monitor at the head of the table. An orogastric tube is introduced for gastric decompression. We generally ask the patient to empty their bladder prior to going back to the operating room and a foley catheter is not routinely placed. Preoperative antibiotics are utilized if there is a suspicion for common duct stones, however in cases of biliary dyskinesia or simple cholelithiasis it can be given at the surgeon's discretion. The abdomen is entered through the umbilicus with the largest trocar usually 10 mm. The standard laparoscopic approach employs three or four trocars. Some newer techniques utilize a reduced number of trocars with suture retraction of the dome and infundibulum of the gallbladder. Single incision techniques utilize either several trocars placed separately through the *fascia* of the umbilicus, a single trocar with several separate stab incisions for instruments, or, a multi-access port. If the three or four port technique is utilized, a 10 mm. trocar is placed in the umbilicus and then a 5 mm. primary working port in the epigastric region for dissection of the gallbladder and placement of clips on the cystic duct and cystic artery. Retraction of the gallbladder is generally performed with the two other sites over the gallbladder and right lower lateral abdominal wall. Either ports or stab incisions with placement of the instruments directly into the abdominal cavity are utilized. Since these instruments are usually not exchanged throughout the procedure a single stab incision is possible and this technique as described by Holcomb has decreased the number of trocars necessary for this procedure and results in significant cost savings.

Reverse Trendelenberg position and rotation of the bed to the patient's left may aid exposure. The gallbladder dome is grasped and retracted superiorly over the liver with the assistant's other instrument grasping the infundibulum and holding it inferiorly as the surgeon separates the adhesions to the duodenum. The cystic duct and artery are dissected free and a clear space identified between these structures and the liver. Three clips are placed on the cystic duct and cystic artery and both divided leaving two clips on the abdominal side. The gallbladder is then separated from the liver in a retrograde fashion. The hook cautery device is generally adequate for removing the rest of the gallbladder from the liver bed although some prefer use of bipolar cautery or energy. Prior to completely separating the gallbladder, the gallbladder bed and triangle of Calot are carefully inspected for bleeding. The gallbladder is extracted through the umbilical port. If large stones are present the *fascia* may need to be enlarged and occasionally the gallbladder can be opened externally and the stones removed from the intraabdominal portion of the gallbladder prior to delivering the entire gallbladder.

All surgeons performing laparoscopic cholecystectomy should be facile in performing intraoperative cholangiograms. This may be necessary in any procedure if there is a question of the anatomy of the common duct or cystic duct and a cholangiogram should be performed to ascertain the exact relationship of the structures. In most children a preoperative ultrasound will determine the presence of common duct stones, however intraoperative cholangiogram may be useful if there is a high index of suspicion including a preoperative episode of gallstone pancreatitis, common bile duct dilatation, a history of preoperative jaundice or known history of previous common duct stones.

In children requiring splenectomy and concomitant cholecystectomy, the patient is positioned with the left side up approximately 30° to aid in the splenectomy portion of the procedure. The trocars for the splenectomy portion are adequate for the cholecystectomy. One additional port or stab incision may be placed to retract the dome of the gallbladder if the surgeon is more comfortable using a low right lateral instrument for this function which may be too far away for the splenectomy. We generally remove the gallbladder first and then proceed with the splenectomy. For the cholecystectomy, the table is rotated to the patient's left and the patient placed in the reverse Trendelenburg position to aid in exposure of the triangle of Calot.

In the presence of known or suspected choledocholithiasis, the options include preoperative ERCP with sphincterotomy and stone extraction, laparoscopic or open duct exploration at the time of laparoscopic or open cholecystectomy or postoperative ERCP with stone extraction. This decision is related to both the surgeon's experience with laparoscopic common duct exploration, as well as the availability of ERCP and sphincterotomy in children and adolescents at the surgeon's institution. Although some pediatric surgeons may be facile with laparoscopic common duct exploration, this is not a common disease treated by pediatric surgeons and for most, adequate experience is probably not present. Cholangiography however should be a routine part of the pediatric surgeon skill set and occasionally flushing of the stones results in clearing of the duct. In most settings however, it is likely that preoperative ERCP with sphincterotomy and stone extraction would be the most reasonable approach. If this is successful, the surgeon can then proceed with laparoscopic cholecystectomy in the next day or two. If the ERCP and stone extraction is not successful, the surgeon is aware at the time of laparoscopic cholecystectomy and can decide to proceed with common duct exploration either on a laparoscpic or open basis depending on the results of the cholangiogram, as well as determining whether flushing of the duct results in stone passage.

OUTCOME

The incidence of cholecystectomy is rising and this is related primarily to biliary dyskinesia. Nearly all cholecystectomies are performed in a laparoscopic fashion. The most devastating complication associated with laparoscopic cholecystectomy is bile duct injury, which has been reported in approximately 0.15% to 0.5% of adults in large database reports. At our institution we perform over 100 cholecystectomies per year and to date have not had a bile duct injury. Patients with symptomatic cholelithiasis generally have improvement with cholecystectomy and many reports note relief of symptoms in 97% of children. Patients with biliary dyskinesia have a somewhat lower success rate with cholecystectomy with complete relief of pain noted in 71–85%. At our institution, we have noted predictors for success with cholecystectomy in children with biliary dyskinesia include the presence of nausea and an ejection fraction less than 15%. The combination of pain, nausea and ejection fraction less than 15% had a positive prediction value of 93%. Children with persistent symptoms after laparoscopic cholecystectomy for biliary dyskinesia may warrant further workup with MRCP or ERCP. Adult data with biliary dyskinesia also notes significant improvement between 89–94% and cure rates between 65–94%.

REFERENCES

1. Rothenberg SS, Shipman K, Yoder S. (2009) Experience with modified single-port laparoscopic procedures in children. *J Laparoendosc Adv Surg Tech* **19**(5):695–698.
2. Melton GB, Lillemoe KD, Cameron JL, *et al.* (2002) Major bile duct injuries associated with laparoscopic cholecystectomy: Effect of surgical repair on quality of life. *Ann Surg* **235**(6):888–895.

3. Carney DE, Kokoska ER, Grosfeld JL, *et al.* (2004) Predictors of Successful Outcome After Cholecystectomy for Biliary Dyskinesia. *J Pediatr Surg* **39**:813–816.
4. Sorenson MK, Fancher S, Lang NP, *et al.* (1993) Abnormal gallbladder nuclear ejection fraction predicts success of cholecystectomy in patients with biliary dyskinesia. *Am J Surg* **166**:672–674 Discussion: 674–675.
5. Al-Homaidhi HS, Sukerek H, Klein M, *et al.* (2002) Biliary dyskinesia in children. *Pediatr Surg Int* **18**:357–360.
6. Michail S, Preud'Homme D, Christian J, *et al.* (2001) Laparoscopic cholecystectomy: Effective treatment for chronic abdominal pain children with acalculous biliary pain. *J Pediatr Surg* **36**:1394–1396.
7. Rescorla FJ. (1997) Cholelithiasis, cholecystitis, and common bile duct stones. *Curr Opin Pediatr* **9**:276–282.
8. Imamoglu M, Sarihan H, Sari A, Ahmetoglu A. (2002) Acute Acalculous Cholecystitis in Children: Diagnosis and Treatment. *J Pediatr Surg* **37**:36–39.

PANCREATIC CYSTS 73

Frederick J. Rescorla

EMBRYOLOGY

The pancreas originates from a ventral and dorsal bud of the embryonic foregut. The ventral bud is closely related to the bile duct and this portion rotates around the duodenum along with the common bile duct to become situated posteriorly and makeup the inferior surface of dorsal pancreatic duct. This brings the common bile duct and ventral (Wirsung) pancreatic duct in close proximity to the dorsal duct. The major papillae is distal to the opening of the dorsal (Santorini) duct. At the seventh week of gestation the ventral duct fuses with the proximal part of the dorsal. Most of the gland rise from the dorsal and this includes the superior and anterior part of the head along with the body and tail. This portion of the pancreas drained by the duct of Santorini through the minor papillae. The ventral bud becomes the posterior and anterior part of the head and is drained to the duct of Wirsung into the major papillae along with the bile duct. With fusion of the ventral and dorsal pancreas the duct of Wirsung becomes the major duct and thus the duct of Santorini becomes the minor drainage system. Failure of the two ductal systems to fuse results in two separate ductal systems referred to as the pancreas divisum. In this disorder the duct of Wirsung drains the embryological smaller ventral process and the duct of Santorini becomes the major ductal system draining into the duodenum through the minor patilla. This anatomic variant is found in 11% of cadavers.

Annular pancreas occurs as a result of abnormal development with incomplete rotation of the ventral pancreas resulting in the pancreas wrapped around an encircling the duodenum. This is often found in association with duodenal atresia.

CONGENITAL AND DEVELOPMENTAL CYSTS

Congenital cysts of the pancreas are very rare and primarily limited to case reports. They appear to be more common in females and occur in the body and tail of the pancreas. Most have been unilocular rather than multilocular and are lined by true epithelium. The cysts contain yellow fluid that has no enzyme activity within it. They have been reported in association with von Hippel–Lindau which is associated with hereditary cerebellar cysts and retinal hemangiomas.

Congenital and developmental cysts can be detected in several findings or detected in the prenatal period with polyhydramnios or prenatal ultrasound. They may be asymptomatic after birth or associated with abdominal distention and symptoms of gastric outlet obstruction with vomiting. Surgical treatment consists of excision if the cyst is located in the body and tail, but internal drainage for those occurring in the head of the pancreas.

RETENTION CYSTS

Enteric Duplication

Enteric duplications involving the pancreas are also very rare and usually associated with gastric duplications. These are most likely due to failure of regression of an enteric diverticulum in the pancreatic duct. Most of the reported cases communicate directly with the pancreatic duct and are lined with gastric type epithelium and contain ectopic pancreas within the wall of the cyst. Abdominal pain is the most common presenting symptom and pancreatitis can be associated with this due to obstruction of the pancreatic ducts by the secretions of the cyst or debris obstructing the main pancreatic duct. The standard treatment is limited resection although some require pancreatico-duodenectomy to establish the internal drainage.

Pancreatic Pseudocyst

Pancreatic pseudocysts are thin walled cysts with collections of pancreatic secretions without a true epithelial lining. These can result as sequalae from any cause of pancreatitis in children with the most common cause being trauma, but also including numerous other causes related to medications, metabolic disorders or cystic fibrosis.

ETIOLOGY

Traumatic pancreatitis is the most common cause of pancreatic pseudocysts in children. This usually occurs due to the result of blunt trauma with crushing of the pancreas against the vertebral body. Child abuse should be considered in children who are young with a vague history and we have seen several cases of this at our institution. In older children, the cause of the trauma is usually blunt with bicycle and all terrain Vehicle (ATV) accidents two of the more common causes. It also occurs with motor vehicle crashes and falls. Endoscopic retrograde cholangiopancreatography (ERCP) pancreatitis is another cause of pancreatitis although many of these children have underlying disorders leading to the diagnostic ERCP. Systemic infections from mumps, Robella or Coxsaky B virus or other infections also are associated with pancreatitis. Various studies have noted that between 6–33% of childhood cases with pancreatitis arise from disorder of the biliary or pancreatic ducts. These can be choledochal cysts leading to obstruction and pancreatitis. Cholelithiasis related pancreatitis is the most common etiology for pancreatic pseudocyst behind trauma at our institution. Cholelithiasis is often associated with hemolytic disorders such as spherocytosis or sickle cell disease and rarely beta thalassmia. It also can be associated with obesity and use of total parenteral nutrition. Pancreatic ductal anomalies can include pancreas divisum. We have had several children with divisum who have presented with severe pancreatitis and pancreatic pseudocyst. Some of these pseudocysts have been treated endoscopically with internal drainage and subsequently needed a ductal drainage procedure such as a Puesto longitudinal pancreatic jejunostomy.

Medications can cause between 8–25% of episodes of pancreatitis and can include L-asparaginase, valproic acid, and Azathioprine. Liver transplantation has also been identified as a risk factor for pancreatitis.

Metabolic abnormalities can include hypertriglyceridemia, hypercalcemia and cystic fibrosis. Certain variants of the cystic fibrosis transmembrane regulation (CFTR gene) and the trypsinogen gene can cause recurrent pancreatitis and should be evaluated in patients with idiopathic pancreatitis.

PRESENTATION

Pancreatitic pseudocysts can be identified as sequalae of pancreatitis and can occur in association with pancreatitis or immediately after blunt abdominal injuries with ductal disruption. Abdominal pain is the most common symptom, but symptoms related to gastric obstruction due to the location of the cyst with associated vomiting and weight loss can also occur. Pancreatic pseudocysts typically reside in the lesser sac behind the stomach and initially represent a collection of fluid surrounded by inflammatory tissue. Early on in the course, this capsule is very thin and ascites may also be noted if the fluid communicates freely with the abdominal cavity. These cases of severe pancreatitis are often undergoing treatment when a fluid collection is noted in the lesser sac and the collection persists after the pancreatitis has been treated with medical measures.

DIAGNOSTIC STUDIES

Ultrasound and Computed Tomography (CT) scan remains the mainstay for diagnostic studies. Magnetic resonance imaging with MRCP is also sometimes useful. Once the cysts are identified, ultrasound is a less expensive test with no radiation exposure to the child while still allowing good visualization of the size of the cyst, as well as evaluation of the thickness of the cys wallt. ERCP is also often useful in order to determine the status of the pancreatic duct and guide surgical intervention. In addition, ERCP often allows an internal drainage procedure which may relieve the cyst if it communicates freely with the pancreatic duct.

MANAGEMENT

The management of pancreatic pseudocysts remains controversial. In general, conservative medical management is utilized initially since a high percentage of pancreatic cysts will resolve during the first 6 wks of treatment. Children with biliary pancreatitis require relief of the obstruction in the biliary tree to allow the pancreas to recover. In many of these, the pancreatic pseudocyst will resolve with time and medical therapy is indicated along with observation even if the cyst is not causing gastric obstruction. If the pancreatic enzymes come back to normal and the pancreatitis resolves to the point that the child can feed, this can be managed with oral feeds and observation at home and the cyst can be followed by serial ultrasound. In general, no intervention is performed prior to six weeks since a high percentage of these will resolve with time.

If the cyst is of such a size that it is causing symptoms which prevent oral intake, then total parenteral nutrition may be required in order to allow the cyst to mature to the point that an internal drainage procedure can be performed. Internal drainage with transgastric cyst gastrostomy or Roux-en-Y cyst jejunostomy are the most common methods for internal drainage. There have been reports of laparoscopic assisted internal drainage and some of these are also using a transgastric procedure. In general, a stapling device is utilized during the transgastric procedure to create the cyst gastrostomy with creation of an opening in the back of the stomach into the cyst and then utilizing the stapling device to create an anastomosis.

For an open cyst gastrostomy a relatively small opening can remain in the abdominal wall. The anterior wall of the stomach is entered and the posterior wall of the stomach examined. A needle can be placed through the posterior wall into the cyst to confirm its location and then cautery used to enter the cyst. A 6–8 cm length opening is created and over sewn with sutures such as 2/0 PDS. The anterior gastrostomy is then closed. Roux-en-Y cyst jejunostomy is the most widely used internal drainage procedure for a pancreatic pseudocyst and does have the lowest rate of complication and recurrence although does require more extensive procedure.

Percutaneous drainage of the cyst has been utilized in some patients and may be useful if the child is unstable. We have generally only utilized this in patients who are unstable and are in need of emergent drainage. This actual drainage does carry a significant risk of fistula formation and a higher recurrence rate than that of internal drainage. Occasionally very small pseudocysts remain and if these are less than 5 cm continued observation may be reasonable if the child does not have symptoms related to the cyst.

Traumatic Pancreatic Pseudocysts

Traumatic pancreatic pseudocysts are somewhat unique in that the onset of the injury is often clearly known and usually the result of a ductal injury. This has been controversial in terms of the management of fluid collections after blunt pancreatic injuries. One option is to perform an early ERCP in order to identify the presence or absence of a ductal injury and communication to the fluid collection. If this is performed within the first 48 hrs after the injury, consideration may be given to early pancreatic resection with distal pancreatectomy and closure of the pancreatic duct with drainage, thus eliminating the possibility of developing a pseudocyst. Another option has been to utilize supportive therapy only and follow the collection. The collection is then allowed to mature and the patient is maintained on total parenteral nutrition until resolution occurs. Some of these groups have also utilized external drainage however this does carry the risk of fistula formation. In general, the management with early resection has had a shorter length of stay, but does carry the morbidity of a major operation. The management process with medical supportive therapy and total parenteral nutrition results in a longer hospital stay, but avoids surgery in a high percentage of patients.

Octreotide acetate which is a long acting analog of somatostatin has been shown to be successful in reducing exocrine secretions after pancreatic surgery and also shown to be useful in the management of pancreatic pseudocysts. There are no prospective randomized studies in children demonstrating this to be effective, however most institutions have relatively small numbers of pancreatic pseudocysts which are treated and therapy with octreotide is often attempted.

The long term outcome is overall good for children, but does vary somewhat based on the etiology. For traumatic pseudocysts treated with internal drainage is usually definitive therapy. Some patients with the etiology related to metabolic disorder or a pancreas divisum may have ongoing difficulties related to an underlying disorder.

REFERENCES

1. Auringer ST, Ulmer JL, Sumner TE, Turner CS. (1993) Congenital cyst of the pancreas. *J Pediatr Surg* **28**:1570.
2. Cotton PB. (1980) Congenital anomaly of pancreas divisum as cause of obstruction pain and pancreatitis. *Gut* **21**:101.
3. Dubay D, Sandler A, Kimura K, *et al.* (2000) The modified Puestow procedure for complicated hereditary pancreatitis in children. *J Pediatr Surg* **35**:343.
4. Gray SW, Skandalakis JE. (1994) The pancreas. *Embryology for Surgeons.* Williams & Wilkins, Philadelphia.

5. Grosfeld JL, Vane DW, Rescorla FJ, *et al.* (1990) Pancreatic tumors in childhood: Analysis of 13 cases. *J Pediatr Surg* **25**:1057.
6. Hough DM, Stephens DH, Johnson CD, Binkovitz LA, *et al.* (1994) Pancreatic lesions in von Hippel–Lindau disease: Prevalence, clinical significance, and CT findings. *AJR Am J Roentgenol* **162**:1091.

Section 9:
Urologic Considerations

UNDESCENDED TESTIS 74

Ethan I. Franke, Kristan Meldrum and Martin Kaefer

CLINICAL PRESENTATION

The undescended testis (UDT) is noted on physical examination in the neonatal period. It may occur in association with other obvious pathologic entities that contribute to maldescent of the testis (Prune Belly Syndrome, gastroschisis, omphalocele, etc.), but it is usually an isolated physical exam finding. Unilateral UDT is twice as common as bilateral UDT and it occurs more frequently on the right. When UDT is associated with genital ambiguity, or in cases where bilateral UDT is identified, an immediate work-up for a disorder of sexual development must be performed to exclude potentially life threatening congenital adrenal hyperplasia. While untreated UDT may predispose to germ cell dysplasia or germ cell neoplasia with time, it is usually a benign neonatal finding that can be addressed sometime within the first year of life.

Incidence

UDT occurs in around 2.8% of term boys. However, prematurity is associated with a 20–30% incidence of UDT and it is an independent risk factor for bilateral UDT. By the age of 12 mths, the incidence of UDT is only 1% as 50–70% of spontaneous descent occurs in the first 3 mths of life in conjunction with a transient physiologic surge in testosterone.

Embryology

The testes develop adjacent to the mesonephros beginning at 6 wks of gestation. Subsequent descent into the scrotum is dependent on several hormonal and potentially mechanical factors that act on the gubernacular ligament. Insulin-like growth factor three derived from the testes induces gubernacular masculinization and outgrowth at 12 wks. This is followed by development of the processus vaginalis as an extension of peritoneum that grows along the gubernaculum into the inguinal canal and scrotum to create a potential space for later testicular descent. At the start of the third trimester, androgen dependent gubernacular regression begins as the testis migrates transinguinally into the scrotum. Failure of complete gubernacular regression to occur leads to patency of the processus vaginalis and an open internal inguinal ring.

Classification

Undescended testes can be broadly classified as palpable and nonpalpable. Palpable testes are found in 80% of cases of UDT while nonpalpable testes make up the remaining 20%. UDTs can be further characterized based on their location. Palpable UDTs are usually canalicular (within the inguinal canal) or are located just distal to the external inguinal ring. These are distinguished from retractile testes which can be brought down to the scrotum but retract cranially due to an overactive cremasteric reflex. Occasionally, palpable UDTs can be in an ectopic location such as the superficial inguinal pouch, or in a femoral, pubic, penopubic, penile, or perineal location. Nonpalpable testes are intraabdominal or canalicular 50% of the time, while the remainder are absent due to intrauterine torsion or agenesis.

DIAGNOSIS/WORK-UP

History should include gestational age, maternal/paternal exposures, and any family history of endocrine/genetic disorders. A prior history of descent may suggest testicular ascent rather than a missed UDT by prior examiners. Prior surgical history, particular inguinal surgery, may prove relevant for secondary cryptorchidism. Diagnosis of the UDT depends on a well performed and careful physical examination. Pressure over the internal inguinal ring with the nondominant hand while gently sweeping the inguinal canal with the dominant hand may reveal a canalicular testis or one located distal to the external inguinal ring. Palpation may be aided by the use of a lubricant such as soap. When a testis is felt, it can often be noted to glide under the examiners fingers as it retracts proximally back to its natural lie. A testis that can be guided to the scrotum and that stays in place for a brief period of time is more consistent with a retractile testis rather than a true UDT. If no testis is felt, one must remember to examine ectopic locations. Additional exam, particularly in the neonate, should focus on the genitalia as UDT may be associated with genital ambiguity. The combined findings of cryptorchidism and hypospadias often indicate the existence of a disorder of sexual development (approximately 25%). If the cryptorchid testis is nonpalpable this number increases to nearly 50%. In the case of bilateral UDT, in addition to an intersex work-up, one may demonstrate the presence of functional testicular tissue with a müllerian inhibiting substance (MIS) assay or a provocative HCG stimulation test for testosterone. Rarely, ultrasonography or Magnetic Resonance Imaging (MRI) may be useful adjuncts to the physical exam, particularly in obese children. However, neither modality is specific enough to rule out the presence of a testis.

Indications for Treatment

The indications for treatment of UDT relate to the issues of preservation of fertility, prevention of malignancy and torsion, and repair of hernia. Although corrected unilateral UDT may not affect paternity rates, bilateral UDT is a risk factor for decreased fertility. Germ cell changes may be noted after 18 mths of age even in unilateral UDT. The risk of a germ cell tumor in either testis is approximately 3–7 fold higher in men with a history of UDT. Scrotal placement of an UDT will allow for subsequent surveillance. Additionally, most UDTs are associated with an inguinal hernia and they are at a higher risk for torsion. With respect to the timing of intervention, most pediatric urologists will observe an UDT up to the age of 6 mths as the majority of testes that will spontaneously descend will do so in the first 3 mths of life. As germ cell histologic changes will manifest at 18 mths, it is prudent to intervene prior to this time.

MANAGEMENT

Medical Treatment

The dependence of testicular descent on a paracrine effect of testosterone forms the basis of medical therapy. The only FDA approved drug in the US for the treatment of UDT is HCG. This drug is similar to luteinizing hormone (LH) in action and induces testicular production of testosterone. The effects are modest in that it may result in testicular descent in 25% of cases.

Surgical Treatment

An UDT that has not descended by the age of 6 mths should be corrected surgically. Careful examination under anesthesia is required to determine which incision to use (palpable vs. nonpalpable). An UDT may be approached via the groin, the scrotum, or transabdominally. An UDT that is palpable is best approached via a groin incision. However, if it can be brought down to the scrotum on examination, consideration may be given to a scrotal approach. When performing an orchidopexy via a groin incision, care should be taken to preserve the ilioinguinal nerve when opening the external oblique *fascia* as it often runs just deep to this *fascia* along the anterior surface of the spermatic cord. When the testis is identified within the canal or at the external inguinal ring, cremasteric fibers and internal spermatic *fascia* are dissected from the cord structures. Distal gubernacular attachments are then divided as the testis and spermatic cord are elevated. Occasionally, a looping vas is encountered and one must identify this prior to division of the gubernaculum. Length is achieved by dissection of the hernia sac from the spermatic cord structures to the level of the internal inguinal ring. Prior to dissection of the posterior wall of the hernia sac from the cord, it is essential to assess whether the testis will likely reach the scrotum. If it appears that it will not reach, one must consider other maneuvers such as a two-stage Fowler–Stephens orchidopexy with high ligation of the gonadal vessels. Further length may be achieved with division of the lateral spermatic *fascia* and additional retroperitoneal dissection by opening the internal ring. Modest additional length may also be achieved with the Prentiss maneuver whereby the testicle and cord are transposed medial to the inferior epigastric vessels. Ligation of the hernia sac at the internal ring is achieved with a silk suture ligature. A transverse scrotal incision and subdartos scrotal pouch are created. The testis is tunneled to the subdartos pouch and secured with a monofilament suture medially and laterally. Prior to securing the testis, inspection of the cord for torsion must be performed to ensure appropriate positioning of the testis. If physical examination reveals a nonpalpable testis and no scrotal nubbin can be appreciated in the canal or near the scrotum, one may proceed with diagnostic laparoscopy or an open abdominal procedure. If there are no contraindications to laparoscopy, a 5 mm infraumbilical trocar may be placed. Inspection of the internal inguinal ring may reveal the following: (1) Open ring with exiting gonadal vessels and vas (compression over the canal may subsequently reveal a canalicular testis), (2) Closed ring with exiting vas and gonadal vessels (inguinal exploration for a testis or nubbin may be performed but the likelihood of finding a viable testis is small), (3) open ring with looping vas and no identifiable gonadal vessels (search pelvis and paracolic gutter up to the kidney for the testis as there is likely epididymal/testicular dysjunction), (4) atretic gonadal vessels ending blindly at the ring (vanishing testis and no further treatment necessary), (5) dysplastic intraabdominal testis necessitating orchiectomy. Two additional lateral 3 or 5 mm trocars may be placed to allow for completion of laparoscopic orchidopexy or for performing the first stage of a Fowler–Stephens orchidopexy. If a staged procedure is to be performed, an additional 5 mm port (rather than a 3 mm port) is necessary to allow for high ligation of the gonadal vessels with an appropriately sized clip applier. A single stage procedure may be accomplished by mobilizing the gonadal vessels retroperitoneally on a strip of peritoneum. Care should be taken to preserve a triangular strip of peritoneum distally near the convergence of the vas and gonadal vessels as potentially important collateral vessels lie in this area. When an adequate length is achieved, the testicle can be tunneled into a scrotal subdartos pouch. A short and direct route into the scrotum can be achieved by creating the tunnel medial to the epigastric vessels or medial umbilical ligament and lateral to the bladder. Of note, testicular microvascular autotransplantation has been performed with reasonable success but has very limited indications (for example; monorchia with very short gonadal vessels, or an intraabdominal testis with short gonadal vessels and an atretic vas that precludes a Fowler–Stephens orchidopexy).

POSTOP CONSIDERATIONS/COMPLICATIONS

Complications of orchidopexy are rare and relate to testicular atrophy and retraction of the testicle. Additional complications related to repair of the associated hernia and complications of laparoscopy have been reported as well. Follow-up should focus on the importance of screening for testicular cancer as UDTs have at least a 3-fold increased risk of malignancy.

REFERENCES

1. Barthold J, Gonzalez R. (2003) The epidemiology of congenital cryptorchidism, testicular ascent and orchiopexy. *J Urol* **170**:2396–2401.
2. Gearhart JP, Rink RC, Mouriquand PD. (2009) (eds.), *Pediatric Urology*, 2nd edition. Elsevier, Philadelphia.
3. Hinmann F, Baskin L. (2009) (eds.), *Hinman's Atlas of Pediatric Urologic Surgery*, 2nd edition. Elsevier, Philadelphia.

URETEROPELVIC JUNCTION OBSTRUCTION 75

Ethan I. Franke, Kristan Meldrum and Martin Kaefer

CLINICAL PRESENTATION

Most cases of neonatal ureteropelvic junction (UPJ) obstruction are found by ultrasound as this is readily available in the United States during routine obstetrical work-up. Maternal ultrasound detects antenatal hydronephrosis in 0.2–2% of all pregnancies. Of these, almost three-fourth are confirmed postnatally. Of the confirmed cases of hydronephrosis, UPJ obstruction as the etiologic entity occurs in a little over 50% of cases. Prior to the advent of maternal ultrasound, UPJ obstruction was found much later in its course and was manifested by flank pain, nausea, a palpable abdominal mass, nephrolithiasis, infection and hematuria.

Incidence

UPJ obstruction affects 1:1500 children. There is a male to female predominance of 2:1 and it more commonly affects the left side (60%). Although usually a unilateral process, it can occur bilaterally in up to 10–40% of cases.

Embryology

The ureteric bud arises from the mesonephric duct at 5 wks of gestation. At about this time, the ureter undergoes a process of fusion to become a solid cord followed by recanalization beginning from the midureter and extending proximally and distally to the UPJ and ureterovesical junction (UVJ) respectively. Meanwhile, the ureteric bud interacts with the metanephric blastema to induce nephrogenesis that continues until the 36th week of gestation. Several generations of branching of the ureteric bud result in the major and minor calyces, and the collecting ducts. Fetal urine is produced beginning from the 10th week onward. At this point, hydrostatic pressure begins to dilate the renal pelvis until rupture of Chwallas membrane allows passage of urine into the bladder.

Pathology/Classification

Obstruction at the UPJ reflects impaired flow of urine from the UPJ to the proximal ureter. It is characterized by a spectrum of severity in that complete obstruction is rare and variable degrees of partial obstruction exist. Obstruction at the UPJ may occur either intrinsically, extrinsically, or secondarily. Intrinsic obstruction is a result of abnormalities of the ureteral wall, with variable alterations in the proportions/arrangement of smooth muscle and collagen. Extrinsic obstruction usually manifests at an older age and is often the result of crossing accessory lower polar vessels to the kidney. Secondary obstruction may be seen in cases of high grade reflux whereby progressive tortuosity of the proximal ureter causes kinking at the UPJ and resistance to outflow. The effects of obstruction on renal development are complex and appear to be related to timing and duration of obstruction. Dysplasia is the histologic end result which may be characterized by reductions in glomerular number, interstitial fibrosis, tubular atrophy, primitive appearing tubular structures and occasionally metaplasia. In addition to possible dysplasia, effects on fetal nephrogenesis and subsequent postnatal development of the kidney, obstruction has a multitude of other possible effects including those on the physical characteristics of the collecting system, growth regulation, response to injury, and renal tubular functional effects.

Associations

UPJ obstruction may be associated with other anomalies. These include VATER syndrome, imperforate anus, cardiac anomalies, renal fusion anomalies, contralateral multicystic dysplastic kidney, and esophageal atresia.

DIAGNOSIS

The clinically relevant definition of obstruction is one in which the impediment to outflow of urine results in progressive renal impairment. Although this may seem to be a straight-forward and obvious definition, in reality it may be difficult to predict which patients with hydronephrosis will ultimately require surgical intervention. The work-up for UPJ obstruction initially involves a careful physical examination and a number of imaging studies. The possibility of a UPJ obstruction usually arises when the urologist is consulted for prenatal hydronephrosis. Important questions to ask relate to the timing of hydronephrosis *in utero*, changes over time on serial imaging, the severity and laterality (unilateral vs. bilateral), gender of the fetus, and other associated sonographic abnormalities such as oligohydramnios and bladder cycling as these may provide clues as to the etiology of the hydronephrosis. As previously stated, over 50% of cases of prenatal hydronephrosis will be due to UPJ obstruction; however, the possibility of other pathologic entities such as posterior urethral valves (PUV), Prune Belly Syndrome, primary megaureter, cloacal/urogenital (UG) sinus anomalies, the exstrophy-epispadias complex, myelodysplasia, and vesicoureteral reflux may exist. Fetal renal anteroposterior (AP) diameter of >20 mm is considered worrisome and may be predictive of the ultimate need for an operative intervention. Physical examination when the baby is born should look for signs/symptoms of myelodysplasia, lower tract dysfunction, cloacal/UG sinus anomalies, and exstrophy. Imaging studies in the immediate neonatal period include a voiding cystourethrogram (VCUG) and renal/bladder ultrasound. As the neonate is relatively dehydrated in the first 48 hrs of life, one may delay sonographic imaging for the first 3–5 days because an ultrasound performed immediately after birth may underestimate the degree of hydronephrosis. A VCUG is also obtained in the postnatal period to look for reflux or lower tract abnormalities such as a neurogenic bladder, ureterocele, ureteral ectopia, and posterior urethral valves. Additional imaging that may provide excellent anatomic and some functional information includes intravenous pyelogram, Computed Tomography (CT) or Magnetic Resonance (MR) urography. Provocative lasix nuclear renography with an appropriate radioisotope such as MAG3 or DTPA provides information regarding differential renal function and degree of obstruction. The interpretation of a nuclear medicine renal scan can be tricky and is dependent on several factors that may alter the results; nonetheless, a general guide regarding the time for 50% of radiotracer to wash out of the renal pelvis (t1/2) is that a t1/2 of greater than 20 mins after infusion of lasix suggests obstruction. Another useful test, albeit invasive, is the pressure-flow study which measures resistance to flow across the UPJ. One iteration of this study involves the infusion of fluid via a needle that is percutaneously introduced into the renal pelvis or via a nephrostomy tube. The fluid is infused at a constant rate (originally suggested as 10 mL/min by Whitaker, but may be adjusted for patient age and size to approximately 10% of GFR) and the renal pelvic pressure is measured. A renal pelvic pressure of >14 cm water is considered obstructive.

MANAGEMENT

The determination of which patients with UPJ obstruction will benefit from surgical intervention is controversial. With the advent of prenatal ultrasound, significant numbers of infants with asymptomatic hydronephrosis were identified. Initial treatment was aggressive surgical management for a large number of these infants due to concern over the possible detrimental effects on renal function over time. Koff and others in 2000 prospectively analyzed the natural history of unilateral hydronephrosis and showed that even in cases of initially severe hydronephrosis, prolonged t1/2 on diuretic renography, or depressed differential renal function, only 25% of infants ultimately required surgery with close follow-up within the first 2 yrs of life. A reasonable approach in light of these data is that closely monitored serial imaging be performed in all infants with suspected UPJ obstruction. The decision to proceed with surgery should be based on changes that occur over time rather than based on the results of a single test. In particular, declining renal function, worsening hydronephrosis, and occasionally the development of the signs and symptoms of urinary obstruction/infection should be viewed as potential indicators that an operative intervention is beneficial.

Surgical Treatment

The correction of UPJ obstruction can be performed by open surgery or endoscopically. Endoscopic approaches have limited use in the treatment of UPJ obstruction in children due to low efficacy and size limitations; these are usually reserved for revision of a failed pyeloplasty. Such approaches can be performed in an antegrade or retrograde fashion and employ the use of balloons, laser, and the hot or cold knife. The most definitive repair of the obstructed UPJ is open pyeloplasty. Before performing pyeloplasty, we routinely perform retrograde pyelography to confirm our diagnosis and to better elucidate the anatomy for surgical planning. Multiple approaches are available to the urologic surgeon for pyeloplasty. The dorsal lumbotomy is a posterior retroperitoneal approach that is primarily used in infants. An incision off the tip of the 12th rib (lateral flank approach) provides excellent extraperitoneal exposure to the dilated renal pelvis. Some authors prefer an anterior extraperitoneal subcostal approach. Minimally invasive approaches with pure laparoscopy or robot assisted laparoscopy may be applicable in older children of the appropriate size. In contrast to open surgery, the minimally invasive approaches are usually performed transperitoneally although a retroperitoneal approach has also been described. Exposure of the renal pelvis can be obtained by colonic reflection or transmesenterically in the appropriate cases (minimal mesenteric fat, easy visualization of mesenteric vessels). Regardless of the approach to the renal pelvis, the steps involved in performing a successful pyeloplasty are the same. These are adequate exposure (often with minimal renal mobilization required), careful identification of aberrant lower pole vessels with anterior transposition of the repair over the vessels, wide spatulation of the proximal ureter to an area of normal caliber, pelvic reduction when appropriate and a funnel shaped, dependently positioned, watertight and tension free anastomosis. Most UPJ repairs can be performed with a dismembered pyeloplasty. This involves transection of the ureter from the renal pelvis. Care is taken to ensure that there is enough ureteral length to allow for a tension free anastomosis. If excessive tension is identified, a renal pelvic flap may be necessary. After ureteral transection at the UPJ, spatulation along the lateral aspect of the proximal ureter to a point of normal caliber is performed. Pelvic reduction is performed with the caudal/lateral extent of the reduction at the most dependent position to allow for a dependent anastomosis. Care must be taken while excising excess pelvis not to enter the infundibula as this may lead to infundibular stenosis. The anastomosis is performed with a 6-0 or 7-0 monofilament absorbable suture (for example, polyglyconate or polydioxanone). We recommend careful placement of interrupted apical sutures followed by a running anastomosis as the apical sutures are critical in creating a widely patent anastomosis. Prior to completion of the anastomosis, a urinary drain may be placed. Multiple options have been described including the option to not leave a drainage catheter. At our institution, we routinely use most forms of previously described urinary drainage; nephrostomy tube, KISS (nephroureteral) stent, and the internalized double-J stent. Each has its own set of advantages and disadvantages and the choice is left to the discretion of the surgeon. Additionally, some form of retroperitoneal drainage may be used. As with urinary drainage, this is left to surgeon preference and is based on individual experience and the complexity of the pyeloplasty.

POSTOPERATIVE CONSIDERATIONS

The majority of patients stay in the hospital for 2–3 days after pyeloplasty. Many variations of the postoperative management of drains, urinary tubes, and antibiotics exist and the exact regimen will depend on the perceived technical outcome of the pyeloplasty, the types of drains and urinary tubes left in place, and surgeon preference. However, most surgeons will continue with treatment and prophylactic doses of antibiotics, and maintenance of bladder drainage for 24–48 hrs. Retroperitoneal drains may be removed prior to discharge from the hospital if no urinary leak is suspected. Urinary drains are usually left in place for at least 10 days. The assessment of surgical success is not standardized. However, repeat ultrasonography and nuclear renography are often employed. Success rates of greater than 95% using nuclear renography has been reported. Regarding the use of sonography, it has been noted that it may take at least 2 yrs for the degree of hydronephrosis to improve even in successfully performed pyeloplasty.

REFERENCES

1. Gearhart JP, Rink RC, Mouriquand PD. (2009) (eds.), *Pediatric Urology*, 2nd edition. Philadelphia, Elsevier.
2. Hinmann F, Baskin L. (2009) (eds.), *Hinman's Atlas of Pediatric Urologic Surgery*, 2nd edition. Philadelphia, Elsevier.
3. Ulman I, Jayanthi V, Koff S. (2000) The long-term followup of newborns with severe unilateral hydronephrosis initially treated nonoperatively. *J Urol* **164**:1101–1105.

VESICOURETERAL REFLUX 76

Brian A. VanderBrink, Martin Kaefer and Kirstan Meldrum

CLINICAL PRESENTATION

Vesicoureteral reflux (VUR) is typically diagnosed following urinary tract infection (UTI). VUR may also be identified during the postnatal radiographic evaluation of antenatally detected hydronephrosis. In these cases the VUR may be detected prior to any clinical symptoms. End stage renal disease secondary to VUR is an extremely uncommon mode of presentation, however significant loss of renal function as a result of repeated episodes of pyelonephritis can occur.

PATHOPHYSIOLOGY

Incidence

The prevalence of VUR in normal children has been estimated to be approximately 1–2%. There does not appear to be gender predominance, although females are detected more often due to the fact that females are more likely to develop UTIs as children. The likelihood of detecting VUR is dependent on the mode of presentation. VUR will exist in up to 40% of patients who undergo a voiding cystourethrogram (VCUG) after suffering a febrile UTI. In contrast, when antenatal hydronephrosis leads to radiographic investigation, only 5% to 15% of patients will be found to have VUR. The severity of the hydronephrosis is an unreliable predictor for the presence or absence of VUR. Up to 50% of siblings and offspring of known individuals with VUR will have VUR.

Pathology

The normal anatomic configuration of the ureter at its entrance into the bladder results in an oblique angle that lengthens its intramural course. This results in a "flap-valve" mechanism whereby increased filling of the bladder results in hydrostatic pressure along the intramural course, compressing the ureter and thus preventing retrograde passage of urine from the bladder to the kidney. The etiology of primary VUR is due to a shorter, more lateral, intramural course of the ureter as it enters the bladder, resulting in an ineffective anti-reflux mechanism. Secondary VUR can be due to bladder outlet obstruction, dysfunctional elimination syndrome or neuropathic conditions which result in higher than normal bladder pressures that can overcome the antireflux mechanism.

Associations

Complete ureteral duplication occurs in approximately 1% of the population. The ureter that drains the lower pole renal moiety is located more lateral than the ureter draining the upper pole. This can predispose the lower pole ureter to reflux. Children with anorectal malformations demonstrate an increased incidence of VUR (15–30%) with higher incidence observed with more severe anomalies (i.e. persistent cloaca, high vs. low imperforate anus). High grade VUR can result in ureteral tortuosity that can result in a kinking at the level of the ureteropelvic junction. This kinking may produce a secondary ureteropelvic junction obstruction with deleterious effects on renal function. This situation may warrant surgical treatment of the proximal obstruction at a higher priority than the VUR, which created it.

DIAGNOSIS

VCUG with fluoroscopy remains the gold standard for the diagnosis of VUR because of its ability to provide high resolution images to allow for categorizing the severity of reflux detected. VUR observed with fluoroscopy is graded according to the International Reflux Classification.

(1) Grade I — reflux into ureter alone
(2) Grade II — reflux into ureter and renal pelvis without distortion of the calyces
(3) Grade III — reflux into ureter and renal pelvis with mild distention of the renal pelvis & calyces
(4) Grade IV — reflux into ureter and renal pelvis with moderate distention of the renal pelvis, calyces and tortuosity of the ureter
(5) Grade V — reflux into ureter and renal pelvis with severe distention of the renal pelvis, calyces, and tortuosity of the ureter

Inspection of the bladder contour (smooth vs. trabeculated), presence of diverticula, and urethral outline (presence of urethral valve or stricture) may raise the clinical suspicion of secondary rather than primary VUR. Radionucleotide cystography, which has the benefits of increased sensitivity and less radiation exposure than fluoroscopy, provides less anatomic detail than standard VCUG. Although this makes it suboptimal for initial diagnosis, it is an excellent modality for subsequent follow up of a previously documented case of VUR. It is advisable to obtain the VCUG after the patient has defervesced and negative urine culture can be documented in order to minimize infectious complications.

MANAGEMENT

Medical Management

Conservative management is the preferred approach in the overwhelming majority of patients upon diagnosis. Spontaneous resolution of VUR can occur as the patient grows older and is attributed to the lengthening of ureterovesical junction in concert with maturation of voiding bladder dynamics. It is important to determine several clinicopathologic factors, as this will impact the prognosis for spontaneous resolution of VUR. A recently published study evaluated over 2,400 children with primary VUR to determine which factors influenced annual resolution rate. They reported the following findings: (1) Age — Patients <1 yr at presentation with VUR resolved more often than older patients, (2) Gender/Laterality — Males with bilateral VUR resolved faster than females with bilateral VUR, (3) Mode of presentation — Reflux identified on postnatal evaluation for prenatal hydronephrosis or sibling screening resolved more frequently than patients whose VUR was diagnosed for UTI, (4) Ureteral anatomy — Single ureters with VUR resolved more frequently than duplicated ureters.

The importance of aggressive treatment of voiding dysfunction and constipation should not be underestimated. Resolution rates increase dramatically by identifying these known factors which can lead to persistence and even failure of treatment. Secondary VUR may be a result of underlying bladder destrusor abnormalities from outlet obstruction or spinal cord pathology. Recognizing and addressing these factors is essential for optimizing therapy. Reevaluation is usually undertaken at 12–18 mth intervals to determine if reflux has resolved. Once, daily antibiotic prophylaxis is typically administered to minimize the risk of UTI during this period of observation. This practice is based on the notion that sterile reflux has not been demonstrated to have deleterious effects to the kidneys while in contrast, urine that refluxes with bacterial colonization resulted in propensity to form renal scars. Antibiotic prophylaxis in the neonate is typically begun with amoxicillin 20 mg/kg. Once hepatic metabolism matures (i.e. 2–3 mths of age) the antibiotic of choice becomes sulfamethoxazole-trimethoprim. Nitrofurantoin is another acceptable alternative in the sulfa-allergic patient. Like any medication, compliance, side effects and complications should be monitored. Sulfonamides can be associated with gastrointestinal upset, skin reactions, and rare instances of leucopenia. Nitrofurantoin has on very rare occasion been associated with pulmonary fibrosis with chronic administration.

Recent prospective, randomized placebo controlled trials are beginning to question the traditional practice pattern of universal antibiotic prophylaxis in patients with all grades of VUR. Rates of febrile UTIs in patients with low grade VUR (grades I–III) comparing placebo and antibiotic have not been significantly different. There have been limitations to and criticisms of these studies (i.e. length of follow-up, assessment of UTI by bagged vs. catheterized specimens), however they provide Level I evidence which brings into question the effectiveness of medical treatment for low grade VUR.

Surgical Management

Certain patients may not be ideal candidates for medical management upon initial diagnosis because of the low likelihood of spontaneous resolution (i.e. high grade bilateral VUR in an 8 yr old with evidence of renal scarring). However more commonly encountered surgical indications for the treatment of VUR are: noncompliance with antibiotic therapy, breakthrough

UTI while on antibiotic therapy and progressive renal scarring or loss of function while on antibiotic therapy.

The surgical approach can be divided into two techniques: endoscopic subureteric injection vs. open or minimally invasive ureteral reimplantation. Endoscopic therapy is based on the concept that injection of a bulking agent into the subureteric space results in adequate coaptation of the ureteral orifice during bladder filling and contraction, thereby preventing the reflux of urine to the upper urinary tract. The benefits of endoscopic therapy include that it is minimally invasive, avoids the morbidity of open surgical incision and can thus be performed on and outpatient basis. Success rates of 65–90% have been reported. Factors predictive of lower success rates include higher grades of reflux, ureteral duplication and neuropathic bladder dysfunction.

Ureteral reimplantation is based on creation of submucosal tunnel that is of adequate length (ideally five times the diameter of the ureteral lumen) to provide an effective antireflux mechanism. This can be achieved by an extravesical technique (i.e. Lich–Gregoir) or intravesically by creating a neohiatus for the ureter (i.e. cross-trigonal reimplantation). Open surgical approach or minimally invasive methods (i.e. laparoscopic or robot-assisted laparoscopic) can be employed to implement both reimplantation techniques. Ureteral reimplantation is successful in 95–99% of cases regardless of VUR severity and has the added benefit of addressing other anomalies at the time of surgery (e.g. ureterocelectomy, excision of bladder diverticulum, bladder neck reconstruction). The disadvantages of ureteral reimplantation include the morbidity of an open surgical incision and the resultant hematuria and bladder spasms that can occur if the bladder is opened.

The significantly dilated refluxing ureter, or megaureter, may need to be tailored to decrease the luminal dimension prior to reimplantation. This can be accomplished by either careful excisional tapering or plication of the distal ureter.

POSTOPERATIVE CONSIDERATIONS

Management

Bladder drainage is helpful in the first 24 hrs, especially if an intravesical or ureteral tapering approach has been utilized. Anticholinergic medications such as oxybutinin assist in minimizing the morbidity of detrusor spasm. It is important to avoid rectal distention from constipation which can exacerbate bladder spasms. Antibiotics should be used to minimize infectious complications following reimplantation and once daily prophylaxis is routinely continued until radiographic follow-up is obtained. Renal ultrasound should be obtained 1 mth postoperatively to asses for hydronephrosis, which if present may indicate distal ureteral obstruction. Given the high success rates of ureteral reimplantation many surgeons may omit a postoperative VCUG to document reflux cessation. If recurrent UTIs arise following an antireflux procedure, a VCUG is generally obtained to assess reflux status.

Complications

It has been reported that persistent VUR following ureteral reimplantation can exist in between 0–5% of patients. A recent meta-analysis of endoscopic therapy for VUR revealed persistent VUR after a single treatment regardless of agent used or grade was 33%. Failure to recognize secondary VUR (e.g. due to bladder dysfunction) is the usual reason for unsuccessful outcome and must be addressed prior to redo surgery. Ureteral obstruction is extremely rare following endoscopic injection but has been described in approximately 1% of ureteral reimplantion series. Abdominal/flank pain, nausea and vomiting are the common signs and symptoms of obstruction. This obstruction is normally transient as a result of the edema from the surgical dissection.

However, obstruction can also result from ureteral kinking, torsion, or ischemia. Persistent symptoms may require ureteral stenting to alleviate the obstruction. Urine leak following standard ureteral reimplantion is exceedingly rare. If extensive ureteral tailoring has been performed a Penrose drain is often left to monitor for the occasional urine leak. Ureteral stent placement may be necessary if leakage persists. Most all leaks will resolve with appropriate drainage procedures.

REFERENCES

1. Estrada CR, *et al.* (2009) Nomograms for predicting annual resolution rate of primary vesicoureteral reflux: Results from 2,462 children. *J Urol* **182**:1535–1541.
2. Hodson EM, *et al.* (2007) Interventions for primary vesicoureteric reflux. *Cochrane Database Syst Rev.*

3. Weiss R, *et al.* (1992) Results of a randomized clinical trial of medical versus surgical management of infants and children with grades III and IV primary vesicoureteral reflux (United States). The International Reflux Study in Children. *J Urol* **148**:1667–1673.
4. Elder JS, *et al.* (2006) Endoscopic therapy for vesicoureteral reflux: A meta-analysis. I. Reflux resolution and urinary tract infection. *J Urol* **175**:716–722.

DISORDERS OF SEXUAL DEVELOPMENT 77

Brian A. VanderBrink, Martin Kaefer and Kirstan Meldrum

CLINICAL PRESENTATION

Disorders of sexual development (DSD) are defined as conditions showing disagreement with chromosomal, gonadal, and phenotypic sex. They were previously referred to as intersex disorders. DSDs are usually identified on newborn physical examination in the delivery room and the genital abnormalities encountered can be quite apparent leading to early recognition. However, a DSD may only become apparent later in life during investigations for primary amenorrhea or infertility. In congenital adrenal hyperplasia (CAH), adrenal crisis may be the initial presentation with vomiting, hypotension, tachycardia, hyponatremia and hyperkalemia.

PATHOPHYSIOLOGY

Normal Embryology

Prior to discussing abnormal development, a brief discussion of normal sexual development is warranted. All developing embryos, regardless of karyotype have indifferent gonads at one point. The *SRY* gene which is normally found on the Y sex chromosome contains the genetic material for testicular organogenesis and subsequent male genital development. The absence of *SRY* gene and its products allows for the normal development of ovaries.

Paired ductal structures (Müllerian and Wolfian) represent internal genital structures and are adjacent to the indifferent gonad. These ducts either develop or regress depending upon the hormonal milieu produced by the ipsilateral gonad and its paracrine effects. Testosterone and Müllerian-inhibiting substance are both products of testicular tissue and influence Wolfian ductal structure development and Müllerian ductal structures regression, respectively. In contrast, ovarian tissue does not produce significant amounts of testosterone. As a result, Wolfian ductal structures such as vas deferens and epididymis regress in the female. The absence of Müllerian-inhibiting substance results in the persistence and development of Müllerian ductal structures such as fallopian tubes and uterus.

External genitalia masculinization is also a testosterone dependent process with a particular form, dihydrotestosterone, playing a more significant role. Transformation of the indifferent genital tubercle and labioscrotal folds into a penis and scrotum are the principal steps of male external genitalia virilization. In the absence of androgen, development of female genital structures such as labia majora, and labia minora distal third of the vagina and introitus proceeds.

Abnormal Development

As with most developmental disorders, a spectrum of abnormalities may be encountered. The phenotype observed is dependent upon what point in the sequence of normal development the defect arises. Obviously an abnormality in gonadogenesis is one way genital development can be affected, however alternate etiologies of DSD occur from enzymatic or receptor defects even in presence of normal gonadogenesis.

DIAGNOSIS

History

A thorough prenatal and family history can be helpful in determining which DSD may be present. Maternal exposure of androgens during pregnancy can virilize the fetal genitalia in the genetic female. Prenatal ultrasonographic findings may or may not be in concordance with physical exam findings. Amniocentesis can alert the physician as to discrepancies between karyotype and phenotype. A family history of sudden infant death might suggest the possibility of CAH, while infertility and amenorrhea suggest potential familial patterns of DSD.

Examination Findings

DSD is recognized in infancy typically as a result of ambiguous genitalia. The spectrum of abnormalities encountered can be quite dramatic. For example, a female with a persistent cloaca will have a single perineal orifice providing the only outlet from the urinary, gastrointestinal and genital systems. In contrast the most severely virilized genetic female with CAH, may have external genitalia that appear as a completely formed penis, scrotum and penile urethra. In such instances, bilateral undescended testicles are the only "abnormality" identified on initial examination leading to further investigation. Yet still another condition, Mayer–Rokatansky–Kuster–Hauser syndrome (MRKH), results in completely normal female external genitalia, however the absence of proximal vagina and uterus can easily elude neonatal detection until primary amenorrhea occurs as an adolescent leading to initial diagnosis.

For genetic males with DSD, the undervirilized genitalia are usually recognized as abnormal. The penile urethra may be underdeveloped resulting in hypospadias that varies in severity; ranging from a distal position of urethral meatus to more proximal (i.e. penoscrotal or perineal) in its location. The phallus itself may be diminutive in size relative to children without DSD. The scrotum may be hypoplastic or bifid in appearance. A critical finding on physical examination is the presence of one or two gonads. Because ovaries do not descend, a distinctly palpable gonad along the pathway of descent is highly suggestive of a testis.

One specific combination of physical findings merits special consideration. The patient with an undescended testis (or testes) and hypospadias should be regarded as having DSD until proven otherwise, whether or not the genitalia appear ambiguous. One study reported the incidence of DSD in patients with cryptorchidism, hypospadias and otherwise nonambiguous genitalia. With a unilateral cryptorchid testis, the incidence of DSD was 30% overall,15% if the undescended testis was palpable and 50% if it was impalpable. In the setting of bilateral undescended testes and hypospadias, the incidence of DSD was quite similar — 32% overall, 16% if both gonads were palpable and 47% if either one or both were impalpable. In addition, a more proximal meatal position was noted to be a strong predictor of DSD in this group of patients — 65%, vs. 5% to 8% with a midshaft or distally located hypospadiac meatus.

Laboratory Studies

In almost all cases of DSD with associated ambiguous genital findings, obtaining a karyotype is the essential first step to avoid potentially catastrophic diagnostic errors. Basic electrolytes demonstrating hyponatremia and hyperkalemia are highly suggestive of adrenal insufficiency. Specific hormone assays that can assist in creating a working diagnosis are testosterone, dihydrotestosterone, Müllerian-inhibiting substance, and 17-Hydroxyprogesterone. An human chorionic gonadotropin (hCG) stimulation test is a dynamic test that can demonstrate normally functioning testicular tissue. In addition to ruling out anorchia, the study can enable diagnosis of 5α-reductase deficiency (by virtue of an increased ratio of testosterone to dihydrotestosterone) and can help distinguish between impaired testosterone synthesis (deficient response to hCG) and androgen insensitivity (normal response to hCG). Müllerian-inhibiting substance is reliable marker of the presence of testes but is not readily available. 17-Hydroxyprogesterone is markedly elevated in patients with CAH as a result of enzymatic deficiencies in cortisol production and an accumulation of this substrate precursor.

Imaging Studies

Imaging studies can be important adjuncts to physical examination findings and metabolic evaluation. Ultrasound of the pelvis can assist in identifying Müllerian structures in the suspected female with virilized genitalia, while imaging the abdomen can obtain important information about bladder and kidneys. Genitography is another imaging modality that can delineate internal genital anatomy by method of instilling contrast into perineal orifice.

CONDITIONS

Disorders of Gonadal Differentiation

Klinefelter's syndrome (XXY)

This is a syndrome characterized by eunuchoidism, gynecomastia, increased gonadotropin levels, and small, firm testes. Secondary sexual characteristics do not develop normally because of decreased androgen production. The gynecomastia typically manifests during puberty and can be marked. There is an increased risk of breast carcinoma, testicular and extragonadal germ cell tumors in these patients.

46 XX male

The result of *SRY* gene translocation from Y chromosome to X chromosome. Phenotypically these patients resemble Klinefelter's Syndrome except they are shorter. Unfortunately almost all patients are infertile.

Gonadal Dysgenesis

Turners syndrome 46 XO

This is characterized by the presence of only one functioning X sex chromosome. The other sex chromosome may be absent or abnormal, or mosaicism may be present. Mosaicism, the presence of two or more chromosomally different cell lines, occurs in 30% to 40% of these patients, the majority (10% to 15%) being 45,X/46,XX and 2% to 5% being 45,X/46,XY. Classic features of 45 XO karyotype are: female phenotype, short stature, lack of secondary sexual characteristics, and a variety of somatic abnormalities. Diagnosis may be made at birth due to lymphedema and webbed neck, however, amenorrhea with short stature is another common presentation. Renal anomalies, such as horseshoe kidneys are present in 33–60% of affected patients. Spontaneous fertility is rare, however advances in treatment of infertility has made pregnancies in affected females a possibility.

Identification of the mosaic patient with an associated Y sex chromosome is critical because the risk of gonadoblastoma, an *in situ* germ cell malignancy, is 7–30%. Therefore, prophylatic excision of the streak gonads in the Y mosaic Turner's patient is advised while the. streak gonads confirmed to be in 45,XO patients need not be removed.

Pure gonadal dysgenesis 46 XX & 46 XY

46 XX patients are closely related to Turner's syndrome however lack the associated somatic signs. Bilateral streak gonads result in elevated

gonadotropins with normal external genitalia. Presentation is usually in adolescence for primary amenorrhea. Treatment in 46 XY patients mandates bilateral gonadectomy because of associated increase risk of germ cell tumor, while in contrast 46 XX do not require gonadectomy as a result of the absence of Y chromosome.

Mixed gonadal dysgenesis

Mixed gonadal dysgenesis (MGD) is characterized by a unilateral testis, a contralateral streak gonad, and persistent müllerian structures associated with varying degrees of inadequate masculinization. Most patients with MGD have a 45,XO/46,XY karyotype. However, it should be kept in mind that there is a wide phenotypic spectrum of patients with XO/XY mosaicism identified prenatally by amniocentesis. Ninety percent of prenatally diagnosed cases will have a normal male phenotype with the remaining ten percent demonstrating some form of genital ambiguity.

In the newborn period, MGD is the second most common cause of ambiguous genitalia (after CAH). The majority of these patients present with varying degrees of phallic enlargement, hypospadias, a urogenital sinus with labioscrotal fusion, and an undescended testis. As in Turner's syndrome, children with Y sex chromosome have increased risk of gonadal tumor. All patients are also at increased risk of Wilm's tumors. Management involves gender assignment and genital reconstruction, appropriate gonadectomy and screening for Wilm's tumors. The potential for normal function of the external genitalia and gonads should guide gender assignment. If the male gender is elected and the testes can be brought to the scrotum, the decision between careful screening for gonadoblastoma vs. prophylactic gonadectomy and androgen replacement must be made.

True hermaphrodite

These are individuals in whom well differentiated ovarian and testicular tissue are both present. Differentiation of external genitalia is variable in true hermaphroditism with hypospadias and phallic enlargement common findings. Differentiation of the internal ducts is also quite variable and is related to the function of the ipsilateral gonad. The most important aspect of management in true hermaphroditism is gender assignment. Sex assignment should be based on the functional potential of external genitalia, internal ducts, and gonads. Unlike patients with most other forms of gonadal dysgenesis, true hermaphrodites have the potential for fertility if raised as female with the appropriate ductal structures. Surveillance of germ cell tumors is essential in all patients however a higher incidence occurs in those with 46 XY.

Masculinized Female — 46, XX DSD

Congenital adrenal hyperplasia

This is the most common cause for ambiguous genitalia in the newborn. This condition results from an enzymatic defect in cortisol production. There are three described deficiencies, but 21-hydroxylase is the most common. Absence of this enzyme results in inability to produce cortisol and aldosterone. These steroids are important in maintaining normal homeostasis with respect to water and salt balance and low levels explain the hemodynamic instability and salt-losing clinical features of these patients. Substrates of cortisol and aldosterone accumulate in the adrenal gland and are shunted towards androgen production. Lack of negative feedback due to deficient cortisol results in increased adrenocorticotropic hormone (ACTH) and further stimulation of the adrenal gland leading to more androgen production. This excess of androgens results in virilzation of the female external genitalia that is typified by clitoromegaly, fusion of labia and persistence of the urogenital sinus.

Females are usually identified in the newborn period, however, more subtle forms lead to diagnosis later in life as a result of amenorrhea or short stature from excess androgen. Males have no ambiguous genitalia and adrenal crisis is the most common neonatal presentation. Fortunately newborn blood screening has detected children with no physical examination findings and decreasing their risk of misdiagnosis. Treatment involves adequate cortisol with or without mineralocorticoid replacement. Genitoplasty, with clitoroplasty, vaginoplasty and labioplasty, can be performed in first months of life in the severely virilized child.

Undermasculinized Male — 46, XY DSD

Disorders of testosterone production

These occur due to rare autosomal recessive conditions. Three of the five enzymes necessary to convert cholesterol to testosterone reside in the adrenal gland and testes. Deficiencies in mineralocorticoid and glucocorticoid can also occur in certain situations.

Disorders of testosterone receptor (androgen insensitivity)

Patients who have decreased organ responsiveness to testosterone can vary in appearance depending on whether the resistance is partial or complete. Patients with complete androgen insensitivity syndrome (CAIS) have normal appearing female external genitalia. Patients are diagnosed either at the time of hernia repair when testicles are identified during surgical procedure or while being investigated later in life for primary amenorrhea. Management of CAIS relates primarily to the optimal timing of gonadectomy given the malignant potential of undescended testes. However because the testes produce estrogen, which results in the appropriate changes for the female phenotype, it is considered by many preferable to leave the testes *in situ* until puberty is complete.

Partial androgen insensitivity syndrome (PAIS) management varies depending on the degree of genital ambiguity. In patients assigned a female gender, gonadectomy and surgical reconstruction of the external genitalia are indicated with hormonal supplementation provided at puberty. Those individuals raised as males would require treatment of their cryptorchidism, reduction of gynecomastia, and genital reconstruction.

Disorders of testosterone metabolism (5α-reductase deficiency)

Individuals present with phenotype that may vary from penoscrotal hypospadias to, more commonly, markedly ambiguous genitalia. Typically, the phallus is quite small, appearing as a normal or enlarged clitoris. A urogenital sinus is present, with separate vaginal and urethral openings and labioscrotal fusion. Remarkably at puberty, partial masculinization occurs with an increase in muscle mass, development of male body habitus, increase in phallic size, and onset of erections as testosterone production increases. This accounts for the "female-to-male" transformation in adolescence associated with this condition. Testes are present and fertility is possible.

Disorders of synthesis, secretion or response to müllerian-inhibiting substance

These are phenotypically normal males. The diagnosis is often incidentally at time of orchiopexy. Wolfian structures such as vas deferens can be in close association with Müllerian structures. Preservation of the necessary Müllerian structures to avoid injury to the vasa at the time of orchiopexy is recommended to preserve fertility.

MANAGEMENT

The neonate with ambiguous genitalia represents a sensitive and emotionally charged clinical situation. An interdisciplinary team approach (typically comprised of a geneticist, endocrinologist, urologist, social worker and neonatologist.) to the care of the child and family has proven helpful in most institutions. Discussions with the family should be clear about the results obtained from imaging studies and blood tests. It can be challenging at times to refrain from using gender pronouns such as "he" or "she" during conversation with the caregivers. However, efforts to avoid such terms can minimize the potential of unintentional confusion of the family during the investigative process.

Given the potential for serious hormone deficiencies in the child with DSD, insuring the medical stability of the child is a chief concern for the physician. Close monitoring of vital signs, urine output and electrolytes should alert the clinician to the possibility of adrenal insufficiency in the salt wasting CAH child. Once again a karyotype should be sent in nearly all cases with ambiguous genitalia. Hormonal assays can be useful and some caveats exist in their interpretation in the immediate neonatal period. 17-hydroxyprogesterone can be elevated secondary to the stress of delivery and some have advocated waiting 3–4 days before sampling. Imaging tests can be performed to add additional important information while constructing a working diagnosis and awaiting blood test results.

Once a diagnosis has been made, family should be informed about reproductive potential. Females with CAH are potentially fertile given the normal internal anatomy. Some males with chromosomal abnormalities will not be able to father children with current assisted reproductive technologies. Retaining gonadal tissue for possible future fertility will need to be balanced with risk of malignancies associated with specific diagnosis.

Parents of children with an increased risk of gonadal tumors must be informed of the need for lifelong surveillance if they choose to decline gonadectomy at an early age. Sexual function and gender identity can be hard to predict based upon neonatal physical examination. As a result, controversy still remains as to the optimal timing for surgical intervention in some of these conditions.

REFERENCES

1. Diamond D. (2007) Sexual differentiation: Normal and abnormal. In: AJ Wein, *et al.* (eds.), *Campbell–Walsh Urology*, 9th edition, pp. 3799–3829. Elsevier.
2. Woodhouse CR. (1994) The sexual and reproductive consequences of congenital genitourinary anomalies. *J Urol* **152**:645–651.
3. Kaefer M, *et al.* (1999) The incidence of intersexuality in children with cryptorchidism and hypospadias: stratification based on gonadal palpability and meatal position. *J Urol* **162**:1003–1006.

VARICOCELE 78

Rahul D. Mehan, Kirstan K. Meldrum and Martin K. Kaefer

CLINICAL PRESENTATION

Most varicoceles are asymptomatic. They typically present as a scrotal swelling discovered by the patient or during routine physical examination. On occasion varicoceles can be painful. In this rare instance, patients can complain of a dull, nagging ache in the scrotum that is often relieved in the supine position.

PATHOPHYSIOLOGY

Incidence

It is believed that testicular enlargement during puberty, with its associated increased blood flow, leads to the formation of most varicoceles. Therefore, varicoceles rarely become clinically evident prior to adolescence. Varicoceles may be identified in as many as 16% of adolescents.

Anatomy

A varicocele is a dilation of the pampiniform plexus and internal spermatic venous system of the scrotum. There are three main blood supplies to the testis: the internal spermatic artery and vein, the vasal artery and vein, and the cremasteric artery and vein. At the testicular level, there is free communication between the arteries as well as between the veins that form the pampiniform plexus.

There is a substantial left-sided predominance of varicoceles (90%). This is likely due to differences of retrograde blood flow from alternate configuration of the right and left internal spermatic veins. Varicocele formation is thought to be due to one of three factors: increased venous pressure in the left renal vein, collateral venous anastomoses, and incompetent valves of the internal spermatic vein.

Classification

Grade 0 (subclinical)
Not visible or palpable; identified only by ultrasound
Grade I
Not visible; palpable in upright position with Valsalva only
Grade II
Not visible; palpable in upright position without Valsalva
Grade III
Visualized and palpable without Valsalva.

Pathology

The main concern with a varicocele is the deleterious effect on spermatogenesis. This effect is felt to arise from several mechanisms including hyperthermia, hypoxia, local testicular hormonal imbalance, and intratesticular hyperperfusion injury. A testis initially determined to be equal in size to the contralateral gonad may sometimes demonstrate progressive growth arrest with time. Furthermore, as puberty progresses, varicoceles may increase significantly in site. In the adult population, the correlation between varicoceles and infertility is well documented. Semen samples from infertile men with varicoceles have demonstrated sperm concentrations less than 20 million sperm/mL in 65% of patients and decreased motility in 90% of patients.

DIAGNOSIS

A diagnosis of a varicocele starts with physical examination. The classic description of a varicocele is the consistency of a "bag of worms". First, it is important that the patient is examined in an upright standing position. When the patient is supine, the dilated veins will collapse which make the diagnosis difficult. Second, a Valsalva maneuver should be elicited which helps transmit increased abdominal pressure to the dilated veins of the scrotum.

When a varicocele is detected, it is important to note the testis volume and consistency. Orchidometry or ultrasonography may be used to more precisely define differences in size. Prader's orchodometry utilizes 12 numbered beads of increasing size to best approximate volume. Testis volume should be compared with measurements in normal boys and also for differences between the patient's own two testicles. Reports show that a volume difference greater than 20% should be regarded as significant and abnormal.

If the varicocele is not appreciated on exam, one may consider Doppler ultrasonography. The indications for imaging include any suspicion about the diagnosis when the varicocele is difficult to feel. Doppler ultrasonography is useful to detect retrograde venous reflux with a Valsalva maneuver. If a patient is found with an unexplained small testis, ultrasound maybe used to diagnose a subclinical varicocele. It has been shown that even small varicoceles may be associated with subfertility later in life.

SURGICAL MANAGEMENT

When varicocele ablation is determined to be appropriate, several therapeutic options are available. All of these techniques have been proven to be effective; however, choice of modality depends largely on individual surgeon experience/comfort and characteristics of the patient. There are relative advantages and disadvantages of each technique. The various procedures are briefly outlined in the following.

Open Repairs

Open transinguinal repair is performed through a standard inguinal incision. The inguinal canal is opened, the spermatic cord is isolated and the varicosities are ligated. Doppler ultrasound is utilized to help appreciate and avoid injury to the testicular artery. It is important to protect the vas deferens and its vessels as these will become the main source for venous return. Care should be given to preserve lymphatic vessels in order to prevent hydrocele formation.

A subinguinal approach involves an incision below the inguinal ring at the level of the pubic tubercle. This approach avoids opening the inguinal canal. Again, the spermatic cord is isolated and the varicosities are ligated. The testicle can be delivered through the incision. As a larger number of veins will be seen in this location, the testicular artery may be more difficult to identify. The utilization of a microscope has improved the results. Under increased (6× to 25×) magnification, spermatic veins, lymphatics, and the testicular artery are more accurately identified.

The Palomo procedure consists of an open repair with high retroperitoneal exposure. A lower-abdominal quadrant muscle-splitting incision is made. The internal spermatic vessels are dissected and mass-ligated close to the internal ring. This approach helps to avoid the vas deferens, but can be somewhat invasive.

Laparoscopic Repairs

At our institution, transperitoneal laparoscopic varicocelectomy is becoming the procedure of choice for varicocele ablation. The laparoscopic approach allows for rapid patient recovery, minimal morbidity, and shorter operative times. The technique offers excellent visualization of the gonadal vessels at a location high above the vas deferens. Its disadvantages are increased cost and the potential for injury of abdominal viscera and vessels resulting from trocar insertion or dissection.

For transperitoneal laparoscopic repair, an infraumbilical incision is made and extended down to the midline *fascia*, which is incised. Pneumoperitoneum is obtained either by Veress needle insertion or a port is placed under direct vision. After a 5-mm video port is established, two additional working ports are inserted. The posterior peritoneum is incised over the internal spermatic vessels, and the spermatic veins are mobilized. A 5-mm automated clip applier is passed through the lowest port, and the veins are elevated, clipped, and divided. Some surgeons clip the entire arterial and venous pedicle. When both vessels are ligated it is important to warn patients against undergoing a vasectomy at a later age.

Other laparoscopic techniques have been reported such as a preperitoneal laparoscopic repair. In this procedure, a subcutaneous plane is developed through an infraumbilical incision over the anterior rectus sheath via a preperitoneal balloon dissector. A 10-mm port is placed and pneumopreperitoneum is established. Two additional ports are placed and the spermatic vessels are identified laterally, grasped, and elevated above the vas deferens and its vessels. The vessels are then clipped and divided.

Angiographic Repair

Angiographic varicocelectomy has a limited role in children. However it can be helpful in refractory situations when traditional repairs fail. These procedures are performed by interventional radiologists often under a general anesthetic. Venous access is initially gained through a groin incision and the internal spermatic veins are ablated by a sclerosing agent or placement of an occluding detachable angiographic coil or balloon. Complications in childhood include difficulty catheterizing the internal spermatic vein, extravasation of contrast material, coil migration, and a significant rate of varicocele persistence.

POSTOPERATIVE MANAGEMENT

Recovery depends largely on which treatment modality is used. Overall, one should assess outcomes by varicocele cure, absence of hydrocele/hernia, observation of satisfactory testicular catch-up growth, and, if available, review of semen parameters.

Complications

Most persisting varicoceles in adolescents are identified within several months after the original surgery. Delayed recanalizations are less common. Clinical diagnosis is made in the same manner as was done initially — that is, by physical examination and complementary ultrasonography, if needed. If recurrence is confirmed, a carefully planned repair is indicated. In these instances, utilization of angiography with radiologic intervention or intraoperative venography at the onset of the reexploration may be helpful. Other complications include hydrocele formation which rarely requires surgical repair.

REFERENCES

1. Schneck FX, Bellinger MF. (2007) Abnormalities of the testes and scrotum and their surgical management. In: AJ Wein, LR Kavoussi, AC Novick, *et al.* (eds.), *Campbell–Walsh Urology*, 9th edition. WB Saunders, Philadelphia.
2. Zelkovic P, Kogan SJ. (2009) The pediatric varicocele. In: JG Gearhart, RC Rink, PE Mouriquand (eds.), *Pediatric Urology*, 2nd edition. WB Saunders, Philadelphia.

Section 10: Vascular Malformations

INFANTILE HEMANGIOMAS 79

Nicole Sharp and Danny Little

CLINICAL PRESENTATION

With an incidence of one in 200 births, infantile hemangiomas (IH) are the most common tumor of infancy. Most IH are small and produce few symptoms. They are more common in Caucasians and children born prematurely. Sexual predilection is strongly female at a ratio of 5:1.

IH commonly appear early in infancy with a median age of onset of 2 wks. In 20–50% of cases, a mild cutaneous sign may be present at birth. Most IH (80%) cause minimal discomfort to the infant and are incidentally detected by caregivers. Spontaneous resolution is expected. Exam reveals a soft, cutaneous mass. Superficial hemangiomas are typically bright red with morphology of a raised papule, nodule or plaque. Deeper hemangiomas are located in the subcutaneous tissues but leave a bluish discoloration at the skin level. The term "cavernous" was previously used to describe a deep hemangioma, but this term is confusing and should not be used. Lesions commonly occur on the face, scalp, trunk or extremity. Visceral hemangiomas are far less likely. Rarely, hemangiomas may be massive. Local complications include bleeding, ulceration (5%) and pain. Life-threatening complications occur in approximately 1% and include massive hemorrhage, platelet-trapping, congestive heart failure, neurologic sequalae, and airway obstruction.

A rare and separate class of hemangiomas that are fully developed at birth include the rapidly involuting congenital hemangioma (RICH) or noninvoluting congenital hemangioma (NICH). The RICH and NICH tumors do not exhibit postnatal growth. RICH tumors fully regress by 8 to 14 mths while surgical excision is often required for NICH tumors.

IH is usually an isolated anomaly. Up to 20% of children will have multiple cutaneous hemangiomas. Hemangiomatosis denotes multiple disseminated hemangiomas and when more than five are present, evaluation for a visceral lesion is indicated. An association with multiple births and internal hemangiomas has been described. Large or midline IH may be discovered along with other congenital anomalies including: cervicothoracic hemangiomas with sternal nonunion, lumbosacral hemangiomas with spinal dysraphism (including meningocele and tethered spinal cord), and pelvic or perineal hemangiomas with urogenital and anorectal anomalies. PHACES Syndrome includes posterior fossa brain malformations (most commonly Dandy–Walker), hemangiomas (most commonly large segmental facial lesions), arterial anomalies, cardiac anomalies and coarctation of the aorta, eye and endocrine abnormalities, and sternal cleft and/or supraumbilical raphe.

PATHOPHYSIOLOGY

IH have a well characterized life cycle consisting of a proliferative phase, plateau, and involuting phase. The proliferating phase is marked by rapid angiogenesis, increasing lesion diameter, and color change from blue to crimson. Stimulators of angiogenesis include fibroblast growth factor (FGF), vascular enthothelial growth factor (VEGF) and matrix metalloproteinases. The tumor is composed of rapidly dividing endothelial cells that form a mass of sinusoidal vascular channels. Markers of mature endothelium including CD-31 and von Willebrand's factor are present. GLUT-1 is a specific marker for endothelial cells of hemangiomas. As the IH begins to stabilize, the plateau phase is entered. The tumor then grows proportionately with the child. Typically this is seen towards the end of first year of life. The involuting phase ensues spontaneously usually around age 12–16 mths with endothelial cell apoptosis and a reduction in angiogenesis. Pro-angiogenic factors like FGF and VEGF decrease while tissue inhibitors of metalloproteinases increase. A pale color initially becomes apparent in the center of the hemangioma and then spreads to the periphery. Likewise, the texture is noted to be softer. As the tumor matures, the endothelial cells flatten while vascular channels dilate. The tumor becomes lobular in structure with a fibrofatty stoma. The process of proliferation and involution vary significantly in length from 2 to 8 yrs. Complete healing occurs spontaneously in approximately 50% without specific therapy. Resolution is independent of initial size or extent of the IH.

The specific causes of IH and the triggers for angiogenesis are largely unknown. Viral causes have been proposed, but no specific link has been established. Additionally, no isolated genetic mutations or inheritance patterns have been elucidated.

DIAGNOSIS

With experience, clinicians can accurately diagnosis IH more than 90% of the time. Radiographic imaging, including Magnetic Resonance Imaging (MRI), can be used to delineate the etiology and extent of this vascular anomaly. During the proliferating phase, MRI reveals a lobulated solid mass with intermediate intensity of T1 sequences and moderate hyperintensity of T2 sequences. Flow voids representing fast-flow and shunting will also be seen. In contrast, during involution the MRI demonstrates decreased flow voids and vascularity within a lobular, fatty background. Ultrasound with color Doppler can be utilized to differentiate between slow and fast-flow anomalies. The proliferative-phase hemangioma exhibits dense parenchyma with a strong fast-flow signal that, even in the hands of an experience ultrasonographer, can often be indistinguishable for the signal of an arterial venous malformation. However, this fast-flow of a proliferative-phase hemangioma can help differentiate it from a venous malformation that would exhibit larger vascular spaces and slow flow vascularity. Operator dependence remains a limitation of ultrasonography. Computed Tomography (CT) is often avoided due to contrast associated radiation exposure. One benefit of CT is that it accurately depicts phleboliths better than MRI and is valuable in the evaluation of possible bone involvement. Endoscopy can be utilized for localization of suspected gastrointestinal hemangiomas. Active bleeding may necessitate the use of visceral angiography for localization and embolization. Localization of visceral hemangiomas, including detection of hemorrhage can also be facilitated by radiolabeled red blood cell scan. Bronchoscopy is used to diagnosis IH of the respiratory system.

CLINICAL MANAGEMENT

Observation and reassurance is usually sufficient for the vast majority of IH due to their tendency to spontaneously resolve. Follow-up appointments, utilizing photography, are necessary to monitor the lesion's evolution. Approximately 20% of IH have serious features that may necessitate treatment including large size, rapid growth, failure to regress, local complications (ulceration, hemorrhage), or life-threatening developments (heart failure, hemorrhage or airway compromise).

Compression therapy can be used for small, uncomplicated lesions. Locations most amendable to this treatment modality include the extremities and trunk. Elastic wraps or graded stocking-type devices limit blood flow and may cause thrombosis leading to increase rate of spontaneous resolution. One must be careful not to create a "tourniquet" effect with this modality.

When medical treatment is indicated, pharmacologic treatment is first-line. Systemic or injected steroids result in accelerated resolution in approximately 30%. Additionally, 40% will show lesion stabilization. Ultimately, 30% fail to respond. Triamcinolone injection is useful for lesions where surgical resection may lead to disfigurement or morbidity, such as the eyelid. Steroid-sensitive hemangiomas show lightening of color, softening, and decreased growth as early as the first week. The mechanism of action is mainly antiangiogenic. Steroids inhibit macrophage production of the pro-angiogenic proteins VEGF and basic fibroblast growth factor (bFGF). Steroids also act to inhibit the pro-angiogenic metalloproteinases and precursors to prostaglandins, phospholipase A2. Dosages of 2–3 mg/kg/day of oral prednisone are commonly administered for approximately 4 to 8 wks followed by every-other-day dosing. Steroids must be gradually tapered as rebound growth may occur. Intralesional steroids are useful for well-localized hemangiomas especially those on the face. A series of three to five injections of triamcinolone (3 to 5 mg/kg) is needed at intervals of 6–8 wks. The response rate is similar to that of systemic steroid therapy. Complications from steroid therapy include hypertension, hyperglycemia, and emotional disturbances. If the child fails corticosteroid treatment, a second line pharmacologic treatment utilizing recombinant interferon α, 2a or 2b (2 to 3 million U/m^2 subcutaneously daily) is instituted. IFN-α2 works to accelerate resolution of IH and kaposiform hemangioendothelioma associated with platelet-trapping. Resistant lesions have been treated with weekly intravenous vincristine (0.5 mmg/m^2 or 0.025 mg/kg in kids less than 20 kg) injections with some success.

High-flow IH with serious complications can be treated by arteriographic embolization in complement with antiangiogenic pharmacotherapy.

This is most commonly used in lesions located in the head, neck, liver, chest wall, and trunk. This should be avoided in the extremities due to risk of compromising the entire limb. Previously, the adequacy of this treatment was thought to be due to embolization of the major feeding vessels. More recent research reveals success is dependent on embolization of the tumor's macrovascular shunts. Repeat embolization can be required.

Surgical resection is considered after failure of nonoperative therapy. Previous concerns over excessive hemorrhage have been dampened by better patient selection, preoperative imaging, and surgical planning. Complete excision is preferable. Well-localized tumors, especially those on the scalp, trunk or extremities, in the proliferative-phase can often be amenable to resection. A small margin is obtained and "feeding" arteries are controlled with absorbable suture. Even in the involuting phase, some large, extrophytic lesions may be considered for resection for cosmetic reasons especially if resection is inevitable. Sometimes surgical resection is undertaken after complete involution due to distortion of the remaining skin. Pneumatic tourniquet devices can be used during excision of extremity hemangiomas to help minimize blood loss. While complete excision is preferred, excessive blood loss (>40 cc/kg) or tumor location may necessitate partial excision with subsequent staged procedures. Redundant, fibrofatty skin can be excised in staged procedures as needed. Rarely, reconstructive procedures are necessary due to extensive tissue destruction.

Visceral hemangiomas may be treated by any combination of the treatment modalities mentioned above. Observation and radiographic follow-up may be sufficient for small asymptomatic lesions. Hemangiomas of the respiratory system are usually treatment with systemic and intralesional steroids. If resection is required, segmental resection of the trachea or bronchus with end-to-end anastomosis is performed. Parenchymal hemangiomas may require lobectomy due to significant risk of hemorrhage. Hemangiomas of the gastrointestinal tract leading to hemorrhage may require endoscopic ligation or enterotomy.

Ulcerated hemangiomas are often treated with wound care and topical antibiotics as necessary. Deep ulceration may require debridement. Punctate bleeding usually responds to pressure. Rarely, placement of a suture may be necessary.

Although popular, laser therapy is not always appropriate for IH. Most cutaneous hemangiomas are actually deeper than the penetration of the flashlamp pulse-dye laser (0.75–1.2 mm). However, there are some instances in which laser therapy is beneficial. Remaining telangiectasias after tumor resolution may benefit from laser treatment. Some studies have indicated that proliferative-phase hemangiomas in the subglottic location may be debulked with endoscopic continuous-wave carbon dioxide laser. Bare fiber neodymium-doped yttrium aluminum garnet (Nd/YAG) lasers have also been shown to be useful in hemangiomas of the upper eyelid when treatment is indicated because of visual obstruction.

Fortunately most IH spontaneously regress. Risks and benefits of all treatment modalities mentioned above must be considered. Parental counseling, frequent clinical visits, and a multidisciplinary approach are recommended.

Kasabach–Merritt Syndrome

Kasabach–Merritt phenomenon is a rare, life-threatening disorder associated with patients affected with tufted angioma or kaposiform hemangioendothelioma. First described in 1940 by pediatricians Kasabach and Merritt, this disorder is characterized by profound thrombocytopenia, microangiopathic hemolytic anemia, consumptive coagulopathy and an enlarging vascular lesion. The lesion traps and destroys platelets. The resultant thrombocytopenia may lead to intracranial, gastrointestinal, peritoneal, pleural, or pulmonary bleeding. Of note, Kasabach–Merritt phenomenon does not occur in children with IH.

Although prenatal and adult cases have been described, this condition generally occurs in early infancy or childhood. There is a slight male predilection. Etiology is unknown. Platelet count may be less than 10,000 cells/mm^3. Fibrinogen levels will be low while prothrombin and partial thromboplastin time are elevated.

Typical the lesion will be found on an extremity and show a blue or reddish- brown hue. The overlying skin will be firm and warm. Rapid evolution leads to a violaceous, bulging mass that is tender. Petechiae and purpura are common. Dangerous internal lesions may present only with skin bruising. Lesion ulceration with infection may occur.

The affected child is hospitalized, and intravenous steroids are begun. If ineffective, the chemotherapy agent vincristine is utilized. Platelet transfusions are usually deferred unless active bleeding is present. Additional regimens include the use of interferon, cytoxan, and amicar. Embolization alone or combined with surgery is reserved for failures of medical therapy. Of note, heparin stimulates tumor growth and should be avoided.

No single treatment is uniformly effective, and responses to therapy are often inconsistent. Early childhood proliferation followed by incomplete regression over 10 yrs is common. Continued musculoskeletal pain is possible, and skin discoloration is expected. Mortality ranging from 20% to 30% is reported and is usually related with viscera involvement including the retroperitoneum or mediastinum. Hemorrhage, infection, and iatrogenic complications add to the morbidity. Due to the complexity of the disease, a multidisciplinary approach is mandatory.

REFERENCES

1. Achauer B, Chany CJ, VanderKam VM. (1997) Management of hemangioma of infancy: Review of 245 patients. *Plast Reconstr Surg* **99**:1301–1308.
2. Klement G, Fishman SJ. (2006) Vascular anomalies: Hemangiomas and malformations. In: JL Grosfeld, JA O'Neill, AG Coran, EW Fonkalsrud (eds.), *Pediatric Surgery*, 6th edition, pp. 2094–2110. Mosby, Philadelphia, PA.
3. Mulliken JB, Fishman SJ, Burrows PE. (2000) Vascular anomalies. *Curr Probl Surg* **37**:519–584.

CONGENITAL ARTERIAL DISORDERS 80

Allen Lee, Gregory A. Stanley and Julie R. Fuchs

CONGENITAL ARTERIAL ANEURYSMS

Clinical Presentation

Congenital aneurysms are typically asymptomatic and discovered incidentally during routine evaluation for a seemingly unrelated problem. They have also been identified on screening prenatal ultrasound. Commonly these lesions are found as isolated arterial aneurysms along the ascending, descending, juxtarenal, or infrarenal aorta, the visceral vessels, and in the extremities. The most common location of congenital aneurysms is the visceral vessels; in descending order of incidence they are splenic, hepatic, renal, and finally abdominal aortic aneurysms. Other vascular beds including the head and neck and proximal and peripheral extremities are reported in the literature.

Signs and symptoms associated with congenital aneurysms include hypertension with renovascular aneurysms, headache with cerebral lesions, and palpable pulsatile abdominal or extremity masses. One case report described feeding intolerance in a newborn secondary to duodenal obstruction from a congenital thoracoabdominal aortic aneurysm. To date there are no documented reports to suggest that aortic or lower extremity aneurysms present with distal embolic stigmata, however abdominal aortic aneurysms may show a tendency to thrombose with extensive collateralization. Most children with congenital aneurysms present by age five, although some visceral aneurysms may go undetected for years. Mycotic aneurysms, while not technically congenital, can present similarly in the early neonatal period after a suspected bacteremic episode from umbilical arterial cannulation.

Rupture of congenital aneurysms is rare but has been reported and depending upon the location, can present with subarachnoid hemorrhage and altered mental status, hypotension with associated hemoperitoneum, retroperitoneal hematoma, or an expanding extremity hematoma.

Pathology

While the etiology of congenital aneurysms is not entirely understood, it is clear that in affected patients, vessel dilatation can begin *in utero* as evidenced by aneurysm detection on prenatal ultrasound. Research by Senzaki and colleagues suggests that arterial wall distensibility decreases with changes in vessel elasticity as a child ages, which may lead to the formation of a saccular or fusiform aneurysm. Histologically, medial dysplasia is a common finding without other significant abnormalities to suggest a developmental cause.

Diagnosis

As with most arterial abnormalities, the differential diagnosis can be narrowed by history and physical examination, however imaging remains the mainstay for confirming the diagnosis. Ultrasound is an inexpensive and noninvasive modality for evaluating some visceral and all extremity aneurysms, however technician dependent limitations apply. Other imaging techniques such as magnetic resonance angiography (MRA), computed tomographic angiography (CTA), and standard angiography are preferable for evaluating visceral aneurysms and can offer more information about the size, specific location, relation to nearby branching vessels, other vascular anatomic variants, and any associated findings such as intraluminal thrombus or saccular dilatation.

Surgical Management

The rarity of primary congenital aneurysms and their unlikelihood to rupture makes the indications for surgical management inexact. All symptomatic lesions should be treated in a timely fashion as dictated by the patient's condition. Asymptomatic aneurysms should be selected for intervention based upon size criteria or enlargement. O'Neill and associates advocate for repair of visceral aneurysms greater than or equal to 2 cm in diameter. The involvement of the visceral vasculature must be taken into account prior to surgical intervention in aortic aneurysms. There is no definitive size criterion for extremity lesions.

Surgical treatment most often includes resection and reconstruction with autogenous or prosthetic interposition graft. There are 12 cases of congenital abdominal or thoracoabdominal aortic aneurysms reported in the literature and of these, seven cases were treated surgically. Short-term results were satisfactory, however there were two deaths reported from cardiac or pulmonary failure. Long-term follow-up results are lacking.

Native tissue is probably the best alternative to allow for size matching and future growth. Arterial ligation is also reported in the literature but relies on collateral vessels and may affect future growth and development. More recently, transarterial embolization techniques have been reported, with varying results, again dependent on collaterals.

ARTERIOVENOUS MALFORMATIONS

Clinical Presentation

Arteriovenous malformations (AVMs) can have a variety of signs and symptoms and depend highly on anatomic location. They are present at birth and become noticeable as an infant or toddler. These lesions are relatively common and surface AVMs can present clinically as skin lesions that have the appearance of variants of hemangiomas, vascular nevi, or aneurysmal varices. Fortunately, the large and life-threatening AVMs are extremely rare. Approximately 50% of all extracranial AVMs present in the lower extremities, however central nervous system AVMs remain the most commonly affected organ system.

Because the bulk of extracranial AVMs occur in the extremities, the most common presentation is localized pain, skin changes, and swelling of the area or affected limb. There may also be hyperemia, a thrill or bruit, prominent varicose veins with or without pulsations, skin ulceration with or without bleeding, and limb hypertrophy due to underlying bone and soft tissue overgrowth. The lesions often grow during puberty or after trauma. A common course for a significant AVM includes pain related to ischemia (decreased oxygen delivery to the surrounding tissue), and hypertrophy of the involved area. Intestinal AVMs are generally multiple and present with hematemesis, melena, or hematochezia depending on the location and severity of bleeding. Liver lesions (hemangioendotheliomas) are often identified in the newborn with high-output cardiac failure. Lesions in the lung may present with rapid-onset heart failure and may also be responsible for infectious brain emboli. Larger AVMs may cause symptoms related to compression of surrounding structures, specifically central nervous system compression leading to seizure activity, focal neurologic deficits, or intracranial bleeding. Significant bleeding with hemodynamic compromise has also been reported during routine tooth extraction or umbilical vein cannulation from an unidentified AVM in these locations.

Pathophysiology

The etiology of AVMs remains elusive but is thought to have both genetic and biochemical influences. Recent research suggests that there may be an over activation of the Notch signaling pathway that controls smooth muscle and endothelial growth in vascular development, although this is not confirmed in humans and remains an area of research. The result is a diffuse or localized collection of arteries and veins with microscopic or macroscopic vascular fistulas lined by normal endothelium. Because there is no capillary bed between the arterial and venous circulation, a functional vascular shunt is created which, depending upon the size of the lesion, can lead to high-output cardiac failure and limb deformities. The surrounding tissue is deprived of the normal oxygen and nutrient providing function of a capillary bed and therefore is friable and prone to bleeding. The formation of abnormal connections between an arterial bed and a venous network allows excess blood to by shunted into the veins, resulting in a expansile, fragile lesion.

AVMs grow proportionally with the child and never regress, differentiating them from hemangiomas, which often involute as the child ages. This is an important distinction to note during the work-up and diagnosis of AVMs because of the significant difference in the treatment pathway of these lesions.

Classification

AVMs are classified and treated based upon the volume of blood flow through the arteriovenous connection. Szilagyi and coworkers coined the terms microfistulous and macrofistulous, while Upton and colleagues use the size and the amount of arterial flow to denote a fast flow or slow flow lesion. This distinction is another important determinant of clinical management and can be demonstrated on imaging studies. Schobinger has described a staging system for the status of an AVM which includes: stage I: a pink-bluish stain and warmth with doppler evidence of arterio-venous shunting, stage II: pulsations, a thrill, and a bruit, stage III: skin changes, pain, bleeding, and stage IV: high-output cardiac failure.

Diagnosis

Similar to other arterial abnormalities, the diagnosis of large AVMs is confirmed by imaging modalities, including computed tomography (CT) and magnetic resonance imaging (MRI). In general, doppler examination is a good screening study, and often shows a continuous signal characteristic of a macrofistulous connection. More recently, MRA has become the noninvasive imaging modality of choice because of the high quality images and ability to determine the speed of arterial and venous filling of the lesion. Traditional angiography is also an important diagnostic and therapeutic modality for visceral and extremity AVMs and should be routinely performed in any patient undergoing surgical resection. Typically on angiography, a tortuous, dilated artery is demonstrated with obvious arteriovenous connections and early filling of the venous system with pooling of dye in the arteriovenous channels. These characteristics are seen in 60% of AVMs. Diffuse microfistulous disease can be missed on arteriography, and the diagnosis can be obtained by observing elevated skin and blood flow determinations with comparative venous blood oxygen saturation levels.

Management

A nonsurgical approach is most appropriate with small, asymptomatic lesions, those that are limited to mild vein dilation, or those that are too extensive to be considered for surgical intervention. In these cases, compression stockings should be prescribed and usually offer stabilization of the lesion or even mild improvement. This is also the primary mode of treatment for microfistulous disease in any location.

For AVMs that are symptomatic and amenable to surgical intervention, there are several treatment options. The goal of surgical treatment remains complete excision of the lesion. Partial excision often leads to recurrence and worsening of symptoms secondary to increasing collateral vessel formation. Large areas of tissue necrosis can be a devastating complication of simple ligation or embolization of the arterial feeding vessel(s) and should be avoided.

Superselective transarterial catheterization and embolization has become an increasingly popular adjunct to surgical management of AVMs. This technique can be used as an adjuvant or neoadjuvant therapy and may also be performed as a series of embolizations in patients who are not amenable to a large operation. It can be used as palliation for pain, bleeding, or cardiac failure, but often does not provide a permanent cure. If embolization is used as a preoperative intervention to help decrease the risk of bleeding, surgery should be performed relatively soon after to minimize collateral vessel formation and maximize the chances of complete excision without recurrence. Many patients with AVMs require several different types of therapy over time (resection, embolization, nonoperative compression), but unfortunately a fair number of patients with significant AVMs of the extremity eventually come to amputation.

ACQUIRED ARTERIAL DISORDERS

ARTERIAL THROMBOSIS AND EMBOLISM

Clinical Presentation

The most common sites of spontaneous arterial thrombosis are the external iliac artery, visceral arteries, and proximal upper extremity arteries. Signs and symptoms of peripheral arterial thrombosis or embolism include absent pulses, coolness, pallor, pain, and decreased motor function. Capillary refill may be prolonged. Skin changes may not be present if there is good collateralization. One should maintain a high index of suspicion in patients with these signs and a history of trauma, external compression, such as a cast or splint, arterial catheterization, or a suspected hypercoagulable state, including sepsis. If unrecognized, peripheral ischemia can progress to gangrene.

Signs and symptoms of visceral arterial thrombosis or embolism are usually more subtle. Visceral ischemia typically presents with nonspecific symptoms including pain, vomiting, and bloody stools. Air-fluid levels can be seen on plain films, and free air can be seen in the setting of bowel infarction which has progressed to perforation. Patients with a low flow state, such as sepsis are most at risk for bowel ischemia. Thrombosis due to low flow states has a propensity to cause skin necrosis of the distal extremities and segmental bowel necrosis. Again, a high index of suspicion should be maintained with critically ill children with vague gastrointestinal symptoms, as bowel ischemia is uniformly fatal if unrecognized.

Pathophysiology

Arterial thrombosis and embolism are often related to a relative hypercoagulable state. Infants in shock, from sepsis or other etiologies, are one susceptible group. Hyperviscosity due to the neonates' relative polycythemia places them at increased risk. Other hypercoagulable states associated with thrombosis and embolism include sickle cell disease, leukemia, among other malignancies, and bacterial endocarditis.

Emboli attributable to bacterial endocarditis can cause peripheral or visceral artery occlusion, followed occasionally by mycotic aneurysm formation. Arterial catheterization has been known to be associated with thrombosis and embolism. Thrombosis and embolism have been reported with umbilical artery catheters. Similarly, arterial puncture for angiography or transluminal angioplasty or stenting are also associated with occlusion. Inadvertent intraarterial administration of large volumes or some medications, such as inotropes, may result in vasospasm and thrombosis. Pediatric patients are at particular risk for iatrogenic vascular injuries leading to thrombosis due to their small vessels and frequency of low flow states.

Diagnosis/Work-up

For both peripheral and visceral occlusive disease, a thorough history including a history suggestive of hypercoagulable disorders or trauma should be obtained. Critical illness or history of arterial catheterization or transluminal interventions are important in hospitalized patients.

After signs of peripheral vascular occlusion are identified, including absent pulses, coolness, pallor, pain, or decreased motor function, a thorough pulse exam should be performed as well as a Doppler exam to attempt to delineate the level of occlusion. It is often difficult to differentiate between vasospasm and a true occlusion. Pulses will be absent on Doppler examination in the setting of occlusion, whereas attenuated pulse waves can be elicited in cases of spasm. Symptoms related to spasm should be self limited and resolve within 4–6 hrs. If evidence of extremity ischemia on serial physical exams and doppler exams persist, treatment should be geared towards treating a thrombotic or embolic event. Angiography is the gold standard to evaluate for thromboembolic events, but is not always possible in an acute setting. Duplex ultrasonography is an acceptable alternative that can be performed at the bedside.

In cases of suspected visceral thromboembolism, there are few definitive diagnostic tests, as findings are often nonspecific. Laboratory abnormalities are not seen until late in the course of the disease. Complete blood count, blood gases, and chemistries should be obtained. Plain films often show only nonspecific findings, such as dilated bowel and air-fluid levels, although a gasless abdomen can also be seen in early stages. Pneumatosis or portal venous air can also be found. CT scan and ultrasound may demonstrate bowel wall edema and free intraabdominal fluid, and may be able to differentiate an arterial occlusion from mesenteric venous thrombosis. Angiography has the potential to be diagnostic as well as therapeutic by facilitating directed lytic therapy.

When the cause of a thrombotic or embolic event is not obvious, a hypercoagulable work-up consisting of protein C, protein S, antithrombin III, and anti-phospholipid antibodies should be performed. Echocardiogram should be performed to evaluate for endocarditis as a source for embolism.

Treatment/Management

Treatment for thrombosis and embolism is varied and depends on the location and extent of disease. Bowel infarction regardless of etiology requires laparotomy and bowel resection. Neonates with limited visceral thrombosis related to low flow states and polycythemia may require plasmapheresis in addition to thrombolysis or thrombectomy. Intraarterial thrombolytics should not be used in those at high risk for intracranial bleeding.

Patients with septic emboli from endocarditis require prompt intervention. Infected emboli must be extracted to prevent mycotic aneurysm formation. Those with catheter associated events should have the offending catheter removed. Systemic anticoagulation should be initiated and directed thrombolysis should be performed once the diagnosis of an arterial thrombosis or embolus is made if the patient is not at excessive risk for hemorrhage. Operative embolectomy or bypass can also be considered.

RENOVASCULAR HYPERTENSION

Clinical Presentation

Symptoms such as headache, irritability, congestive heart failure, and encephalopathy may prompt a work-up that may reveal a diagnosis of hypertension. Commonly, asymptomatic hypertension is discovered incidentally during a preoperative evaluation for an elective surgical procedure. In cases of bilateral renal artery stenosis, malignant hypertension may present with evidence of end organ dysfunction, including congestive heart failure, retinopathy, or renal failure. Prior to evaluation for an intervention, medical management of the severe hypertension has often been initiated. Characteristically, the hypertension associated with renovascular disease is very difficult to control medically and is still often present despite intensive drug regimens. About half of the patients will have audible abdominal bruits and those with the midaortic syndrome variant can have diminished lower extremity pulses.

Incidence

The incidence of hypertension is estimated to be between 1 to 5% in children, the presence of which is often indicative of underlying pathology. Approximately 80% of those 0 to 5 yrs of age will have a surgically correctable cause of hypertension. This incidence declines with age, approaching approximately 44% in the 6- to 10-yr age group, and 20% in the 11- to 20-yr age group. In cases of surgically correctable hypertension, renovascular hypertension is the most common cause and comprises up to 10% of cases.

Pathology

Renal artery stenosis results in a relative renal ischemia which then causes elevated renin levels and then hypertension through the activation of the renin-angiotensin axis. The causes of renovascular hypertension are varied, but a specific cause is usually identifiable. The most common form of acquired renal artery stenosis is fibromuscular dysplasia, thought to be an autoimmune vasculitis which causes fibrous hypertrophy of the muscularis as well as intimal fibrous dysplasia. A variety of syndromes can be associated with renal artery stenosis, the most frequent being neurofibromatosis. A cuff of hypertrophied neural tissue around the ostia of the renal arteries that can extend to the surrounding aorta is found in these patients.

Renovascular hypertension is also noted with many vasculitides, with Takayasu's most commonly. Extrinisic compression from a nearby tumor or retroperitoneal fibrosis after radiation therapy can rarely constrict the renal artery. Trauma leading to renal artery disruption and umbilical artery catheters causing thrombosis can also lead to renal artery stenosis (Table 1).

Diagnosis

Children with renovascular hypertension generally present with very high blood pressures. Systolic pressures are often greater than 200 mm Hg, and the hypertension is often very difficult to control medically. Renovascular etiologies should be investigated as part of the hypertension work-up.

Evidence of end organ damage should be investigated, including EKG, chest X-ray, and echocardiography (left ventricular failure). Fundoscopy should be performed to assess for retinopathy. Up to two thirds will have evidence of left ventricular hypertrophy, 60% will have retinopathy, and 10% will have renal dysfunction.

Several imaging studies can be helpful in establishing the diagnosis. Duplex ultrasonography can be a valuable noninvasive modality. Peak systolic velocities can be increased or decreased distal to a stenosis. False positive and false negatives are not uncommon. This modality is currently poor at detecting branch vessel or accessory renal artery stenoses.

CTA and MRA are both useful for diagnosing renal artery stenoses and can provide detailed three dimensional reconstructions. They may eventually replace angiography, but both currently have limitations in children with small renal vessels. Presently, angiography with selective renal arteriography remains the gold standard for diagnosis and adds the benefit of potential therapeutic intervention. Angiography is the best method to detect small branch vessel lesions and collaterals.

Table 1. Causes of pediatric renovascular hypertension.

Fibromuscular dysplasia
Congenital
Neurofibromatosis type I
Tuberous Sclerosis
Coarctation of the aorta
Arterial hypoplasia
William's syndrome
Marfan's syndrome
Other syndromes
Vasculitis
Kawasaki's disease
Takayasu's disease
Polyarteritis nodosa
Midaortic syndrome
Other vasculitides
Extrinsic compression
Wilm's tumor
Neuroblastoma
Other tumors
Other causes
Thrombosis/embolism
Hemolytic uremic syndrome
Radiation
Umbilical artery catheters
Trauma
Nephritis/Pyelonephritis
Obstructive Uropathy
Transplant renal artery stenosis

Treatment/Management

Endovascular

Antihypertensives should be initiated as soon as the diagnosis of hypertension is made. Modest improvements may be seen, but difficult to control hypertension is the rule with renovascular hypertension. Most commonly, a combination of α and β adrenergic blockers and a thiazide diuretic are used. Angiotensin-converting-enzyme (ACE) inhibitors are generally avoided, as these can worsen renal function by dilation of the efferent arteriole, further reducing the GFR.

Percutaneous transluminal renal angioplasty can be a valuable treatment if medical management of hypertension is inadequate or poorly tolerated. When angioplasty with a standard balloon is unable to abolish the waist, a high pressure or cutting balloon can be used. Stent placement is recommended in cases where the residual stenosis is greater than 50%. Flow limiting dissections can usually be treated by reinflation or stent placement if unsuccessful. Arterial rupture can also be successfully treated by repeated reinflation and covered stent placement. Long-term outcomes of renal artery stenting in children are unknown. Their use is generally limited to inadequate dilation due to recoil after angioplasty, treating dissections and to treat early restenoses after a clinically successful angioplasty. Balloon angioplasty has the most success for a renal artery branch vessel stenosis, and less so for ostial stenoses.

Balloon expandable stents are preferred as they can be postdilated as a child grows. In-stent stenosis due to intimal hyperplasia or thrombosis can usually be treated with repeat angioplasty. Notably, the use of stents may adversely affect future surgical options.

Surgical

Open surgical techniques are indicated when hypertension is refractory to medical and endovascular approaches. Complete evaluation of the aortoiliac system is needed as aortic, iliac, as well as celiac, SMA, and IMA abnormalities are frequently seen. Surgical options consist of bypass or nephrectomy.

An optimal conduit must be taken into careful consideration. Saphenous vein is generally contraindicated, as it has a tendency for aneurysmal degeneration in children. Some have had success using this conduit by supporting the area with a Dacron wrap to prevent aneurysm formation. Other options include the use of an internal iliac artery as an interposition graft, or transposing the splenic artery on the left and gastroduodenal or hepatic arteries on the right if there is no celiac involvement as an end-to-end bypass. Autogenous conduits are often not feasible in most children, who will then require prosthetic grafts. Ideally, these definitive procedures with prosthetic grafts should be delayed until adolescence by temporizing renal perfusion with endoluminal techniques.

Nephrectomy, the only surgical option in the past to manage renovascular hypertension, is now reserved as a last resort. It may however be the only option in very small infants, those with diffuse renal artery disease, failed open bypass, or for whom reconstruction is not feasible. Total nephrectomy is indicated for atrophic, poorly functioning kidneys. Some segmental intrarenal lesions may lend themselves to a partial nephrectomy.

Special Considerations

Midaortic syndrome, a variant of fibromuscular dysplasia associated with more widespread vascular involvement beyond the renal arteries, is often associated with renal artery stenosis. Midaortic syndrome has a variable pattern of stenosis. It can be suprarenal, infrarenal, or pararenal. Pure infrarenal lesions are rare. All have aortic narrowing. Most stenoses begin at the aortic hiatus to just above the IMA. Most patients with midaortic syndrome have bilateral renal artery involvement and are severely symptomatic, presenting with malignant hypertension, congestive heart failure, renal failure, or even lower extremity claudication.

Reconstruction options include patch aortoplasty and bypass grafts. Frequently, an aorto-aortic bypass graft using a synthetic graft is needed. Renal arteries can then be directly implanted into normal infrarenal aorta, if present, or into the tube graft. In cases of extensive renal artery involvement, explantation and back table reconstruction of the segmental renal vessels with orthotopic or heterotopic autotransplantation is an option.

Outcomes

Results of percutaneous transluminal renal angioplasty for renovascular hypertension are highly variable. In part, this variability is due to differences in the extent of disease. Tullus *et al.* have reported improvements in 55% of children overall and in 85% with more limited disease in one or both renal arteries.

In a series of 17 operative cases of midaortic syndrome, 12 patients were cured. Four renal bypasses alone were performed. One primary nephrectomy was done and, 12 aortoaortic bypasses were performed, with

9 of those undergoing bilateral renal artery reconstruction and the remaining undergoing unilateral renal bypass. Mortalities after open procedures are extremely rare, as these are relatively well tolerated in children. Surgical reconstruction is associated with cure in a reported 36–70% and partial improvement in 26–50%.

ACQUIRED ARTERIAL ANEURYSMS

Acquired aneurysms continue to be relatively rare and are caused by accidental or iatrogenic trauma to the artery, infection of the artery, an underlying connective tissue disorder, or an arteritis such as Kawasaki's disease. The aneurysms caused by trauma (blunt, penetrating, or iatrogenic such as arterial puncture for dialysis, arterial line, or cardiac catheterization) are typically false aneurysms with progressive enlargement. They may be treated with embolization or compression. Thrombin injection may be an option in larger aneurysms with a narrow neck. Resection with or without interposition graft is sometimes required.

Patients with infective endocarditis and septic emboli may also present with aneurysms most commonly in the thoracic aorta and also the abdominal aorta. These lesions should be resected and replaced as they have a high rupture rate without surgical intervention. The highest risk patients are those with a history of umbilical artery catheter and those with coarctation of the aorta. Staphylococcus aureus is the most common organism.

Kawasaki's disease is also associated with acquired aneurysms that may be present in any part of the body, with 15% developing coronary artery aneurysms. Large coronary artery aneurysms can result in myocardial ischemia and require coronary artery bypass. Peripheral arterial aneurysms can also form and they are usually small, multiple and fusiform and generally do not require surgical treatment unless they are symptomatic or enlarging, with the axillary artery being the most common peripheral site.

There are several connective tissue disorders that are associated with the development of arterial aneurysms, including Marfan's syndrome, Ehlers–Danlos syndrome, tuberous sclerosis, familial cystic medial necrosis, and rarely neurofibromatosis, polyarteritis nodosa, giant-cell arteritis, cystinosis, melorheostosis, and sarcoidosis.

Marfan's syndrome is a hereditary autosomal dominant disorder characterized by arterial cystic medial necrosis with intimal rupture secondary to a genetic defect in the fibrillin gene. Aortic root dilation and dissecting aneurysms of the ascending aorta with aortic ring or coronary vessel involvement are common manifestations of this syndrome and often require emergent operation.

Ehlers–Danlos syndrome is another hereditary disorder that can have extensive vascular involvement. Type IV most commonly presents with arterial manifestations because of the absence or abnormal amount of type III collagen. Aneurysmal disease may involve the abdominal aorta, iliac arteries, and extremities.

Doppler ultrasound and angiography are generally used for diagnosis and surgical planning. Once the aneurysm is diagnosed, surgical treatment involves resection with prosthetic interposition graft. Ehlers–Danlos type IV is an important exception to this algorithm because of the exceedingly poor collagen matrix in this disease. Angiography is contraindicated and a noninvasive study such as MRA or CTA is preferable. In addition, the proximal and distal clamping required for vessel reconstruction can cause disruption of the vessel wall, making surgical intervention extremely difficult and dangerous such that it should only be undertaken in the most ominous circumstances.

ARTERIOPATHIES OF CHILDREN/OCCLUSIVE DISEASES

Intracranial

Strokes and transient ischemic attacks occur in 1–3/100,000 children per year, the cause of which is identified in about 75% of patients. Association with hereditary prothrombotic risk factors leads to a 10% recurrence rate. The causes of strokes include: congenital heart disease, hematologic diseases, such as sickle cell disease or hypercoagulable states, vasculitis, infection, intracranial vascular diseases, meningitis, neurofibromatosis, radiation, and trauma. Arteriopathies such as Moyamoya disease are becoming increasingly recognized and associated with 50–80% of strokes. Carotid or vertebral dissection following manipulation or trauma is noted in up to 20%. Varicella zoster infections are associated with a threefold increase in ischemic strokes by causing a characteristic ICA, MCA, and ACA stenosis. Angiographic work-up in some children after stroke will reveal an arteriopathy of unknown etiology. A few of these will represent early Moyamoya disease which includes many disorders that involve multiple stenoses of the intracranial arteries (mainly Circle of Willis). Moyamoya disease is progressive and is defined as bilateral distal ICA stenoses with the formation of collateral arteries, giving rise to the typical "puff of smoke" appearance on angiography. Stroke treatment is generally supportive. Anticoagulation and thrombolytics are appropriate in select cases. Treatment for Moyamoya disease also includes surgical revascularization, including encephaloduroarteriomyosyangiosis (EDAMS) and superficial temporal to MCA bypass. These treatments have mixed success, as in most cases, the treatment is performed after a significant stroke has already occurred.

Extracranial

Several vasculidites or inflammatory arteriopathies are associated with arterial occlusion. Takayasu's arteritis is a progressive large and medium vessel vasculitis associated with aortitis and occlusion of the great vessels. One common presenting symptom of Takayasu's arteritis is renovascular hypertension secondary to renal artery occlusion, which is in turn secondary to the inflammatory process in the vessel wall. It can also involve occlusive disease of the aortic arch branches and an elevated ESR. It can be progressive with eventual fibrotic narrowing. In late stages of the Takayasu's, fibrotic changes lead to stenotic or aneurismal degeneration as the disease "burns out". Generally, operative intervention should be strongly considered in cases of renovascular hypertension, coronary or cerebral ischemia, or severe claudication. Mortality is 16–20% long-term.

Other inflammatory disease processes, such as Kawasaki's disease, Behcet's syndrome, rheumatoid arthritis, giant-cell arteritis, syphilis, and tuberculosis can account for large vessel arteritis. Kawasaki's disease is characterized as an inflammatory illeness affecting children in the first year of life. It presents with high fever, conjunctivitis, truncal erythema, adenopathy, and elevated ESR, thrombocytosis. The disease can also present with the development of coronary artery aneurysms in 15% of patients. Treatment includes aspirin and steroids. Some patients benefit from high dose gamma globulins. Coronary artery surgery is sometimes required. Aortic, brachial, axillary, renal, and mesenteric aneurysms can also be seen.

Williams syndrome is a hereditary disorder characterized by occlusion of extracranial vessels. It often is associated with congenital heart disease (pulmonary stenosis), arterial stenoses (mainly subclavian and renal), and a characteristic facies. Often patients present with renovascular hypertension. Balloon angioplasty is often performed for subclavian and upper extremity stenoses, and reconstruction is offered for renal artery stenosis, as the lesions are often ostial.

SMALL ARTERY DISEASE AND VASOSPASTIC DISORDERS

Several entities are associated with nonatherosclerotic occlusion of small arteries in children. While symptoms, depending on the disease process can range from mild to severe, progressive occlusion of small arteries can lead to ulceration, gangrene, and ultimately amputation of fingers or toes. Conditions associated with small vessel disease include: scleroderma, lupus erythematosus, dermatomyositis, juvenile rheumatoid arthritis, polyarteritis nodosa, and purpura fulminans. The primary pediatric vasospastic disorders are Raynaud's syndrome and reflex sympathetic dystrophy. Other conditions that can be associated with vasospasm include frostbite, cryoglubulinemia, and antiphospholipid antibody syndrome.

Raynaud's syndrome causes temporary digital artery spasm with cold or emotional stress. Patients may describe cyanosis, numbness, pain, or redness of the fingers. Symptoms can range from mild to severe. When severe, atrophy and even ulceration may be seen. Thoracic outlet syndrome, viral infections, and sympathomimetic use must be excluded. Treatment includes avoiding cold exposure, calcium channel blockers, or prostacyclins in extreme cases. Sympathectomy is reserved for intractable pain, but has poor long-term results.

Reflex sympathetic dystrophy is a disorder which may follow trauma in which patients have severe pain on touching the skin. This syndrome is associated with stress and psychosomatic problems. Physical therapy and pain medication are the main therapies. Antiphospholipid antibody syndrome is often associated with lupus. The syndrome can result in vascular thrombosis that may require surgical intervention, but patients are generally treated with coumadin for anticoagulation.

SELECTED REFERENCES

1. O'Neill JA. (2006) Arterial disorders. In: JL Grosfeld, AA Caldamone, AG Coran, EW Fonkalsrud, JA O'Neill (eds.), *Pediatric Surgery*, 6th edition, pp. 2111–2123. Mosby, St. Louis, MO.

2. Sheppard G, *et al.* (2000) Syndrome of idiopathic childhood aneurysms: A case report and review of the literature. *JVIR* **11**:997–1004.
3. Zhuge Q, *et al.* (2009) Notch-1 signalling is activated in brain arteriovenous malformations in humans. *Brain.* **132**(Pt 12):3231–3241.
4. Klement G, Fishman SJ. (2006) Vascular anomalies: Hemangiomas and malformations. In: JL Grosfeld, AA Caldamone, AG Coran, EW Fonkalsrud, JA O'Neill (eds.), *Pediatric Surgery,* 6th edition, pp. 2094–2110. Mosby, St. Louis, MO.
5. Guzetta PC. (1994) Congenital and acquired aneurysmal disease. *Semin Pediat Surg* **3**(2):97–102.
6. Oğuzkurt P, Senocak ME, Ciftci AO, Tanyel FC, Büyükpamukçu N. (2000) Mesenteric vascular occlusion resulting in intestinal necrosis in children. *J Pediatr Surg* **35**(8):1161–1164.
7. Price V, Massicotte MP. (2003) Arterial thromboembolism in the pediatric population. *Semin Thromb Hemost* **29**(6):557–565.
8. Sparks SR, Chock A, Seslar S, Bergan JJ, Owens EL. (2000) Surgical treatment of Takayasu's arteritis: Case report and literature review. *Ann Vasc Surg* **14**(2):125–129.
9. Tullus K, Brennan E, Hamilton G, Lord R, McLaren CA, Marks SD, Roebuck DJ. (2008) Renovascular hypertension in children. *Lancet* **371**(9622):1453–1463.
10. Dean RH and Robaczewski D. (1994) Arteriopathies of childhood. *Semin Pediat Surg* **3**(2):103–113.
11. Athreya BH. (1994) Vasospastic disorders in children. *Semin Pediat Surg* **3**(2):70–78.

PEDIATRIC VENOUS DISORDERS

81

Paul R. Crisostomo and Michael C. Dalsing

INTRODUCTION

This review of pediatric *venous* disorders focuses on congenital venous malformations (VM) as well as the growing problem of pediatric venous thromboembolism (VTE).

PERIPHERAL CONGENITAL VENOUS MALFORMATIONS

The difference between a vascular hemangioma and a congenital vascular malformation (CVM), both of which are commonly called "birth marks" is important to recognize. Vascular hemangiomas account for the vast majority of pediatric vascular anomalies and characteristically grow rapidly during the first year of life, plateau, and involute slowly during childhood. In contrast, CVMs have no endothelial proliferation and do not go away. CVMs occur in approximately 1% of the general population.[1,2] They occur sporadically and are rarely genetically transmitted. CVMs are classified as predominately: (1) arterial; (2) venous; (3) arteriovenous; (4) lymphatic; and (5) mixed or combined anomalies.[3,4] Each is further classified into one of two groups based on the embryonal stage at which the developmental arrest occurred: extratruncular or truncular. The extratruncular arrests at an early embryonal stage and retains characteristics of the mesenchymal cells which allow the lesion to grow when stimulated during puberty, pregnancy or surgery. Because growth was stunted prior to differentiation into main channels, no true vessels are present but rather primitive vascular channels form the connections present. It can be further divided into diffuse, infiltrating or limited, localized. In contrast, the truncular form has development arrested at a later stage and lack the ability to rapidly grow when stimulated. The main channels have developed and the problem noted is either aplasia or obstruction and alternatively dilatation (localized or diffuse). It is helpful to note that fast-flow lesions generally have an arterial component while venous and lymphatic defects are slow-flow lesions.

VMs account for nearly 50% of all CVMs and have a slight female predominance.[4–6] The truncular form appear most frequently in the lower extremities while the extratruncular forms (diffuse and localized) are most commonly noted in the head and neck.[1] As the name implies, VM are present at birth but are often not recognized until the late teens with a predilection for the lower extremity.[5] Symptoms common to all venous disorders (acute thrombosis or chronic venous disease) eventually brings the patient to the attention of the clinician and must initially be treated as any acute venous thrombosis or symptomatic chronic state. Furthermore, because of an association with other congenital VM, symptoms uncommon to more routine venous disorders may be observed. Early diagnostic studies should involve Magnetic Resonance Imaging (MRI) which aids in the embryologic staging and anatomic associations.[7] A venous duplex evaluation will aid in determining anatomy and hemodynamic parameters. Venography may be required to clearly demonstrate venous connections and avert misadventures during interventional procedures.[7,8]

Truncular VM may present as simple varicose veins with abnormal dilatation and tortuosity of the peripheral veins probably due to vein wall defects. There can be phlebectasia, an abnormal dilation of a vein involving a long segment of the venous trunk. If only involving the superficial system, treatment ranges from compression stockings to sclerotherapy and/or ablative surgery (laser, radiofrequency or open stripping) when the child is sufficiently mature.

Obstructive deep truncular VMs may be seen by pediatricians and pediatric surgeons. Aplasia / hypoplasia of the deep veins occurs in approximately 8% of patients with peripheral venous anomalies,[2] and in as many as 50% with specific disorders (e.g. Klippel–Trenaunay syndrome). Because superficial veins may be the main or sole route for venous drainage from these limbs it is critical to avoid ablation of superficial veins prior to completely defining the anatomy. Commonly, these patients develop a "marginal vein" on the lateral extremity which is an abnormal superficial outflow vein derived from a remnant embryonal vein. Narrowing of the *left* common iliac vein (i.e. May–Thurner syndrome, Cockett's syndrome, and iliac compression syndrome) is seen in approximately 20% of the general population but is exceedingly rare in children. Compression and repetitive trauma of the left common iliac vein occurs as the overlying right common iliac artery contacts the fifth lumbar vertebra. In children, the majority of patients are teenage females on oral contraceptives with symptomatic left leg venous outflow obstruction. Diagnosis is suspected by duplex ultrasonography but confirmed by Magnetic Resonance Venogram (MRV), Computed Tomography (CT), or venography. Treatment of symptoms begins with compression stockings and anticoagulation if deep vein thrombosis (DVT) is present. These patients might well benefit from catheter-directed thrombolysis and/or stenting as appropriate.

Dilated deep truncular VMs are also seen in children. Avalvulia, is seen in 7% of deep veins in patients with venous CVMs.[2] Avalvulia or congenital vein valve aplasia is the virtual absence of venous valves in all deep and superficial veins. This autosomal-dominant anomaly often presents in adolescence after the child begins to walk. Significant venous reflux and sustained venous hypertension lead to severe orthostatic leg swelling, edema and varicose veins often before puberty. Treatment varies from graduated compression stockings to deep vein axillary vein valve transplantation. A venous aneurysm can occur in as many as 20% of patients with concomitant venous CVMs and is a *localized* area of deep venous dilation.[9,10] Abdominal venous aneurysms may affect the inferior vena cava, the superior mesenteric vein, the splenic vein, the portal vein, and the iliac veins. Presentation varies from pulmonary embolism to abdominal pain or intestinal bleeding secondary to fistula formation. Calligaro and colleagues reported that 41% of patients with abdominal venous aneurysms developed life-threatening complications if the aneurysms are managed conservatively, and these authors recommend prophylactic complete or partial excision with bypass or aneurysmorrhaphy in low-risk patients.[11] Others favor ultrasonographic surveillance of small asymptomatic aneurysms. Thoracic vena caval aneurysms are incidental findings on radiographs with little risk of spontaneous rupture and nonoperative treatment is the norm.

The extratruncular variety of VM has little formal venous structure and can involve bone and muscle. The anatomy must be well defined to prevent unwanted damage to the involved bone or muscle and require advanced imaging with MRI and more invasive diagnostics. VMs are sometimes amenable to endovascular management, a technique in which venous drainage become a very important consideration. A classification introduced to address this specific interventional need has been proposed with venous drainage described as absent, into normal veins, into dysplasic veins or the lesion is described as venous ectasia.[8] The last two situations make embolic agents difficult to use since the agents are prone to enter the systemic circulation. However, when large draining veins are accessible, they can be percutaneously embolized to prevent later egress of the liquid sclerosants or embolic agents injected into the VM. Surgery is useful in rare cases.[12] In some cases, the most prudent treatment is therapeutic compression and elevation.

Complex VMs are rare but clinically severe disorders. Some venous disorders are so well known that they deserve comment. Complex VMs are divided into those without (Maffucci syndrome, Proteus syndrome, Klippel–Trenaunay syndrome) and those with arteriovenous shunting (Parkes–Weber syndrome). The Maffucci syndrome is the coexistence of a VM (often large and subcutaneous), cartilage growth, and bone deformities. About 20% of patients suffer malignant change, commonly chondrosarcoma, and require dedicated surveillance with serial radiographs and biopsy of suspicious lesions. Surgical excision is required since radiation therapy is of no therapeutic value.[6–13] The Proteus syndrome is characterized by a combination of capillary, venous and lymphatic malformations with disproportionate growth of bones, muscles, and fatty tissues. Children are usually born without obvious deformity. As they age; tumors, skin, and bony growths appear and progressively worsen and may encompass more than half the body. Connective tissue nevi on the plantar surface, abdomen, hands, or nose are pathognomonic. VMs play a significant role in the risk of DVT, pulmonary emboli, and premature death. No cure exists. The Klippel–Trenaunay syndrome is a mixed capillary, venous, and lymphatic *low flow* malformation. Symptoms vary from mild varicosities to massively enlarged unilateral lower limb involvement.[14] A skin blemish or hyperpigmented area is commonly seen. Radiographic findings may include iliofemoral vein abnormalities and persistent sciatic vein.[15] Mild varicosities should be managed with compressive garments and leg elevation. Raised verrucous capillary malformations with repeated bleeding can be treated with sclerotherapy. Although recurrence of venous varicosities is as high as 50%, significant superficial venous pathology may be treated with ablative techniques after diagnostic studies confirm patency of the deep venous system.[16] The Parkes–Weber syndrome is distinguished by *high-flow* arteriovenous fistulas and consequent hemodynamic complications. Brightly stained skin which is warm with the presence of a bruit, and thrill are characteristic. Cardiovascular problems usually present later in life. However, rare fistulas in central locations arising from major branches of the aorta may present as infantile high-output congestive heart failure. Most lesions are surgically inaccessible or cause significant morbidity with operative intervention. Thus, endovascular sclerotherapy has become the palliative mainline treatment for large symptomatic malformations and may be used as an adjunct to surgery in select cases.[5,17]

Embolization with liquid embolic agents such as n-butyl cyanoacrylate of venous CVMs was previously advocated. However, embolization was marked by poor efficacy due to incomplete obstruction, recanalization, high recurrence, and embolic complications such as inadvertent embolization of normal tissues and pulmonary emboli.[18] Endovascular ultrasound guided sclerotherapy has instead become the main treatment for CVMs. Absolute ethanol is the most effective and preferred sclerosing agent for CVMs and is applicable to the VM as well.[19,20] Ethanol sclerotherapy results in complete obliteration of the most distal vessels rather than simple obstruction of the vessel lumen. However, ethanol sclerotherapy causes significant pain which requires general anesthesia. Complications include local tissue injury, thrombophlebitis, and pulmonary embolism, which can theoretically occur from thrombus dislodgment from the sclerosed CVM. There are less caustic sclerosants which can be used especially in more superficial locations such as sodium morrhuate or sodium tetradecylsulfate. In some instances, surgical extirpation is the optimal approach for localized lesions.[21]

PEDIATRIC VENOUS THROMBOEMBOLISM

VTE in children occurs significantly less often than in adults. Proposed factors include decreased exposure to prothrombotic risk factors (e.g. smoking, oral contraceptives), decreased prevalence of vascular diseases (e.g. diabetes, hypetension), decreased levels of vitamin K dependent clotting factors, and increased levels of thrombin inhibitor alpha 2 macroglobulin. Nevertheless, VTE still represents a substantial pediatric burden with an incidence 0.05–0.14/10,000 children and a mortality of 2.2%.[22–24] In hospitalized children, the incidence of VTE/DVT is even higher at about 5 to 10/10,000 admissions and appears to be increasing.[25] Approximately 60% of DVT in hospitalized children is related to the use of central venous access.[25,26] Central venous lines were found to be directly associated with extremity DVT and correlates with increasing frequency of central venous line use. In contrast to predominant lower extremity VTE in adults, only 50–60% were documented in the lower extremity in hospitalized children and is a reflection of the impact of CVL on upper extremity and caval DVT in children. CVL related VTE most commonly remains asymptomatic (66%) but can present as loss of CVL patency and prominent collateral circulation in the skin.[27,28] If the catheter is the nidus for DVT in the lower extremity, it is removed. Whether catheter related or not, duplex evaluation is often used to confirm the diagnosis. Therapeutic anticoagulation is instituted with treatment for 3 to 6 mths, and symptoms are treated conservatively with elevation, rest, and elastic support. Patients in whom venous access or major vessel occlusion is a concern should be evaluated for the more aggressive approach of catheter-directed thrombolysis. Thrombolytic therapy for central venous line-related DVT and pulmonary embolism (PE) has been attempted in neonates and children with mixed results.[29]

The true incidence of PE is not known but is likely considerably higher than reported in the literature. PE accounts for 17% of pediatric VTE and in the presence of DVT, the incidence varies between 30 to 60%. Mortality directly attributable to PE occurred in 2.2% of children.[29]The available options for treatment of PE are anticoagulation, thrombolysis, or surgery.[30] Clinical trials on the management of PE in children have not been completed, so guidelines are extrapolated from studies done in adults. In children older than 2 mths of age without inherited coagulation disorders, anticoagulation for 6 mths after the thrombotic episode is recommended. Children with hereditary coagulation disorders and pulmonary embolus should be placed on lifelong anticoagulation. Surgical placement of an inferior vena cava (IVC) filter should be considered in larger patients with DVT and any contraindication to anticoagulation. Consideration of catheter-directed thrombolytic therapy is appropriate for pulmonary embolism with hemodynamic compromise and severely symptomatic large proximal venous thrombosis. Pulmonary artery embolectomy must be considered on an individualized basis.

Inherited anomalies of the coagulation system predispose infants and children to thrombotic and thromboembolic disease. However, the impact of these coagulation disorders on VTE in children remains unclear. The most frequent coagulation disordes found with VTE include Factor V Leiden (4.7–13%), Prothrombin gene mutation (2–3%), Antithrombin deficiency (1%), Protein C/S deficiency (1%). Less common are primary antiphospholipid syndrome, presence of lupus anticoagulant, hyperhomocysteinemia, and familial hyperlipidemia. Thrombotic disorders were also associated with significant risk of VTE recurrence.[31] Infants with homozygous protein C or S deficiency require lifelong anticoagulation. Other thrombotic disorders should be considered for prophylactic anticoagulation in high risk situations.

The post-thrombotic syndrome (PTS), the development of chronic venous insufficiency after acute DVT due to residual thrombus and venous fibrosis, commonly occurs despite adequate anticoagulation.[32] Although not as common as in adults, PTS is seen in up to one third of children with prior VTE.[33] In patients with congenital peripheral venous abnormalities, complications are seen at a younger age than that of the general population. Symptoms include pain, swelling, stasis pigmentation, and ulcers of the affected limb. Unlike adults, the American College of Chest Physicians make no recommendation for thrombolysis after DVT in prevention of PTS.[29] Judicious use of central venous catheters is the best method yet known for reducing the incidence of VTE and preventing PTS in children.

Primary venous thrombosis of the upper extremity most commonly occurs as a result of thoracic outlet syndrome. Venous thoracic outlet syndrome (Paget–von Schroetter syndrome, Effort thrombosis) may be caused by compression of the vein between the first rib and clavicle with possible contributions from hypertrophied muscles or anomalous axillopectoral muscles. Effort thrombosis presents as pain or swelling usually in the dominant arm of male athletes and is not uncommon in adolescence. Without decompression of the thoracic outlet, endovascular techniques to open the vein (balloon angioplasty, stent placement) fare poorly due to fracture or stent deformation. Surgical decompression of the thoracic outlet is required with or without vein patch/bypass or subsequent endovascular venous interventions which then are more successful.

Renal vein thrombosis is the most common manifestation of thrombosis in the neonate and almost always accompanied by concurrent severe illness and genetic prothrombotic risk. The thrombosis starts at the level of intrarenal venules and is symptomatic (hematuria, thrombocytopenia) in more than 40% of cases. The prognosis remains grave among newborns with renal vein thrombosis (mortality ~ 10%). Treatment is supportive therapy and anticoagulation. Use of systemic thrombolytics is recommended only in cases of bilateral renal vein thrombosis with renal failure.[29]

Portal vein thrombosis is one of the most common causes of portal hypertension. Children present with sequelae of portal hypertension, such as gastrointestinal bleeding. Congenital malformations, malignancies, thrombophilia, umbilical vein catheterization, abdominal operations, sepsis and omphalitis in the neonatal period, and trauma are some of the potential causes of portal vein thrombosis. However, in up to 40% of cases, the etiology is unknown.[34] Treatment involves measures directed toward the portal vein thrombosis itself, the resulting portal hypertension, and its complications. Anticoagulation has proven to be effective in treatment of acute portal vein thrombosis. An endovascular or open portosystemic shunt may be considered depending on the child's age and anatomy.

REFERENCES

1. Tasnadi G. (1993) Epidemiology and etiology of congenital vascular malformations. *Semin Vasc Surg* **6**(4):200–203.
2. Eifert S, Villavicencio JL, Kao TC, *et al.* (2000) Prevalence of deep venous anomalies in congenital vascular malformations of venous predominance. *J Vasc Surg* **31**(3):462–471.
3. Lee BB, Laredo J, Lee TS, *et al.* (2007) Terminology and classification of congenital vascular malformations. *Phlebology* **22**(6):249–252.
4. Belov S. (1993) Anatomopathological classification of congenital vascular defects. *Semin Vasc Surg* **6**(4):219–224.
5. Lee BB. (2004) Critical issues in management of congenital vascular malformation. *Ann Vasc Surg* **18**(3):380–392.
6. Mulliken JB, Young AE. (1998) *Vascular Birthmarks: Hemangiomas and Malformations.* Saunders, Philadelphia.
7. Lee BB, Laredo J, Lee SJ, *et al.* (2007) Congenital vascular malformations: General diagnostic principles. *Phlebology* **22**(6):253–257.
8. Puig S, Aref H, Chigot V, *et al.* (2003) Classification of venous malformations in children and implications for sclerotherapy. *Pediatr Radiol* **33**(2):99–103.
9. Gillespie DL, Villavicencio JL, Gallagher C, *et al.* (1997) Presentation and management of venous aneurysms. *J Vasc Surg* **26**(5):845–852.

10. Sfyroeras GS, Antoniou GA, Drakou AA, *et al.* (2009) Visceral venous aneurysms: Clinical presentation, natural history and their management: A systematic review. *Eur J Vasc Endovasc Surg* **38**(4):498–505.
11. Calligaro KD, Ahmad S, Dandora R, *et al.* (1995) Venous aneurysms: Surgical indications and review of the literature. *Surgery* **117**(1):1–6.
12. Meissner MH, Gloviczki P, Bergan J, *et al.* (2007) Primary chronic venous disorders. *J Vasc Surg* **46** (Suppl S):54S–67S.
13. Lobo-Mueller E, Amaral JG, Babyn PS, *et al.* (2009) Complex combined vascular malformations and vascular malformation syndromes affecting the extremities in children. *Semin Musculoskelet Radiol* **13**(3):255–276.
14. Samuel M, Spitz L. (1995) Klippel–Trenaunay syndrome: Clinical features, complications and management in children. *Br J Surg* **82**(6):757–761.
15. Gloviczki P, Hollier LH, Telander RL, *et al.* (1983) Surgical implications of Klippel–Trenaunay syndrome. *Ann Surg* **197**(3):353–362.
16. Noel AA, Gloviczki P, Cherry KJ, Jr, *et al.* (2000) Surgical treatment of venous malformations in Klippel–Trenaunay syndrome. *J Vasc Surg* **32**(5):840–847.
17. Lee BB, Bergan JJ. (2002) Advanced management of congenital vascular malformations: A multidisciplinary approach. *Cardiovasc Surg* **10**(6):523–533.
18. White RI, Jr., Pollak J, Persing J, *et al.* (2000) Long-term outcome of embolotherapy and surgery for high-flow extremity arteriovenous malformations. *J Vasc Interv Radiol* **11**(10):1285–1295.
19. Lee BB, Kim DI, Huh S, *et al.* (2001) New experiences with absolute ethanol sclerotherapy in the management of a complex form of congenital venous malformation. *J Vasc Surg* **33**(4):764–772.
20. Rosenblatt M. (2007) Endovascular management of venous malformations. *Phlebology* **22**(6):264–275.
21. Loose DA. (1993) Surgical treatment of predominantly venous defects. *Semin Vasc Surg* **6**(4):252–259.
22. Stein PD, Kayali F, Olson RE. (2004) Incidence of venous thromboembolism in infants and children: Data from the National Hospital Discharge Survey. *J Pediatr* **145**(4):563–565.
23. Andrew M, David M, Adams M, *et al.* (1994) Venous thromboembolic complications (VTE) in children: First analyses of the Canadian Registry of VTE. *Blood* **83**(5):1251–1257.
24. van Ommen CH, Heijboer H, Buller HR, *et al.* (2001) Venous thromboembolism in childhood: A prospective two-year registry in The Netherlands. *J Pediatr* **139**(5):676–681.

25. Sandoval JA, Sheehan MP, Stonerock CE, *et al.* (2008) Incidence, risk factors, and treatment patterns for deep venous thrombosis in hospitalized children: An increasing population at risk. *J Vasc Surg* **47**(4):837–843.
26. Kuhle S, Massicotte P, Chan A, *et al.* (2004) Systemic thromboembolism in children. Data from the 1–800-NO-CLOTS Consultation Service. *Thromb Haemost* **92**(4):722–728.
27. Glaser DW, Medeiros D, Rollins N, *et al.* (2001) Catheter-related thrombosis in children with cancer. *J Pediatr* **138**(2):255–259.
28. Journeycake JM, Buchanan GR. (2006) Catheter-related deep venous thrombosis and other catheter complications in children with cancer. *J Clin Oncol* **24**(28):4575–4580.
29. Monagle P, Chalmers E, Chan A, *et al.* (2008) Antithrombotic therapy in neonates and children: American College of Chest Physicians Evidence-Based Clinical Practice Guidelines (8th Edition). *Chest* **133**(6 Suppl):887S–968S.
30. Babyn PS, Gahunia HK, Massicotte P. (2005) Pulmonary thromboembolism in children. *Pediatr Radiol* **35**(3):258–274.
31. Goldenberg NA, Knapp-Clevenger R, Manco-Johnson MJ. (2004) Elevated plasma factor VIII and D-dimer levels as predictors of poor outcomes of thrombosis in children. *N Engl J Med* **351**(11):1081–1088.
32. Meissner MH, Eklof B, Smith PC, *et al.* (2007) Secondary chronic venous disorders. *J Vasc Surg* **46** (Suppl S):68S–83S.
33. Goldenberg NA. (2005) Long-term outcomes of venous thrombosis in children. *Curr Opin Hematol* **12**(5):370–376.
34. Sarin SK, Agarwal SR. (2002) Extrahepatic portal vein obstruction. *Semin Liver Dis* **22**(1):43–58.

LYMPHATIC DISORDERS 82

Scott A. Engum

LYMPHEDEMA

Clinical Presentation

The epidemiology of lymphedema has received little attention and the number of children suffering is unknown with the situation compounded further by a general lack of professional awareness and knowledge. It is an abnormal collection of interstitial lymph fluid due to either congenital maldevelopment of the lymphatics or secondary lymphatic obstruction.

The most common cause is a primary congenital abnormality affecting the lymphatics of the lower extremities. In Milroy's disease, one notes congenital onset of swelling with large caliber leg veins (23%), hydrocele in men (37%), and family history of the disease.

Other causes of lower limb lymphedema include chronic infection, filariasis, insect bites, neoplasms, inguinal or axillary surgery, irradiation, and trauma. Unilateral leg swelling can arise from a retroperitoneal tumor or lymphoma compressing the veins. In addition, lymphedema can occur in patients with chronic diseases such as spina-bifid, rheumatoid arthritis and stroke. Children may develop this condition as a part of other disorders such as Turner's syndrome.

Incidence

Lymphedema is recognized as a major health care problem affecting 1.3/1000 general population. Primary lymphedema occurs predominantly in girls (65%). Milroy's disease affects boys and girls equally. Affected families have single nucleotide substitutions at the chromosomal locus 5q35.3.

Classification

Primary lymphedema has three categories that are based on age and onset. Congenital lymphedema is usually present at birth, while lymphedema praecox appears in early adolescence and may be influenced by hormonal factors. Lymphedema tarda occurs spontaneously in middle age (>30 yrs). Lymphatic impairment can be genetically inherited such as Milroy's congenital familial lymphedema which accounts for less than 2% of all cases and is asscociated with an autosomal inheritance of a single gene. The location of a gene responsible for at least some cases of the disorder was discovered on chromosome 5q35.3, and the mutated gene identified as coding for vascular endothelial growth factor receptor 3.

At the pediatric age, secondary lymphedema is mainly caused by inflammatory or traumatic injuries. Obstructive mechanisms (pelvic tumor, compressive lymph nodes) are less frequent than in the adult population. In developing countries, secondary lymphedema is most frequently caused by lymphatic filariasis.

Pathology

The underlying pathology in most cases is an absence (aplasia) or hypoplasia of the subcutaneous lymphatic channels. With hypoplasia, lymph nodes and vessels are small and few in number. Hormonal factors have been implicated and are involved in lymphedema praecox. The system is divided into a valveless superficial system and a valved deep system. Fluid pools in the subcutaneous tissues and production exceeds drainage capabilities. The protein rich fluid increases the oncotic pressure and worsens the edema. The deep system beneath the *fascia* and in the muscle component is separate and unaffected.

Diagnosis

For many parents, the realization that their child has lymphedema is an insidious one. What appears to be a small swelling of one of the limbs of their child is often dismissed by professionals with a lack of knowledge and skills and the lesion is attributed to other cause such as trauma. For others, the condition may be recognized during an ultrasound examination during pregnancy. For many families, there is a considerable delay before a correct diagnosis and treatment is offered for this condition.

Diagnosis is usually made clinically. Noninvasive Doppler studies and plethysmography can rule out arterial or venous disease. Radionuclide imaging using technetium 99m sulfur colloid after subcutaneous injection usually demonstrates lymphatic channels and sites of obstruction. Ninety percent of children have hypoplasia of the superficial lymphatics with distal rather than proximal involvement. An Magnetic Resonance Imaging (MRI) may be of value in differentiating disease processes.

Unilateral leg swelling can arise from a retroperitoneal tumor or lymphoma compressing the veins. Bilateral lower extremity edema should lead to an evaluation to exclude causes of hypoalbuminemia, (nephritic syndrome, venous obstruction) while upper extremity edema is unusual in children.

Surgical Management

In the event of lower extremity disease, the initial treatment requires attentive foot care and hygiene. It is important to use antibiotics to treat and prevent cellulitis. If suspected, topical antifungal therapy may be warranted. Weight control and loss is of benefit, however, diuretics do not play a role in therapy. Warfarin has been shown to decrease edema volume by as much as 50% by what is postulated to be its stimulatory effect on cutaneous macrophages and protein absorption is unknown. Prolonged standing without compression accelerates accumulation, where exercise slows the process. The patient should wear compression stockings during the day and keep legs elevated at night to reduce swelling.

The management of genital lymphedema is challenging. There are three options which involve conservative measures such as elevation, diuretics, and compressive devices. For primary lymphedema, these techniques have been generally unsuccessful. Lymphangioplasty may be performed in an attempt to reconstitute or bypass the diseased lymphatic glands and is most applicable in the cases of secondary lymphedema. The option most frequently elected for primary lymphedema is excision of all lymphedematous tissue.

Complications

Primary complications involve persistent swelling, brawny edema with skin thickening and discoloration, cellulitis, and lymphangitis. Children frequently suffer from veruccas and infections secondary to in-growing toe nails. Access to services such as podiatry is important. Making sure families have access to adequate supply of hosiery is critical. Provisions of shoes are a major challenge for parents and children and if a facility is making orthotics, this can take significant time to accomplish. Sporting activities can be a constant challenge as one needs staff available to take off or reapply hosiery after activities and some schools do not actively embrace children with disabilities. Lastly, parents live in constant tension between giving the child freedom to undertake normal childhood activities and the fear of harm from injury or infection.

LYMPHANGIOMA

Clinical Presentation

Lymphatic malformations account for approximately 5% of all benign neoplasms in infants and children. These tumors typically appear in children younger than 2 yrs (90%). In a significant number of cases they are already present at birth (50%).

Lymphangiomas are congenital lesions that are characterized by multiple communicating lymphatic channels and cystic spaces which can occur anywhere on the body, but most frequently in the head, neck, axilla, and oral cavity. The natural history is the presence of a mass with a variable growth rate. One typically sees slow progression; however, one can see rapid growth or engorgement with lymph or blood when associated with direct infection, trauma or a secondary respiratory or skin infection. Spontaneous regression is unlikely with most enlarging and occasionally extending into adjacent structures. Most involve the skin and subcutaneous tissues and can be associated with venous malformations. These lesions may occur with disfigurement, dysphagia, dysphonia, and dyspnea. Lingual lesions can cause obstruction, bleeding, pain, feeding problems, edema, lingual extorsion, dental problems, breathing problems, and jaw deformities. The introduction of prenatal ultrasound has allowed for the *in utero* detection of this disease process in a high percentage of infants.

Incidence

The incidence of lymphangiomas has been reported to range from 1.2 to 2.8/1000 newborns. The international incidence has been approximated to be anywhere from 1 in 6000 to 1 in 16,000 live births. No racial or sexual predilections have been demonstrated.

Classification

Lymphangiomas have been classified as microcystic (capillary lymphangiomas), macrocystic (cavernous lymphangiomas) and cystic hygromas according to the size of the lymphatic cavities incorporated. A commonly used classification classifies these lesions into capillary lymphangioma/ lymphangioma simplex, cavernous lymphangioma, and cystic lymphagioma/ cystic hygroma.

When a lymphangioma is confined to fairly dense tissue, such as the tongue and floor of mouth, it presents as a cavernous lymphangioma. Cystic lymphangioma (cystic hygroma) are usually soft and compressible and will transilluminate when a light is applied. These lesions may occur anywhere on the body, but are more common in the neck, axilla, mediastinum, and groin and account for approximately 90% of the lymphangiomas in the head and neck region. They arise from lymphatic tissue in areas where expansion can occur and large multi-loculated cystic spaces can develop. These lesions can be singular, but most have multiple noncommunicating loculations.

Pathology

During the embryonic development, blood vessels originate from mesodermally derived endothelial cell precursors (vasculogenesis). These vessels grow and remodel into mature network by endothelial sprouting and splitting (angiogenesis). The lymphatic vasculature appears after the blood vasculature forms, which was the first indication that lymphatics might have a blood vasculature origin. The lymphatic system is composed of a vascular network of blind-ended, thin-walled capillaries and larger vessels that drain protein-rich interstitial fluid (lymph) from the extracellular spaces within organs into larger collecting ducts. The lymphatic system is crucial for maintaining the colloid osmotic volume (or pressure).

Three theories have been proposed to explain the origin of lymphangiomas. One suggests that a blockage or arrest of normal growth of the primitive lymph channels occurs during embryogenesis. Other postulates that the primitive lymphatic sacs do not reach the venous system. Lastly, some believe that during embryogenesis, the lymphatic tissue lies in the wrong area.

Histologically, these lesions are composed of dilated lymphatic channels with one or two endothelial layers, with or without an adventitial layer. These dilated lymphatics can vary in size depending on the location and surrounding tissue.

Diagnosis

The most prominent sign or symptom of all lymphangiomas is the presence of a mass. The mass may be small and not noticed at birth only to present later. Most lesions are recognized early on because of symptoms related to respiratory obstruction or problems with feeding. Difficulty swallowing can be due to extension of the lesion into the oral cavity or oropharynx. Isolated tongue disease can lead to macroglossia and have associated dysfagioa or even airway obstruction.

A physical examination is the primary method of diagnosis. There is usually a soft, compressible, loculated and ill-defined mass. The lesions are not attached to the skin and readily transilluminates. Ultrasound may be used to confirm as it provides size and extension of the lesion. If extension of the lesion is noted into deeper structures, a Computed Tomography (CT) scan with contrast can show the full extent of the lesion. An MRI is not uncommon, especially with complex vascular lesions that involve the lymphatic system or an extremity.

Surgical Management

Surgical resection still remains the best treatment for lymphangiomas. Indications for treatment include disfigurement, large size, chronic leakage of lymph fluid, and frequent infections. Whenever possible, a lymphagioma should be completely excised, although staged resection may be necessary. It is rarely possible to completely excise this type of lesion unless it is a cystic hygroma and vital structures should not be compromised due to the benign nature of these lesions. Infiltrative lesions usually splay out and surround nerve branches. Dissection may be lengthy and technically tedious. When the lesion extends into deep and vital structures, the major portion of the lesion should be removed.

Treatment of unresectable lesions has been accomplished with percutaneous sclerotherapy to reduce the impact and complications of surgery. Various products, such as sodium morrhuate, 50% dextrose, tetracycline, doxycycline, bleomycin, ethibloc, alcohol and OK-432 have been used as sclerotherapeutic agents. Intralesional injection of OK-432, a monoclonal antibody, has shown a response rate upward of 60%. Apart from OK-432, the other agents have been reported to cause perilesional fibrosis and may complicate eventual surgical excision. Giant lymphangiomas of the head and neck with significant microcystic components have had challenged responses to injection therapy.

A systematic review demonstrates a high level of effectiveness for the nonsurgical treatment of lymphatic malformations with the use of percutaneous sclerotherapy. The most experience was reported with OK-432 and bleomycin, with both producing good to excellent responses in a majority of patients.

Lingual localization present specific therapeutic problems because of the almost exclusively microcystic character of the lesion and the marked functional problems they cause. Complete surgical exeresis is not possible because of the unacceptable degree of mutilation it would entail. Partial glossectomy is a serious operation with a high rate of relapse or secondary growth and often results in a morphological modification of the tongue with postoperative painful healing that is relatively long and thus sclerotherapy and the use of low radiofrequency treatment are primary options.

Complications

The most common complication of lymphangioma is recurrent bouts of inflammation. Lymphangitis can be noted with swelling, pain, and cellulitis. With each bout of infection, the lesion develops fibrosis. It is not uncommon to have rupture of the cutaneous cyst with associated leakage of the lymphatic fluid and blood. Streptococcal and staphylococcal organisms can cause a rapidly progressive cellulitis and require prompt treatment.

Complications are more common in lesions involving the midline. Recurrence rates vary depending upon the complexity of the lesion and the completeness of the excision. Simple hygromas that are completely excised seldom recur. Complex lesions that are completely excised might recur in 10–27%, whereas partially resected lesions may recur in 50–100%. Persistent involvement of the skin may result in recurrence or weeping cutaneous lesions.

Major complications from sclerotherapy are infrequent, however, there has been report of pulmonary complications as a result of bleomycin therapy.

LYMPHANGIECTASIA

Clinical Presentation

Lymphangiectasia can affect multiple organs and tissues including the intestine, lung, and bone. Intestinal lesions occur in children younger than 3 yrs and presents with diarrhea, vomiting, growth failure, and a protein-losing enteropathy. The degree of protein loss may range from mild to severe. Fat absorption can also be affected. Lymphopenia and hypoproteinemia are commonly present. One can see coexistent pitting edema of the lower extremities.

Pulmonary lymphangiectasia may be present with respiratory distress in the newborn or in infancy with obstruction of lymphatics draining the lung. This obstruction leads to pulmonary edema (diffusely affected) and pleural effusion (usually bilateral). This condition can be associated with congenital heart disease. Some infants may have spontaneous resolution; however, most progress rapidly to fatal respiratory failure. Clubbing, dyspnea, and hemoptysis may be noted.

Bone lymphangiectasia is often associated pain, along with a deformity or pathologic fracture. Lesions can be seen in most bones except the skull and digits. This can coexist with other lymphangiomas. These lesions gradually increase in size and eventually destroy the bone and can lead to collapse of the bone structure.

Classification

Pulmonary lymphangiectasia can be divided into three groups: generalized lymphangiectasia, pulmonary venous obstruction with secondary lymphangiectasia, and primary pulmonary lymphatic development anomaly. Others have placed the cases into two categories, cardiac and non cardiac. In the generalized form, associated intestinal lymphangiectasia, hemi hypertrophy, and angiomatosis are seen. The pulmonary disease is less severe, and children have a better prognosis. In children with pulmonary lymphangiectasia associated with congenital heart disease, the cardiac anomalies are characterized by obstruction of the pulmonary venous return and by pulmonary venous hypertension. Primary congenital pulmonary lymphangiectasia that is isolated without other heart or lymphatic abnormalities is thought to be caused by primary failure of normal regression of the pulmonary lymphatics after the 16th week of gestation. This group has the highest perinatal mortality.

Intestinal lymphangiectasia is classified as primary when the dilation is related to a disorder of the lymph vessels or secondary due to obstruction of the lymph flow through the mesenteric lymph channels.

Pathology

The bowel histology shows dilatation of lymphatic channels in the intestinal villi, with obstruction in the lamina propria alone; more generalized involvement of the lamina propria, submucosal, serosa, and mesentery; or, occasionally, involvement of the mesentery alone.

Congenital pulmonary lymphangiectasia has subpleural, interlobar, perivascular, and peribronchial lymphatic dilation.

Diagnosis

Intestinal lymphangiectasia can result from many diverse pathologic processes, ranging from congestive heart failure and lymphoma to Crohn's disease and retroperitoneal fibrosis. Primary lymphangiectasia is less well understood and if the involved area is within the reach of the endoscope, a biopsy can be diagnostic. Otherwise, lymphangiography or surgery may be required for diagnosis. Recently, video capsule endoscopy and wireless capsule endoscopy have been utilized to easily view the mucosa of the entire small bowel and to make an educated guess based on gross appearance, and to exclude other disorders. The diagnosis is made by small bowel mucosal biopsy.

In pulmonary lymphangiectasia, the chest radiograph may show interstitial fluid and a pleural effusion. The typical radiographic findings are bilateral pulmonary hyperinflation and reticulonodular increased interstitial markings. The increased interstitial markings likely represent dilated pulmonary lymphatics. The diagnosis of congenital pulmonary lymphangiectasia is difficult, often being made at autopsy. The differential diagnosis includes causes of both nonimmune hydrops and congenital chylothorax. It is not uncommon to have pleural fluid output of greater than 150 mL/kg/day in the first week of life. Although definitive diagnosis can be made on lung biopsy, there are no definitive criteria as to when this procedure should be performed. If surgical intervention is performed to manage persistent drainage from a chylothorax, a biopsy should be performed at that time. High resolution CT offers an accurate noninvasive means to diagnosis this condition. One will see smooth, thickened intralobular septa which contain dilated pulmonary lymphatics and with the clinical presentation, the diagnosis can usually be made.

The diagnosis of bone lesion is usually confirmed by radiograph and subsequent biopsy to rule out other lesions.

Surgical Management

Treatment of intestinal lymphangiectasia includes a high-protein, low-fat diet with the addition of medium-chain triglycerides and vitamin supplements. This disease process is usually too extensive for surgical resection. Interferon alpha has been used with variable effects.

Pulmonary lymphangiectasia treatment in the newborn period is supportive, including prompt recognition of respiratory failure, assisted ventilation, surfactant administration, pleural decompression, and replacement of fluid and protein losses. Use of high mean airway pressure was suggested to assist in controlling effusions. Nutritional support consists of total parenteral nutrition, and when pleural drainage ceases, gradual introduction of a low-fat, high-protein diet involving a medium-chain triglyceride formula. Methods of pleurodesis may prevent the reaccumulation of fluid. Unfortunately, the outcome in congenital pulmonary lymphangiectasia is uniformly fatal.

There is no specific treatment for diffuse lymphangiectasia of the bone, although some have used curettage and autologous bone chips to fill the defect.

CHYLOUS ASCITES

Clinical Presentation

This is a rare clinical condition that occurs as a result of disruption of the abdominal lymphatics with associated extravasations of milky chyle into the peritoneal cavity. There are multiple causes of this condition and include abdominal surgery, blunt abdominal trauma, malignant neoplasm, spontaneous bacterial peritonitis, cirrhosis, pelvic irradiation, peritoneal dialysis, abdominal tuberculosis, carcinoid syndrome, and congenital defects of lacteal formation.

In children, the most common causes are congenital abnormalities, such as lymphangiectasia, mesenteric cyst, and idiopathic "leaky lymphatics." Neoplasia is an uncommon cause. Abdominal distension is the most common symptom in patients with chylous ascites and unfortunately, this disease process can be unrelenting and fatal due to malnutrition, hypoproteinemia, dehydration, and sepsis.

Incidence

Early studies reported an incidence of 1 case per 187,000 adult hospital admissions. However, with more aggressive retroperitoneal and cardiothoracic surgical procedures, the incidence has increased to 1 case in 11,000 adult hospital admissions; however, the pediatric data is limited. This condition has no difference in sex distribution and can occur in children of all age groups, although most are infants and toddlers.

Classification

The disease process is divided into three groups with (1) true chylous ascites where the fluid has a high triglyceride content, (2) chyliform ascites where the fluid has lecithin-globulin complex due to fatty degeneration of cells, and (3) Pseudochylous ascites where the fluid is milky in appearance due to the presence of purulent material.

Pathology

The most common cause (45–60% of cases) is idiopathic and in the pediatric patient population, usually a result of aplastic, hypoplastic, or absent connections between the mesenteric lymphatic and the thoracic duct. It is most likely a manifestation of generalized hypoplasia of the lymphatic system, with reflux of chyle into the intestinal lymphatics. Rupture of enlarged intestinal lymphatics into the intestinal lumen can occur, with subsequent enteral loss of protein and fat. This can also occur with chyluria with rupture into the renal pelvis.

The next most common cause is thought to be related to obstruction of lymphatic channels by conditions such as intussusception, malrotation, incarcerated hernia, primary or metastatic cancer, tuberculosis, gastroschisis, and inflammatory lesions causing nodal enlargement.

Lastly, injury to the lymphatics is responsible for an additional 15–20% of cases.

Diagnosis

In addition to abdominal distention, patients may complain of abdominal pain, respiratory compromise, anorexia, weight loss, edema, weakness, nausea, dyspnea, weight gain, lymphadenopathy, fever, diarrhea, inguinal hernia, and night sweats. Routine laboratory evaluation may show hypoalbuminemia, lymphocytopenia, hyponatremia, anemia, and it is not uncommon to see a normal triglyceride level.

The diagnosis is made by peritoneocentesis and analysis of the ascetic fluid. The fluid will usually be white or milky with a triglyceride level that is greater than 110 mg/dL. One will likely see an elevated leukocyte count within the fluid and a marked lymphocytic predominance (70–90%). One may also see an elevated cholesterol and total protein concentration within the fluid. When cultured, there is no bacterial growth.

Determining the cause of chylous ascites can be challenging and studies such as ultrasound, CT, and gastrointestinal contrast studies may be helpful. Lymphangiography is described, however, difficult to perform in children and may not add much to the treatment strategy.

When a neoplasm is considered, a CT scan of the abdomen and pelvis, lymph node biopsy, and possible laparoscopy/laparotomy carry the highest yield of diagnostic information.

Surgical Management

Treatment consists of a low-fat or medium-chain triglyceride, high-protein enteral diet. Repeated paracentesis may be required to improve comfort for the patient. If the chylous ascites persists despite dietary management changes, bowel rest and total perenteral nutrition is instituted. There are case reports describing the use of octreotide, a somatostatin analog, in the management of chylous ascites as somatostatin receptors have been described in the lymphatic vessels of the intestine.

Surgical intervention is warranted if nonoperative therapy is not successful after 6 wks. Identification and ligation of the leak is curative in 85% of patients. Peritoneovenous shunting has been used successfully in a small number of patients, however, shunt failure is not uncommon.

In the event there is a correctable lesion is identified such as malrotation, intussusception, mesenteric cyst, or incarcerated hernia, these should be dealt with expeditiously. If a postsurgical lymphatic leak is identified and the site is known, early reoperation is indicated and the use of preoperative ingested butter or cream will aid in finding the leak.

Malignant chylous ascites requires therapy directed at the primary cause and this may include laparotomy with biopsy of lesion, ligation of leaking lymphatic, resection of small bowel segment, and removal of obstructing tumor. In addition, chemotherapy and radiation treatment may be required.

CHYLOTHORAX

Clinical Presentation

Chylothorax is the accumulation of chyle-containing lymphatic fluid within one or both pleural spaces. This condition is the most common form of pleural effusion in the first few days of life with 50% of newborns developing symptoms within 24 hrs of birth. Birth trauma was formerly thought to be the cause of many neonatal chylothoraces, but the increasing use of prenatal ultrasonography has changed the perspective as this condition has been noted prior to delivery. In the neonate, whether acquired or congenital present a clinical challenge.

Chyle causes symptoms related to respiratory compromise secondary to compression of the lung from the pleural effusion leading to progressive pulmonary insufficiency, nutritional failure, immunologic depletion contributing to sepsis, metabolic acidosis, and renal failure secondary to the loss of fats, protein, and lymphocytes. Associated anomalies include trisomy 21 syndrome, Noonan syndrome, congenital pulmonary lymphangiectasia, tracheoesophageal atresia, extralobar pulmonary sequestration, thoracic duct hypoplasia, and polyhydramnios.

Classification

Historically, chylothorax has been classified according to etiology. In the neonatal period it is usually categorized as either congenital (idiopathic) caused by lymphatic malformation, or acquired, which is typically postoperative due to trauma (surgical or birth related). Chylothorax in older children is rarely spontaneous and occurs almost invariably after trauma or cardiothoracic surgery; however, some patients with thoracic lymphangioma may present in this older age group.

Pathology

The thoracic duct develops from outgrowths of the jugular lymphatic sacs and the cisterna chyli. During embryonic life, bilateral thoracic lymphatic channels are present, however; the upper third of the left and the lower two thirds of the right persist. The thoracic duct originates in the abdomen at the cisterna chyli located over the second lumbar vertebra. The duct then extends into the right thorax and posterior mediatstinum before shifting toward the left at the level of the fifth thoracic vertebra. From this location it ascends into the posterior left neck to the junction of the subclavian and internal jugular veins. The chyle contained in the thoracic duct conveys approximately three fourths of the ingested fat from the intestine to the systemic circulation.

Chylothorax can occur because of overproduction of chyle, failure of communication of the lymphatic vessels, minimal reabsorption of lymph, abnormalities of the pulmonary lymphatics, or injury in the newborn during a difficult delivery. Chyle has classically been described as a white, milky, or opalescent appearing fluid; however, this characteristic color is seen in less than one half of patients with a chylous effusion.

Diagnosis

The fluid may have one or more of the following inclusion criteria: (1) a pleural fluid triglyceride level of 110 mg/dL or greater, (2) the presence of chylomicrons in the pleural effusion that stain for fat, or (3) a chylous leak into the pleural cavity documented on lymphangiography or during surgery. If a cell count of the fluid is performed, typically there are more than 60% lymphocytes and is diagnostic of chylothorax. The protein content averages 40 g/L and the electrolyte and glucose levels match that of plasma levels.

Surgical Management

Patients are initially treated with restriction of dietary fats using total parenteral nutrition or enterally administered medium-chain triglycerides.

Drainage of the pleural fluid is accomplished either by thoracentesis or tube thoracostomy. In most cases, these simple measures are successful. Opinions vary on how long to continue nonoperative management; however, if drainage persists at 50 mL/kg/day, an attempt at surgical therapy should be considered.

Surgical therapy is undertaken with the goal to relieve the respiratory embarrassment with drainage of the pleural space and allowing the lung to reexpand, followed by minimizing the loss of the nutritional elements and immunologic cells present in chyle. The surgical options for refractory chylothorax include chemical pleurodesis, apical pleurectomy, thoracotomy with thoracic duct ligation, thoracoscopy, and the use of a pleuroperitoneal shunt.

Thoracotomy with thoracic duct ligation remains a major procedure in an already compromised neonate. When performed, use of cream before surgery is helpful in identifying the site of the leak and ligation above and below the leak is effective in most cases. Apical pleurectomy or pleurodesis increases the possibility of pulmonary lymphedema, fibrosis, and further pulmonary demise. Video-assisted procedures are becoming more popular; however, the infant's size and pulmonary status may limit it use. Because of the limited treatment options, the use of a pleuroperitoneal shunt has been very attractive due to it ease of performance and limited postoperative complications.

Outcome

Nutritional complications were a major source of mortality from chylothorax in the era proceeding parenteral nutrition. Loss of lymphocytes through a thoracic duct fistula may lead to an immunocompromised state. Chyle appears to have a bacteriostatic property, which accounts for the rare occurrence of infection complicating chylothorax. Overall, most patients with chylothorax can be cured with conservative measures, nutritional support, and occasional operative intervention. Patients with diffuse lymphatic malformations remain a challenge.

REFERENCES

1. Engum SA, Rescorla FJ, West KW, *et al.* (1999) The use of pleuroperitoneal shunts in the management of persistent chylothorax in infants. *J Pediatr Surg* **34**:286–290.

2. Caserio S, Gallego C, Martin P, *et al.* (2010) Congenital chylothorax: From fetal life to adolescence. *Acta Pediatrica* **99**:1571–1577.
3. Das A, Shah PS. (2010) Octreotide for the treatment of chylothorax in neonates. *Cochrane Db Syst Rev* **9**.
4. Gellini C, Boccardo F, Corradino C, *et al.* (2008) Lymphatic dysplasias in newborns and children: The role of lymphoscintigraphy. *J Pediatr* **152**:587–589.
5. Moffatt CJ, Murray SG. (2010) The experience of children and families with lymphedema — a journey within a journey. *Int Wound* **7**:14–26.
6. Saijo M, Munro IR, Manger K. (1975) Lymphangioma: A long-term follow-up study. *Plastic Recontr Surg* **56**:642–651.
7. Karago BS, Zenciroglui A, Gokce S, *et al.* (2010) Therapeutic management of neonatal chylous ascites: Report of a case and review of the literature. *Acta Pediatr* **99**:1307–1310.
8. Cochran WJ, Klish WJ, Brown MR, *et al.* (1985) Chylous ascites in infants and children: A case report and literature review. *J Pediatr Gastro and Nutr* **4**:668–673.
9. Burrows PE, Mitri RK, Alomari A, *et al.* (2008) Percutaneous sclerotherapy of lymphatic malformations with doxycycline. *Lymphatic Research and Biology* **6**:209–216.
10. Boardman SJ, Cochrane LA, Roebuck D, *et al.* (2010) Multimodality treatment of pediatric lymphatic malformations of the head and neck using surgery and sclerotherapy. *Head and Neck Surg* **136**:270–276.
11. Harsha WJ, Perkins JA, Lewis CW, *et al.* (2005) Pediatric admissions and procedures for lymphatic malformations in the United States: 1997–2000. *Lymphatic Research and Biology* **3**:58–65.
12. Esther CR, Barker PM. (2004) Pulmonary lymphangiectasia: Diagnosis and clinical course. *Pediatr Pulm* **38**:308–313.
13. Bouchard S, Di Lorenzo M, Youssef S, *et al.* (2000) Pulmonary lymphangiectasia revisited. *J Pediatr Surg* **35**:796–800.

Section 11: Special Considerations

CONGENITAL HEART DISEASE

83

Mark Rodefeld

CLINICAL PRESENTATION

Congenital heart disease is frequently encountered by the physician caring for children. Diagnosis is typically made shortly after birth when dynamic changes in circulatory status occur. With prenatal screening, fetal diagnosis of cardiac disease is becoming much more common. Infrequently, an infant or child will present at a later age with occult congenital heart disease. Surgical treatment of congenital heart disease has improved markedly since the advent of cardiopulmonary bypass in 1953; mortality of repair is now less than 5% for all categories combined. Although the spectrum of defects can be morphologically classified into 37 individually recognized categories, many can be subclassified into groups which share similar clinical presentation and management. In this chapter, general considerations are discussed with a focus on issues germane to the pediatric general surgeon encountering these patients. Special consideration is given to single ventricle patients who represent an increasingly common and high-risk group, and who require complex and paradoxical management strategies.

PATHOPHYSIOLOGY

Incidence/Epidemiology

Congenital heart defects are the most common defects of birth. They are estimated to occur in 0.5–1.25% of live births. Genetic factors may be responsible, although most defects are felt to be due to a malformation during embryogenesis. The most serious form is Hypoplastic Left Heart Syndrome in which the left ventricle fails to form: It is the leading cause of death from any birth defect in the first year of life. Single ventricle disease is the fifth most common diagnosis at centers treating infants with congenital heart disease, and constitutes the most enigmatic, high-risk patient population encountered in a children's hospital. With improvement in medical and surgical management, for the first time ever, there are now more adults alive with congenital heart disease than children.

Embryology

Cardiac development begins as cardiac tube formation. In early gestation, the tube undergoes a complex series of folds with rotation and septation to arrive at the final cardiac morphology. Disruptions in this process result in a variety of anomalies seen clinically. The physiologic circumstances of fetal life allow these anomalies to exist to term where they may have had no prior hemodynamic consequence. Postnatally, however, marked physiologic shifts unmask their appearance. The perinatal shifts which are most significant include expansion of the lungs, marked increase in pulmonary blood flow, closure of the foramen ovale, and oxygen-mediated closure of the ductus arteriosus. Fetal intervention to ameliorate term expression of cardiac disease has been investigated in depth, but clinically meaningful fetal intervention is not yet integrated into practice at this time.

Pathology/Classification

Congenital heart defects have been historically classified into cyanotic and acyanotic groups (Table 1). While this is helpful, more current classification schemes consider each defect based on its particular anatomy and physiologic behavior. For many defects, early repair is preferable to avoid damaging consequences of unchecked maladaptive pathophysiology. This especially

Table 1. Representative cardiac lesions.

Cyanotic	**Acyanotic**
Tetralogy of Fallot	Ventricular Septal defect
Transposition of the great arteries	Atrial septal defect
Tricuspid atresia	Atrioventricular Canal
Total anomalous pulmonary venous return	Patent ductus arteriosus
Truncus arteriosus	Aortic stenosis
Hypoplastic left heart syndrome	Pulmonic stenosis
Ebstein's anomaly	Coarctation of the aorta

applies to defects in which pulmonary overcirculation is a predominant component. Left unchecked, pulmonary overcirculation will induce hypertensive pulmonary vasculopathy which can complicate efforts at subsequent physiologic repair and impact quality and duration of life. On the other hand, pulmonary undercirculation — manifesting as severe hypoxemia — may require urgent intervention. Prostaglandin infusions have moderated this problem to a great extent. Ductal patency can be maintained in the neonatal period until a definitive source of pulmonary blood flow can be secured. In other cases, optimum timing for repair can be deferred to a later age.

A significant "other" category of heart defects comprises single ventricle defects, in which one of the ventricles (right or left) has failed to form in a way that will ever be functional. These children are committed to a palliative repair pathway known as staged Fontan palliation. In a series of staged operative procedures, the circulation is ultimately reconstructed to a single ventricle series circulation in which blood flow through the lungs and body is in a series arrangement, but there is no subpulmonary power source to drive pulmonary blood flow.

Associations

The majority of congenital heart disease is not associated with a syndromic cause — most occur as an isolated defect. Conversely, however, a number of syndromes are associated with concomitant congenital heart disease. Common genetic syndromes with a heart defect component include Down syndrome/trisomy 21 (atrioventricular canal), VACTERL syndrome (conotruncal anomalies: tetralogy of Fallot, transposition of the great vessels, truncus arteriosus), trisomy 13, Turner syndrome (aortic coarctation),

Williams syndrome (supravalvar aortic stenosis/pulmonary stenosis), Noonan syndrome, and Marfan syndrome. Other agents have been associated with increased incidence of congenital heart disease including drugs (retinoic acid), chemical toxicities, maternal alcohol abuse, and maternal infection (Rubella).

DIAGNOSIS/WORKUP

Once suspected, further evaluation should include a careful physical examination and assessment for the presence of other congenital disease. Three extremity blood pressure assessments may be diagnostic. Further workup, however, inevitably includes an echocardiographic evaluation. Nearly all congenital heart defects can be readily diagnosed with this noninvasive procedure which yields important anatomic and physiologic details which guide further management. Whether a cardiac catheterization is indicated depends on the defect in question, the chronicity of the defect, and the nature of the repair contemplated. In some cases, additional information is required including direct physiologic pressure, vascular resistance, and shunt calculations. The anatomic detail that an angiogram can provide may assist planning for optimal surgical repair. In the current era, repair of the majority of defects are safely based on echocardiography alone.

In left-to-right shunts, blood shunted to the right-sided circulation results in increased pulmonary blood flow, possibly at the expense of systemic perfusion. Patients may present with respiratory insufficiency and features of heart failure. Chest radiograph may show evidence of pulmonary vascular engorgement and cardiomegaly. Right heart chamber enlargement may be seen on echocardiogram. In right-to-left shunts, patients will present with variable degrees of cyanosis. Assessment of cardiac output may be difficult in the setting of shunts, but traditional markers of systemic perfusion — urine output, acid/base status, warmth, and capillary refill of extremities — are usually reliable.

MANAGEMENT

Preoperative

Principals of preoperative management of congenital heart disease vary markedly from other surgical lesions not involving the heart or lungs. As a general rule, patients who are being prepared to undergo surgical repair are preferably managed "dry". This optimizes their pulmonary status prior to repair, especially in cases with pulmonary overcirculation, and smoothes the intraoperative and early postoperative course. Other management issues often include maintenance of ductal patency with prostaglandins, and optimization of systemic perfusion, acid/base status, etc. Manipulation of ventilator status may be a key component of preoperative management. For example, patients with single ventricle are optimally managed on FiO_2 0.21 despite low systemic oxygen saturations. Pulmonary vascular resistance is acutely sensitive to variation in pO_2 and pCO_2 and this can be used advantageously in preoperative management and optimization prior to surgical repair. In transposition of the great vessels, a transvenous balloon atrial septostomy performed at bedside with echo guidance is often used to promote intracardiac mixing and improve systemic oxygen saturations prior to elective repair.

Surgical Considerations

Closed-heart repairs are typically performed via posterolateral thoracotomy. Common lesions repaired in this way include coarctation repair, patent ductus arteriosus ligation, pulmonary artery band placement (temporarily restrict pulmonary blood flow), or construction of a systemic-to-pulmonary artery shunt (temporarily increase pulmonary blood flow). Often, these procedures may be part of a staged approach prior to definitive intracardiac repair at a subsequent time. Open-heart repairs require cardiopulmonary bypass and are nearly always performed via median sternotomy. Several considerations of importance to the general surgeon are the presence of tunneled central venous lines exiting the skin on the anterior chest wall, and the location of gastrostomy tubes near the subcostal margin, both of which may increase risk of mediastinal contamination and mediastinitis. Patients are cooled systemically while on cardiopulmonary bypass (18–28°C depending on the magnitude of the repair), which is neuro- and cardio-protective. Topical hypothermia (4°C) is used for myocardial protection. Cardioplegic arrest is induced by hyperkalemic blood delivered to the coronary arterial system via the aortic root after placement of an aortic cross-clamp. Reversal of cardiac arrest is accomplished by removal of the cross-clamp, and reperfusion of the myocardium with normokalemic blood. After repair, chest tube(s) are placed for mediastinal/pleural drainage. Transthoracic pressure lines are commonly placed to monitor right or left atrial pressure to guide postoperative management. Occasionally, a pulmonary arterial line is placed. Infants may be managed with an open sternum after complex repairs. This facilitates rapid reentry in the event of sudden instability or need for extracorporeal membrane oxygenation (ECMO) support. Delayed sternal closure is performed once the acute perioperative phase is complete, edema has resolved, and relative stability is assured. Venoarterial ECMO may be required for postoperative mechanical circulatory support, most frequently using the same arterial and venous cannulation sites as used for cardiopulmonary bypass. Postoperative bleeding in patients requiring mechanical circulatory support is a common problem and may be difficult to manage.

POSTOPERATIVE CONSIDERATIONS

Management

Postoperative management of the patient with congenital heart disease can be challenging and must be tailored to the particular patient. Management priorities may differ in several key ways from the management of other noncardiac surgical diseases. Perhaps, the greatest difference is a conservative fluid management strategy in the perioperative period. The rationale for this stems from the physiology of cardiopulmonary bypass, in which a capillary leak state exists for 12–36 hrs after the insult, and which subsequently resolves in a process of interstitial fluid mobilization and increase in circulating blood volume. For this reason, patients are optimally managed by maintaining relatively negative fluid balance in the first 2–4 days after repair. This results in improved pulmonary function, and minimizes risk of pleural and pericardial effusions and issues related to systemic edema formation. With this strategy, systemic and renal perfusion must be carefully monitored; the clinician should be vigilant for signs of prerenal azotemia, although fortunately renal failure is now a relatively rare event. An intravenous fluid management strategy of one-half to two-thirds maintenance intravenous fluids is utilized. In closed-heart repairs (coarctation repair, patent ductus arteriosus ligation), an aggressively conservative fluid management strategy may not apply as the patient has not been exposed to cardiopulmonary bypass; however, many of these patients still benefit from a negative fluid balance due to preexisting pulmonary congestion and heart failure symptoms that exist as a component of their disease presentation.

Depending on the management preferences of the surgeon, diuretic therapy may be instituted immediately after repair, or within 12–24 hrs of repair. Some believe that the first 12–24 hrs are associated with third-spacing, and therefore diuretic therapy during this phase is premature. However, if diuretic therapy is delayed beyond fluid mobilization, risk of prolonged recovery and morbidity (prolonged chest tube drainage, etc.) from the sequelae of volume overload is increased. Fluid mobilization is a clinical indicator of systemic recovery and improvement in hemodynamic status; its timing correlates grossly with the magnitude of the repair and the severity of illness. Fluid mobilization for straightforward cases (atrial septal defect repair) will occur earlier than more complex cases with residual hemodynamic lesions or associated pathophysiology (hypoxemia, etc.)

Other postoperative management considerations are unique to the individual patient. Thorough understanding of the postrepair circulatory physiology is mandatory for optimal management. Traditionally, beneficial support practices may be harmful in some circumstances. For example, some patients may require maintenance of hypoxemia to maintain circulatory balance; supplemental oxygen to address low systemic arterial oxygen saturations may be destabilizing. Pulmonary hypertension is less of a problem in the current era with early corrective repair; however, it is encountered in patients with preexisting unrestricted pulmonary blood flow or large left-to-right shunts (atrioventricular canal). Physiologic management strategies or medications to deal with this problem are readily utilized (blood gas management, phosphodiesterase-5 inhibitors, inhaled nitric oxide) in management. Systemic blood pressure management must balance concern for suture line bleeding vs. adequate perfusion of both systemic and pulmonary capillary beds (if systemic shunt dependent). Rhythm disturbances may occur in patients, particularly after the repair of ventricular septal defects (VSD). The His-Purkinje conduction system is located near the poster-inferior margin of perimembranous VSD, the most common anatomic subtype of VSD. Most perioperative arrhythmias are transient and resolve within a short time. Postoperative hemodynamic instability which is not addressed by first-line intervention should prompt consideration of an urgent echocardiogram to assess myocardial function and cardiac status/intracardiac shunt. Pericardial tamponade requires a high index of suspicion.

The single ventricle patient: This common and highly complex category of patients merits special consideration. Increasingly, children born with functional single ventricle are offered a series of three-staged palliative open-heart repairs which culminate in a final palliative physiologic state known as a univentricular Fontan circulation.

The first procedure, performed in infancy, has two primary objectives: (1) Establish unobstructed outflow from the single (morphologically right or left) ventricle to the systemic circulation, and (2) Secure a reliable, but metered, source of pulmonary blood flow. The source of pulmonary blood flow may be constructed as a Blalock–Taussig systemic-to-pulmonary arterial shunt (for insufficient pulmonary blood flow) or as a pulmonary artery band (for excessive pulmonary blood flow) depending on the anatomic/physiologic circumstances. The resulting stage-I physiology is highly unstable due to four potentially lethal characteristics: (1) The systemic and pulmonary circulations are arranged in an inherently unstable parallel arrangement. Circulatory "balance" must be maintained: Overperfusion of the lungs or body occurs at the expense of the other vascular bed; (2) The patient is exposed to severe hypoxemia (pO_2 30–40 mm Hg) necessary to maintain circulatory balance. Goal oxygen saturation is 75–85%; higher is undesirable. Supplemental oxygen or hyperventilation may be destabilizing; (3) The single ventricle is subjected to twice normal volume load, as it must pump blood to both systemic and pulmonary circulations; (4) Coronary perfusion is compromised due to reduced diastolic blood pressure from shunt run-off. The mortality and instability risk of these patients is notoriously high, and the risk of interstage (between stages I and II) death is also exceedingly high (10–24%). In general, elective noncardiac surgical procedures should not be performed in these patients unless necessary and only if the patient is supported in a setting of advanced perioperative cardiac care. At this point, knowledge of the precise intracardiac anatomy is inconsequential — regardless of the anatomy of the defect, the ventricle is committed to serve as a single systemic ventricle. Regardless of intracardiac anatomy, the patient is entered into the staged single ventricle palliation pathway with the end goal of a Fontan circulation.

The second operation (stage-II, Hemi–Fontan or Bidirectional Glenn) is typically performed at 4–6 mths of age. The systemic-to-pulmonary arterial shunt is taken down, and the superior vena cava (SVC) is connected to the pulmonary arteries. The SVC now serves as the sole source of pulmonary blood flow, and SVC pressure is elevated 2–3 fold. Hypoxemia is partially improved, but not normalized, because inferior vena cava (IVC) flow continues unabated into the single ventricle. Systemic arterial oxygen saturations of ~85% are expected. The SVC pressure required for adequate transpulmonary blood flow (12–15 mm Hg) is directly dependent on pulmonary resistance. Interestingly, hyperventilation does not improve transpulmonary blood flow (expected secondary to reduced pCO_2) after stage-II conversion because hypocarbia concurrently increases cerebral vascular resistance (in the infant, 90% of SVC flow is cerebral in origin), thus reducing total SVC flow. Therefore, these patients are often managed with "permissive hypercapnia". The placement of subclavian or internal jugular venous access is frequently a source of concern in these patients, as it presents a thrombogenicity risk in the pathway which serves as the sole source of pulmonary blood flow with potential for lethal consequences. In general, however, lines can be carefully placed, and patients can be managed with cautious anticoagulation.

In the third operation (stage-III, Fontan completion), the IVC is connected to the pulmonary arteries. This procedure is performed anywhere from 18 mths to 5 yrs of age depending on institutional preference. The circulation is returned to a series arrangement identical to a normal 2-ventricle circulation, with the exception that there is no right-sided ventricular power source to pump blood through the lungs. Therefore, the Fontan circulation is characterized by concurrent elevated systemic venous pressure and subnormal preload and low cardiac output (the so-called Fontan paradox). These problems underlie subsequent Fontan-related disease for life. Hypoxemia is no longer a problem, and supplemental oxygen is no longer deleterious. Hemodynamic stability is markedly improved. Patients are at high risk of "Fontan failure" early or late after repair. Similar to heart failure, this manifests as sequelae of increased tissue water and decreased tissue perfusion, although systolic ventricular function is not typically the underlying cause. Typical manifestations include lower extremity edema, ascites, pleural effusions, hepatic/gut dysfunction (secondary to splanchnic venous hypertension), hypercoagulability, and protein losing enteropathy. In the current era, management is expectant; there is no direct therapy for these problems short of cardiac transplantation.

Fontan conversion is staged in two separate procedures because it provides a greater margin of safety. Although technically feasible in one-stage, the hemodynamic impact of exposing the SVC and IVC territories to 2–3x venous pressure elevation in one-stage places too much physiologic stress on the highly complaint systemic venous circulation. The early postoperative volume requirement may lead to tissue edema and malperfusion superimposed on low cardiac output. Fontan conversion is not considered possible in the neonatal period due to persistence of the fetal pulmonary circulation and risk of elevated pulmonary resistance which would prohibit adequate transpulmonary blood flow from a low-pressure systemic venous source alone. In normal neonates, the pulmonary arterial smooth muscle layer involutes within 6–8 wks of life, after which time the risk of a pulmonary hypertensive response is considerably decreased.

Complications/Morbidity

Complications after cardiac repair can often be attributed to a suboptimal technical repair with residual hemodynamic pathology (stenosis, regurgition, and shunt) within the limits of the anatomic substrate of that particular patient. Technically perfect repairs without residual lesions result in optimal physiology and high likelihood of recovery without incident. Cardiac surgical patients are at high risk for postoperative bleeding after cardiopulmonary bypass, which contributes to a coagulopathic state. Aggressive blood product replacement may be necessary, and complete resolution of coagulopathy occurs in a similar time frame to postoperative fluid mobilization. More serious morbidities which stem from cardiopulmonary bypass may include risk of stroke, seizure, and end-organ dysfunction: fortunately, these are relatively rare. Other complications mirror those of any other type of invasive procedure (infection, would dehiscence), and are relatively uncommon with meticulous management.

OUTCOMES/FOLLOW-UP

For nearly all lesions, both anatomic and physiologic repair is achieved and outcomes are excellent. Depending of the lesion type, patients will require longitudinal follow-up as they may outgrow valves and require replacement. In certain subsets, additional procedures will almost certainly be required. This includes patients with complex left ventricular outflow tract obstruction, and valve pathology. Patients with univentricular Fontan physiology are considered to be chronically palliated and are expected to eventually present with sequelae of elevated systemic venous pressure (ascites, pleural effusions, gut/hepatic dysfunction) for which there is little known direct therapy at this time. The long-term outcome of univentricular Fontan patients is still unknown.

SPECIAL CONSIDERATIONS FOR NONCARDIAC SURGICAL PROCEDURES IN PATIENTS WITH CONGENITAL HEART DISEASE

A thorough understanding of the physiology of patients with uncorrected or corrected heart disease is required when considering interval noncardiac operative interventions. Even minor procedures may be associated with excessive risk depending upon the status of the patient. Of particular importance are infants who have been palliated with a stage-I Norwood procedure for Hypoplastic Left Heart Syndrome; these patients are prone to sudden instability, and can have adverse reactions to anesthetic induction or other seemingly benign stimuli. Cardiac surgical patients may be anticoagulated or put on aspirin therapy which may increase bleeding risk with other corrective surgery. Residual cardiac shunts or stenoses increase the risk of bacterial seeding and endocarditis. Recent cardiac surgery may also be relative contraindication to other surgical procedures. Careful consultation with the cardiologist and cardiac surgeon is prudent when contemplating other surgical procedures in patients prior to or after repair of congenital heart disease.

REFERENCES

1. Jonas RA. (2004) *Comprehensive Surgical Management of Congenital Heart Disease.* Oxford University Press, London.
2. Grosfeld JA, O'Neill JA, Coran AG, Fonkalsrud E. (2006) *Pediatric Surgery*, 6th edition. Mosby, St. Louis.

PEDIATRIC NEUROSURGICAL CONSIDERATIONS 84

Laurie L. Ackerman

NEURAL TUBE DEFECTS

Neural tube defects are a diverse group of disorders resulting from an opening in the spinal cord or brain occurring in the early stages of fetal development. These disorders are reported to occur as frequently as 1 in 1000 live births and are one of the most common birth defects. Neural tube defects may be either open (e.g. myelomeningocle) or closed (e.g. lipomyelomengingocele, lipomeningocele, and spina bifida occulta) (Table 1).

Clinical Presentation

Clinical presentation is varied, depending on the type and severity of the lesion. Open neural tube defects are often diagnosed prenatally on ultrasound, or are obvious at birth. Closed defects can be much more subtle. In the infant, close attention must be paid to an examination of the midline neuroaxis from the nasion, over the top of the head and all the way down to the top of the gluteal cleft. Any cutaneous abnormality in this region should be noted, and evaluated by a neurosurgeon. The size, shape, symmetry, and motion of the limbs are also evaluated. Decreased gluteal bulk or foot abnormalities may signal abnormalities in the distal cord, and their workup should include neuroimaging of the spine and neurosurgical consultation. In the older child, presence or development of an abnormal gait,

Table 1.

Open spinal dysraphism

Meningocele

Meninges or dura protrudes from the spinal opening

May be skin covered (and considered closed spinal dysraphism)

Symptoms vary

Myelomeningocele

Meninges and neural elements protrudes from the spinal opening

Usually partial or complete paralysis below spinal opening

Occult (closed) spinal dysraphism

Spina bifida occulta

Vertebral malformation

Rarely causes disability or symptoms

Split cord malformations (diastematomyelia)

Type I — two hemicords in separate dural sheaths separated by an osteocartilaginous septum

Type II — two hemicords in a single dural sheath separated by a fibrous septum

Tight filum terminale

Abnormally tight filum causes caudal traction on the spinal cord with variable symptoms

May cause the conus to be abnormally low

Lipomatous filum

Abnormal fat in the filum — functions as a "tight filum"

Lipomyelocele/Conus lipoma

Abnormal fat extending from the subcutaneous plane through spinal and dural defects to abut or terminate on the spinal cord

Lipomyelocystocele

Similar to lipomyelocele or conus lipomas with terminal hydromyelia or CSF collection in the distal spinal cord

Meningocele manque (dorsal bands)

Meningocele that scarred and did not fully develop.

May have adherent nerve roots or dorsal root ganglia.

Dermal sinus tracts

Epithelial-lined tracts from skin structures that can terminate intradurally on neural elements

(*Continued*)

Table 1. (*Continued*)

Terminal syrinx
Cystic dilatation of the lower spinal cord — can occur with other forms of occult dysraphism
Anterior sacral meningocele
Meninges herniated anteriorly
Frequently associated with rectal anomalies, malformations of the uterus and vagina, urologic abnormalities including duplicated ureters and renal pelvis, bony pelvic, and vertebral anomalies and inclusion tumors

back and leg pain, asymmetrical motor and sensory function, upper motor neuron signs such as hyperreflexia, delay, or regression in toilet training, frequent urinary tract infections or delay in meeting developmental milestones may be symptoms of a tethered spinal cord or some form of occult spinal dysraphism (Table 2).

Pathophysiology

Embryology

Most neural tube defects have their genesis in some disorder of embryonic development. Defects in primary neurulation occur at 3–4 wks as the neural plate, groove and folds are formed. The neural folds fuse at 22 days to form the neural tube, with the proximal two-thirds forming the brain and the distal one-third the spinal cord. Closure occurs in both directions with the anterior neuropore closing at 24 days and the posterior neuropore closing at 26 days. Defects from faulty closure include neural tube defects such as myelomeningoceles. Secondary neurulation occurs at 4–5 wks as the mesoderm forms the dura, skull, and spine. Between the third and eight week of gestation, the cutaneous ectoderm that ultimately forms the skin and dermal appendages separates from the neuroectoderm, which forms the spinal cord. This process, referred to as dysjunction, allows for the insertion of mesoderm, which then forms the dura, vertebral column and paraspinous muscles. When a focal failure of dysjunction occurs, a persistent connection or dermal sinus tract is established between the skin elements and the underlying neural structures. If this separation occurs too early (premature dysjunction), mesenchyme enters the neural tube

Table 2. Physical exam findings of occult spinal dysraphism/neural tube defects.

Cutaneous markings over the midline neuroaxis
Skin pits or dimples
Sinus ostea with a cephalically oriented tract
Angiomata
Hypertrichosis
Skin tags
Caudal appendage
Abnormal pigmentation
Subcutaneous lipomas
Symptoms of infection such as erythema or induration
Forked or assymetrical gluteal cleft
Orthopedic abnormalities
Foot and leg asymmetry or abnormalities
Scoliosis
Neurologic
Motor weakness
Altered sensation
Abnormal reflexes
Abnormal gait
Spasticity
Altered sensation
Decreased gluteal bulk
Developmental delay in meeting milestones
Genitourinary
Urinary frequency/incontinence
Frequent urinary tract infections
Bowel incontinence
Decreased sphincter tone
Other
Back or leg pain

and can form lipomas or lipomyeloceles. The caudal spinal cord is formed by retrograde differentiation at 4–8 wks as the caudal cell mass forms and cavitates; defects in this process result in a tight or fatty filum.

Associated conditions

Most children with myelomeningocele require placement of a shunt for treatment of associated hydrocephalus, which will be discussed in a later section of this chapter. Myelomeningoceles are frequently accompanied by displacement of the medulla and some of the cerebellum into the spinal canal. This malformation known as a Chiari II malformation can cause obstruction of cerebrospinal fluid (CSF) at the foramen magnum and lead to a syrinx (collection of fluid within the spinal cord), syringobulbia (collection of CSF in the brainstem), or hydrocephalus. A syrinx can lead to decrement in neurologic function in the portion of the spinal cord in which it is associated. For instance, a cervical syrinx may lead to motor weakness and sensory loss in the hands and arms, while a lumbar syrinx may affect lower extremity movement and sensation as well as bowel, bladder, and sexual function. Syringobulbia can lead to respiratory difficulty and cranial nerve dysfunction. Altered bowel, bladder, and sexual function frequently occur, and most children also require urologic care. Orthopedic follow-up is necessary to evaluate for needs for bracing, and ongoing assessment for scoliosis. Latex precautions should be observed in all children with neural tube defects.

Diagnosis/Work-up

Diagnosis of open neural tube defects is usually made prenatally on ultrasound, or at birth on clinical examination findings. Supporting radiographic images are obtained as deemed necessary by the neurosurgeon. The diagnosis of occult spinal dysraphism may be more subtle. Anterior–posterior (AP) and lateral spine films of appropriate levels document vertebral abnormalities and assist with surgical planning. Computed tomography (CT) may be utilized to better characterize complex anatomy, with three dimensional (3-D) reconstructions. Magnetic resonance imaging (MRI) is the procedure of choice for imaging occult spinal dysraphism. T1-weighted images are good for identifying the level of the conus (normally L1–2 in older children, and L2–3 in infants), as well as identification of abnormal fat in the spinal cord or filum. T2-weighted images are good in identifying abnormal fluid collections such as a syrinx or meningocele. Tumors may also be identified. Ultrasound is of limited use as the resolution is not as good as MRI (Table 3). Urodynamic studies are useful in the evaluation of bladder function, particularly in the nonverbal, nontoilet

Table 3. Radiographic signs/symptoms of occult spinal dysraphism/neural tube defects.

Plain films/CT
Butterfly or block vertebrae
Laminar defects or fusion
Hemivertebrae
Missing vertebrae
Sacral agenesis
Scoliosis, kyphosis or exaggerated lordosis
MRI
Low lying or abnormally positioned conus*
Syrinx
Chiari II malformation
Split cord malformation
Mass lesions**

*Below L2.
**e.g. lipomas, dermoids, or inclusion cysts.

trained infant. Although potentially difficult to interpret, they remain the best objective test of bladder function. Bladder capacity has defined age/size specific values. Deviation from these values or evidence of early contractions on bladder filling may suggest a neurogenic bladder. Also, it is important to assess bladder emptying, to avoid or assist in early detection of hydronephrosis and hopefully avoid renal damage.

The neurological examination should identify the motor and sensory level of functioning for the patient. In contrast to the older child, in the infant it is best to evaluate function in the lowest levels first, and move more proximally as one is usually interested in the lowest level of functioning. Any muscle atrophy or asymmetry or diminished gluteal bulk should be noted. In the newborn, evaluation of head circumference, fontenelle turgor and evaluation of the degree of cranial suture separation (if present) is important for diagnosing hydrocephalus. All infants with open neural tube defects should have some form of neuroimaging of the brain such as a head ultrasound, CT or MRI at birth to look for hydrocephalus. CT and MRI are better in terms of characterizing the Chiari malformations and other abnormalities that may accompany both open and closed neural tube defects.

Management

Surgical management is the treatment of choice. Open neural tube defects are usually closed on the first day or two after birth with the goal of preserving neural function and preventing infection. At birth, the malformation is covered with sterile saline-soaked gauze dressings, and the infant is positioned prone or side-lying to avoid pressure upon or further damage to neural structures. Prophylactic antibiotics such as ampicillin and gentamicin are administered and continued for several days. When the infant is stable, s/he is taken to the operating room for closure of the defect. The goal is restoration of normal anatomy, closure of the dura to prevent CSF leakage, and hopefully to achieve a closure that minimizes risk of future tethering. The placode is dissected free of other tissues (to prevent future tethering or dermoid tumors), and if possible the pial surface is sutured back into a tube with a fine suture. The dura is mobilized and closed over the placode in a patulous, water tight fashion as much as possible. Available fascial and muscle components are closed over this, and the skin is undermined and closed as well. With very large defects, rotation of tissue flaps to obtain closure may be necessary.

Closed neural tube defects may be addressed at a later time. The presence of one of these lesions is generally an indication for surgery. Timing of the surgery is dependent on the surgeon's degree of comfort and skill, as well as the individual characteristics of each lesion. Absence of neurologic findings does not exclude the need for intervention, as problems may surface many years later, and the neurologic changes may not be reversible at that time. Goals of surgery are largely restoration of as normal anatomy as possible, and untethering to prevent traction upon neural structures. These procedures may be done with intraoperative electromyography (EMG) or somatosensory evoked potentials (SSEP's) to assist the surgeon in identifying neural structures. The child is placed prone, and whenever possible, a midline incision is utilized. The anatomy can be challenging as tissue planes may be indistinct. Dermal sinus tracts are traced down to their intradural termination and dissected free from or truncated at neural structures. Tethered cords are dissected free from scar tissue, and a good dural closure is attempted either with native dura or dural substitutes. Fatty filums are sectioned intradurally. Lipomyeloceles, anterior sacral meningoceles, and split cord anomalies are particularly challenging. In the lipomyeloceles, the lipomatous tissue is resected as aggressively as the surgeon can accomplish without injuring neural tissue. The descriptions of these operations are beyond the scope of this chapter and the reader is referred to the excellent text published by Albright *et al.*

Outcomes/Follow-up

The most feared operative complications of these procedures are worsened neurologic status, infections and CSF leak. If there is altered neurologic status postoperatively, the patient should be reimaged to exclude a compressive lesion such as a clot or herniated nerve root that might be amenable to surgery. Aggressive physical and occupational therapy are also indicated. Infection and CSF leak usually present in the first few weeks after surgery. Infections are treated with appropriate antibiotics. CSF leaks can be challenging to manage. The wound may initially be oversewn if there is a leak, but often reexploration is required. Watertight closure is particularly difficult in patients with myelomeningoceles or lipomyeloceles as the dural quality may be poor. Patients are often kept supine for a period of time postoperatively to decrease pressure on the recently closed wound. If reexploration does not solve the leak, the patient may require CSF diversion such as a shunt to decrease CSF fluid pressure on the closure. Recurrent tethering of the spinal cord is an all too frequent complication that may occur months to years after procedures. Back and leg pain, decrement in motor and sensory function, and loss of bowel and bladder function may ensue. There may be development of a syrinx or scoliosis. Treatment is reexploration and untethering. Chiari malformations may also be symptomatic and require operative decompression. Hydrocephalus will be discussed in the subsequent section.

HYDROCEPHALUS

Hydrocephalus is one of the most commonly encountered problems in pediatric neurosurgery. Etiologies for hydrocephalus are numerous in the pediatric population and include intraventricular hemorrhage, aqueductal stenosis, Dandy–Walker malformation, infection, hydrocephalus associated with neural tube defects or brain tumors and idiopathic hydrocephalus. It is a condition that requires life-long care. Failure to recognize and appropriately treat hydrocephalus may result in neurologic injury or death. As the number of children living with hydrocephalus continues to increase, it is incumbent upon pediatric practitioners in all disciplines to be familiar with this condition.

Clinical Presentation

There are illnesses that by definition will include a possible diagnosis of hydrocephalus, and screening for this condition is necessary. Premature infants with germinal matrix hemorrhage or the presence of an open neural tube defect are commonly associated with hydrocephalus. The presenting symptoms can vary by age (Table 4). In the infant, increasing head circumference, a full or bulging fontanelle, split sutures and "sunset eyes" (a downward deviation of gaze) are commonly seen in symptomatic hydrocephalus. Poor feeding, irritability, and excessive sleepiness or lethargy is also seen. In the older child, complaints of headache, nausea and vomiting, papilledema, VIth nerve palsy, loss of milestones and

Table 4. Signs and symptoms of hydrocephalus/shunt malfunction.

Infant	***Child***
Full or bulging fontanelle	Headache
Split sutures	Nausea/vomiting
Rapid head growth with crossing of percentiles	Lethargy and sleepiness
	Sunset eyes or loss of upgaze
Feeding intolerance and vomiting	VIth nerve palsy
Irritability	Visual changes or papilledema
Lethargy and sleepiness	Loss of developmental milestones
Sunset eyes or loss of upgaze	Decline in academic performance
Prominent scalp veins	Gait abnormalities
Swelling along the shunt tract	Swelling along the shunt tract
VIth nerve palsy	Neck pain*
New seizure or change in seizure pattern	New seizure or change in seizure pattern
Additional symptoms suggestive of shunt infection	
Fever (Particularly after a recent shunt revision)	
Stiff neck	
Abdominal pain or swelling	
Redness or drainage from the incisions	

*May be a symptom of shunt fracture.

worsened academic performance may be also seen. Presentation may be acute, or slowly progressive and quite subtle. In the child with an existing shunt, close attention must be paid to previous patterns of malfunctions (if known), and to the parent's report of the child's symptoms.

Pathophysiology

CSF is produced mainly by the choroid plexus with a smaller contribution from blood vessels. The CSF flows into the ependymal surfaces, generally moving from the lateral ventricles, through the intraventricular foramen to the third ventricle, through the Sylvian aqueduct to the fourth ventricle, and then CSF exits the ventricular system via the foramen of Magendie and the paired foramina of Luschka. It then flows into the spinal subarachnoid space and over the cerebral convexities and passes through the arachnoid granulations into the venous sinus system. Hydrocephalus is often described as obstructive or noncommunicating hydrocephalus (implies a blockage in the CSF circulation before it reaches the arachnoid granulations) or communicating hydrocephalus (implies a problem at the level of the arachnoid granulations). Germinal matrix hemorrhage is a frequent cause of hydrocephalus. The germinal matrix is formed at 7 wks gestation and gives rise to future neurons and glia, and then usually involutes around 30 wks gestation. This area is prone to hemorrhage in premature infants.

Diagnosis/Workup

Neuroimaging is obtained when there is suspicion of hydrocephalus. In the infant, ventricular size can be assessed by head ultrasound. In most cases however, CT and MRI are the most common imaging modalities, as they allow assessment of ventricular size, configuration and anatomy, as well as potentially aiding in identification of an underlying etiologic problem.

In the patient with an existing shunt, scans are used to serially follow the patient's ventricular size and catheter location. When a question of shunt failure exists, standard workup generally includes neuroimaging and a shunt series. A shunt series consists of plain radiographs of the shunt including skull, chest and abdominal films. This is examined for any discontinuity or fracture of the shunt system, adequacy of abdominal tubing length, and location of proximal and distal catheters. Fluid density noted around the catheter tip with lack of bowel gas may signal a "CSFoma", which is indicative of infection or impaired CSF absorption. A neurosurgeon may perform a shunt tap in which a 23 or 25 gauge needle is inserted under sterile conditions into a reservoir or other access chamber in the shunt. This allows for measurement of the CSF opening pressure, and allows for removal of fluid to temporize the increased intracranial pressure seen in acute shunt failure issues or to submit CSF for analysis in an infectious workup. CSF laboratory studies should include measurement of the total protein, glucose, cell counts and culture, and sensitivities. In some cases, the neurosurgeon may also obtain a nuclear medicine shunt study (shunt-o-gram) in which a radioisotope is injected into the shunt and serial images allow assessment of the speed in which the isotope moves down the shunt system and disperses through the abdomen. Lack of dispersion in the abdomen could indicate the presence of a CSF pseudocyst or CSFoma.

Management

In the child with an open fontanelle, the neurosurgeon may perform a ventricular tap to remove CSF. This is done in emergency situations or serially to temporize an infant who is either to small or too ill to undergo shunt or reservoir placement. Lumbar puncture is *contraindicated* in obstructive or noncommunicating hydrocephalus as a herniation syndrome may ensue. There is no medical management of hydrocephalus, other than administration of acetazolamide, a carbonic anhydrase inhibitor given in doses of 25–100 mg/kg/day divided TID as a temporizing measure. It is important to monitor the patient for electrolyte imbalances when using this medication.

Hydrocephalus remains a primarily surgically treated condition, either via implantation of a shunt or by performing a third ventriculostomy. Shunts consist of a proximal catheter, a valve mechanism and a distal catheter. Most common is the ventriculoperitoneal (VP) shunt which allows for insertion of extra tubing in the abdomen to "pull up" and keep the shunt positioned in the abdomen as the child grows. The ventriculoatrial (VA) shunt requires lengthening in the growing child as it may not function well as the tubing pulls out of the atria. The VA shunt is often utilized in patient with abdominal pathology that impairs CSF absorption such as scarring from previous surgeries or infection such as necrotizing enterocolitis in preterm infants. Less common termini include the pleural cavity, gallbladder, and on rare occasions the sagittal or transverse sinus.

Pleural shunts may cause hydrothorax and are not recommended in children less than 7 yrs of age. A lumboperitoneal (LP) shunt may be used only in patients with communicating hydrocephalus, usually pseudotumor cerebri (AKA idiopathic intracranial hypertension) or in patients with communicating hydrocephalus and very small ventricles. There are numerous valves commercially available today, including both fixed pressure valves which open and drain at a given pressure and adjustable valves that allow different opening pressures based on the valve settings. It is important to know what kind of valve the patient has, as most programmable valves must be reset after an MRI.

Third ventriculostomy is used in patients with obstructive hydrocephalus and favorable anatomy for entering the third ventricle. A small perforation is made in the floor of the third ventricle, allowing movement of CSF into the interpenducular cistern to bypass the site of CSF flow obstruction.

Postoperative Considerations

Management

Postoperatively, the patient is usually treated with 24 hrs of antibiotics. Practice varies widely, but most practitioners will obtain a shunt series, head CT/MRI, or both to confirm correct shunt placement and to document adequate resolution of enlarged ventricles. However, it may take several months to reach steady-state ventricular size after an intervention.

Complications and morbidity

Potential complications of shunt implantation are myriad (Table 5). The major concerns with any shunting procedure are malfunction and infection. Malfunction can occur immediately after surgery or months to years later. Symptoms of shunt infection or malfunction are summarized in Table 4. Catheter blockage is a common cause of shunt malfunction and is diagnosed on the basis of clinical examination in conjunction with worsened CT or MRI findings and an abnormal shunt tap. Ventricular (proximal) catheters can occlude with blood, or choroid plexus. Tumor cells, blood, or high CSF protein can obstruct the valve mechanism. Distal catheters can obstruct with debris or extrude from the planned distal terminus into other tissues. A catheter tip may very rarely migrate into a hollow

Table 5. Complications of shunting.

Hardware complications
Incorrect placement of shunt components requiring reoperation and repositioning
Obstruction
Proximal at the catheter tip by choroid plexus, blood, or debris
Valve mechanism failure (Mechanical or debris associated)
Distal
Shunt disconnection
Shunt fracture
Erosion of shunt components through the skin
Migration of catheter tip out of the planned terminus or into a viscus such as the intestine, stomach or scrotum
Infections
VP shunt: peritonitis
VA shunt: sepsis
CSFoma: accumulation of CSF in the abdomen secondary to infection
Other
Overdrainage
Slit ventricle syndrome
Subdural hematoma formation
Development of a trapped fourth ventricle from aqueduct collapse
Underdrainage
Hardware failure such as obstruction or disconnection
Need for a different valve opening pressure
Inguinal hernia
Volvulus
Failure of the absorptive surface to absorb CSF (CSF ascites or hydrothorax)
Potential conduit for extraneural metastasis of tumors
Shunt emboli (VA shunt)
Shunt nephritis
LP shunt:
Acquired Chiari I malformation
Lumbar nerve root irritation
Scoliosis

viscus such as the stomach, intestine or bladder. It may also (particularly in premature infants) migrate into the scrotal sac, and a shunted patient with a hydrocele should have plain radiographs to exclude migration of the catheter into the scrotum as the source of the hydrocele. Plain radiographs (shunt series) will show fractured or disconnected shunt catheters. This most commonly occurs in high motion areas such as the neck, and patients present with swelling over the course of the shunt or persistent neck pain. If a disconnection or fracture is noted, neurosurgical consultation should be obtained, even if the patient is asymptomatic as they may present later with acute onset of shunt failure when the pseudotract bridging the fracture or disconnect fails.

If infected, the shunt hardware must be removed. The shunt is tapped to evaluate patency and to obtain CSF to check for infection in the proximal catheter and valve. If the proximal shunt is free from infection, but abdominal infection is known or suspected, the shunt is externalized below the valve. If the infection has spread to the proximal catheter or valve, all shunt components are removed and a ventriculostomy catheter (AKA external ventricular drain or EVD) is placed for continued CSF drainage until the infection has cleared and a new shunt can be implanted. There is always a risk that the previous shunt terminus site may have been rendered unable to absorb CSF after infection, and failure of the shunt in the abdomen after infection may necessitate placement of a VA shunt instead. A VA shunt may also be placed in patients with recurrent or prolonged abdominal infections that would necessitate long term shunt externalization or ventriculostomy, which also carry an increased risk of infection. Shunt hardware may also be semi-electively externalized in situations such as a ruptured appendix in order to prevent retrograde infection of the CSF via migration up the peritoneal catheter. Shunted patients with large abdominal fluid collections are suspicious for "CSFoma" or CSF ascites and even with negative shunt and peritoneal fluid cultures these collections are generally regarded as low grade infections and are treated as previously described.

Endoscopic third ventriculostomy (ETV) can be a technically challenging procedure. Potential complications include injury to the hypothalamus, transient IIIrd or VIth nerve palsies, and the devastating complications of memory deficit following injury to the fornices, basilar artery puncture, or aneurysm formation. The success of this technique is about 56%. ETV failures are usually treated with conventional shunting.

Outcomes/follow-up

Patient with shunts need continued neurosurgical follow-up throughout their lifetimes. A "well" head CT is often utilized as a baseline study to compare future films with, as many children do not have normal ventricular anatomy. Not all shunt malfunctions present with large ventricles — some children are in failure with very small, normal appearing ventricles and previous scans are essential to make the diagnosis. There should be a low threshold to obtain neurosurgical evaluation if there is any question of malfunction. Increasingly, many practitioners chose to obtain a "fast spin" or limited T2-weighted MRI for evaluation of ventricular anatomy as a way of limiting radiation exposure in these children who are frequently imaged.

REFERENCES

1. Albright AL, Pollack IF, Adelson PD (eds.), (2008) *Principles and Practice of Pediatric Neurosurgery*, 2nd edition. Thieme, New York.
2. McComb JG, Mittler MA. (2001) Myelomeningoceles and Meningoceles. In: AL Albright, IF Pollack PD Adelson (eds.), *Operative Techniques in Pediatric Neurosurgery*, pp. 75–88. Thieme, New York.
3. Oakes WJ. (2001) Spina bifida occulta. In: AL Albright, IF Pollack, PD Adelson (eds.), *Operative Techniques in Pediatric Neurosurgery*, pp. 89–102. Thieme, New York.
4. Iantosca M, Drake JM. (2001) Cerebrospinal fluid shunts. In: AL Albright, IF Pollack, PD Adelson (eds.), *Operative Techniques in Pediatric Neurosurgery*, pp. 3–15. Thieme, New York.
5. Greenberg MS. (2006) *Handbook of Neurosurgery*, 6th edition. Thieme, New York.

ORTHOPEDIC DEFORMITIES 85

Christine Caltoum

INTRODUCTION

Pediatric orthopedic deformities are wide and varied. The included selection presented below is by no means an all inclusive list but rather a selection of malformations which can be encountered in the newborn. Most importantly, many of these anomalies may be associated with pathology in other systems making them especially important to be recognized by other medical practitioners and not just the Pediatric Orthopedic Surgeon.

CONGENITAL SPINAL DEFORMITIES

Congenital scoliosis results from failure of normal vertebral development in early embryogenesis. To date, most disruptions result from a spontaneous occurrence. Disruption of normal somitogenesis results in failures of formation and segmentation seen in congenital scoliosis.[1] The time period for somitogenesis between the 5th and 7th week of gestation is the same as organogenesis for the auditory, renal, cardiac and visceral systems. It is therefore not surprising that there is an association between vertebral malformations and abnormalities within these other organ systems.[2] 20% of patients will have an abnormality of the genitourinary system (GU) and 12%, the cardiac system.[3] 40 % of patients will have an associated neural axis abnormality with diastematomyelia being the most frequently recognized. Diplomyelia, syringomyelia, Arnold–Chiari malformations and spinal tumors are also seen. Other abnormalities include radial hypoplasia, imperforate anus, foot deformities and dislocated hips (VACTERL syndrome).

Congenital scoliosis is classified into failure of formation or failure of segmentation. When both types of anomalies are present it is considered a mixed type of deformity. Examples of failure of formation include wedge vertebrae and hemivertebrae while block vertebrae and unilateral bars are examples of failures of segmentation. Curve progression tends to occur during the two major growth spurts: the first during the first 2 yrs of life and the second during the adolescent growth spurt.[4] McMaster and Ohtsuka found that in 143 patients with congenital scoliosis followed past the age of ten, 10% had a minimally progressive curve, 26% had a moderately progressive curve while 64% had significant curve progression. Of the 58 patients remaining untreated by skeletal maturity, 20% developed curves of >60°.[5] The rate of curve progression is dependent on the type of congenital scoliosis, the age of the patient at the time of diagnosis, as well

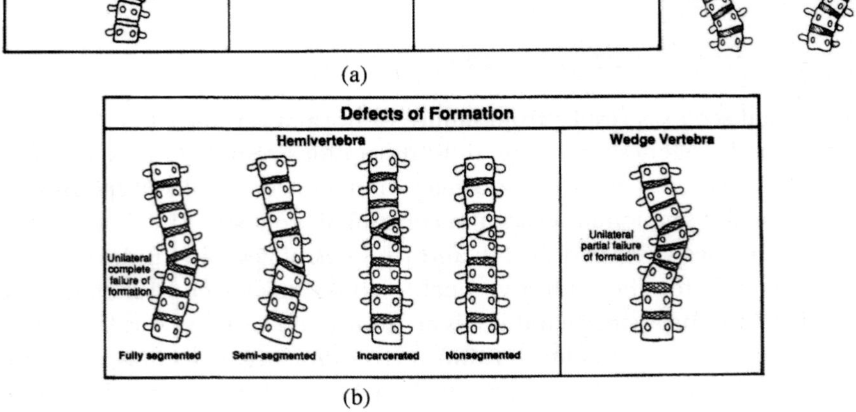

Figure 1. Congenital scoliosis: Defects of segmentation and formation. With permission from Ref. 4.

as the location of the curve. Regardless of location, the highest rate of curve progression is seen in patients with a unilateral unsegmented bar with a contralateral hemivertebrae at the same level. This is closely followed by patients with a unilateral unsegmented bar or double hemivertebrae. Patients with single hemivertebrae, a wedged vertebra or a block vertebra have decreasing rates of curve progression.[6] Patients with curves with high risk of progression need to be diagnosed early, with surgical intervention offered at an early age prior to the development of a large curve. Patients with curves with low risk of progression can be followed with sequential radiographs.

As congenital scoliosis is a potentially serious condition with multiple associated anomalies and the high risk of curve progression, it is important to recognize the vertebral anomalies early. This affords the possibility of appropriate treatment prior to the onset of a large deformity.

CONGENITAL TALIPES EQUINOVARUS

Congenital talipes equinovarus, or clubfoot, is one of the most common birth defects affecting the lower extremity. The incidence is 1/1000 live births overall[7] but this varies from 0.6/1000 in the Asian population to as high as 7/1000 in Hawaiians, Polynesians and Maoris. The condition is present bilaterally 50% of the time with boys being affected from 2–4 times more often than girls.

The clubfoot deformity is typically an isolated defect and is considered idiopathic; however, it can be associated with other congenital anomalies or neural-axis abnormalities. The most common association is with myelomeningocele and with distal arthrogyrposis, and disorders which specifically affect the central nervous system are most often seen.[8] Other syndromes associated with clubfoot include Larsen syndrome, diastrophic dwarfism, Streeter's dysplasia and tibial hememilia. Infants identified with clubfeet must therefore always be carefully examined for evidence of other associated anomalies.

The etiology of clubfoot is considered multifactorial. There is clearly a genetic component: 25% of all patients with clubfeet have a positive family history and there is a 33% twin concordance rate.[9] Wynne also found that there is a 17 times higher rate of clubfoot in first degree relatives than in the population at large.[10] However, environmental factors have also been implicated. Exposure to cigarette smoke *in utero* has been shown to be an independent risk factor for the development of clubfoot (odds ratio of 1.34). When combining exposure to cigarette smoke and family history, the odds ratio increases to over 20 suggesting a complex interaction between genetics and environmental factors.[11] Early amniocentesis (<13 wks) has also been linked to increased risk of clubfoot.[12] This has not been the case with amniocentesis performed later in the pregnancy and data has not supported a uterine compressive theory.

In a clubfoot deformity, the forefoot is supinated with the hindfoot in equinus and varus. The navicular is displaced medially and only articulates with the medial aspect of the head of the talus while the talus is shortened and plantar-flexed. The posterior tibialis tendon is shortened and thickened as is the calcaneonavicular ligament. The calcaneofibular ligament is also shortened causing medialization of the calcaneus under the talus. There are associated deep medial and posterior creases. Also noted is a decrease in the size of the calf associated with the clubfoot with a predominance of type I muscle fibers and an increase in intracellular connective tissue within the posterior and medial muscle groups.[13] The affected side may also demonstrate a growth disturbance resulting in leg length discrepancy of over 0.5 cm predominantly in the tibia[14] for which these children need to be followed to maturity. The vascularity within a clubfoot has also been shown to be abnormal: abnormalities within the dorsalis pedis artery

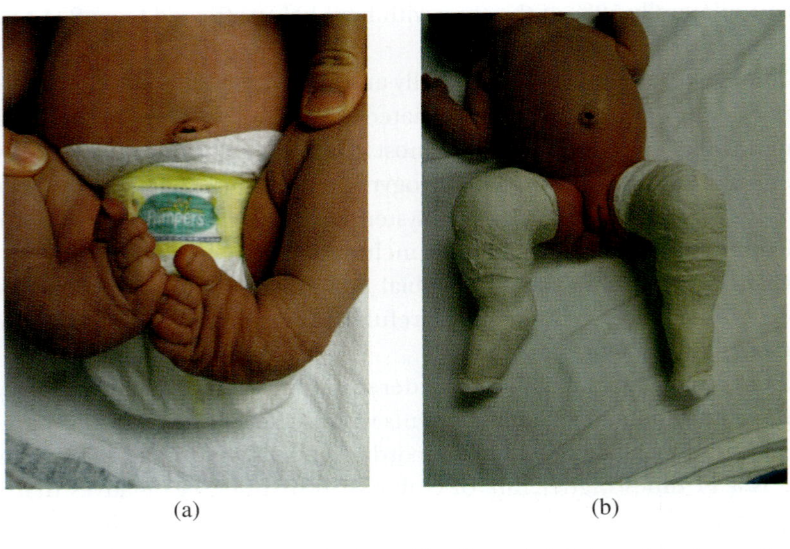

(a) (b)

Figure 2. Clubfoot. (a) 1-wk old infant with bilateral clubfoot. (b) s/p application of bilateral clubfoot cast.

can be present 20–55% of the time with the more severely affected feet being more often compromised.

Treatment of clubfeet was initially with some form of positional correction. However, due to poor results with initial casting techniques in the 1930's and 1940's, treatment turned to extensive surgical releases through a variety of incisions. It was during this time period that Ponseti developed and perfected the method that is the standard of care for the treatment of clubfeet in the United States and worldwide. Ninety five percent of all clubfeet can be successfully treated with serial manipulation and casting. The Ponseti method of clubfoot casting consists of sequential manipulation of the foot with cast application on a weekly basis. The foot is gradually manipulated over a 6–8-wk period during which time long leg casts are applied to hold the correction. The cavus component is corrected first by supination of the first ray. Next the forefoot is abducted with counterpressure applied over the head of the talus. Once the forefoot and midfoot correction is achieved, the equinus is corrected. The equinus deformity is the last deformity to be corrected in order to prevent a secondary rocker bottom deformity from being created. Ninety percent of clubfeet will require a percutaneous Achilles tenotomy to correct the equinus deformity. The patient is then placed in the last cast for 2–3 wks. The patient will then require prolonged splinting with bar and shoes to avoid a recurrence. This is maintained full time for 3 mths followed by night time splinting until age three to four. Seventy percent of feet will recur without long-term splinting therefore compliance with brace wear is extremely important. Relapses can be treated with repeat casting. Patients over the age of three with supination during the swing phase of the gait cycle may be a candidate for a full transfer of the anterior tibialis tendon to the lateral aspect of the foot. This is done once all other deformities are corrected.

Surgical treatment of clubfoot still has a role. Most idiopathic clubfeet can be treated with serial casting and heel cord tenotomy. Resistant clubfeet, syndromic and neurogenic clubfeet may need more extensive surgical releases although even these more severe clubfeet may respond to serial casting. Only those structures that remain tight after casting need be surgically lengthened with an "à la carte" approach utilized.

CONGENITAL VERTICAL TALUS

Congenital vertical talus is a rare disorder that can occur as an isolated entity, however 50% of cases are associated with an underlying genetic or neuromuscular entity. There is bilateral involvement 50% of the time with equal occurrence in male and females. Congenital vertical talus is associated with meylomenigocele, arthrogryposis, sacral agenesis as well as trisomy 13 and 18. Given the high frequency of associated neuroaxial abnormalities with congenital vertical talus, MRI evaluation of the spine is indicated in patients found with isolated vertical talus.[15]

Congenital vertical talus, also known as congenital convex pes planus, is characterized by a fixed dorsal dislocation of the navicular on the head of the talus. The hindfoot is in equinus with contractures of the anterior soft tissues including the anterior tibialis tendon, the extensor hallicus longus and digitorum longus as well as the peroneals. The Achilles is also always contracted with varying degrees of dorsal cuboid dislocation.

Diagnostic imaging is with radiographs of the foot. In the infant these are in the neutral position; if the child is able to stand, standing AP and lateral X-rays are preferable. The diagnostic X-ray in a congenital vertical talus is a forced plantarflexion lateral. The long axis of the talus should line up with the first metatarsal in normal alignment. Since the navicular does not begin to ossify in a child until 3–4 yrs of age, the collinear alignment of the talus and the metatarsal implies reduction of the talus and the navicular. In a congenital vertical talus, the long axis of the talus does not line up with the long axis of the first metatarsal, but passes dorsal to it.

Without treatment, congenital vertical talus will lead to significant disability with difficulty with shoe wear, poor push off strength and gait abnormalities. Treatment is typically surgical, in most cases with a one stage surgical release. Prior to surgery, a series of casts may be applied in order to stretch the dorso-lateral structures. Surgical release involves lengthening the contracted anterior structures including the anterior tibialis tendon

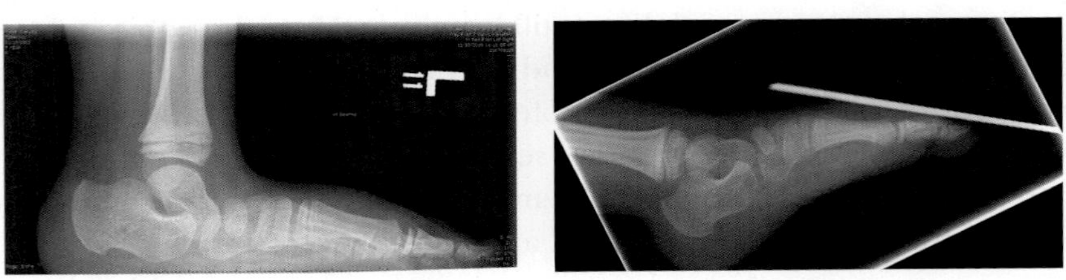

(a) (b)

Figure 3. (a) and (b) 7-yr old female with CVT.

Note: Long axis of talus that passes dorsal to long axis of metatarsal on both standing lateral and plantarflexion lateral X-ray.

and toe extensors as well as the tight peroneals and Achilles tendon. The talo-navicluar joint is also reduced and pinned. This can be done through a posterior Cincinnati incision or a dorsal incision. In older children, a salvage operation may be required. This includes procedures such as talectomy, naviculectomy, subtalar arthrodesis and triple arthrodesis.

More recently, Dobbs *et al.* has reintroduced serial casting as a primary method of treatment much as the Ponseti technique is utilized to treat clubfeet. This method involves manipulation of the foot with casting at weekly intervals to gradually reduce the dislocated talo-navicular joint. Once this is achieved and confirmed on plantar-flexion lateral radiograph, the patient is taken to the operating room for pinning of the talo-navicular joint and percutaneous Achilles tenontomy. Early reports with this technique are promising in patients with idiopathic congenital vertical talus.[16]

CALCANEOVALGUS FOOT

Calcaneovalgus foot is a positional foot deformity seen in infancy. It is reported to have an incidence of 1/1000 live births, more commonly seen in first born girls. In this condition, the foot is flexible with the dorsum of the foot often positioned against the anterior aspect of the tibia. The hyperflexed position of the foot will resolve usually by the age of 6 mths. The parents should be taught stretching exercises to relax the anterior structures as these can speed the recovery of the condition. Most importantly the condition should be differentiated from other foot deformities.

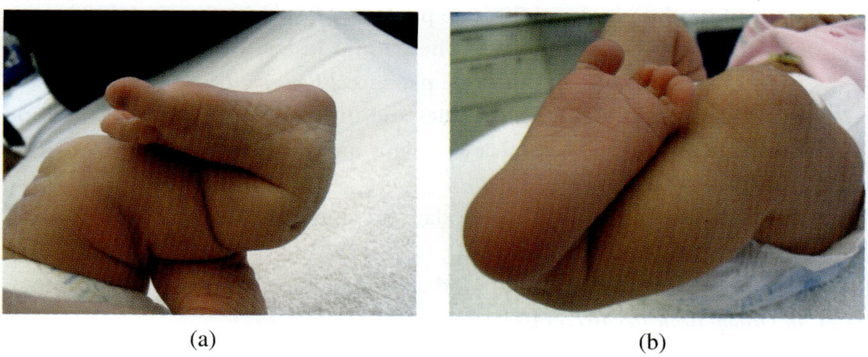

(a) (b)

Figure 4. (a) and (b) 4-day old infant with calcaneovalgus foot and posteromedial bowing of the tibia.

A positional calcaneovalgus foot must be differentiated from a congenital vertical talus or a paralytic calcaneus. This can be done on the basis of the foot's flexibility. If there is any doubt radiographs including a plantar flexion lateral should be obtained.

A calcaneovalgus can be associated with posteromedial bowing of the tibia. When posteromedial bowing of the tibia is present, a calcaneovalgus foot is always seen, however, bowing of the tibia is seen in a very small percentage of calcaneovalgus feet. Posteromedial bowing of the tibia is a benign condition which straightens over time. However, it may result in leg length discrepancy at skeletal maturity for which these patients must be followed. Furthermore, there is a direct relationship with the initial degree of bowing and the severity of leg length discrepancy.[17]

REFERENCES

1. Erol B, Tracy MR, Dormans JP, *et al.* (2004) Congenital scoliosis and vertebral malformations: Characterizations of segmental defects for genetic analysis. *J Pediatr Orthop* **24**(6):674–682.
2. Emans, JB. (2002) Congenital scoliosis. In: RT Morrissy & SL Weinstein (eds.), *Lovell and Winter's Pediatric Orthopedics*, 6th edition, pp. 765–795. Lippincott Williams & Wilkins.
3. Herring, *et al.* (2002) Scoliosis. In: JA Herring (eds.), *Tachdjian's Pediatric Orthopedis*, pp. 282–283. Saunders.
4. McMaster, MJ. (2001) Congenital scoliosis. In: SL Weinstein (ed.), *The Pediatric Spine: Principles and Practice*, p. 167. Lippincott.
5. McMaster MJ, Ohtsuka K. (1982) The natural history of congenital scoliosis: A study of two hundred and fifty-one patients. *J Bone Joint Surg* **64-A**:1128.
6. McMaster MJ, Ohtsuka K. (1982) The natural history of congenital scoliosis: A study of two hundred and fifty-one patients. *J Bone Joint Surg* **64-A**:1128.
7. Wynne-Davies R. (1964) Family studies and the cause of congenital club foot, talipes equinovarus, talipes calcaneo-valgus and metatarsus varus. *J Bone Joint Surg Br* **46**:445–463.
8. Dobbs MB, Gurnett CA. (2009) Update on clubfoot: Etiology and treatment. *Clin Orthop Relat Res* **467**:1146–1153.
9. Dobbs MB, Gurnett CA. (2009) Update on clubfoot: Etiology and treatment. *Clin Orthop Relat Res* **467**:1146–1153.
10. Wynne-Davies R. (1964) Family studies and the cause of congenital club foot, talipes equinovarus, talipes calcaneo-valgus and metatarsus varus. *J Bone Joint Surg Br* **46:**445–463.

11. Honein MA, Paulozzi LJ, Moore CA. (2000) Family history, maternal smoking and clubfoot: an indication of a gene-environment interaction. *Am J Epidemiol* **152**:658–665.
12. Tredwell SJ, Wilson D, Wilmink MA. (2001) Review of the effect of early amniocentesis on foot deformity in the neonate. *J Pediatr Orthop* **21**:636–641.
13. Gray DH, Katz JM. (1981) A Histochemical study of muscle in club foot. *J Bone Joint Surg Br* **63**:417–423.
14. Spiegel DA, Loder RT. (2003) Leg-length discrepancy and bone age in unilateral idiopathic talipes equinovarus. *J Pediatr Orthop* **23**:246–250.
15. Kasser JR. (2006) The foot. In: RT Morrissy & SL Weinstein (eds.), *Lovell and Winter's Pediatric Orthopedics,* 6th edition, pp. 765–795. Lippincott Williams & Wilkins.
16. Dobbs MB, Purcell DB, Nunley B, Morcuencde JA. (2006) Early results of a new method of treatment for idiaopathic congenital vertical talus. *J Bone Joint Surg* **88**:1192–1200.
17. Hofmann A, Wenger DR. (1981) Posteromedial bowing of the tibia. Progression of discrepancy in leg lengths. *J Bone Joint Surg* **63**:384–388.

CENTRAL VENOUS LINES 86

Sarah C. Oltmann and David T. Schindel

INTRODUCTION

Central venous (CV) access in the form of an indwelling catheter, obtained with minimal morbidity, has significantly improved the care of ill children over the last four decades. Multiple catheter formats exist to provide central access for safe infusion of medications and nutrition, provide routes for hemodialysis or pheresis, as well as allow for frequent blood draws. With the numerous applications for use, placement of a CV catheter is one of the most frequently performed procedures by the pediatric surgeon.

TYPES OF CATHETERS AND INSERTION TECHNIQUES

Lines for CV access can be classified in several different ways: Location of insertion (peripheral vs. central), mechanism of insertion (cut down vs. percutaneous), and catheter characteristics (temporary vs. tunneled vs. implanted).

Peripherally Inserted Central Venous Catheters (PICC)

Peripherally inserted central venous catheters (PICC) lines have grown in use over the last 10 to 15 yrs. Catheters come in a range of sizes (2 to 7 Fr) with one to three lumens available. These lines have become particularly useful within the neonatal population. PICC lines can be inserted at the bedside with local sedation via a peripheral vein and advanced into a central location using a modified Seldinger technique. Both ultrasound (US) and fluoroscopy can be used as adjuncts, to assist in vein location, as well as to visualize the tip of the catheter during insertion, respectively. Typically, the antecubital fossa is the preferred site of insertion, although the superficial saphenous, basilic, and cephalic veins are also commonly used. These catheters are particularly useful when a patient needs CV access but is otherwise an unacceptable risk for a general anesthetic. Unfortunately, their usefulness is often limited by their small lumen diameter impeding infusion speeds.

Centrally Inserted Central Venous Catheters

The most common CV access sites are the internal jugular, subclavian, and femoral veins. These sites are usually accessed via a percutaneously placed needle, using the Seldinger technique. Other commonly used sites include the external jugular, saphenous, facial, and cephalic veins. These sites are accessed via a cut-down allowing direct catheter insertion into the vein. The catheter is then advanced centrally under fluoroscopic guidance. The azygos, hemizygous, intercostals, inferior epigastric, gonadal and lumbar veins, are additional sites reserved when typical access sites are exhausted. Access to the azygos, hemizygous and intercostal veins generally requires a thoracotomy or thoracoscopic approach. Some larger centers employ interventional radiologists capable of using image guidance to obtain line placement in these locations. Typically used as a last resort, the right atrial appendage can also be directly cannulated via a thoracotomy or thoracoscopy.

Permanent Percutaneous Tunneled Central Venous Catheters

Tunneled CV catheters considered to be "permanent" are made of a soft plastic material having a cuff, typically made of Dacron, located along its length. The cuff allows for ingrowth of host tissue, resulting in catheter fixation and likely creates a protective barrier preventing bacteria migration along the catheter. Catheter placement should take in consideration such concerns as the child's body habitus, clothing and activities, thereby reducing the likelihood of catheter dislodgement and risk of infection.

Totally Implantable Venous Access Devices

These devices consist of an implantable metal or plastic reservoir or "port" having an overlying silicone membrane allowing for repeated penetration with a side-fenestrated, noncoring (Huber) needle. These devices come in a variety of sizes and shapes. All are Magnetic Resonance Imaging (MRI) compatible. Some port models accommodate high pressure/high flow injections without causing damage to the catheter or dislodgement. This characteristic allows their use for intravenous contrast MRI or Computed Tomography (CT) studies. Implantable devices are generally preferred for those children who require long term, intermittent access. The device is placed anteriorly, in a subcutaneous cuff, typically between the clavicle and breast against the rib or, alternatively, just above the costal margin. Because the port is implanted in the subcutaneous tissue deep to the skin, infection is less common, dislodgment is unlikely and activities such as swimming can be allowed.

PATIENT EVALUATION

The authors stress the point that, as a matter of routine, the indication for line placement should be discussed with the child's referring physician. Such discussions should elucidate what route/type of CV access is needed and provides insight to future access needs and goals. A complete history and physical exam is of paramount importance. Scars from previous CV access or potentially complicating surgeries, such as a previous sternotomy, concerns of an obstructing mediastinal mass, signs suggestive of venous obstruction or stenosis, as well as evidence of vasculature or limb hypoplasia should be sought. A history of having previous difficulties with obtaining access as noted in prior operative reports or history of a previous line infection at a given site should also be sought. Such histories are often suggestive of a complicated access site, whereby subsequent cannulation may be difficult, complicated or impossible. In such circumstances, it is recommended to obtain an imaging study preoperatively to further investigate the anatomy, and evaluate a site's appropriateness for cannulation. A vascular US with doppler is, in most centers, easily obtained and performed without the need for sedation or a general anesthetic. US can be an excellent study to determine if a central vein is patent at the site of insertion. It is the author's experience, however, that US often under appreciates the degree of CV obstruction or stenosis more proximal to the insertion site. It is the author's practice to employ magnetic resonance venography (MRV) when possible to investigate all central access sites simultaneously if there is doubt to which access sites are appropriately patent in children with potentially complicating issues identified preoperatively.

Additional history should be sought that might identify the infant or child whom is at risk for bleeding. A history of medication usage, such as aspirin or wafarin, which might affect bleeding time should be aggressively sought. Thrombocytopenia, as a result of chemotherapy or disease, or abnormal coagulation parameters, resulting from disease processes such as total parenteral nutrition (TPN)-induced cholestasis and subsequent liver diseases, are common issues in children needing CV access. A platelet count of at least $50,000/mm^3$ has been recommended to reduce the risk of hemorrhage, especially when the insertion technique of choice is by needle insertion. Abnormal coagulation parameters (protime, prothrombin time, INR) should be corrected preoperatively if possible and is accomplished most commonly by fresh frozen plasma (FFP) infusion. However, some disease states make such goals difficult. In such cases, a concurrent transfusion of platelets and/or FFP, if appropriate, can be given during the procedure effectively reducing the risk of bleeding.

LINE PLACEMENT PEARLS

Prior to proceeding to the operating room, the operative surgeon must complete the following: discuss with the requesting physician purpose of CV line and what type and size is needed, thoroughly assess access sites available for cannulation, and carefully prepare for anesthesia and bleeding risks. It is the author's practice to involve the child and family in discussions regarding catheter placement, in addition to the explanation of risks and benefits constituting appropriate consent. Great consideration must be given to line location to avoid impingement on clothing and accessories, such as wheelchairs or braces, as well positions that might impact the child's quality of life.

After the child is asleep, a shoulder roll is placed. This allows the shoulders to fall away from the clavicles, and effectively widen the space needed to percutaneously access the subclavian vein. This roll also should allow the head to gently extend, widening the window at the apex of the clavicular head of the sternocleidomastoid muscle and thus exposing the internal jugular vein. Similarly, a roll is placed under the pelvis when a percutaneous femoral line is contemplated. This roll straightens the femoral/iliac junction which, in the author's experience, allows easier advancement of the J-wire induced via the modified Seldinger technique. Contingency plans for alternative access sites should be considered when the patient is prepped, and subsequently draped.

When available, the author's favored CV access site is direct cut down on the external jugular vein, and cannulation using fluoroscopy to advance the catheter centrally. This technique greatly diminishes the risk of a pneumo- or hemothorax, arterial injury, and vascular injury secondary to a guidewire or dilator, not so uncommonly noted when using a modified Seldinger technique, even when done with US guidance. The newborn's external jugular vein can be easily cannulated with a 2.7 or 3.0 Fr silastic catheter. In older children, age-appropriate soft silastic catheters are easily advanced centrally from the external jugular vein, although some external compression of surrounding structures may be necessary to guide the catheter. The external jugular vein is easily accessed through a small incision and is typically noted to be superficial in the majority of children. Care should be taken when handling the vein, as it is prone to vasospasm, making cannulation more difficult. Additionally, when vasospasm occurs, the author bathes the vessel in 2% Lidocaine which effectively inhibits vasospasm, allowing the vessel to accommodate larger catheter diameters. One limitation of the external jugular vein, however, is that the angle which the external jugular inserts into the proximal internal jugular can act to impede the central advancement of larger, stiffer catheters needed for hemodialysis or plasmapheresis.

The cut down technique requires circumferential control of the desired vein which is established with either suture or vessel loops, both proximal and distal to the proposed venotomy site. Using an inverted 11 blade, a transverse venotomy is made. Tension is kept on the proximal and distal sutures to minimize back bleeding. The catheter is beveled at its end, and is then gently inserted into the vein to the desired depth. The proximal suture is then tied gently to secure the catheter in place without occluding the lumen.

The facial vein and saphenous vein are also excellent options, especially in newborns, allowing direct vascular control of the vessel. These vessels are easily found in most children. These veins accommodate passage of a relatively large catheter without risk of hemo- or pneumothorax and, because the catheter is inserted into a branch of a central vessel, the risk of thrombosis of the vein is, at least theoretically, reduced. The right internal jugular vein is also a favored access site by the author because of the anatomical predictability, straight access to the right atrial junction with the superior vena cava, and the ability to obtain direct vascular control of the vein if needed. It is the author's preference to access the internal jugular vein percutaneously by the modified Seldinger method assisted by a sterile vascular US transducer (5–13 Hz) placed at the base of the neck. This technique allows full visualization of the needle insertion and passage of the J-wire into the vein, thereby reducing the risk of injury to the carotid artery. This method still requires the passage of a dilator to widen the subcutaneous path of the J-wire to allowing catheter advancement and as a result, complications can arise secondary to the stiff dilator and sheath.

The infraclavicular, percutaneous approach to the subclavian vein is one of the primary methods to gain central access, regardless of patient age or size. After placing the patient in the Trendelenburg position, the author's technique is to place the thumb of the hand not holding the access needle on the clavicle and the finger tip of the fifth digit of the same hand at the sternal notch. After these landmarks are fully appreciated, the needled syringe, held in the opposite hand, is kept on gentle aspiration while it is inserted at the deltopectoral groove, and advanced both slowly and parallel to the rib, to pass just underneath the second portion of the clavicle. The thumb of the hand holding the landmarks assists the needle's passage by depressing the soft tissues as the needle is advanced towards the under surface of the clavicle and toward the sternal notch. In neonates and infants, the path of the subclavian vein is more arched, requiring a trajectory aimed cranial to the sternal notch. Keeping the needle parallel to the rib reduces the risk of the needle entering the pleura. Passing the needle parallel to the undersurface of the clavicle reduces the likelihood of entering the subclavian artery which is usually found just posterior and inferiorly to the subclavian vein in relationship to the clavicle. If the vein is not encountered, the author will move the needle more medial along the clavicle toward the sternum but redirect the needle at an angle more superiorly at a slight angle away from the sternal notch. This typically results in successful cannulation of the subclavian vein while limiting potential needle insertion into the great vessels of the mediastinum. After ensuring free aspiration of blood into the syringe, the syringe is removed, and the J-wire gentle inserted through the needle, using the modified Seldinger technique.

The authors employ fluoroscopy while passing the J-wire to confirm appropriate wire positioning at the right atrial junction with the superior vena cava which is marked by the junction of the right mediastinal strip and the right bronchus on anteroposterio (AP) views of the chest. After the catheter has been appropriately sized and tunneled subcutaneously, positioning the cuff of permanent lines just deep to the tunnel's entrance, the dilator is then passed over the J-wire while maintaining firm control of the J-wire. Inappropriate handling of the J-wire can result in the J-wire being lost intravascularly. When passing the dilator, the patient should be maintained in the Trendelenberg position to avoid air embolism, and the wire should be freely mobile to ensure entrance into the vessel. The authors stress that the dilator is to be passed only to the extent where it enters into the vessel, thereby only dilating the subcutaneous tissue along the J-wire as it inserts into the vein. After the dilator and J-wire are withdrawn and the sheath is left in place, the catheter, were it exits the subcutaneous tunnel is then advanced through the sheath. The sheath is then withdrawn once the catheter is appropriately positioned, as confirmed by fluoroscopy Once the catheter is appropriately positioned, the line is secured with a nonabsorbable suture. While seemingly elemental, much frustration can be avoided by securing the line adequately without over tightening the stitch which may result in occlusion or the stitch cutting through the skin from necrosis, causing dislodgement of the catheter. The catheter is typically aspirated, then flushed, and heparinized saline is left indwelling in the line. Upon arrival to the postanesthesia care unit (PACU) an upright chest radiograph is obtained to confirm line placement, and document the absence of pneumo- or hemothorax or a widened mediastinum.

For port insertion, venous control is obtained as previously described for the tunneled catheter. Instead of selecting a catheter exit location, a port insertion site is chosen. Ideally, this site is located along the rib cage so that there is a firm surface to support the port when accessed. It is important to ensure there is enough subcutaneous tissue to cover the port without undue tension on the skin, as skin necrosis is possible. In addition, consideration should be made to port placement in regards to the shoulder and breast. Poor planning in this regard can injure the developing breast bud and cause undue pain with movement, irritation from clothing straps, or difficulty with port access. A skin incision slightly larger than the port is made and carried down through the subcutaneous tissues to the underlying muscle *fascia*. Blunt dissection is used to create an adequate pocket to accommodate the port. A minimum of three, nonabsorbable sutures are placed to secure the port to the *fascia*; they are left untied until the catheter has been tunneled to the venous access site and cut to length.

The port is then inserted into the pocket and sutures tied, thereby insuring against port malposition within the port pocket. The catheter is placed into the vein as previously described. The port is accessed with a Huber needle to ensure blood return, and flushed to assess for good flow. Fluoroscopy is used to visualize the catheter through its entirety, evaluating for kinks in the tubing and location of the tip. Skin incision at the port insertion site is closed in two layers with absorbable suture. Sterile dressings are applied over the incisions, allowing for port accessibility in the postoperative period if needed. Once again, a postoperative chest X-ray is obtained to verify tip location and evaluate for complications.

COMPLICATIONS

Complications after placement of central lines in children can be grouped into two main categories based on the timing of occurrence, early vs. late. In general, early complications arise either during the placement of the line, or become evident in the following 24 hrs, while late complications occur thereafter.

Early Complications

Early complications are the ones most often discussed while obtaining consent for line placement with the child's parents, and can be fatal if not immediately recognized and corrected. Intraoperative cardiac monitoring, use of fluoroscopy, and a postoperative chest X-ray can help detect these early complications, and allow for prompt intervention.

Early complications can be further grouped by etiology. Cardiac injuries can range from a simple dysrhythmia due to endocardial irritation from the wire or catheter, to perforation or cardiac tamponade. Dysrhythmias can quickly become a fatal arrhythmia in a patient with an electrolyte abnormality, in a patient with underlying cardiac anomalies, or if the offending wire or catheter is not promptly pulled back out of the heart. Direct perforation of the cardiac wall can occur secondary to the catheter, the dilator or sheath, and even by the soft J-wire used for Seldinger technique. It is the author's opinion that these complications are best avoided by performing such maneuvers under fluoroscopic visualization, as well as avoidance of excessive force during insertion. Injuries caused by the stiffer dilator are most likely, and can be minimized by understanding that the tissue needing dilation is the subcutaneous tissue along the path of the wire, and where the wire enters the vein. Inserting the dilator more proximal to the venotomy and into the vessel places the soft, great vessels of the mediastinum at undue risk. These perforation injuries, and the potential subsequent cardiac tamponade, are life-threatening, and require quick recognition and surgical correction. Patients may demonstrate hypotension, low oxygen saturation, increased CV pressures, distended neck veins, muffled heart sounds or bradycardia. Fluoroscopy may reveal a widened mediastinum, and if echocardiogram is available, a pericardial effusion may be visualized.

If tamponade alone is suspected, pericardiocentesis can be both diagnostic and therapeutic. However, if concern exists for a free perforation of the myocardium, prompt surgical exploration is required, preferably via a median sternotomy to allow the fastest approach to the heart, and excellent exposure. Control of bleeding from the heart is best done with digital pressure/occlusion to minimize any further damage to the surrounding myocardium. Pledgeted, horizontal mattress stitches with a permanent suture are then used to seal the injured area, without strangulating the tissue.

Pericardial effusion may also have a delayed presentation, with symptoms developing over the days to weeks following insertion. In these instances, it is thought that perforation results from repeated or continuous contact of the catheter tip with the myocardium. Hyperosmolar fluids infused through the catheters, like TPN, can also cause an osmotic injury to the tissues, allowing fluid to diffuse transmurally and an effusion subsequently develops. Catheter tips can also migrate through the cardiac wall without tissue necrosis, resulting in infusions flowing directly into the pericardial space, instead of into the heart. Any time a patient develops chest pain at the beginning of an infusion through a central line, perforation should be suspected, and the infusion stopped immediately. The patient should then undergo further work-up to evaluate the catheter placement should they otherwise remain hemodynamically stable.

Vascular injuries can also occur during catheter placement, and can range from a simple arterial puncture to laceration or perforation of a major vessel. Inadvertent arterial punctures are not necessarily problematic, so long as they are promptly recognized, and direct pressure is held to avoid hematoma formation. The unrecognized arterial puncture becomes life-threatening if a line placement continues with dilation of the arterial wall and/or catheter placement.

Lacerations can be avoided by ensuring needle trajectory is only altered while the needle tip is immediately under the skin. Careful advancement of the dilator/sheath pair over the wire is also crucial to avoid vascular injury, as the stiff plastic will not always conform to the curve of the vessel and/or wire resulting in back wall injuries if the surgeon is not diligent to ensure the wire always passes freely.

Vascular injuries may be detected in an asymptomatic patient on postoperative chest X-ray as an apical cap, a widened mediastinum or a hemothorax. Chest tube thoracostomy should be placed for any blood or fluid detected in the pleural cavity to provide drainage. Venous injuries will likely seal due to the low intravascular pressures, and not require further intervention. Ongoing blood loss via the chest tube, hypotension or other hemodynamic instability requires intervention, either endovascularly or with open surgical repair.

Air embolism can theoretically occur at time of catheter insertion, during use, as well as at time of removal. Incidence is unknown. Patients will have acute onset of dyspnea, hypoxia, wheezing, tachypnea, tachycardia, altered mental status, lightheadedness, and eventual cardiovascular collapse. A "millwheel" cardiac murmur may be appreciated, but is not always present. Air embolism can be avoided during insertion by placing the patient in Trendelenburg position, and by holding ventilation or Valsalva maneuver during venipuncture. At time of catheter removal, the patient should also be flat or in Trendelenburg position, a Valsalva maneuver performed, and direct pressure held over the insertion site. An occlusive dressing should remain in place for 48 hrs after removal.

Guidewire positioning is crucial for correct placement of the catheter. With the use of fluoroscopy either during guidewire insertion or to verify its placement, malposition of the wire can be caught and corrected. Tactile feedback during wire advancement should give the surgeon clues of possible malposition, and if resistance is felt, fluoroscopy used immediately to determine the wire location. Even with proper wire placement, the catheter tip can end up migrating after insertion. In the immediate postoperative period, change in patient positioning can result in tip migration either down into the heart, across midline to the contralateral subclavian vein or into the pleural space. Catheters inserted via cutdown technique can also end up malpositioned, heading away from the heart. Again, intraoperative use of fluoroscopy can detect this problem when it is still possible to correct it without the need for a second procedure.

Complications reported in the literature from catheter malposition include subdural hematoma, quadriplegia secondary to TPN infusion into the epidural space, arterial placement (as previously mentioned), pleural effusion, seizure activity, intraabdominal hemorrhage, abscess and intraabdominal infusions.

The lung can also be injured during catheter insertion, seen as a resultant pneumothorax, hemothorax, or pleural effusion. Acute hypotension during line placement should always raise suspicion of a pneumothorax or hemothorax, and a chest tube placed on the ipsilateral side. A small pneumothorax noted on postinsertion chest X-ray, in an otherwise asymptomatic, stable patient not requiring positive pressure ventilation can be managed expectantly.

Placement of an internal jugular catheter may result in phrenic nerve paresis. While this may be well tolerated in larger children or adults, a neonate with underlying pulmonary immaturity, phrenic nerve paresis can severely complicate the ability to wean from the ventilator. Diaphragmatic placation may be necessary.

Additional nerve injuries seen acutely after line placement include a brachial plexus injury or a femoral nerve injury.

Late Complications

Late complications are numerous, and vary in severity. Underlying patient factors, as well as duration of catheter insertion, greatly influence these late arising issues.

Infectious complications are common; these can range from minor tract infections to life-threatening bacteremia and sepsis. Meticulous catheter care, as well as sterile technique when accessing the catheter or port must be used. The use of antibiotic lock solutions (ABL) or ethanol lock solutions have been investigated for both the prevention of, as well as treatment of, catheter related blood stream infections with mixed results. Simple exit site infections involve localized erythema, induration, tenderness and possible discharge from the skin around the catheter. These can be managed with antibiotics and aggressive local wound care. The catheter does not need to be removed in these instances. A tunnel or pocket infection involves erythema, induration and tenderness along the tunneled path, or around the implanted port. These patients may also have a fever. These patients need to have blood cultures drawn, intravenous antibiotics initiated, and prompt surgical removal of the catheter. Any purulence noted should be sent for culture, and the pocket and/or tunnel should be opened and allowed to drain, as with any other type of abscess.

Systemic signs of infection should raise suspicion for line sepsis, whether or not there is microbiological evidence for bacteremia or fungemia. Blood cultures should be drawn peripherally, as well as through the catheter. Use of quantitative vs. qualitative cultures to determine the presence of infection varies by institution. The use of catheter tip cultures is debatable in use, as the catheter may become contaminated during the process of removal. Temporary catheters should be removed, however, those surgically placed may be attempted to be salvaged using a combination of systemic intravenous antibiotics, and locking solutions containing antibiotics, ethanol and/or thrombolytic agents. Should patients fail conservative management, the line must ultimately be removed. Conservative management is of the utmost importance in those patients with long term catheter needs for TPN, but must be balanced with the severity of the patient's clinical picture secondary to sepsis. The most common pathogen involved in line infections is *Staphylococcus epidermidis,* although other organisms commonly seen include *Staphylococcus aureus, Escherichia coli, Pseudomonas* sps, *Streptococcus* sps, *Bacillus* sps, *Enterobacteriaceae,* and *Candida* sps.

Thrombotic and/or embolic phenomena are also late arising complications from prolonged catheter placement. Small thrombi can form on the tip of the catheter, affecting function by acting as a ball valve allowing infusion of fluid but restricting or preventing withdrawal of blood. Thrombi can also grow anywhere along the length of the catheter, and can ultimately cause occlusion of the vessel if left in place. Thrombosis of the vessel wall adjacent to the catheter can result in the incorporation of the line to the vein wall. This makes for a difficult removal, and may require the catheter to be tied off at the vessel entrance and left behind or retrieved by interventional radiologists with intravascular approaches. Reports of intravascular attempts to retrieve these segments have noted variable success.

Management of vessel thrombosis varies, depending on the severity of symptoms and the underlying reason for catheter placement. Patients only requiring short term line placement, or with severe clinical symptoms should have the catheter removed, and anticoagulants initiated as needed. Those patients with long term need for central access and/or minimal symptoms may be treated with anticoagulants while leaving the catheter in place. The risk of pulmonary embolism from catheter related thrombus is unknown.

Signs and symptoms of thrombosis are relative to line location. Neck and extremity access points are at risk to cause superior vena cava syndrome, and/ or central stenosis. Lumbar and femoral veins can potentially cause thrombosis of veins at the level of the spinal cord, with resultant paralysis. Patients can also develop thrombophlebitis, incompetent venous valves, or infection of the thrombus with subsequent septic emboli.

Mechanical problems with the device can also arise over time. External portions of both PICC lines and tunneled catheters can develop small cracks, resulting in a leak from the catheter tubing. These can often be visualized and subsequently repaired with commercially available patch kits. Subclavian lines placed too medially can become pinched between the clavicle and first rib, and over time, this can result in catheter breakage. Patients will present with localized pain upon infusion, extravasation, or inability to draw back blood from a previously working line. The distal portion of the catheter is often lost intravascularly, and may require intravascular retrieval by interventional radiology. If adherent to the vessel wall, it may be left *in situ*. The proximal catheter is promptly removed. Subcutaneous ports can become cracked, or broken, with either the diaphragm or the posterior wall of the port involved. Again, pain during infusion and/or extravasation at the port site will be noted. These must be removed and replaced. Lines frequently become occluded. This can be secondary to thrombosis within the catheter when used for frequent blood draws, or due to crystallization within the catheter when used for infusion of TPN and lipid mixtures, or certain chemotherapy agents. Recombinant tissue plasminogen activator or dilute hydrochloric acid can be instilled in the catheters in attempts to restore patency, respectively. Catheters with externalized components are also at risk for inadvertent removal, and careful catheter fixation along with an occlusive dressing over the skin entry site is mandatory to minimize this complication.

For those patients dependent on TPN, the gradual loss of central access sites due to vessel thrombosis and stenosis poses a serious problem. Alternative sites, as previously discussed here, may tide the patient over until definitive management of small bowel failure is performed by way of small bowel and/or liver transplantation. However, as these alternative sites are associated with their own risks, they should be reserved for only those patients with no alternative options.

REFERENCES

1. Askegard-Giessmann JR, Caniano DA, Kenney BD. (2009) Rare but serious complications of central line insertion. *Sem Pediatr Surg* **18**:73–83.
2. Nuchtern JG. (2005) Vascular access. In: KT Oldham, PM Colomani, RP Foglia, MA Skinner (eds.), *Principles and Practice of Pediatric Surgery*, 2nd edition, pp. 1705–1722. Lippincott Williams & Wilkins, Philadelphia, PA.
3. Stringer MD. (1995) Vascular access. In: L Spitz, AG Coran (eds.), *Rob & Smith's Operative Surgery Pediatric Surgery*, 5th edition, pp. 25–37. Chapman & Hall, London, UK.
4. Turner CS. (2005) Vascular access. In: KW Ashcraft, GW Holcomb, JP Murphy (eds.), *Pediatric Surgery*, 4th edition, pp. 105–111. Elsevier Saunders, Philadelphia, PA.
5. Whiteman ED. (1996) Complications associated with the use of central venous access devices. *Curr Probl Surg* **33**:300–388.
6. Onder AL, Kato T, Simon N, Rivera-Hernandez M, Chandar H, Montane B, Francoeur D, Salvaggi G, Tzakis AG, Zilleruelo G. (2007) Prevention of catheter-related bacteremia in pediatric intestinal transplantation/short gut syndrome children with long-term central venous catheters. *Pedatr Transplantation* **11**:87–93.
7. Maiefski M, Rupp ME, Hermsen ED. (2009) Ethanol lock technique: Review of the literature. *Infect Control Hosp Epidemiol* **30**:1096–1108.

SKIN AND SOFT TISSUE INFECTIONS 87

Mustafa Kabeer and Alan P. Ladd

INTRODUCTION

Despite the aspirations of most, if not all, of the children's hospitals to provide ground breaking care using the latest in technological breakthroughs in tertiary and quaternary care settings, we must all face the reality and the necessity of taking care of the routine and sometimes mundane problems. Skin and soft tissue infections consist of a spectrum of diseases that can range from the minor cellulitis to the major and the devastating necrotizing fasciitis. These infections often are due to minor abrasive injuries to the skin and the offending organisms are usually related to skin flora. Many of these patients require the same aptitude of care with the same attention to detail as any other patient requiring hospitalization. The clinician's ability to properly assess the problem and treat it appropriately according to evidence based practice is of utmost importance.

It is necessary to develop an algorithm in assessing and treating children with varying severities of skin and soft tissue infections. The first step is to properly identify the severity of the infection. This, in turn, will dictate the level and intensity of intervention. Finally, there should be follow up for resolution and monitoring for recurrence.

CLINICAL PRESENTATION

Minor infections that are localized to the epidermis and superficial dermis with no concomitant collections of pus are best classified as erysipelas. This is most often seen as a patchy raised area of erythema. Cellulitis is often a similar diffuse skin infection but it affects the deeper dermis (Figure 1). Some cellulitis can occur in areas where there may be concern for compartment syndrome. These patients should be imaged to rule out any undrained fluid collections. Cellulitis associated with an underlying fluid collection is most often due to Staphylococcus species; whereas if it is not associated with an abscess, it is usually a Streptococcus species. Periorbital cellulitis which is common in children is usually due to Haemophilus influenzae. The clinical severity dictates the level of aggressive intervention. New onset skin infections that are minor and small can be treated with oral medication in an outpatient setting. Most of the time, skin aspiration for culture and blood cultures to identify causal organisms are not useful. For outpatient treatment, the patient should have no clinical instability, high fevers, or evidence of systemic toxicity. Any

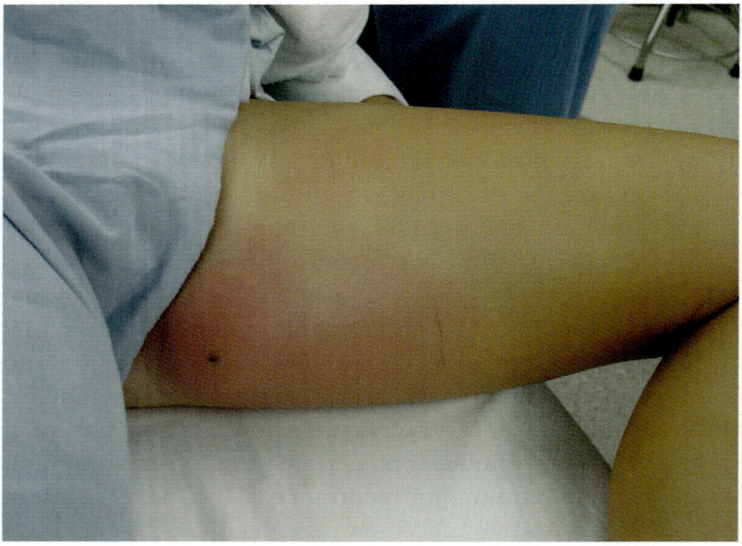

Figure 1. Depiction of clinical cellulitis.

evidence of the aforementioned signs requires hospital admission for intravenous antibiotic treatment.

PATHOPHYSIOLOGY

Recent trends in the care of soft tissue infections in pediatrics have demonstrated a huge surge in the identification of community-acquired methicillin resistant *Staphylococcus aureus* (MRSA). Although erythromycin- or macrolide-resistant *Streptococcus pyogenes* is also an emerging pathogen, it is not highlighted as often as MRSA by institutions tracking resistant strains. *Staphylococcus aureus* has different subtypes, with certain gene expressions, that make it more or less likely to cause abscess formation. The Panton–Valentine Leukocidin (PVL) gene often leads to expression of this PVL protein that implicates these isolates to more likely cause abscess but not bacteremia.[1–3] The SCCmec IVa subtype constitutes the majority of the PVL positive strains and account for 70% of the abscesses.[2] These differences influence the natural history and evolution of the infectious process and may even determine whether or not an abscess forms.

A deeper soft tissue infection with an associated fluid collection should be suspected if there is lack of improvement with appropriate antibiotic treatment. These abscesses are collections of pus adjacent to or underlying an area of entry or breakdown of the skin barrier. These collections are often painful, tender and fluctuant with an erythematous rim. The fluctuance is the soft area in the center or skin entry region that is usually related to the fluid nature of the superficial collection. The area may appear whitish if it is superficial but many are deeper to the dermis and may just appear as swollen or tense areas. The clinical picture for MRSA infections is often similar to classic presentations, but the occurrence of fluctuance may not be apparent until significant subcutaneous tissue destruction and necrosis has occurred.

MANAGEMENT

Most of these minor skin infections can be treated with semisynthetic penicillin, first or second generation cephalosporins, macrolides, or clindamycin.[1] Uncomplicated cellulitis can be treated with a 5–10 day treatment of antibiotics. It is worthwhile to keep in mind that 50% of methicillin-resistant

Staphylococcus aureus (MRSA) have an inducible or constitutive clindamycin resistance.[1] Most community-acquired MRSA is sensitive to Bactrim. Any evidence of progression of illness despite therapy should escalate therapy by broadening the spectrum of microbial coverage. If illness has progressed while the patient has been on oral medications at home, the patient should be hospitalized for intravenous antimicrobial treatment. And if illness has progressed while on intravenous antibiotics, consideration should be made for broader microbial coverage or coverage for resistant organisms in addition to prompt imaging and perhaps even surgical intervention. Linezolid, Daptomycin, and Vancomycin are excellent for skin and soft tissue infections, especially those due to MRSA.

Surgical Treatment

The classic treatment for skin and soft tissue abscesses is wide incision, drainage, irrigation and packing. It is important to probe the cavity and completely break up any loculations and completely drain the area. The commonly used technique of daily packing removal and repacking, which is often practiced in adult settings, is not routinely utilized in the pediatric setting. Successful outcomes are able to be achieved with small abscesses by packing strips of iodoform gauze into the wound and then daily removal of a small segment of packing until all of the packing has been removed. This greatly decreases the trauma and fear associated with repacking. The caregiver must be taught packing removal since a portion of the packing always needs to remain protruding through the wound to prevent skin annealing and recurrence. Once the packing is completely out, the skin edges can be gently separated daily following warm soaks or baths with cotton tipped swabs allowing time for the cavity to contract and obliterate.

A new technique obviating the need for any packing with very good results was recently described whereby the infected cavity is traversed by a one-fourth inch penrose drain or Silicone vessel-loop material secured to itself and left in place with minimal care required by the caregiver (Figure 2).[4,5] Topical cleansing of the wound and a cover dressing is performed twice a day, while the underlying cavity decompresses, collapses, and slowly obliterates and contracts over a 5–7 day period. The drain can then be removed without difficulty in the office once the cavity is nearly healed as evident by no further evidence of cellulitis and limited drainage. These patients may be discharged home with oral antibiotics and parental

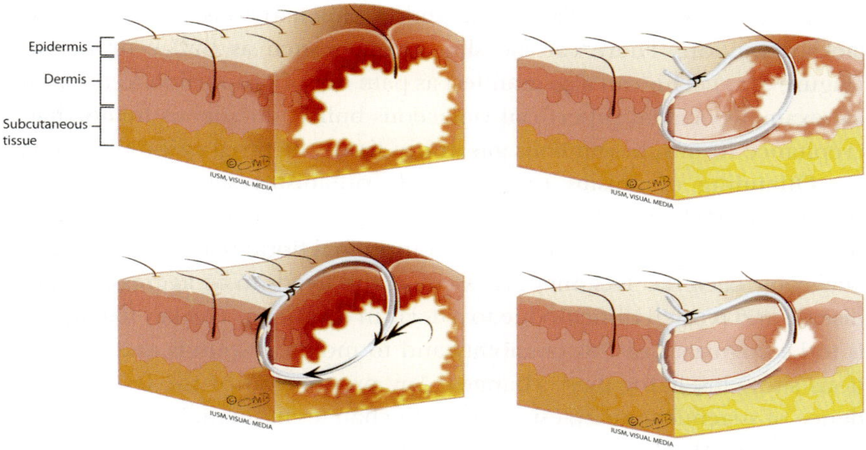

Figure 2. Minimally invasive technique for operative drainage (used by permission).

understanding of wound care. Follow-up should be within a week to ensure proper wound healing and for drain removal.

NECROTIZING FASCIITIS

Fluid collections can be purulent or of a thin, serous type. Although abscesses are collections of thick, purulent fluid, thin serous-type fluid may represent necrotizing fasciitis and has a brown, murky appearance. Necrotizing fasciitis represents an infection that is usually deeper than the subcutaneous tissues. It tends to track along fascial planes and is often identified by subtle cutaneous changes resembling ecchymosis with a rapid progression and wider involvement of the subcutaneous tissues. The fasciitis process may occasionally present with bacteremia and myonecrosis. The superficial appearance can be spreading erythema, blistering, tenderness, and induration (Figure 3(a)). Many times, onset is initiated by a superficial skin infection that appears cellulitic but progresses much more aggressively depending on its pathogenicity. One particular association has been seen with patients having varicella infections and then treated with NSAIDS. This infection is usually due to invasive group A Streptococcus. Other risk factors for necrotizing infections are in settings of omphalitis or perianal/perineal abscesses. The characteristic features are cellulitis, edema, discoloration, anesthesia of the overlying skin, and a subcutaneous induration that lacks definition. There can be skin changes such as bullae or necrosis (Figure 3(a)). This can also manifest as pain out of proportion to the physical exam, associated superficial violaceous bullae, cutaneous hemorrhage, crepitance from subcutaneous gas within tissue, or progression of illness.

Offending organisms can be single organisms such as *Streptococcus pyogenes* or *Staphylococcus aureus* or Peptostreptococcus species but often can be polymicrobial and are usually gastrointestinal flora such as coliforms and anaerobic bacteria. Treatment is essential and needs to be aggressive in this disease and is often difficult due to a delay in diagnosis. The key to diagnosis is to be cognizant of this possibility and to monitor wounds and/or infectious sites closely for these changes. Any progression of the lesion or evidence of systemic toxicity, especially with changes in mental status, requires aggressive medical and surgical intervention. In addition to recognition and diagnosis, the electrolyte panel and complete blood cell count with a type and cross should be obtained. Sometimes, severe hypocalcemia may be encountered due to the massive soft tissue necrosis and fat saponification.

The operative treatment for necrotizing fasciitis has to be timely and include wide debridement of all affected tissue (Figure 3(b)). Upon initial incision, there is usually a thin, murky, brown fluid that is released that has a characteristic "mousy" odor. The subcutaneous tissues tend to be swollen and may exhibit necrosis. Vasculature is often thrombosed, further compromising tissue viability. Debridement needs to be complete and all boundaries must be free of infection. This is secured by having healthy bleeding tissue at the margins of the entire debridement bed. Release of collagenases, proteases and other enzymes from these infections cause necrosis and more rapid invasion by these offending organisms. Additional debridements may be necessary until all devitalized tissue is removed. Postoperative care involves fluid resuscitation, antibiotic coverage, wound coverage (Figure 3(c)), prevention of hypothermia, local wound care and nutritional support. The best choice of antibiotics coverage is Unasyn (Ampicillin–Sulbactam), Clindamycin and Ciprofloxacin, or Clindamycin and Gentamicin. Clindamycin can actually provide good anaerobic coverage as well as coverage for aerobic gram positive cocci but can also suppress toxin and modulate TNF production in animal studies.[1]

Imaging for necrotizing fasciitis is unnecessary and may prove to be life threatening by delaying operative intervention. The best evaluation is by the trained surgeon's eyes and sequential evaluation of the lesion over time.

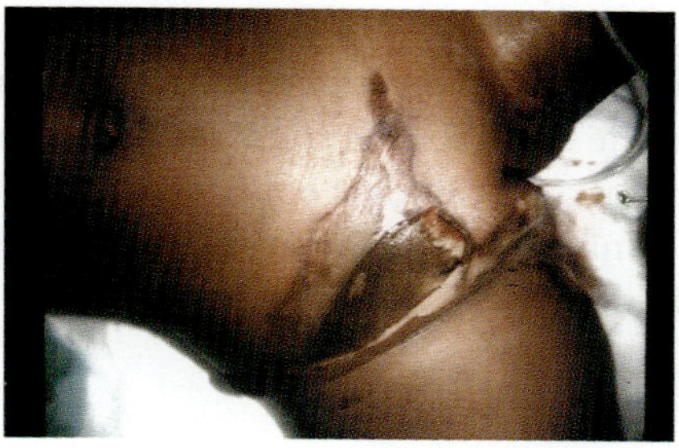

(a)

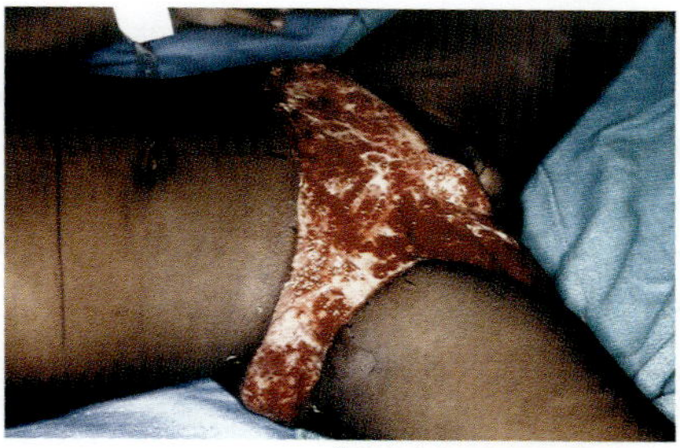

(b)

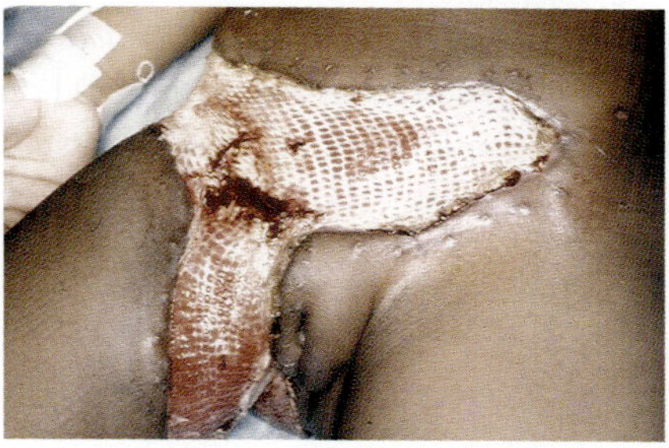

(c)

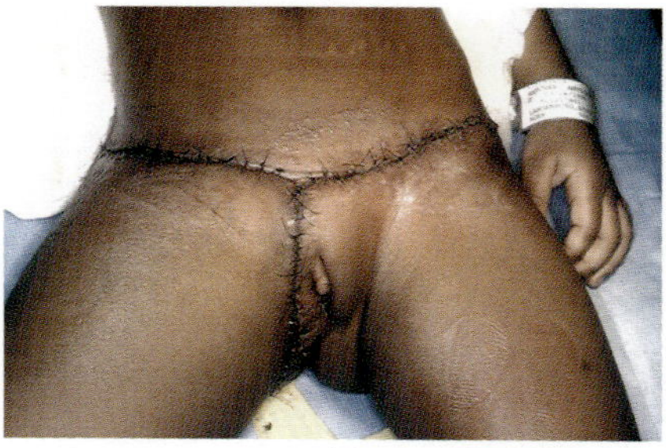

(d)

Figure 3. Necrotizing fasciitis. (a) Blistering, skin necrosis, (b) Wide debridement, (c) Wound coverage, (d) Final wound coverage and closure.

Hyperbaric oxygen has not proven to be beneficial and the use of immunoglobulin to decrease the intensity of toxic shock symptoms has shown little value in the treatment of these patients. There is also no need to obtain frozen section or pathologic confirmation to determine extent of debridement. The limits of debridement are determined by visualizing healthy, live, bleeding tissue.

REFERENCES

1. Stevens DL, Bisno AL, Chambers HF, *et al.* (2005) Practice guidelines for the diagnosis and management of skin and soft tissue infections. *Clinical Infectious Diseases* **41**:1373–1406.
2. Jahamy H, Ganga R, Raiy BA, *et al.* (2008) Staphylococcus aureus skin/soft tissue infections: The impact of SCCmec type and Panton–Valentine leukocidin. *Scand J Infect Dis* **8**:1–7.
3. Faden H, Rose R, Lesse A, *et al.* (2007) Clinical and molecular characteristics of staphylococcal skin abscesses in children. *J Pediatrics* **151**(6):700–703.
4. Ladd AP, Levy MS, Quilty J. (2010) Minimally invasive technique in treatment of complex, subcutaneous abscesses in children. *J Pediatr Surg* **45**(7):1562–1566.
5. McNamara WF, Hartin Jr, CW, Escobar MA, *et al.* (2011) An alternative to open incision and drainage for community-acquired soft tissue abscesses in children. *J Pediatr Surg* **46**(3):502–506.

INDEX